Handbook
of Anaesthesia
&
Peri-operative
Medicine

Edited by
Cyprian Mendonca

Chandrashekhar Vaidyanath

i

tfm Publishing Limited, Castle Hill Barns, Harley, Nr Shrewsbury, SY5 6LX, UK. Tel: +44 (0)1952 510061; Fax: +44 (0)1952 510192
E-mail: nikki@tfmpublishing.com; Web site: www.tfmpublishing.com

Design & Typesetting: Nikki Bramhill BSc Hons Dip Law
First Edition: © 2017
Background cover image © Comstock Inc., www.comstock.com
Paperback   ISBN: 978-1-910079-19-5
E-book editions: 2017
ePub   ISBN: 978-1-910079-20-1
Mobi   ISBN: 978-1-910079-21-8
Web pdf   ISBN: 978-1-910079-22-5

Printed by Cambrian Printers, Llanbadarn Road, Aberystwyth, Ceredigion, SY23 3TN.
Tel: +44 (0)1970 627111; Web site: www.cambrian-printers.co.uk

Contents

Section 2 — Peri-operative medicine

Section 3 — Airway management

Section 4 — Specialty-specific procedures

Section 5 — Peri-operative emergencies

Section 6 — Critical care medicine

Section 7 — Pain medicine

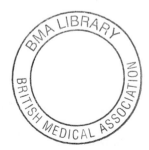

Contributors

Anuji Amarasekara, MBBS FRCA
Consultant Anaesthetist
University Hospitals Coventry & Warwickshire NHS Trust, UK

Vassilis Athanassoglou, MA MB BChir FRCA
Consultant Anaesthetist
Oxford University Hospitals NHS Trust, UK

Mohammed Auldin, MB ChB FRCA
Speciality Registrar
Warwickshire School of Anaesthesia, UK

Ranjna Basra, MBChB MRCEM
Advanced Respiratory & ECMO Fellow
Guy's and St Thomas' NHS Foundation Trust, UK

Tom Billyard, FRCA FFICM
Consultant Anaesthetist & Intensivist
University Hospitals Coventry & Warwickshire NHS Trust, UK

Kate Bosworth, MB ChB FRCA
Speciality Registrar
Warwickshire School of Anaesthesia, UK

Alistair Burns, BSc MB ChB FRCA
Speciality Registrar
Warwickshire School of Anaesthesia, UK

Narotham R. Burri, MD FRCA
Consultant Anaesthetist
University Hospitals Coventry & Warwickshire NHS Trust, UK

Shefali Chaudhari, MBBS FRCA
Consultant Anaesthetist
George Elliot Hospital NHS Trust, UK

Kavitkumar Dasari, BSc (Hons) MB ChB
Speciality Registrar
Warwickshire School of Anaesthesia, UK

Gemma Dignam, BMedSc BMBS FCAI FRCA FFICM
Consultant Anaesthetist and Intensivist
University Hospitals Coventry & Warwickshire NHS Trust, UK

Llewellyn Fenton-May, MB ChB FRCA
Consultant Anaesthetist
Heart of England NHS Foundation Trust, UK

Alastair Fairfield, BSc FRCA
Speciality Registrar
Warwickshire School of Anaesthesia, UK

Alireza Feizerfan, MD FRCA FANZCA
Fellow in Anaesthesia
Royal Perth Hospital, Australia

Mahul Gorecha, MBChB FCAI FRCA
Speciality Registrar
Warwickshire School of Anaesthesia, UK

Peeyush Kumar, MBBS FRCA FCAI
Consultant Anaesthetist
University Hospitals Coventry & Warwickshire NHS Trust, UK

George Madden, BMedSc MB ChB MAcadMEd FRCA
Speciality Registrar
Warwickshire School of Anaesthesia, UK

Laith Malhas, MB ChB FRCA
Speciality Registrar
Warwickshire School of Anaesthesia, UK

Antonia Mayell MBChB (Hons) MRCP FRCA
Consultant Anaesthetist
University Hospitals Coventry & Warwickshire NHS Trust, UK

Cyprian Mendonca, MD FRCA
Featherstone Professor, AAGBI (2016-18)
Honorary Associate Professor, Warwick Medical School
Consultant Anaesthetist, University Hospitals Coventry & Warwickshire NHS Trust, UK

Ahmed Mesbah, MB BCh FCAI FRCA
Locum Consultant Paediatric Anaesthetist
Great Ormond Street Hospital for Children NHS Foundation Trust, UK

Vinesh Mistry, BSc (Hons) MB ChB
Speciality Registrar
Warwickshire School of Anaesthesia, UK

Aleksandra Nowicka, FRCA
Speciality Registrar
Warwickshire School of Anaesthesia, UK

Charles Pairaudeau, BMedSci BMBS FRCA
Speciality Registrar
Warwickshire School of Anaesthesia, UK

Mark Pais, MB ChB FRCA
Speciality Registrar
Warwickshire School of Anaesthesia, UK

Anuja Patil, FRCA
Speciality Registrar
Warwickshire School of Anaesthesia, UK

Alexander Philip, MBBS DA FRCA PGCert Med Ed
Consultant Anaesthetist
Colchester General Hospital, UK

Nagendra Prasad, MD DNB FRCA
Locum Consultant Anaesthetist
Derby Teaching Hospitals NHS Foundation Trust, UK

Ilyas Qazi, MBBS DA FRCA FCAI
Speciality Registrar
Warwickshire School of Anaesthesia, UK

Melanie Sahni, BSc (Hons) MBChB (Hons)
Speciality Registrar
Birmingham School of Anaesthesia, UK

Rathinavel Shanmugam, FRCA
Consultant Anaesthetist
South Warwickshire NHS Foundation Trust, UK

Meghna Sharma, MBBS DA FCPS FRCA
Consultant Anaesthetist
University Hospitals Coventry & Warwickshire NHS Trust, UK

Nick Talbot, MB ChB BSc (Hons) FRCA
Speciality Registrar
Warwickshire School of Anaesthesia, UK

Christina Tourville, MBBS BSc FRCA
Speciality Registrar
Warwickshire School of Anaesthesia, UK

Narcis Ungureanu, MD DESA FRCA
Consultant Anaesthetist
Burton Hospitals NHS Foundation Trust, Burton-upon-Trent, UK

Chandrashekhar Vaidyanath, MBBS MD FCPS FRCA
Consultant Anaesthetist
University Hospitals Coventry & Warwickshire NHS Trust, UK

Akilan Velayudhan, FRCA FCARCSI FIPP
Consultant in Anaesthesia and Pain Specialist
Mildura Base Hospital, Victoria, Australia

Preface

The feedback and constant encouragement received from senior medical students and junior doctors on the *Handbook of Anaesthesia* for the Warwick Medical School inspired us for the challenge of writing this book. Over the years the role of the anaesthetist has been redefined as it extends much beyond the intra-operative management of the surgical patient. A holistic approach to patient management necessitates the anaesthetist's involvement in the pre-operative preparation and postoperative care of the surgical patient; therefore, a basic knowledge of common surgical and medical presentations is essential for the practising anaesthetist.

This book consists of seven sections covering applied science, peri-operative medicine, airway management, specialty-specific procedures, peri-operative emergencies, critical care medicine and pain medicine. The section on peri-operative medicine particularly focuses on the significance of problems that impact on the peri-operative management of surgical patients. After reading any topic in medicine, it is always important for the reader to self-assess their knowledge gained and to reflect on how to improve this knowledge and skills further. The case scenarios at the end of each chapter are additionally helpful in this self-assessment and understanding the topic in greater depth.

This book is aimed at senior medical students and foundation doctors who wish to develop an interest in the fields of anaesthesia and intensive care, and peri-operative medicine. This book will be a good companion for postgraduate trainees in anaesthesia, intensive care and allied specialties. It will also serve as an invaluable educational tool for practising anaesthetists and intensive care specialists; however, the advanced specialty skills and more detailed knowledge of applied science need to be supplemented from review articles and specialty textbooks.

We believe that the book, despite its possible omissions, provides a depth of knowledge of anaesthesia and peri-operative care of surgical patients.

Cyprian Mendonca, MD FRCA
Chandrashekhar Vaidyanath, MBBS MD FCPS FRCA

Abbreviations

%	percent
2,3-DPG	2,3-diphosphoglycerate
6MWT	Six-minute walk test
AAGBI	Association of Anaesthetists of Great Britain & Ireland
ABG	Arterial blood gas
ABW	Actual body weight
ACC	American College of Cardiology
ACCP	American College of Chest Physicians
ACE	Angiotensin-converting enzyme
ACEI	Angiotensin-converting enzyme inhibitor
AchE	Acetylcholinesterase
ACS	Acute coronary syndrome
ACT	Activated clotting time
ACTH	Adrenocorticotropic hormone
ADH	Antidiuretic hormone
ADP	Adenosine diphosphate
AF	Atrial fibrillation
AHA	American Heart Association
AICD	Automatic implantable cardioverter defibrillator
AIP	Acute intermittent porphyria
ALA	Aminolevulinic acid
ALS	Advanced life support
APL	Adjustable pressure limiting
APTT	Activated partial thromboplastin time
AR	Aortic regurgitation
ARB	Angiotensin receptor blocker
ARDS	Acute respiratory distress syndrome
AS	Aortic stenosis
ASA	American Society of Anesthesiologists
ATIII	Antithrombin three
ATLS®	Advanced Trauma Life Support®

ATP	Adenosine triphosphate
AV	Aortic valve
AVA	Aortic valve area
AVNRT	Atrioventricular nodal re-entrant tachycardia
AVPU	Alert, verbal, pain or unresponsive
AVRT	Atrioventricular re-entrant tachycardia
BBB	Bundle branch block
BD	*Bis die*
BIS	Bispectral Index
BiVAD	Biventricular assist device
BMI	Body mass index
BMS	Bare metal stent
BNP	Brain natriuretic peptide
BP	Blood pressure
bpm	Beats per minute
CABG	Coronary artery bypass graft
cAMP	Cyclic adenosine monophosphate
CAPD	Continuous ambulatory peritoneal dialysis
CBF	Cerebral blood flow
CBG	Capillary blood glucose
CBV	Cerebral blood volume
CBT	Cognitive behavioural therapy
CCB	Calcium channel blocker
CCS	Canadian Cardiovascular Society
CCU	Critical care unit
CDH	Congenital diaphragmatic hernia
CK	Creatine kinase
cmH_2O	Centimetre of water
$CMRO_2$	Cerebral metabolic rate of oxygen consumption
CMV	*Cytomegalovirus*
CN	Cranial nerve
CNB	Central neuraxial blockade
CNS	Central nervous system
CO	Cardiac output
CO_2	Carbon dioxide
COPD	Chronic obstructive pulmonary disease
COX	Cyclo-oxygenase
CPAP	Continuous positive airway pressure
CPB	Cardiopulmonary bypass
CPDA	Citrate phosphate dextrose adenine
CPET	Cardiopulmonary exercise testing

CPP	Cerebral perfusion pressure
CPR	Cardiopulmonary resuscitation
CRP	C-reactive protein
CRT	Cardiac resynchronisation therapy
CSDH	Chronic subdural haematoma
CSE	Combined spinal-epidural
CSF	Cerebrospinal fluid
CSL	Compound sodium lactate
CSOM	Chronic suppurative otitis media
CT	Computed tomography
CTEPH	Chronic thromboembolic pulmonary hypertension
CVA	Cerebrovascular accident
CVC	Central venous catheter
CVP	Central venous pressure
CVS	Cardiovascular system
CVVH	Continuous veno-venous haemofiltration
CXR	Chest X-ray
DAPT	Dual antiplatelet therapy
DAS	Difficult Airway Society
DC	Direct current
DES	Drug-eluting stent
DHCA	Deep hypothermic circulatory arrest
DI	Diabetes insipidus
DIC	Disseminated intravascular coagulation
DINAMAP	Device for indirect non-invasive automated mean arterial pressure
DKA	Diabetic ketoacidosis
DLCO	Diffusing capacity of the lungs for carbon monoxide
DLT	Double-lumen tube
DMR	Depolarising muscle relaxant
DNA	Deoxyribonucleic acid
DO_2	Oxygen delivery
DPG	Diphosphoglycerate
DVT	Deep vein thrombosis
ECG	Electrocardiogram
ECMO	Extracorporeal membrane oxygenation
ECT	Electroconvulsive therapy
EDD	End-diastolic dimension
EEG	Electroencephalogram
EF	Ejection fraction

EMG	Electromyography
EMLA	Eutectic mixture of local anaesthetic
ENT	Ear, nose and throat
EPAP	Expiratory positive airway pressure
ERAS	Enhanced recovery after surgery
ERV	Expiratory reserve volume
ESC	European Society of Cardiology
ESD	End-systolic dimension
ESICM	European Society of Intensive Care Medicine
$EtCO_2$	End-tidal carbon dioxide
EtO_2	End-tidal oxygen concentration
ET	Endotracheal
EVD	External ventricular drain
F_A	Alveolar concentration
FAST	Focused assessment with sonography for trauma
FBC	Full blood count
FEMG	Frontal electromyography
FESS	Functional endoscopic sinus surgery
FEV_1	Forced expired volume in first second
FFP	Fresh frozen plasma
FG	French gauge
FGF	Fresh gas flow
F_I	Inspired concentration
FiO_2	Fraction of inspired oxygen concentration
FOI	Fibreoptic intubation
FRC	Functional residual capacity
FTc	Corrected flow time
FVC	Forced vital capacity
g	Gram
g/hr	Gram/hour
g/kg/day	Gram/kilogram/day
g/L	Gram/litre
GA	General anaesthesia
GABA	Gamma aminobutyric acid
GCS	Glasgow Coma Scale
GDT	Goal-directed therapy
GFR	Glomerular filtration rate
GH	Growth hormone
GI	Gastrointestinal syatem
GTN	Glyceryl trinitrate

GU	Genito-urinary
Hb	Haemoglobin
HCP	Hereditary coproporphyria
HDU	High dependency unit
HELLP	Haemolysis, elevated liver enzymes, low platelets
HES	Hydroxyethyl starches
HIV	Human immunodeficiency virus
HME	Heat and moisture exchange
HOCM	Hypertrophic obstructive cardiomyopathy
HONKC	Hyperosmolar non-ketotic coma
HPA axis	Hypothalamic-pituitary-adrenal axis
HPV	Hypoxic pulmonary vasoconstriction
HR	Heart rate
HRT	Hormone replacement therapy
IABP	Intra-aortic balloon pump
IASP	International Association for the Study of Pain
IBP	Invasive blood pressure
IBW	Ideal body weight
ICP	Intracranial pressure
ICU	Intensive care unit
IL	Inflammatory interleukins
ILMA	Intubating laryngeal mask airway
IMA	Internal mammary artery
INR	International Normalised Ratio
IPAP	Inspiratory positive airway pressure
IPPV	Intermittent positive pressure ventilation
ITU	Intensive therapy unit
IV	Intravenous
IVC	Inferior vena cava
IVRA	Intravenous regional anaesthesia
J	Joule
JVP	Jugular venous pressure
K^+	Potassium
kcal/kg	Kilocalorie/kilogram
kg/m^2	Kilogram/square metre
kJ/L	Kilojoule/litre
kPa	Kilopascal
LA	Local anaesthetic
LABA	Long-acting beta agonist
LAD	Left anterior descending
LAMA	Long-acting muscarinic agonists

LBBB	Left bundle branch block
LBW	Lean body weight
LED	Light-emitting diode
LEDP	Left end-diastolic pressure
LIMA	Left internal mammary artery
LMA	Laryngeal mask airway
LMS	Left main stem
LMWH	Low-molecular-weight heparin
LTOT	Long-term oxygen therapy
LV	Left ventricle
LVAD	Left ventricular assist device
LVEDP	Left ventricular end-diastolic pressure
LVH	Left ventricular hypertrophy
LVRS	Lung volume reduction surgery
M3G	Morphine 3-glucuronide
M6G	Morphine 6-glucuronide
MAC	Minimum alveolar concentration
MAO	Monoamine oxidase
MAOI	Monoamine oxidase inhibitor
MAP	Mean arterial pressure
Max	Maximum
MEN	Multiple endocrine neoplasia
MET	Metabolic equivalent of task
MEWS	Modified Early Warning Score
µg	Microgram
mg	Milligram
Mg	Magnesium
µg/kg	Microgram/kilogram
mg/kg	Milligram/kilogram
mg/kg/hr	Milligram/kilogram/hour
µg/min	Microgram/minute
mg/min	Milligram/minute
$MgSO_4$	Magnesium sulphate
MH	Malignant hyperthermia
MHRA	Medicines and Healthcare products Regulatory Agency
MI	Myocardial infarction
MILS	Manual in-line stabilisation
ml	Millilitre
ml/kg	Millilitre/kilogram
ml/kg/hr	Millilitre/kilogram/hour
ml/kg/min	Millilitre/kilogram/minute

ml/L	Millilitre/litre
MLT	Microlaryngeal tube
mmHg	Millimeters of mercury
mmol/L	Millimole/litre
MPAP	Mean pulmonary artery pressure
MR	Mitral regurgitation
MRC	Medical Research Council
MRI	Magnetic resonance imaging
MRSA	Methicillin-resistant *Staphylococcus aureus*
MS	Mitral stenosis
ms	Millisecond
MST	Morphine sulphate
mV	Millivolt
MVP	Mitral valve prolapse
N.B.	*Nota bene* (note well)
Na$^+$	Sodium
nAchR	Nicotinic acetylcholine receptor
NAP	National Audit Project
NAPQI	N-acetyl-p-benzoquinone imine
NBM	Nil by mouth
NCEPOD	National Confidential Enquiry into Patient Outcomes and Death
Nd-YAG	Neodymium-yttrium aluminium garnet
NDMR	Non-depolarising muscle relaxant
NEC	Necrotising enterocolitis
NG	Nasogastric
NHS	National Health Service
NIBP	Non-invasive blood pressure
NICE	National Institute for Health and Care Excellence
NICU	Neonatal intensive care unit
NIST	Non-interchangeable screw thread
NIV	Non-invasive ventilation
NMDA	N-methyl-D-aspartate
NMDR	Non-depolarising muscle relaxant
NMJ	Neuromuscular junction
N$_2$O	Nitrous oxide
NPPV	Non-invasive positive pressure ventilation
NSAID	Non-steroidal anti-inflammatory drug
NSTEMI	Non-ST elevation myocardial infarction
NYHA	New York Heart Association
O$_2$	Oxygen

OCP	Oral contraceptive pill
OD	*Omne in die*
ODM	Oesophageal Doppler monitor
ODP	Operating department practitioner
OPA	Ordinary physical activity
ORIF	Open reduction and internal fixation
OSA	Obstructive sleep apnoea
P/F	PaO_2/FiO_2
PA	Alveolar partial pressure
PA_{agent}	Alveolar partial pressure of anaesthetic agent
PABA	Para-aminobenzoate
PAc	Pulmonary artery catheter
$PaCO_2$	Partial pressure of carbon dioxide in arterial blood
PAH	Pulmonary artery hypertension
PAN	Primary afferent neuron
PaO_2	Partial pressure of oxygen in arterial blood
PAOP	Pulmonary artery occlusion pressure
PAP	Pulmonary artery pressure
PBW	Predicted body weight
PCA	Patient-controlled analgesia
PCI	Percutaneous coronary intervention
PCO_2	Partial pressure of carbon dioxide
PCWP	Pulmonary capillary wedge pressure
PDE	Phosphodiesterase
PDPH	Post-dural puncture headache
PE	Pulmonary embolism
PEA	Pulseless electical activity
PEEP	Positive end-expiratory pressure
PEG	Percutaneous endoscopic gastrotomy
PET	Positron emission tomography
PG	Prostaglandin
PGE_2	Prostaglandin E_2
PGI_2	Prostaglandin I_2
PNB	Peripheral nerve block
PNS	Peripheral nerve stimulator
PO_2	Partial pressure of oxygen
PONV	Postoperative nausea and vomiting
PPH	Post-partum haemorrhage
PPI	Proton pump inhibitor
ppo	Predicted postoperative
PRIS	Propofol-related infusion syndrome

PRN	*Pro re nata*
PSS	Plume scavenging system
PT	Prothrombin time
PTC	Post-tetanic count
PV	Peak velocity
PVC	Polyvinyl chloride
PVR	Pulmonary vascular resistance
QDS	*Quater die sumendum*
RA	Regional anaesthesia
Ra	Right atrium
RAA	Renin-angiotensin-aldosterone
RAE	Ring-Adair-Elwyn
RCA	Right coronary artery
RCOA	Royal College of Anaesthetists
RCOG	Royal College of Obstetricians & Gynaecologists
REM	Rapid eye movement
RIMA	Right internal mammary artery
RoTEM®	Rotational thromboelastometry
RSI	Rapid sequence intubation
RUL	Right upper lobe
RV	Right ventricle
RVAD	Right ventricular assist device
SAD	Supraglottic airway device
SAG-M	Saline, adenine, glucose and mannitol
SAM	Systolic anterior motion
SAN	Secondary afferent neuron
SC	Subcutanoeus
SIADH	Syndrome of inappropriate antidiuretic hormone
SIGN	Scottish Intercollegiate Guidelines Network
SIRS	Systemic inflammatory response syndrome
SLR	Straight leg raise
SLT	Single-lumen tube
SOL	Space-occupying lesion
SORT	Surgical Outcome Risk Tool
SpO_2	Pulse oximeter oxygen saturation
SSRI	Selective serotonin reuptake inhibitor
STEMI	ST elevation myocardial infarction
SV	Stroke volume
SVC	Superior vena cava
SVR	Systemic vascular resistance
SVT	Supraventricular tachycardia

TAP	Transversus abdominis plane
TAVI	Transcatheter aortic valve implantation
TB	Tuberculosis
TBI	Traumatic brain injury
TCA	Tricyclic antidepressant
TCI	Target-controlled infusion
TDS	*Ter die sumendum*
TED	Thromboembolic deterrent
TEG®	Thromboelastography
TENS	Transcutaneous electrical nerve stimulation
TFT	Thyroid function test
TIA	Transient ischaemic attack
TIVA	Total intravenous anaesthesia
TKR	Total knee replacement
TLCO	Transfer factor for carbon monoxide
TNM	Tumour node metastasis
TOE	Transoesophageal echocardiography
TOF	Train of four
TSH	Thyroid-stimulating hormone
TTE	Transthoracic echocardiography
U&E	Urine and electrolytes
UK	United Kingdom
US	Ultrasound
USRA	Ultrasound regional anaesthesia
VAD	Ventricular assist device
VAP	Ventilator-acquired pneumonia
VATS	Video-assisted thoracoscopic surgery
VC	Vital capacity
VF	Ventricular fibrillation
VL	Videolaryngoscope
VP	Venous pressure
VP	Variegate porphyria
VP	Ventriculoperitoneal
V/Q	Ventilation/perfusion
VRIII	Variable rate intravenous insulin infusion
VT	Ventricular tachycardia
VTE	Venous thromboembolism
WHO	World Health Organisation

Acknowledgements

We are indebted to Nikki Bramhill, Director of tfm publishing for her help and commitment in reviewing the manuscript and also for her permission to use some of the illustrations from the textbooks, *The Structured Oral Examination in Clinical Anaesthesia* (ISBN 978-1-903378-68-1) and *The Objective Structured Clinical Examination in Anaesthesia* (ISBN 978-1-903378-56-4).

We thank Paul Sweeney, ACPS, Clinical Perfusion Manager, Cardiothoracic Surgery, UHCW NHS Trust, for supplying Figure 25.3, Jason McAllister, Graphic Designer, University Hospitals Coventry & Warwickshire NHS Trust, for his help with the illustrations and Dr Rashmi Rebello, SHO, Kettering General Hospital, for critically reviewing the chapters in this book.

1 Intravenous agents

Mohammed Auldin

Introduction

Intravenous anaesthetic agents were developed more recently than inhalational agents. Of the commonly used agents, thiopental is the oldest having been introduced in 1934, the most recent being propofol which was introduced in 1986.

Induction of anaesthesia is most commonly achieved by intravenous agents. In this chapter we will discuss the following drugs:

- Propofol (phenol derivative).
- Thiopental (barbiturate).
- Ketamine (phencyclidine derivative).
- Etomidate (imidazole).
- Midazolam (benzodiazepine).

These drugs are of different classes but they can all be used to induce general anaesthesia, although they also have other indications such as sedation and maintenance of anaesthesia.

Intravenous anaesthetics have a wide array of effects, the extent of which are dependent upon the individual drug pharmacology and concomitant use of other drugs, as well as patient physiology. It is therefore important to select a drug or a combination of drugs based on each individual patient and to be prepared for adverse events.

Propofol

Clinical uses and indications

Propofol is the most commonly used induction agent in the United Kingdom. The induction dose is 1.5-2.5mg/kg and loss of response to verbal command is a good indicator for onset of anaesthesia. It is also used for maintenance of anaesthesia as part of a total intravenous anaesthesia (TIVA) technique and sedation either intra-operatively or in critical care.

Structure and physical properties

Propofol is highly lipid-soluble and is presented as an oil-water emulsion in concentrations of 1% and 2%. It is a phenolic derivative and is chemically named 2,6 di-isopropyl phenol. The formulation also contains 10% soya bean oil, 2.25% glycerol and 1.2% egg phosphatide. Propofol can be used in patients with an egg allergy because these patients are usually allergic to egg protein or albumin, not the phosphatide. Patients with a soya bean allergy do not appear to be allergic to propofol, as the protein component of soya bean oil is removed. The solution has a characteristic white colour that makes it easily recognisable and may contribute to safety in terms of reducing drug administration errors.

Propofol tends to be painful on injection, particularly when given into a smaller vein. This effect can be reduced by adding lidocaine to the mixture (10mg for every 100mg of propofol). Most formulations contain medium-chain triglycerides, which have reduced pain on injection.

Mechanism of action

Propofol predominantly acts on $GABA_A$ and glycine receptors by potentiating their inhibitory effects. The exact mechanism of action is unclear although it is thought to act by a different mechanism to benzodiazepines and thiopental.

Pharmacokinetics

Propofol has a pKa of 11 and is 98% protein bound. It is highly lipid-soluble. Following an initial intravenous dose, the plasma concentration rises immediately and then falls in an exponential fashion (Figure 1.1). The initial fall in concentration is rapid (a redistribution half-life of 1-3 minutes) and is due to the redistribution from the central compartment. It is for this reason that the duration of action is short following a single induction dose. When given as an infusion, propofol begins to accumulate in the central and peripheral compartments.

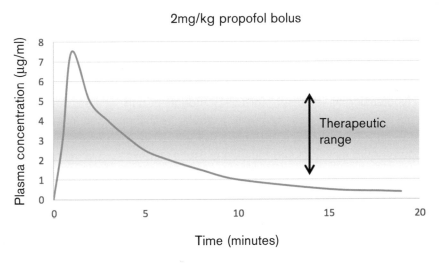

Figure 1.1. Plasma concentration following a single bolus dose of propofol (the y axis shows the plasma concentration and the x axis shows the time in minutes).

Propofol undergoes hepatic metabolism to inactive compounds. Clearance of propofol is 30ml/kg/min, which exceeds the hepatic blood flow and therefore this suggests that some of the propofol is metabolised extrahepatically. The kidneys excrete it as glucuronide and sulphate conjugates. It has a variable elimination half-life of between 10 to 70 minutes. Propofol does not accumulate to the same extent as thiopental following prolonged intravenous infusion.

Clinical effects

Central nervous system

During induction some patients may experience involuntary movements. These movements are not epileptiform in origin; however, some anaesthetists avoid propofol in epileptics as the social implications on driving and occupation following a seizure can be significant for the patient. Propofol has been used for status epilepticus although thiopental is a more suitable induction agent. It reduces cerebral blood flow, intracranial pressure and intraocular pressure.

Cardiovascular system

Hypotension is common following induction and occurs due to a combination of reduced systemic vascular resistance and myocardial depression. This effect is sometimes exaggerated in hypertensive patients, those on ACE inhibitors and the elderly. Reflex tachycardia is uncommon, possibly because of resetting of the baroreceptor reflex.

Respiratory system

Respiratory depression is marked and most patients will become apnoeic following an induction dose. It also depresses laryngeal reflexes to a greater extent than other induction agents, which allows for easy placement of the supraglottic airway device.

Other effects

The use of propofol for maintenance of anaesthesia has shown an antiemetic effect. This may be in part due to the avoidance of volatile anaesthetics. Prolonged infusion, particularly on the intensive care unit, can lead to propofol-related infusion syndrome (PRIS). It consists of progressive myocardial failure, metabolic acidosis and hyperkalaemia.

Biochemically, creatinine kinase and lactate rise and there is associated hyperlipidaemia. PRIS has a high mortality and treatment is supportive. Propofol doses of more than 4mg/kg/hr should not be exceeded when using it for long-term sedation.

Thiopental

Clinical uses and indications

Thiopental is used for the induction of anaesthesia at a dose of 3-7mg/kg depending on the patient's haemodynamic status. It can be administered in the form of a pre-calculated dose as a rapid bolus but the downside of this is the more pronounced adverse side effects. Alternatively, the induction dose can be carefully titrated to minimise adverse effects. It was more commonly used for rapid sequence induction along with suxamethonium in patients at risk of aspiration, although propofol is gaining popularity as part of the 'modified' rapid sequence induction. It rapidly produces its effects, in one arm brain cycle — about 30 seconds and onset of anaesthesia is indicated by the loss of the eyelash reflex. It is also used in status epilepticus refractory to benzodiazepines and conventional anticonvulsants.

Structure and physical properties

Thiopental is the sulphur analogue of pentobarbitone. It is available in a glass vial as a yellow powder. To optimise its solubility in water, the vial also contains sodium carbonate, which dissolves in water to give a strong alkaline solution. It also contains nitrogen in place of air. This is to prevent carbon dioxide from dissolving in the water and making the solution acidic.

The vial contains 500mg of thiopental and this is reconstituted in 20ml of water for injection, giving a concentration of 25mg/ml.

Thiopental exists in two forms when in solution, depending on the pH of the solution it is in. The reconstituted solution has a pH of 10.5, which makes it bacteriostatic. At this alkaline pH most of thiopental is in the ionised form and therefore water-soluble. At physiological pH it becomes predominantly unionised and therefore lipid-soluble. This is important to note, as mixing thiopental with acidic drugs will result in precipitation, e.g. opioids and neuromuscular blocking agents.

Mechanism of action

Thiopental is a barbiturate and is thought to exert its effect by inhibiting the release of neurotransmitters from presynaptic nerve terminals. It also reduces the sensitivity of the postsynaptic membrane to neurotransmitters. This occurs centrally, particularly in the reticular activating system.

Pharmacokinetics

Eighty percent of thiopental is bound to plasma proteins and this fraction does not exert an effect. Of the remaining fraction, just over half is in the unionised form at physiological pH and able to cross lipid membranes and exert its effect.

Pathophysiological factors leading to a low protein state or acidaemia will lead to more drug in the unbound and unionised form able to exert its effect. Therefore, it is important to adjust the dose depending on the patient's clinical condition.

The plasma concentration of thiopental decreases in a tri-exponential fashion following a bolus dose. The initial decline in plasma concentration is rapid and leads to rapid emergence within 5-10 minutes; this is due to redistribution to well-perfused tissues, such as the liver, rather than metabolism. It then redistributes to the skin and muscle.

Thiopental is metabolised in the liver by oxidation. During prolonged administration the hepatic enzymes become saturated and metabolism will follow zero order kinetics. The elimination half-life is 4 to 20 hours.

Clinical effects

Central nervous system

There is a fall in cerebral oxygen consumption, cerebral blood flow and intracranial pressure. An isoelectric EEG trace indicates maximally reduced cerebral oxygen consumption. It is used for cerebral protection in various situations such as circulatory arrest during cardiac surgery.

Cardiovascular system

Thiopental causes a reduction in stroke volume and systemic vascular resistance. There is usually a compensatory tachycardia but cardiac output falls. As this is a dose-dependent effect, reducing the dose or titrating the drug in unstable patients will result in a more stable induction.

Respiratory system

Minute volume falls and a period of apnoea is occasionally seen following induction. Unlike propofol laryngeal reflexes are not depressed to the same degree and there is a possibility of laryngospasm to occur. Hence, insertion of a supraglottic airway device without muscle relaxation should not be attempted.

Other effects

Renal perfusion is decreased and antidiuretic hormone (ADH) release is stimulated. This leads to a reduction in urine output. Severe anaphylactoid reactions are rare occurring in around 1 in 20,000 administrations. Thiopental is contraindicated in patients with porphyria as it may induce an acute porphyric crisis.

Intra-arterial injection

Accidental intra-arterial injection of thiopental is a medical emergency as it is limb-threatening. As alkaline thiopental solution enters arterial blood at a pH of 7.4, it begins to precipitate. In the venous system, the drug is diluted by ever increasing blood as it travels towards the heart. In the arterial system, however, blood vessels branch and become narrower and the precipitated crystals become wedged in small blood vessels causing obstruction to blood flow with local inflammatory mediator release and noradrenaline release which leads to ischaemia. This is an emergency and treatment should begin immediately with the two priorities being optimising distal blood flow and analgesia. The cannula should be left in the artery and saline should be injected to dilute the drug. Vasodilators such as papaverine and a local anaesthetic such as procaine that also has vasodilatory properties should be injected. Heparinisation will prevent superimposed thrombosis. A sympathetic upper limb block such as a stellate ganglion block will enhance vasodilation and a brachial plexus block will provide analgesia.

Ketamine

Clinical uses and indications

Ketamine is used for the induction of anaesthesia, at a dose of 2mg/kg intravenously or 5-10mg/kg intramuscularly, particularly in patients who are hypotensive or have bronchospasm. It takes 30 seconds to work after an intravenous dose and 2-8 minutes following an intramuscular dose.

It is also used for sedation, peri-operative analgesia, analgesia for patients with chronic pain and for the treatment of bronchospasm in severe asthma.

It can be used intrathecally or epidurally to augment central neuraxial blockade; however, only the preservative-free mixture can be used for this purpose which is not currently produced in the UK.

Structure and physical properties

Ketamine is a phencyclidine derivative and is presented as a racemic mixture of S(+) ketamine and R(-) ketamine. It is available in concentrations of 10, 50 and 100mg/ml.

S(+) ketamine is also available on its own. It is twice as potent and has less of a direct depressant effect on the myocardium compared to the racemic mixture.

Mechanism of action

Ketamine non-competitively antagonises N-methyl-D-aspartate (NMDA) receptors. It also interacts with opioid, monaminergic, nicotinic and muscarinic receptors. It is because of this complex interaction with a wide number of receptors that ketamine has a number of beneficial and some unpleasant effects.

Pharmacokinetics

Onset of action is slower than thiopental and propofol at around 1-5 minutes. The duration of action following an intravenous induction dose is around 5-10 minutes. The plasma concentration falls in a bi-exponential manner, the initial fall occurring due to redistribution across lipid membranes and the second phase occurring due to hepatic metabolism. Ketamine is metabolised by the cytochrome P450 system to the potent metabolite, norketamine. It is further metabolised to inactive metabolites and excreted by the kidneys.

Clinical effects

Central nervous system

Ketamine produces a 'dissociative anaesthesia'; this means a profound analgesic effect with light anaesthesia. The eyes remain open and nystagmus occurs; therefore, the endpoint for onset of anaesthesia is not clearly defined. Cerebral blood flow, cerebral metabolic oxygen requirement, intracranial pressure and intraocular pressure are all increased.

Cardiovascular system

Cardiac output is increased due to tachycardia and increased blood pressure following an increase in sympathetic tone. Ketamine is used in shocked patients for these reasons; however, in severely hypovolaemic patients, cardiac output can fall. A mild degree of direct myocardial depression occurs and ketamine use is contraindicated in patients with severe ischaemic heart disease.

Respiratory system

Minute volume increases slightly and laryngeal reflexes are preserved. It is a potent bronchodilator and should be considered when inducing anaesthesia in patients with bronchospasm. Occasionally, it is used for the treatment of refractory asthma at sub-anaesthetic doses as an infusion.

Other effects

Salivation increases but the gastrointestinal tract motility is not affected. Uterine tone is increased. Ketamine is associated with the emergence phenomenon. Emergence delirium and hallucinations are relatively common, but the coadministration of benzodiazepines reduces the incidence. In chronic drug abusers, ketamine causes bladder dysfunction but this has not been seen in clinical use.

Etomidate

Clinical uses and indications

Etomidate is used for induction of general anaesthesia, given intravenously at a dose of 0.3mg/kg. It is the most cardiostable of the intravenous induction agents, but its use has fallen because of increased morbidity and mortality said to be associated with adrenocortical suppression.

Structure and physical properties

Etomidate is an ester as well as an imidazole derivative. It is presented as a white lipid emulsion at a concentration of 2mg/ml. It is also available as a clear solution in 35% propylene glycol.

Mechanism of action

Only the R(+) enantiomer produces anaesthesia. It acts on $GABA_A$ receptors to potentiate inhibitory transmission within the central nervous system.

Pharmacokinetics and pharmacodynamics

Etomidate acts rapidly following an induction dose and wears off after 6-10 minutes. The initial offset of effect is due to redistribution; however, it is rapidly metabolised as is the case with most esters. It undergoes ester hydrolysis by plasma and hepatic esterases. It does not accumulate following repeated doses.

Clinical effects

Central nervous system

A fifth of patients show generalised epileptiform activity on EEG.

Cardiovascular system

The most desirable property of this drug is its cardiovascular stability. It has little effect on autonomic tone and heart rate. A small decrease in systemic vascular resistance occurs with a slight decrease in blood pressure and cardiac output. It does not increase myocardial oxygen demand.

Metabolic system

Etomidate inhibits the steroid synthesis pathway by inhibiting the enzymes 11-β-hydroxylase and 17-α-hydroxylase. This results in reduced circulating cortisol and aldosterone levels up to 48 hours after a single dose. There is conflicting evidence on whether a single induction dose is safe; however, a continuous infusion for sedation does increase mortality. It may have a role in selected patients. Two new drugs, methoxy-carbonyl-etomidate and carboetomidate, are in the early stages of development. Both drugs cause significantly less adrenocortical suppression in animal studies but clinical trials are awaited.

Midazolam

Clinical uses and indications

Midazolam is predominantly used as a sedative agent either for short procedures or on the intensive care unit. However, it can be used for induction of anaesthesia as a sole agent at a dose of 0.3mg/kg or more commonly as a co-induction agent to reduce the required dose of the primary induction agent.

It is also used for premedication in the paediatric age group at a dose of 0.5mg/kg orally and also in the treatment of chronic pain.

Structure and physical properties

Midazolam is presented as a clear solution containing 1, 2 or 5mg/ml. It is usually diluted with saline to a concentration of 1mg/ml.

Mechanism of action

It works in a similar way to other benzodiazepines, by acting on benzodiazepine receptors within the central nervous system. They are related to GABA receptors.

Pharmacokinetics

Midazolam has a slow onset when used for induction of anaesthesia and a slow emergence. It has a bioavailability of approximately 45% when administered orally. It is metabolised in the liver almost completely to active metabolites and is excreted in the urine.

Midazolam demonstrates tautomerism. The structure of its 'diazepine' ring opens to form an ionised water-soluble isomer in an acidic solution. At a higher pH, the ring closes so it becomes unionised and lipid-soluble. It has a pKa of 6.5, so at a physiological pH of 7.4 around 90% is unionised.

Clinical effects

Central nervous system

The principal effects of midazolam are hypnosis and anterograde amnesia. Cerebral oxygen consumption and cerebral blood flow are decreased. It also has anticonvulsant effects. A buccal formulation is available for the treatment of seizures. It decreases the minimum alveolar concentration (MAC) of inhaled anaesthetic agents by 15%.

Cardiovascular and respiratory systems

It leads to a fall in blood pressure and reflex tachycardia occurs. Tidal volume falls but the respiratory rate increases and minute volume remains stable. Apnoea can occur either due to its central effects or airway obstruction. The dose this occurs at is variable between patients.

Other effects

Withdrawal phenomena may occur after prolonged infusion. The effects of midazolam can be reversed with flumazenil.

Total intravenous anaesthesia (TIVA)

. TIVA is the delivery of anaesthetic by a continuous infusion of intravenous agent. There are many drugs which can be used, but the two most common are propofol and remifentanil.

The two fundamental differences in TIVA and inhalational anaesthesia are the inability to measure the plasma concentration of anaesthetic in TIVA and the dissociation of anaesthesia from the respiratory system. The obvious disadvantage of not being able to monitor plasma concentration is the risk of underdosing or overdosing the patient. Safety mechanisms have been developed to prevent accidental awareness during TIVA and these are related to the pharmacokinetic models incorporated in the infusion pumps and special infusion lines that maintain unidirectional flow.

Target-controlled infusion (TCI) pumps are able to predict the plasma concentration and adjust the infusion rate accordingly. They are programmed with a range of pharmacokinetic models for different drugs. The detailed pharmacokinetics of the algorithms is beyond the scope of

Table 1.1. The advantages and disadvantages of TIVA.

Advantages	Disadvantages
Reduce incidence of postoperative nausea and vomiting	Relatively expensive
Less environmental pollution	Higher incidence of accidental awareness
Rapid recovery	Special infusion pumps required
Rapidly titratable	

this book. The algorithms have been developed by using pharmacokinetic data from healthy volunteers. The TCI pump requires patient details such as height, weight, age and sex, as well as the desired plasma concentration and it will then adjust the infusion rate over the course of the anaesthetic to maintain that concentration. At the end of the anaesthetic the infusion is stopped and the drug effects wear off due to redistribution, metabolism and excretion. The drug cannot be removed any other way unlike inhalational agents where increasing ventilation will increase drug clearance. The advantages and disadvantages of TIVA are shown in Table 1.1.

Case scenario 1

You are planning to anaesthetise a 51-year-old male for a craniotomy. He has a brain tumour and signs of raised intracranial pressure (ICP).

Which agent would you choose for induction and maintenance of anaesthesia?

The Monroe Kellie doctrine states that as intracranial volume increases due to an increase in one of its constituents, i.e blood, cerebrospinal fluid or brain parenchyma, the pressure will initially remain stable due to a compensatory decrease in one of the other constituents but after a critical point, ICP will rise exponentially. Volatile anaesthetic agents cause cerebral vasodilatation and therefore an increase in cerebral blood volume (CBV). In patients with signs of intracranial hypertension, this small increase in volume could lead to significantly raised pressure and ischaemia. Propofol and remifentanil are ideal agents in this situation, as they do not increase intracranial pressure; in fact, propofol decreases CBV. They are also rapidly-acting so can be titrated quickly to the surgical stimulus to prevent swings in blood pressure and heart rate.

Although the physiological evidence for using TIVA and avoiding volatile anaesthetics seems strong, this has not translated into measurably significant clinical outcomes. This may be due to multiple factors determining neurological outcome. The CBV increases secondary to volatile anaesthetics in a dose-dependent effect.

Case scenario 2

You are called to help in the emergency department. A 20-year-old female has been admitted following multiple episodes of seizures. She has no other medical history. She is now disorientated, combative and uncooperative. Following your assessment your plan is to get a CT head scan to rule out serious intracranial pathology.

How would you proceed?

The seizures could be due to a multitude of reasons and getting a timely CT scan is essential to aid diagnosis. Her neurological status may be due to an underlying pathology or due to the treatment received to control the seizures. It will not be possible to get a CT scan in her current state. There are two options. The first is to provide sedation; however, there are a number of risks with this option. The airway will be unprotected, there is no control over ventilation and once the patient is in the CT scanner it will be difficult to monitor vital signs. If the patient was to vomit it may not be detected.

The second option is to secure the airway with a cuffed endotracheal tube following a rapid sequence induction. The use of an anaesthetic machine would be impractical to maintain anaesthesia during transfer. The ideal method would be to use TIVA, as the equipment required is portable and can be run on batteries. By giving a continuous infusion of propofol the effects of anaesthesia can be reversed relatively quickly, which is useful when waking the patient up and assessing the patient's neurological function.

Further reading

1.   Dinsmore J. Anaesthesia for elective neurosurgery. *Br J Anaesth* 2007; 99: 68-74.
2.   Khan SK, Hayes I, Buggy DJ. Pharmacology of anaesthetic agents I: intravenous anaesthetic agents. *Br J Anaesth CEACCP* 2014; 14: 100-5.
3.   Henrik E, Raeder J. Total intravenous anaesthesia techniques for ambulatory surgery. *Curr Opin Anesthesiol* 2009; 22: 725-9.
4.   Academy of Medical Royal Colleges. Safe sedation practices for healthcare procedures: standards and guidance, 2013. http://www.rcoa.ac.uk/document-store/safe-sedation-practice-healthcare-procedures-standards-and-guidance.

2 Inhalational agents

Mohammed Auldin

Introduction

Inhalational anaesthetic agents can be used for the induction and maintenance of anaesthesia. They are also known as volatile anaesthetic agents because at room temperature they are in a liquid state with low boiling points. Early inhalational anaesthetics have now been phased out for a number of reasons. Chloroform was introduced in the mid 1800s but quite soon it became apparent there were safety issues with its use. Others such as ether and cyclopropane were flammable. Newer agents have similar favourable properties without the risk profile.

The delivery of anaesthetic agents to the patient has evolved. Early methods involved soaking gauze or cloth with the anaesthetic and having the patient breathe through it. Modern anaesthetic machines are able to deliver gas mixtures with accurate concentrations of gases and anaesthetics, with the ability to rapidly adjust the various concentrations. Monitoring allows the inspired and expired concentrations of oxygen and anaesthetic agents to be measured. Collectively, these advances have increased the safety of delivering inhalational anaesthesia and improved the cost efficiency of using relatively expensive agents.

In this chapter we will discuss the commonly used anaesthetic agents and their clinical effects, with particular attention placed on the aspects that influence clinical decisions. The mechanism of action for inhalational agents will be reviewed along with their pharmacokinetics.

Mechanism of action

The main clinical effect desired from an inhalational anaesthetic is loss of consciousness or hypnosis. Other beneficial effects are amnesia, analgesia and immobility. A number of theories for the molecular mechanism of action have been proposed but detailed understanding is lacking.

Volatile anaesthetics are unique in that they are inhaled continuously for the duration of the anaesthetic. Very few drugs are administered in this way and therefore a number of terms need to be defined in order to aid the understanding of the unique pharmacokinetics.

Potency

Potency in orally or intravenously administered medications is the dose needed to lead to an equivalent effect. Knowing the potency of drugs allows us to decide the dose required to achieve a given effect — unconsciousness in the case of anaesthetics. For inhaled anaesthetics, potency is discussed in terms of the minimum alveolar concentration (MAC). MAC is the alveolar concentration of an inhaled anaesthetic that prevents movement in response to a standard surgical incision in 50% of subjects. This definition assumes that no other sedative or analgesic drugs are administered and the volatile is mixed in oxygen so that the only drug contributing to unconsciousness and immobility is the volatile anaesthetic.

MAC is inversely related to potency. It is measured as a percentage at atmospheric pressure and is therefore not affected by altitude. However, there are a number of factors that will affect MAC and these are listed in Table 2.1.

In the 19th century, Meyer and Overton independently described that the potency of an inhalational anaesthetic was directly proportional to its lipid solubility, i.e. a highly lipid-soluble agent such as halothane has a lower MAC than a poorly lipid-soluble agent such as nitrous oxide. Two different agents mixed together will provide an additive effect, for example,

Table 2.1. Factors affecting the minimum alveolar concentration (MAC).

Increase MAC	Decrease MAC	No effect
Children	Opioids	Duration
Hyperthermia	Benzodiazepines	Sex
Hyperthyroidism	Nitrous oxide	Blood pH
Chronic alcohol use	Hypothermia	pCO_2
	Hypoxia	
	Hypotension	
	Pregnancy	
	Extremes of age	

0.5% MAC of nitrous oxide with 0.5% MAC of isoflurane will have the same anaesthetic effect as either agent at 1% MAC.

Inhalational anaesthetics have a relatively rapid onset of action and the effect is easily reversible. It is therefore likely that the mechanism of action is related to temporary forces either due to the physical property of the anaesthetic or reversible intermolecular forces. Meyer and Overton's theory on the relationship between potency and lipid solubility led to the lipid theory of anaesthesia. The hypotheses suggested inhalational anaesthetic agents worked by dissolving into the phospholipid bilayer of neuronal cells and altering the membrane structure.

Further work disproved this. The concentration of anaesthetic required to alter phospholipid structure is many times the amount administered clinically. Recent theories show the site of action to be ligand gated ion channels, in particular the $GABA_A$ and glycine receptors, the effect being a potentiation of their inhibitory actions. Inhalational anaesthetics bind to specific lipophilic sites within the protein structure and neuronal cell membranes. The primary effect is on a number of proteins, ligand gated receptors and ion channels within the central nervous system rather than a simple interaction at one site, but the final pathway is to potentiate inhibitory receptors to prevent postsynaptic action potentials.

Onset of action

A quick onset and offset of action is a desirable property for an anaesthetic agent. It ensures patient comfort, early mobilisation and efficient turnover in theatre. Loss of consciousness occurs when the partial pressure of the inhalational agent in the CNS reaches a level that is unique to each agent. This is proportionate to the alveolar partial pressure of the anaesthetic agent (PA_{agent}), which is relatively easy to measure. Therefore, factors which promote the rapid increase of partial pressures of anaesthetic agents in the alveoli will lead to a rapid equilibrium being established with the CNS and therefore a rapid onset and offset.

The speed at which equilibrium is established is dependent on three factors, the concentration delivered in the fresh gas flow, lung ventilation and rate of uptake from alveoli. These factors are a combination of patient physiology, specific properties of the agent and the dose administered by the anaesthetist.

Concentration delivered

A high-inspired concentration will ensure a steep concentration gradient and, theoretically, very high concentrations could be delivered but this is limited by the vapouriser design. All vapourisers have a maximum concentration that can be delivered. The term 'overpressure' is used to describe the technique of using high concentration settings to rapidly increase the alveolar partial pressure and therefore the CNS partial pressure. The maximum percentage setting selectable on a vapouriser is dependent on the agent it is designed for and it is a safety measure to prevent overdose.

Lung ventilation

As the inspired gas mixture enters the lung, the anaesthetic concentration is diluted by the gases already in the functional residual capacity. This effect can be overcome in part by increasing the tidal volume. In a spontaneous breathing patient, tidal volume is dependent on central respiratory drive; however, as depth of anaesthesia increases, the respiratory drive is depressed and this acts as a negative feedback mechanism limiting a rapid increase in alveolar anaesthetic concentration. During controlled ventilation, higher tidal volumes can be delivered and this will result in a quicker rise in alveolar anaesthetic agent concentration.

Rate of uptake from the alveoli

Once the anaesthetic agent has reached the alveoli it moves into the alveolar capillaries and equilibrium is achieved across the alveolar-capillary membrane. Somewhat paradoxically, as more anaesthetic agent dissolves across into the pulmonary capillaries, the longer it takes for loss of consciousness to occur. This can be explained by understanding that it is the partial pressure of anaesthetic agent in the blood stream that determines its effect not the total amount dissolved in blood. Therefore, a high cardiac output will encourage more agent to dissolve by maintaining a concentration gradient and increase the time for the partial pressure to rise. Hence, in a high cardiac output state, such as anxiety or sepsis, it takes longer for loss of consciousness to occur when using an inhalational technique.

Blood:gas solubility

The blood:gas solubility of an agent relates to the solubility of the anaesthetic agent in blood as compared to its solubility in air. If a 10ml container was filled with 5ml of blood, 5ml of air and a small amount of inhalational anaesthetic and then sealed, the anaesthetic would dissolve in blood and eventually an equilibrium would develop where the partial pressure of the anaesthetic was the same in blood and air. The ratio of the content of anaesthetic in the blood and air at this point is the blood:gas partition coefficient. An agent with high blood:gas solubility will be more soluble in blood and the partial pressure will take longer to rise, thereby slowing its onset. Nitrous oxide and desflurane have low blood:gas solubility and both these agents have a quick onset and offset of action. Conversely, halothane has a high blood:gas solubility and so the onset is slower.

This can be demonstrated experimentally by administering a fixed concentration of anaesthetic agent (inspired concentration, F_I) to a subject and measuring the expired agent concentration (alveolar concentration, F_A) over a period of time. Plotting the F_A:F_I ratio against time shows that agents with a low blood:gas solubility reach equilibrium more quickly than the agents with high solubility (Figure 2.1).

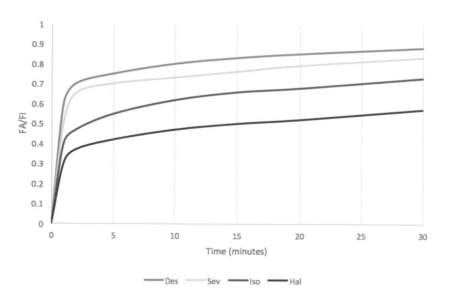

Figure 2.1. The effect of blood:gas solubility on the relationship between time and the F_A:F_I ratio. Inhalational agents with low blood:gas solubility show a rapid rise in alveolar concentration and achieve a higher F_A:F_I ratio quickly.

Obesity leads to an increase in onset and offset time. This is due to the large lipid compartment which acts as a reservoir for inhalational anaesthetics. It takes longer for the concentrations to equilibrate across tissues on induction and emergence. Volatile agents with lower lipid solubility, such as desflurane, reduce this effect.

Concentration effect

The concentration effect is uniquely seen with nitrous oxide because it is the only agent currently used in high concentrations. When nitrous oxide is delivered at high concentrations, the rate in rise of alveolar pressure is disproportionately rapid when compared to delivering nitrous oxide in low concentrations. Although nitrous oxide is relatively insoluble in blood when compared to other volatiles, it is twenty times more soluble than nitrogen (nitrogen has a blood:gas partition coefficient of 0.014). More nitrous oxide diffuses out into the blood than nitrogen diffuses into the alveoli. So the pressure in the alveoli falls slightly and this draws more gas in from the respiratory tree increasing the alveolar concentration of nitrous oxide.

Second gas effect

The second gas effect leads on from the concentration effect. When an inhalational agent is given with high flows of nitrous oxide, the alveolar partial pressure for the agent will rise disproportionately quickly. Again, as the nitrous oxide diffuses out quicker than nitrogen diffuses into the alveolus, the resultant smaller volume in the alveoli will lead to the anaesthetic agent exerting a greater partial pressure.

Metabolism of inhalational anaesthetics

Halogenated anaesthetic agents contain a carbon-halogen bond (C-Cl, C-F, C-Br) and these bonds are metabolised to some extent in the liver by the cytochrome p450 system. The C-F bond is extremely stable and is not metabolised to any significant extent; the C-F bond is present in isoflurane, sevoflurane, desflurane and halothane. The C-Br (halothane) and C-Cl (isoflurane, halothane) bonds are metabolised to a greater extent. The carbon-halogen bond is broken down to a halogen ion (F⁻, Cl⁻, Br⁻) and other reactive metabolites. Toxicity is associated with the extent of metabolism. Twenty percent of halothane is metabolised and its use, especially in patients requiring frequent anaesthetics, has been associated with hepatic and renal toxicity. Since newer fluorinated (C-F) agents have been in use, toxicity is rare.

Metabolism of nitrous oxide

A minimal amount of nitrous oxide is metabolised to nitrogen by gut bacteria and during the oxidation of vitamin B12. However, nitrous oxide can have toxic effects when inhaled at high concentrations for a prolonged period of time. This puts healthcare workers at risk when they are working in an unscavenged environment. Megaloblastic changes occur in the bone marrow and these can progress to agranulocytosis. These changes occur over a time period of hours to days. Chronic exposure in unscavenged areas can lead to neurological syndromes similar to subacute combined degeneration of the spinal cord. The pathophysiology behind these changes is impaired DNA synthesis. Nitrous oxide oxidises the vitamin B12 molecule. Subsequently, it cannot act as the cofactor for methionine synthase and the enzyme is inhibited. This results in reduced production of methionine, which has an effect on DNA synthesis. It is important to note that these effects are rarely seen clinically and a recent large randomised controlled trial has not shown an increase in 30-day mortality with nitrous oxide use.

Metabolism of sevoflurane

Around 3.5% of sevoflurane is metabolised; patients on drugs that induce cytochrome p450 will metabolise slightly more. Sevoflurane is metabolised in the liver to inorganic fluoride ions and hexafluoroisopropanol. Fluoride is toxic to the kidneys; however, high plasma concentrations of fluoride ions have not been detected even after prolonged administration of sevoflurane in humans. There is no evidence that patients with chronic kidney disease are at increased risk with sevoflurane.

The physical properties of inhalational anaesthetic agents are shown in Table 2.2.

Table 2.2. Physical properties of inhalational anaesthetic agents.

Agent	Molecular weight	Saturated vapour pressure at 20 (kPa)	MAC (% volume) Adult	Blood:gas partition coefficient	Oil:gas partition coefficient
Nitrous oxide	44	5300	105	0.47	1.4
Isoflurane	184.5	33	1.28	1.4	97
Sevoflurane	200	21	2.5	0.69	53
Desflurane	168	88	5-10	0.42	19
Halothane	197.4	32	0.76	2.4	225
Xenon	131	-	71	0.14	1.9

Nitrous oxide

General properties

Nitrous oxide is used as an adjunct to inhalational anaesthetic agents. It is also used for analgesia in obstetric patients and in the emergency department as Entonox®, a 50:50 mixture with oxygen.

At room temperature and atmospheric pressure, nitrous oxide is colourless and sweet smelling. It is stored in French blue-coloured cylinders. It has a low blood:gas solubility of 0.47, which results in rapid onset and offset, and a low oil:gas solubility of 1.4, which explains its poor potency and a MAC of 105%.

Despite its low blood:gas solubility, nitrous oxide is twenty times more soluble than oxygen and nitrogen. It enters air-filled spaces faster than air can diffuse out and expands these spaces, which can worsen pneumothorax and bowel obstruction. The use of nitrous oxide in these conditions is contraindicated.

Clinical effects

Central nervous system

As well as the anaesthetic effect, nitrous oxide has a relatively potent analgesic effect. It has agonist activity at opioid and adrenergic receptors. It slightly increases cerebral blood flow, cerebral metabolism and intracranial pressure, and for this reason is avoided in patients with serious intracranial disease.

Respiratory system

The minute volume remains unchanged, although the tidal volume falls and the respiratory rate increases.

Cardiovascular system

Compared to volatile anaesthetic agents, nitrous oxide is relatively cardiostable. It does exert a slight depressant effect directly on the myocardium, but centrally it increases sympathetic activity and therefore in most healthy patients the cardiovascular system is unchanged. Its use is not contraindicated in patients with cardiac disease.

Gastrointestinal system

Its use is associated with postoperative nausea and vomiting; distension of bowel and action on opioid receptors are possible mechanisms. Recent evidence suggests that this effect can be negated with antiemetics.

Isoflurane

General properties

Isoflurane is widely used in the UK and is significantly cheaper than desflurane and sevoflurane. It is a non-flammable liquid with a pungent odour. It is more potent than desflurane and sevoflurane with a MAC of 1.1% in a 40-year-old; however, it has a slower onset. It has been used for analgesia for changing burn dressings and labour analgesia as a commercial preparation called Isoxane® (mixture of Entonox® and 0.25% isoflurane). Isoflurane vapourisers and bottles are colour-coded purple.

Clinical effects

Central nervous system

Isoflurane acts centrally to relax skeletal muscles and enhance the action of non-depolarising muscle relaxants. It depresses EEG activity, acting as an anticonvulsant and at 2% MAC it produces an isoelectric EEG.

It increases cerebral blood flow because of vasodilation and as a result it increases intracranial pressure. This effect is somewhat offset by the reduced cerebral metabolic oxygen requirement which can be reduced by up to 50%.

Respiratory system

Isoflurane is an irritant and is likely to cause coughing and breath holding and for this reason it is rarely used for inhalation induction. It is a respiratory depressant, the minute volume falls and $PaCO_2$ rises; this is mainly due to a fall in tidal volume. The respiratory rate increases slightly but not enough to compensate. It also causes bronchodilatation in higher concentrations.

Cardiovascular system

Isoflurane causes vasodilation and as a result hypotension and compensatory tachycardia. It causes a relatively small amount of direct myocardial depression. Myocardial oxygen demand decreases but some areas of the myocardium may have a reduced supply due to coronary steal, although more recent research has shown regional ischaemia does not occur as long as coronary perfusion is maintained. It is not contraindicated in ischaemic heart disease.

Other effects

Isoflurane causes a dose-dependent relaxation in uterine smooth muscle tone; this needs to be kept in mind when managing uterine atony and haemorrhage.

Sevoflurane

General properties

Sevoflurane has a low blood:gas solubility (fast onset) and a pleasant smell; this makes it an ideal agent for inhalation induction. It is commonly used in paediatrics but over the last few years its use has become widespread for the maintenance of anaesthesia although it is significantly more expensive than isoflurane. Sevoflurane reacts with strong bases and water to produce toxic breakdown products. These are called compounds A, B, C, D and E. Clinically, compounds A and B are of interest. In experimental concentrations of more than 50ppm, compound A may cause renal tubular acidosis, but in clinical use much lower concentrations of compound A and B are detected. The hydrolysis reaction producing these compounds is accelerated by high temperatures, high concentration of sevoflurane, and low-flow anaesthesia. Baralyme® also accelerates the reaction when compared to soda lime, possibly because the temperatures in Baralyme® are higher.

Clinical effects

Central nervous system

Sevoflurane has similar effects on the EEG and skeletal muscles as isoflurane. Compared to other inhaled anaesthetics, studies suggest cerebral vascular autoregulation is preserved in patients with cerebrovascular disease, making it the volatile of choice for neuroanaesthesia. It provides smooth and rapid induction of anaesthesia when inhaled at concentrations of 4-8% mixed with nitrous oxide. Its use has been associated with immediate postoperative delirium mainly in children, unlike isoflurane.

Respiratory system

Ventilatory effort is depressed with a resulting drop in minute volume and rise in $PaCO_2$. It causes bronchodilatation and minimal airway irritation. This makes it useful for the treatment of asthma refractive to conventional treatment.

Cardiovascular system

Sevoflurane affects systemic vascular resistance and therefore blood pressure falls. However, unlike isoflurane, there is usually no compensatory tachycardia.

Other effects

Sevoflurane causes uterine smooth muscle relaxation but can be used in obstetric patients at low concentrations.

Desflurane

General properties

Desflurane was introduced into UK clinical practice in 1994 despite first being synthesised in the 1960s. It is a colourless liquid with a pungent smell. It has a blood:gas solubility of 0.42, which means it has a rapid onset and offset of action. It has an oil:gas solubility of 19 and a MAC of 5-7% in adults. Desflurane is delivered by a special vapouriser due to its boiling point of 23°C and saturated vapour pressure of 88kPa at 20°C. The vapouriser heats the desflurane so it is in the gaseous state and then injects it into the fresh gas flow.

Clinical effects

Central nervous system

It has the same effects as isoflurane. It is useful in spinal and brain surgery because its quick offset allows early examination of neurological function.

Respiratory system

It has the same physiological effects as isoflurane. It is markedly irritant to the respiratory tree in high concentrations and may cause coughing on induction or emergence. It is not an ideal agent for inhalation induction.

Cardiovascular system

Desflurane causes a decrease in myocardial contractility and systemic vascular resistance but sympathetic tone is preserved leading to reflex tachycardia. The coronary steal phenomenon does not occur.

Halothane

General properties

Halothane has not been routinely available in the UK since 2007; however, it is still used in some parts of the world albeit rarely. It is presented as a clear liquid in 0.01% thymol and is protected from sunlight to prevent degradation. It has a blood:gas solubility of 2.5, an oil:gas solubility of 225 and a MAC of 0.76%. It has a C-Br bond that is metabolised in the liver.

Clinical effects

Central nervous system

Halothane has anticonvulsant properties and it increases cerebral blood flow.

Respiratory system

Due to its pleasant smell and early abolition of laryngeal reflexes, it is an ideal agent for inhalation induction. It is possible to intubate the trachea without the use of muscle relaxants in patients spontaneously breathing halothane.

Cardiovascular system

Halothane shares the adverse effects on the cardiovascular system with other inhalational agents. In addition, it sensitises the myocardium to catecholamines making arrhythmias more common.

Other effects

Repeated and frequent administration of halothane may cause halothane hepatitis; this can vary from mild impairment of liver function to gross hepatic failure.

Xenon

General properties

Xenon is a noble gas with anaesthetic properties and has been used experimentally for the last 50 years in clinical anaesthesia. It is present in the atmosphere but is extremely rare, making up just 0.09ppm. Its production is by fractional distillation and is relatively expensive especially when considering the quantities required for its use in a conventional anaesthetic circuit.

There is considerable interest in the use of xenon because of several advantages over nitrous oxide and other inhalational anaesthetic agents:

- Its blood:gas partition coefficient is only 0.12 leading to a rapid onset and offset. Inhalational induction times for xenon have been reported on average as 71 seconds compared to 147 seconds for sevoflurane.

Table 2.3. Anaesthetic effects of inhalational agents.

Properties	Nitrous oxide	Halothane	Isoflurane	Sevoflurane	Desflurane
Onset/offset of action	+++	+	++	+++	+++
Analgesic properties	+++	+	+	+	+
Respiratory					
Respiratory rate	↑	↑	↑	↑	↑
Tidal volume	↓	↓↓	↓↓	↓↓	↓↓
$PaCO_2$	No effect	↑	↑	↑	↑
Irritation	Non-irritant	Pleasant smell	Irritant	Sweet smell	Pungent and irritant
Cardiovascular					
Heart rate	No effect	↑↑	↑↑	↑↓	↑
Blood pressure	Minimal effect	↓↓	↓↓	↓↓	↓↓
Cardiac sensitivity to catecholamines	Minimal effect	↑↑↑	↑	↑	↑
CNS					
Cerebral blood flow	↑	↑↑↑	↑	↑	↑
EEG	No effect	Decreased voltage	Decreased voltage	Decreased voltage	Decreased voltage

Table 2.3 *continued*. Anaesthetic effects of inhalational agents.

Properties	Nitrous oxide	Halothane	Isoflurane	Sevoflurane	Desflurane
Metabolism %	<0.01	20	0.2	3.5	0.02
Toxicity	Inactivation of vitamin B12, bone marrow suppression	Hepatitis	None	Renal toxic?	None

- It has remarkable cardiovascular stability. Studies have noted no clinically significant change in blood pressure or heart rate when using xenon for anaesthesia or sedation. This is thought to be due to less autonomic effects. These effects are also seen in patients with impaired cardiac function undergoing cardiac surgery.
- Xenon has potent analgesic effects. When compared to nitrous oxide (the only other inhalational agent with analgesic efficacy), less intra-operative fentanyl supplementation was required. The analgesic effect is mediated by inhibition of N-methyl-D-aspartate (NMDA) receptors.

The main disadvantages to the use of xenon are:

- Cost is the major barrier to using xenon. Special closed delivery systems have been developed which keep the amount used to a minimum, the most being used during the initial flushing of the system.
- It has a relatively high MAC value of between 60-70% that precludes its use as a sole anaesthetic agent in some instances.

A summary of anaesthetic effects of inhalational agents is outlined in Table 2.3.

Case scenario 1

A 3-year-old boy is brought into the emergency department by ambulance. You are asked to see him, as there are concerns about his airway. On assessment he looks unwell and is in respiratory distress. He has stridor and is drooling from his mouth. The working diagnosis is acute epiglottitis.

How would you manage this child's airway?

Acute epiglottitis is a life-threatening emergency due to infection of the epiglottis usually secondary to *Haemophilus influenzae* and complete airway obstruction may be precipitated.

The main concerns in this scenario are:

- The risk of airway obstruction due to the large epiglottis and airway oedema. To protect against complete obstruction, the trachea will need to be intubated.
- With an anxious child, disturbing the child further will likely worsen airway obstruction. It would be unwise to attempt intravenous cannulation.
- In a difficult airway situation, the child is likely to have difficult direct laryngoscopy as well as difficult or impossible bag mask ventilation.

Taking the above points into consideration, the aim is to anaesthetise and intubate this child whilst minimising distress. Gaining intravenous access can cause anxiety and is best avoided. Spontaneous ventilation will need to be maintained because of the likelihood of difficult bag mask ventilation. To achieve this, a suitable technique would be to do an inhalational induction with sevoflurane in 100% oxygen. Sevoflurane is non-irritant and has a relatively quick onset of action. Inducing anaesthesia in whichever position they are comfortable will minimise distress. A senior ENT surgeon must be present and ready to perform an emergency tracheostomy if intubation and bag mask ventilation are impossible.

Whilst inducing with sevoflurane the child will continue breathing spontaneously. Laryngoscopy must only be attempted once a deep plane of anaesthesia is achieved. With regard to the pharmacokinetics, this will take some time because the child is breathing spontaneously and the minute ventilation will be relatively low. He will also have a high cardiac output, which will prolong the time taken for the alveolar partial pressure of sevoflurane to equilibrate with the CNS. Once the child has reached a deep plane of anaesthesia, direct laryngoscopy may be attempted and the trachea intubated. Further management will be to treat the underlying infection and supportive intensive care treatment. Sedation will be required to allow tolerance of the endotracheal tube, and extubation is usually possible after a few days once the airway oedema has settled.

Further reading

1.   Myles PS, Leslie K, Peyton P, *et al.* The safety of addition of nitrous oxide to general anaesthesia in at-risk patients having major non-cardiac surgery (ENIGMA-II): a randomised, single-blind trial. *Lancet* 2014; 384(9952): 1446-54.

2.   Hudson AE, Hemmings HC. Are anaesthetics toxic to the brain? *Br J Anaesth* 2011; 107(1): 30-7.

3.   Sellers WFS. Inhaled and intravenous treatment in acute severe and life-threatening asthma. *Br J Anaesth* 2013; 110(2): 183-90.

4.   Perks A, Cheema S, Mohanraj R. Anaesthesia and epilepsy. *Br J Anaesth* 2012; 108(4): 562-71.

5.   Schifilliti D, Grasso G, Conti A, *et al.* Anaesthetic-related neuroprotection. *CNS Drugs* 2010; 24(11): 893-907.

3 Neuromuscular blocking drugs

Meghna Sharma

Introduction

The use of neuromuscular blocking drugs in anaesthesia has changed the practice of general anaesthesia (GA) over the years. Neuromuscular blocking drugs can be classified into many categories but in anaesthetic practice they are primarily divided into depolarising and non-depolarising muscle relaxants. In order to understand these drugs we need to have a fair idea about the neuromuscular junction (NMJ).

In humans the NMJ has a terminal nerve axon, synaptic cleft and muscle membrane. Acetylcholine is the main neurotransmitter that is responsible for initiation of a sequence resulting in muscle contraction. The acetylcholine is stored in the terminal nerve axon in synaptic vesicles. A nerve action potential is responsible for rapid release of acetylcholine into the synaptic cleft. This in turn acts on the nicotinic acetylcholine receptor (nAchR) that is present in higher concentration on the shoulders in the synaptic cleft. When two molecules of acetylcholine are bound to a nAchR, it results in calcium and sodium influx into the muscle membrane thereby depolarising it and leading to muscle contraction. Following this the acetylcholine is acted upon by the acetycholinesterase (AchEs) present in the cleft and metabolised to choline and acetyl CoA. These are used to regenerate new molecules of acetylcholine to be stored in synaptic vesicles. The muscle relaxants tend to act on the nAchR and based on whether they cause depolarisation or behave as an antagonist on the alpha subunits of nAchR, they can be classified as depolarising or non-depolarising muscle relaxants.

Depolarising muscle relaxants (DMR)

These are short- to moderate-acting muscle relaxants and are used as an accompaniment for GA. The two main drugs in this class are suxamethonium and decamethonium. We shall only discuss suxamethonium in this chapter as this drug is the more widely used of the two.

Suxamethonium

Indications

- Suxamethonium helps to facilitate endotracheal intubation for rapid sequence induction especially in patients with a full stomach or in pregnant women undergoing GA.
- It is also used in low doses quite frequently in patients undergoing electroconvulsive therapy (ECT).

Structure and physical properties

Suxamethonium is structurally made up of two molecules of acetylcholine joined together through their acetyl groups. It is available as a colourless solution of suxamethonium chloride in ampoules of 50mg/ml. The dose required for endotracheal intubation is 1.5-2mg/kg. It must be stored at 4°C.

Mechanism of action

Suxamethonium tends to cause depolarisation of the membrane, as it is structurally similar to acetylcholine by binding to the nAchR. It cannot be metabolised by AchEs, hence the duration of action lasts for a few minutes. There is contraction followed by muscle relaxation, which is clinically seen as twitches all over the body when it is administered intravenously.

Pharmacokinetics

Suxamethonium is metabolised in the body by plasma cholinesterase. It is hydrolysed to form choline and succinylmonocholine which is further metabolised to succinic acid and choline.

Clinical effects

Suxamethonium has variable effects on body systems. It may cause ventricular arrhythmias or bradycardia. It is known to cause a rise in intracranial, intraocular and intragastric pressure. It is also known to cause a rise in serum potassium concentration by 0.2-0.4mmol/L. Hence, it should be used with caution in patients with renal failure as well as in patients with burns and neuromuscular disorders. There is a potential for prolonged block with suxamethonium when it is given as a second dose.

In susceptible individuals with a plasma cholinesterase deficiency, it may lead to suxamethonium apnoea. This is possible in patients with liver disease, hypoproteinaemia, carcinomatosis, cardiac or renal failure and also in pregnancy. Based on the genetic makeup of the individual, the response to suxamethonium is variable.

Non-depolarising muscle relaxants (NDMR)

All non-depolarising muscle relaxants act as compotitive antagonists of acetylcholine at the alpha subunit of the nAchR on the postsynaptic membrane of the NMJ. Experimental evidence suggests that 75-80% of receptors on the postsynaptic membrane should be occupied before there is any effect on neuromuscular transmission. NDMRs can be divided into two classes: benzylisoquiniliniums and aminosteroids. The common examples amongst these classes of drugs include vecuronium and rocuronium, which are aminosteroids, and atracurium and mivacurium, which are benzylisoquiniliniums that are discussed below.

Vecuronium

Indications

- Vecuronium helps to facilitate endotracheal intubation in patients undergoing GA.
- It can also be used for controlled ventilation in an intensive care setting.

Structure and physical properties

Vecuronium is a monoquarternary aminosteroid compound, available in ampoules as a 10mg white powder containing mannitol and a buffer. On dilution with water it forms a clear colourless solution. The dose required for endotracheal intubation is 0.1-0.15mg/kg. It can be stored at room temperature.

Mechanism of action

Vecuronium is a competitive antagonist of acetylcholine at the alpha subunit of the nAchR on the postsynaptic membrane of the NMJ.

Pharmacokinetics

Vecuronium is 10-20% protein bound and does not cross the placental or blood brain barrier. It undergoes deacetylation in the liver to form various metabolites, of which the 3-hydroxy metabolite has muscle relaxant properties. It is excreted in urine and bile, unchanged to a large extent.

Clinical effects

Vecuronium is an extremely cardiostable drug and does not lead to hypotension, as there is very low potential for histamine release. It does not cause a rise in intracranial, intraocular and intragastric pressure. Vecuronium can be safely used in patients susceptible to malignant hyperthermia. Its duration of action can be prolonged due to acidosis, hypercapnia, hypokalaemia and hypocalcaemia.

Rocuronium

Indications

- Rocuronium can provide rapid intubating conditions to facilitate endotracheal intubation. Hence, it can be used for modified rapid sequence induction, especially in patients with a full stomach undergoing GA.

Structure and physical properties

Rocuronium is a monoquarternary aminosteroid compound. It is available in vials as a clear and colourless solution of 10mg/ml rocuronium bromide. Rocuronium is physically incompatible with diazepam and thiopentone. The dose required for endotracheal intubation is 0.6-1.2mg/kg. At higher doses, intubation can be attempted at 60 seconds. It must be stored at 2-8°C.

Mechanism of action

Rocuronium is a competitive antagonist of acetylcholine at the alpha subunit of the nAchR on the postsynaptic membrane of the NMJ. It is also known to have some action on the presynaptic membrane.

Pharmacokinetics

Rocuronium is 10-20% protein bound and is known to undergo deacetylation in the liver. It is excreted in bile unchanged to a large extent and to a lesser extent can be found in urine.

Clinical effects

Rocuronium is painful on injection intravenously. It is cardiostable and does not lead to hypotension. It may cause an increase in mean arterial pressure and heart rate. Its duration of action can be prolonged due to acidosis, hypercapnia, hypokalaemia and hypocalcaemia. Amongst all aminosteroids, rocuronium is said to be associated with a higher incidence of anaphylactic reactions.

Atracurium

Indications

- Atracurium helps to facilitate endotracheal intubation in patients undergoing GA.
- It can be used in an intensive care setting as a continuous infusion occasionally.

Structure and physical properties

Atracurium is a benzylisoquinolinium ester compound. It is a mixture of ten different stereoisomers. It is available as a clear and colourless solution of atracurium besilate of 10mg/ml in ampoules of 2.5, 5 and 25ml. The dose required for endotracheal intubation is 0.3-0.6mg/kg. It must be stored at 4°C.

Cisatracurium is one of the stereoisomers, which is also available as a clear and colourless solution. It is three to five times more potent than the parent drug. The dose required for endotracheal intubation is 150μg/kg. It should also be stored at 4°C.

Mechanism of action

Atracurium is a competitive antagonist of acetylcholine at the alpha subunit of the nAchR on the postsynaptic membrane of the NMJ.

Pharmacokinetics

Atracurium is 82% protein bound and does not cross the placental or blood brain barrier. It undergoes hydrolysis by non-specific esterases to quaternary alcohol and quaternary acid. It also undergoes spontaneous breakdown at body pH and temperature (Hofmann elimination) to form laudanosine and quaternary monoacrylate. Laudanosine is known to cross the blood brain barrier and cause convulsions.

Clinical effects

Intravenous atracurium is associated with histamine release in high doses and may cause bronchospasm, hypotension, erythema and wheals; hence, it is best avoided in asthmatics. Atracurium may also cause bradycardia. It has no effect on intracranial or intraocular pressure. Its duration of action can be prolonged due to acidosis, hypercapnia, hypokalaemia and hypocalcaemia.

As cisatracurium does not undergo direct hydrolysis but is mainly metabolised by Hofmann elimination, it can be used effectively in patients with end-stage renal failure and hepatic disease.

Mivacurium

Indications

• Mivacurium is indicated for short procedures where tracheal intubation is required.

Structure and physical properties

Mivacurium is a bisquarternary benzylisoquinolinium diester compound. It is a mixture of three different stereoisomers: cis-cis=6%, trans-trans=58%, cis-trans=36%. It is available in the form of mivacurium chloride as a clear and colourless solution of 2mg/ml in 5 and 10ml ampoules. The dose required for endotracheal intubation is 0.1-0.25mg/kg. It must be stored below 25°C.

Mechanism of action

Mivacurium is a competitive antagonist of acetylcholine at the alpha subunit of the nAchR on the postsynaptic membrane of the NMJ.

Pharmacokinetics

Mivacurium is up to 10% protein bound and undergoes hydrolysis by plasma cholinesterase to quaternary alcohol and quaternary monoester metabolite.

Clinical effects

Since its introduction mivacurium was used in day-case procedures requiring endotracheal intubation. Over a period of time this has reduced. It has no significant effects on the cardiovascular system. It may cause histamine release. In patients with hepatic failure, the duration of action may be prolonged due to reduced levels of plasma cholinesterase. Edrophonium is more suitable to reverse neuromuscular block secondary to mivacurium.

Reversal agents

The neuromuscular blocking drugs used in anaesthetic practice are muscle relaxants acting at the NMJ. In order for an individual to gain control of ventilatory effort and muscle strength, recovery from neuromuscular blockade should be adequate. This is possible by increasing the activity of acetylcholine at the nAchR present at the NMJ. Thus, logically, drugs belonging to the anticholinesterase group are commonly used. More recently, a modified alpha cyclodextrin, sugammadex, is now used for reversal of rocuronium-induced neuromuscular blockade.

Anticholinesterases

Drugs belonging to this group antagonise AchEs, thereby increasing the availability of acetylcholine at the NMJ. This group can be further subdivided into three categories based on how they antagonise AchEs:

- Reversible inhibition, e.g. edrophonium.

- Formation of carbamylated enzyme complex, e.g. neostigmine, physostigmine, pyridostigmine.
- Irreversible inactivation, e.g. organophosphorus compounds.

Neostigmine

Indications

- Neostigmine in combination with glycopyrrolate is most commonly used for the reversal of non-depolarising neuromuscular blockade.
- Neostigmine is also used in the treatment of myasthenia gravis and urinary retention.

Structure and physical properties

Neostigmine is a quaternary amine, which is an ester of alkyl carbamic acid. It is available as a clear and colourless solution in combination with glycopyrrolate in 1ml ampoules (500µg of glycopyrrolate and 2.5mg of neostigmine metisulfate). They can be stored at room temperature.

Mechanism of action

Neostigmine being a carbamate ester forms a carbamylated enzyme complex with AchEs; thus, it prevents AchEs from hydrolysing acetylcholine. This eventually leads to a higher concentration of acetylcholine at the NMJ and subsequent neuromuscular transmission. However, the action of neostigmine is not specific to the NMJ. It has autonomic cholinergic effects; hence, an anticholinergic like glycopyrrolate is used in combination to counter these effects.

Pharmacokinetics

Neostigmine has a bioavailability of less than 1% after oral administration and is minimally protein bound up to 6%. It is highly ionised and does not cross the blood brain barrier. It is metabolised by plasma esterases to quaternary alcohol. The majority of the drug is excreted in the urine unchanged.

Clinical effects

The effects of neostigmine include bradycardia, a fall in cardiac output, hypotension, nausea, vomiting, sweating, lacrimation and increased salivation. It often leads to miosis and failure of accommodation. It can also lead to an increase in bronchial secretions and thus precipitate bronchospasm.

Sugammadex

Indications

- Sugammadex is used for the reversal of non-depolarising neuromuscular blockade induced by rocuronium.

Structure and physical properties

It is a modified alpha cyclodextrin consisting of eight oligosaccharides. They are spatially arranged to form a toroid. It is available as a clear and colourless solution as 100mg/ml in vials. They can be stored at room temperature.

Mechanism of action

Sugammadex encapsulates plasma rocuronium molecules in a ratio of 1:1. It has no effect on AchEs and it is ineffective against depolarising muscle relaxants and benzylisoquinolinium compounds. The dose of sugammadex depends on the degree of neuromuscular block. For immediate reversal the dose is 16mg/kg. In the presence of two twitches of a train-of-four (TOF) response, then the dose required is 2mg/kg. In the event of a more profound block, the dose is 4-8mg/kg.

Pharmacokinetics

Sugammadex has minimal protein binding. It does not cross the blood brain barrier and placental transfer is minimal. The parent drug and its complex are eliminated unchanged by the kidneys.

Clinical effects

Sugammadex has been known to cause prolongation of the QT interval in some patients. In extremely high doses (32mg/kg), it has caused hypotension. Sugammadex has also been used to treat patients who have developed anaphylaxis to rocuronium.

Newer muscle relaxants

Gantacurium is a diester derivative belonging to the tetrahydro-isoquinolinium group. It is undergoing phase III trials in the USA. It has an onset of action of 90 seconds with spontaneous recovery in 10-14 minutes. It could be a potential replacement for succinylcholine. It is associated with less histamine release and its effects can be reversed by edrophonium.

Case scenario 1

A 48-year-old male with a history of poorly controlled asthma is scheduled for an urgent exploration and repair of an obstructed inguinal hernia. He has had a previous lumbar spinal fusion. Following clinical examination of the lumbar spine, it was decided that spinal anaesthesia is not possible; hence, general anaesthesia with tracheal intubation has been planned.

What would be your choice of muscle relaxants for this procedure?

This patient has an increased risk of aspiration; therefore, rapid sequence induction using suxamethonium or a modified rapid sequence induction using rocuronium is ideal. If suxamethonium is used for initial tracheal intubation, then for further muscle relaxation, vecuronium or rocuronium can be used. The aim is to avoid using atracurium, which is known to cause histamine release and can induce bronchospasm.

In this case, rocuronium was used. But intra-operatively, part of the bowel was found to be ischaemic and a bowel resection and anastomosis was performed.

What reversal agent would you use for reversing the muscle relaxant?

It is important to monitor neuromuscular blockade using train-of-four (TOF) monitoring, and an objective method where the TOF ratio can be recorded is most ideal. A reversal agent should be preferably administered in the presence of at least two twitches of a TOF response. Considering the fact that the use of neostigmine has been found to be associated with gastrointestinal anastomotic breakdown, it makes good sense to use sugammadex in this case. The dose would be 2mg/kg.

Case scenario 2

A 56-year-old female patient with hypertension and end-stage renal disease is scheduled for insertion of a continuous ambulatory peritoneal dialysis (CAPD) catheter under general anaesthesia. Pre-operative assessment revealed that there is no risk of aspiration.

What would be the muscle relaxant of choice?

This patient has renal failure. It is important to check the pre-operative electrolytes; potassium is likely to be at the higher side of the normal range. Therefore, suxamethonium should be avoided. As the elimination of atracurium does not depend on hepatic and renal function, it is the muscle relaxant of choice.

Further reading

1. Farooq K, Hunter JM. Neuromuscular blocking agents and reversal agents. *Anaesth Intens Care Med* 2014; 15: 295-9.

2. Khirwadkar R, Hunter JM. Neuromuscular physiology and pharmacology: an update. *Br J Anaesth CEACCP* 2012; 12: 237-44.

3. Eikermann M, Houle TT. Antagonism of neuromuscular block: all things are poison; only the dose makes a thing not a poison. *Br J Anaesth* 2016; 116: 157-9.

4. Fortier LP, McKeen D, Turner K, *et al*. The RECITE Study: a Canadian prospective, multicenter study of the incidence and severity of residual neuromuscular blockade. *Anesth Analg* 2015; 121: 366-72.

4 Analgesic drugs

Shefali Chaudhari and Cyprian Mendonca

Introduction

Postoperative pain depends on many factors such as the anatomical location of surgery, surgical technique, level of postoperative care and psychological preparation of the patient. Various techniques have been used for postoperative pain relief including local infiltration, regional anaesthetic techniques and peripheral nerve blocks.

Multimodal analgesia involves using smaller doses of different analgesic drugs in an additive or synergistic way to achieve maximum analgesic effect with minimum side effects.

Commonly used analgesics for peri-operative pain management are outlined below.

Simple analgesics:

- Paracetamol, non-steroidal anti-inflammatory drugs.

Opioid analgesics:

- Naturally occurring: morphine, codeine.
- Semisynthetic: diamorphine, dihydrocodeine, naloxone.
- Synthetic: pethidine, fentanyl, alfentanil, sufentanil and remifentanil.

Paracetamol

Paracetamol is the first-line treatment for pain and pyrexia with an excellent safety profile. It was introduced in clinical practice in 1883 and became the preferred analgesic from the 1950s when phenacetin was withdrawn because of renal toxicity.

Mechanism of action

The exact mechanism of action of paracetamol is still to be elucidated. It is believed that it acts by:

- Inhibition of cyclo-oxygenase-mediated production of prostaglandins.
- Activation of serotonergic pathways (part of the descending pain system), which arise from brain stem nuclei, the hypothalamus and cortex, and interact with pain afferents in the dorsal horn.
- Increasing the cannabinoid receptor activation by inhibiting the reuptake of endocannabinoids, such as anandamide, from the synaptic cleft. This action causes relaxation and tranquility.

Presentation

Oral tablets, suppositories and intravenous preparations.

Dose

In adults, over 50kg of body weight, 1g 4-6 hourly (maximum 4g/day). In patients with renal impairment, the dose interval should be 6 hours.

In children weighing ≤10kg, the dose is 7.5mg/kg and >10kg, it is 15mg/kg.

Pharmacokinetics

Paracetamol is well absorbed orally, mainly from the small intestine with a bioavailability of 70-90%. It does not cause gastric irritation or bleeding.

Paracetamol is metabolised by hepatic enzymes to glucuronide, sulphate and cysteine conjugates, which are pharmacologically inactive. A small amount of N-acetyl-p-benzoquinone imine (NAPQI) is also formed by N-hydroxylation and conjugated with glutathione to form a non-toxic compound.

Drug interactions

Paracetamol interacts with the following drugs:

- Metoclopramide: increases absorption by increasing gastric emptying.
- Opioids: decreases absorption by decreasing gastric emptying.
- Cholestyramine: reduces the absorption if administered within 1 hour by ion-exchange resin.
- Carbamazepine, phenytoin, barbiturates, isoniazid: increase the risk of toxicity by inducing enzymes.
- Oral anticoagulants: leads to a slight alteration in the International Normalised Ratio (INR).

Toxicity

This drug is generally safe, but in acute overdose or, rarely, even after a therapeutic dose in the presence of subclinical risk factors such as fast metaboliser status or glutathione deficiency, it causes fatal liver, kidney and brain damage.

N-acetyl-p-benzoquinone imine (NAPQI), a toxic metabolite formed in small amounts during normal metabolism, reacts with sulphydryl groups in glutathione to form a non-toxic compound. In paracetamol overdose, hepatic reserves of glutathione are conjugated and depleted. This toxic metabolite combines with sulphydryl groups of liver cell proteins leading to sub-acute hepatic necrosis. This may also occur secondary to inadequate nutrition, cytochrome P450 enzyme induction by chronic alcohol excess or by the use of drugs such as barbiturates or carbamazepine.

The initial presentation of toxicity is nausea, vomiting, and abdominal pain. Signs of liver damage are usually delayed for 2-5 days. Treatment involves gastric lavage (if within 4 hours of ingestion), i.v. fluids and cautious use of antiemetics if there is persistent nausea and vomiting. Immediate administration of N-acetyl cysteine (sulphydryl donor) by infusion is essential. The plasma paracetamol levels should be monitored to assess the severity and effectiveness of treatment. Coagulation is monitored and corrected with vitamin K and other clotting factors.

Adverse effects

Although paracetamol causes adverse effects mainly in overdose, chronic consumption may lead to headache, skin rashes, analgesic nephropathy, chronic nephritis and renal papillary necrosis. Haematological effects include thrombocytopenia, leucopenia and neutropenia. Methaemoglobinaemia and haemolytic anaemia are other rare side effects.

Clinical uses

- Paracetamol is the drug of choice for analgesia and antipyretic actions.
- It prevents remifentanil-induced hyperalgesia.

Non-steroidal anti-inflammatory drugs (NSAIDs)

These are simple analgesics, which also possess anti-inflammatory activity. They are mainly used for mild or moderate pain.

Commonly used NSAIDs are outlined below:

- Enolic acids: piroxicam, meloxicam.
- Carboxylic acids:
  - acetic acids: indomethacin, ketorolac, diclofenac;
  - salicylates: aspirin;
  - propionates: ibuprofen, naproxen.

- Coxibs: celecoxib, etoricoxib, lumiracoxib.

Mechanism of action

NSAIDs inhibit prostaglandin synthesis (Figure 4.1) from arachidonic acid by inhibiting the enzyme, cyclo-oxygenase (COX).

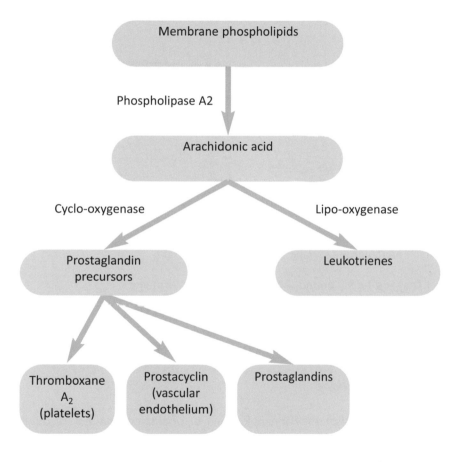

Figure 4.1. Synthesis of prostaglandins.

COX exists in two forms: COX-1 regulates prostaglandin synthesis in the gastric mucosa and renal vascular bed, and also thromboxane A_2 in platelets; COX-2 is present in the brain, spinal cord and macula densa of the glomerulus. It is also produced in cells induced in the process of inflammation, such as endothelial cells and fibroblasts.

Inhibition of COX-1 causes side effects such as gastrointestinal ulceration, impaired renal function and bleeding.

Presentation

As oral tablets, suppositories, and intravenous and intramuscular preparations.

Pharmacokinetics

NSAIDs are well absorbed orally or intramuscularly. They are weak organic acids and mainly unionised in the acid medium of the stomach, which facilitates absorption. However, absorption from the small intestine which has a larger surface area is more important.

They are highly bound (95-99%) to plasma proteins.

NSAIDs are metabolised by hepatic biotransformation, and conjugation followed by renal excretion.

Drug interactions

NSAIDs modify the pharmacokinetics or pharmacodynamics of other drugs.

NSAIDs are highly protein bound (90-99%) and have the potential to displace oral anticoagulants, anticonvulsants, lithium and oral hypoglycaemic agents, leading to supratherapeutic plasma concentration of these drugs.

A pharmacodynamic interaction may occur with antihypertensive drugs regardless of the mechanism of action. The inhibition of COX-2 results in the reduced production of the vasodilator prostaglandin I_2 (PGI_2) in the renal cortex and natriuretic prostaglandin E_2 (PGE_2) in the medulla. This leads to vasoconstriction, and sodium and water retention causing an increase in blood pressure. This action has not been described with low-dose aspirin.

Adverse effects

- Gastrointestinal: dyspepsia, nausea, bleeding from gastric or duodenal vessels, mucosal ulceration, perforation, and diarrhoea.
- Respiratory: bronchoconstriction, pulmonary eosinophilia and can exacerbate asthma (in 5-10% of patients).
- Renal: reduction in glomerular filtration and sodium excretion leading to the retention of fluid. This effect is significant in patients with impaired cardiac function and can lead to heart failure. In the presence of impaired renal function, NSAIDs can precipitate acute renal failure. They can cause hyperkalaemia by inhibiting renin release from the kidney, which decreases aldosterone concentration. Aldosterone regulates potassium concentration and this elevates the potassium.
- Rarely, it can cause papillary necrosis or interstitial fibrosis.
- Haemostasis: NSAIDs reduce platelet aggregation by inhibiting thromboxane A_2. This increases the risk of bleeding.

Other side effects

- Hepatic damage.
- Pancreatitis.
- Stevens-Johnson syndrome.
- Toxic epidermal necrolysis.
- Aseptic meningitis.

Contraindications of NSAIDs

- Past history of gastrointestinal bleeding or peptic ulcer.
- Aspirin-sensitive asthma.
- Renal impairment.
- Hypovolaemia.
- Hyperkalaemia.
- Circulatory failure.
- Severe liver dysfunction.
- Uncontrolled hypertension.
- Pre-eclamptic toxaemia.
- Systemic inflammatory response syndrome.

NSAIDs should either be avoided or used with caution in the elderly population because of altered pharmacokinetics.

Clinical uses

NSAIDs are useful in treating mild to moderate pain such as musculoskeletal and dental pain.

They are administered peri-operatively to spare opioid dosing by 30-40%.

Opioids

Opioids are naturally occurring, semi-synthetic or synthetic compounds that produce agonist or antagonist activity at opioid receptors.

The term "opioid" includes all natural and synthetic drugs, which act on opioid receptors in the central and peripheral nervous system. The term "opiate" is limited to the natural alkaloid found in the resin of the opium poppy.

They are clinically useful in the management of continuous, dull, poorly localised moderate to severe pain arising from deeper structures.

Opioid receptors

Opioids act on opioid receptors that are mainly present in the central nervous system, particularly in the peri-aqueductal grey area and the substantia gelatinosa of the spinal cord. They are also present in the gastrointestinal tract and other peripheral sites.

There are mainly three types of opioid rceptors: μ, κ and δ:

- μ (mu) receptors or OP_3 are found in the brain stem and medial thalamus. They are responsible for supraspinal analgesia, respiratory depression, euphoria, sedation, decreased gastrointestinal motility and physical dependence.
- κ (kappa) or OP_2 receptors are found in limbic and other diencephalic areas, the brain stem and spinal cord. They are responsible for spinal analgesia, sedation, dyspnoea, dependence, dysphoria and respiratory depression.
- δ (delta) or OP_1 receptors are located mainly in the brain. They are responsible for psychomimetic and dysphoric effects.

Opioid analgesics act at the supraspinal and spinal level and decrease the release of substance P, glutamate and other neurotransmitters.

Analgesic potency of opioids is dependent on their affinity for μ recceptors. Only a small degree of receptor occupancy by opioids is required for an analgesic effect. The rest of the drug produces additional pharmacological effects such as respiratory depression, constipation, and increased biliary tract pressure.

Opioids can have a different affinity and efficacy for receptors. On the basis of this, opioids are classified as agonists, partial agonists or antagonists.

Affinity is a measure of the strength of interaction between the drug and receptor. Efficacy is the measure of the strength of activity after binding with the receptor.

Mechanism of action

After binding with opioid receptors, they:

- Inhibit calcium entry into the cell which prevents excitatory neurotransmitter release.
- Potentiate potassium efflux which causes hyperpolarisation making the cells less excitable.
- Inhibit adenylate cyclase reducing cyclic adenosine monophosphate (cAMP). cAMP is associated with phosphorylation of membrane proteins and alteration of ion channels.

Pharmacokinetics

Opioids are well absorbed from the gastrointestinal tract. They are weak bases, ionised in the acidic gastric environment; therefore, absorption is delayed till they reach the alkaline small intestine where they become unionised and absorbed. Oral bioavailability is low due to considerable first-pass metabolism. Opioids are metabolised in the liver by conjugation to both active and inactive metabolites. The metabolites are excreted in urine or bile.

Clinical effects

Central nervous system

Opioids provide analgesia by acting on μ receptors. In the absence of pain, opioids act on κ receptors and cause restlessness and agitation. Stimulation of 5HT3 and dopamine receptors in the chemoreceptor trigger zone of the area postrema causes nausea and vomiting. Miosis is due to stimulation of μ and κ receptors in the Edinger-Westphal nucleus of the occulomotor nerve. Opioids also cause hallucinations.

Respiratory system

Opioids suppress the sensitivity of the brain stem to carbon dioxide causing a fall in respiratory rate. Opioids such as morphine, codeine and pholcodine have an antitussive effect.

Cardiovascular system

Opioids cause mild bradycardia but no other arrhythmia. Hypotension results due to histamine release and a reduction in sympathetic tone.

Gastrointestinal system

Opioids decrease the motility of the gastrointestinal tract and constricts the sphincters causing constipation. Constriction of the sphincter of Oddi raises the biliary pressure.

Renal system

Opioids increase the tone of the bladder's detrusor and vesical sphincters and precipitate urinary retention.

Other effects

Morphine releases histamine from mast cells causing urticaria, itching, bronchospasm and hypotension. Intrathecal administration of opioids causes pruritis which can be reversed by naloxone.

Following the long-term use of opioids, patients can develop tolerance and drug dependence.

Contraindications

Opioids should be avoided in acute respiratory depression, raised intracranial pressure and in head injury (as they interfere with pupillary responses vital for neurological assessment). They should be avoided or used in reduced doses in patients with hepatic and renal impairment.

Side effects

- Central nervous system: euphoria, dysphoria, mood changes, dependence, dizziness, confusion, drowsiness, sleep disturbances, headache, miosis, hallucinations, vertigo.
- Respiratory system: respiratory depression.
- Gastrointestinal tract: nausea, vomiting, constipation, dry mouth, biliary spasm.
- Cardiovascular system: hypotension, bradycardia.
- Renal system: difficulty with micturition, urinary retention, ureteric spasm.
- Other: sweating, flushing, rash, urticaria, pruritis.

Commonly used opioids for peri-operative analgesia

Morphine

Morphine is a naturally occurring opioid. It is the opioid of choice for severe pain and is the standard against which other opioids are compared. It is widely available and can be administered by a variety of routes.

It is available as tablets, suspensions, suppositories and parenteral preparations.

Oral bioavailablitiy is 30% due to hepatic first-pass metabolism.

Morphine is metabolised in the liver to morphine 3-glucuronide (M3G) and morphine 6-glucuronide (M6G), which are excreted in urine. M6G is an agonist at μ receptors and is more potent than morphine.

Elderly patients have a reduced volume of distribution leading to higher plasma levels of morphine. In neonates, a reduced hepatic conjugating capacity increases the sensitivity to morphine.

Fentanyl

Fentanyl is a synthetic opioid, which is widely used in anaesthetic practice. It is 100 times more potent than morphine. It is available as a colourless solution containing 50µg/ml, transdermal patches which release 25-100µg/hour over 3 days, lozenges releasing 200µg to 1.6mg over 15 minutes and as a nasal spray. It is used at a dose of 1-2µg/kg for analgesia during minor surgery, 10 to 25µg to augment intensity of spinal anaesthesia and 25-50µg to augment epidural anaesthesia.

Pharmacodynamics
It is a µ receptor agonist and shares morphine's effects. In high doses, it can cause chest wall rigidity and bradycardia.

Pharmacokinetics
Fentanyl has a quick onset of action, as it is highly lipid-soluble, crossing the membrane easily. The drug has strong protein binding.

The offset of effect is due to redistribution. It is metabolised in the liver to inactive metabolites, hydroxyfentanyl and norfentanyl.

It has a poor oral bioavailabilty due to high first-pass metabolism (70%).

When administered intrathecally, it diffuses rapidly from the cerebrospinal fluid into the spinal cord because of lipid solubility. This prevents the drug being transported to the midbrain causing respiratory depression.

It is used for intra-operative analgesia, to obtund the stimulation of laryngoscopy, and to augment the effects of local anaesthetics, such as in spinal and epidural anaesthesia.

Alfentanil

Alfentanil is a synthetic opioid that is structurally related to fentanyl and has 10-20% of its potency. It is available as a colourless solution as 500µg/ml or 5mg/ml.

Pharmacodynamics
It is a μ receptor agonist.

Pharmacokinetics
Alfentanil has a rapid onset and offset of action compared to fentanyl. This is because 89% of alfentanil is present as a non-ionised form in the plasma compared to 9% fentanyl. Complete recovery from alfentanil is rapid as it has a short distribution half-life and shorter terminal half-life than fentanyl.

Metabolism
Alfentanil is metabolised in the liver by N-demethylation to noralfentanil. Less than 2% of the drug is excreted unchanged.

It is used for attenuating the cardiovascular responses during intubation in a dose of 10μg/kg, and for sedation in the intensive care unit at a loading dose of 25-50μg/kg followed by an infusion of 0.5-2μg/kg/min.

Remifentanil

Remifentanil is an ultra-short-acting opioid. It is a synthetic phenylpiperidine derivative of fentanyl with approximately equal potency. It is available as crystalline white powder in glass vials containing 1, 2 or 5mg of remifentanil. The drug is formulated in glycine, therefore it is not suitable for epidural or intrathecal administration.

Pharmacodynamics
It is a pure μ receptor agonist.

Pharmacokinetics
Remifentanil is highly protein bound and has a low volume of distribution compared to other opioids. The clearance is 45-50ml/kg/min; much greater than other opioids leading to a very short elimination half-life (3-10 minutes).

Metabolism
Remifentanil is metabolised by non-specific plasma and tissue esterases resulting in an elimination half-life of 3-10 minutes. The context-sensitive half-life is not affected by the duration of the infusion.

The metabolism is not affected by genetic abnormalities of cholinesterase or administration of anticholinesterase drugs.

The main metabolite is an inactive carboxylated derivative, which is excreted by kidneys.

For induction of anaesthesia it is used at 0.5-1µg/kg/min and for maintenance of anaesthesia 0.05-2µg/kg/min.

Side effects
Severe muscle rigidity or apnoea with a higher dose or rapid administration.

Clinical uses
Remifentanil is the preferred opioid for intra-operative use in:

- Short-lasting surgery with intense stimulation, e.g. bronchoscopy.
- Prolonged surgery where a rapid recovery is indicated, e.g. neurosurgery.
- Surgery where hypotensive anaesthesia is required, e.g middle ear surgery.
- Total intravenous anaesthesia.
- Labour analgesia as patient-controlled analgesia.

Case scenario 1

A 25-year-old fit and healthy male patient is undergoing inguinal hernia surgery as a day case.

How would you manage his intra-operative and postoperative pain?

Inguinal hernia surgery is superficial soft-tissue surgery performed as a day-case procedure.

The pain associated with this is generally managed using a multimodal approach involving non-steroidal anti-inflammatory drugs, paracetamol and short-acting opioids such as fentanyl or alfentanil. This is supplemented with local anaesthetic infiltration or an inguinal field block.

Postoperative analgesia is provided by regular paracetamol and non-steroidal anti-inflammatory drugs such as ibuprofen. Some patients may additionally need a weak opioid such as codeine.

Case scenario 2

A 64-year-old female patient is presenting for an elective total knee replacement. She is a known asthmatic and is on regular inhalers.

What are the options for postoperative pain management in this lady?

Total knee replacement (TKR) surgery involves operating on a joint/bone tissues as well as muscles, which are richly innervated by nerves. Therefore, TKR is commonly associated with severe postoperative pain.

Intra-operative and immediate postoperative pain is well managed by the use of paracetamol, short-acting strong opiates and local anaesthetic techniques (either infiltration around the joint tissues or femoral nerve block/adductor canal block) or intrathecal administration of an opiate (diamorphine).

Management of postoperative pain by regular paracetamol, NSAIDs (ibuprofen), gabapentin and opiates, such as oxycontin or morphine, enables patients to undergo physiotherapy effectively with minimal pain. Regular physiotherapy is essential after TKR surgery for regaining optimum joint movements.

NSAIDs can be contraindicated in asthmatics, as approximately 10% of individuals with asthma may have bronchospasm after taking NSAIDs.

If a patient has already had NSAIDs in the past without any bronchospasm, then it is safe to administer. If a patient with asthma has never had NSAIDs in the past or had bronchospasm after taking NSAIDs, then it is best to avoid them.

Case scenario 3

A 70-year-old male patient has been admitted with abdominal pain and vomiting. A CT scan is suggestive of intestinal obstruction. The patient is known to have chronic obstructive pulmonary disease (COPD) and hypertension. The blood results show a normal full blood count and deranged renal function. The patient is undergoing an emergency laparotomy.

What are the options for analgesia?

The laparotomy involves a large abdominal incision and therefore postoperative pain is a significant issue. The abdominal movements during breathing increase the pain and this leads to alveolar hypoventilation. Patients also avoid coughing and this leads to retention of secretion and chest infection. For this reason, effective pain control is very important.

NSAIDs are contraindicated in this case as the patient is elderly and has deranged renal function.

Opioids are also not appropriate in this case as the patient has COPD.

Epidural analgesia is the best option for pain relief in these patients. The epidural is sited before induction of general anaesthesia to provide intra-operative and postoperative analgesia. This is supplemented with regular paracetamol.

Effective analgesia reduces pulmonary complications such as atelectasis, hypoxaemia and infection, and enhances recovery. It also reduces thromboembolic complications.

Further reading

1. Pathan H, Williams J. Basic opioid pharmacology: an update. *Br J Pain* 2006; 6: 11-6.
2. Trescot A.M, Datta S, Lee M, Hansen H. Opioid pharmacology. *Pain Physician* 2008; 11: s133-53.
3. Husband M, Mehta V. Cyclo-oxygenase 2 inhibitors. *Br J Anaesth CEACCP* 2013; 13: 131-5.
4. Shankar R, Wilson JA, Colvin L. Non-opioid based adjuvant analgesia in perioperative care. *Br J Anaesth CEACCP* 2013; 13: 152-7.
5. Sharma CV, Mehta V. Paracetamol: mechanisms and updates. *Br J Anaesth CEACCP* 2014; 14: 153-8.
6. Ong CK, Lirk P, Seymour RA, Jenkins BJ. The efficacy of preemptive analgesia for acute postoperative pain management: a meta-analysis. *Anesth Analg* 2005; 100: 757-73.

5 Local anaesthetics

Vinesh Mistry and Cyprian Mendonca

Introduction

Anaesthetic practice favours reducing the side effects of anaesthesia, such as drowsiness and postoperative nausea and vomiting, much of which can be attributed to strong analgesics such as opioids. The use of local anaesthetic drugs for peri-operative analgesia allows a reduction for the need to use opioids. There are different local anaesthetic drugs that can be used for a variety of applications.

Local anaesthetic mechanism of action

Local anaesthetic action is dependent on blockade of the voltage-gated Na^+ channel. An unionised lipid-soluble drug passes through the phospholipid membrane where in the axoplasm it is protonated (reduced). In this ionised form it binds to the internal surface of a Na^+ channel, preventing it from leaving its inactive state. The degree of block is proportional to the rate of nerve stimulation due to attraction of local anaesthetic to 'open' Na^+ channels. More molecules enter the sodium channels when they are open and this results in inactivation of more channels resulting in a greater degree of block. This is known as use-dependent (phasic) block.

Local anaesthetics produce reversible blockade of neural transmission in autonomic, sensory and motor nerve fibres, depending on concentration and dose of the local anaesthetic. They are active both peripherally and within the CNS. They bind to the fast Na^+ channels in the axon membrane, preventing Na^+ entry during depolarisation. The threshold potential is thus not reached and the action potential is not propagated (stabilising the membrane). Local anaesthetics diffuse into the axons, hence they are more effective nearer to the nerve fibre.

Commonly used local anaesthetics (Table 5.1) can be divided into two classes based on the structure. The basic structure includes an aromatic ring linked to a terminal amine. The intermediate linkage is the ester in esters and the amide in amides. Esters are hydrolysed by plasma esterases whereas amides are biotransformed in the liver.

Table 5.1. Commonly used local anaesthetics.

Esters	Amides
Procaine	Lidocaine
Amethocaine	Prilocaine
Cocaine	Bupivacaine
	Levobupivacaine
	Ropivacaine
	Dibucaine

Pharmacodynamics

Local anaesthetics are weak bases. They exist predominantly in ionised forms at a neutral pH, since their pKa is greater than 7.4.

Structure

- Ester group: ester bond between the aromatic lipophilic group and terminal hydrophilic amine group.

- Amide group: amide bond between the aromatic lipophilic group and terminal hydrophilic group.
- Esters: unstable in solution.
- Local anaesthetics with an ester structure have an inherently more potent action than those with an amide structure.

Potency

- Related to lipid-solubility mainly, but also vasodilator properties and tissue distribution.

Duration of action

- Related to extent of protein binding.
- The more protein binding, the longer the duration of action.

Onset of action

- Related to pKa.
- The higher the pKa, the more the ionised form which is unable to penetrate the membrane; therefore, it has a longer onset of action, and the converse also applies.

Vasodilation and vasoconstriction

- They cause vasodilation at low concentrations and vasoconstriction at high concentrations.
- Vasodilation effect: prilocaine > lidocaine > bupivacaine > ropivacaine.
- Cocaine causes pure vasoconstriction (inhibiting neuronal uptake of catecholamines and inhibiting mono-amine oxidase enzymes).

Cardiovascular system

- Lidocaine may be used to treat ventricular tachyarrhythmias, whilst bupivacaine should not be used.
- Both block cardiac Na^+ channels and decrease the maximum rate of increase of phase 0 of the cardiac action potential.

- They also have direct myocardial depressant properties.
- The PR and QRS intervals are prolonged and the refractory period is prolonged.
- However, bupivacaine is ten times slower at dissociating from the Na^+ channels, resulting in persistent depression and precipitating re-entry arrhythmias and ventricular fibrillation (VF). Tachycardia may enhance frequency-dependent blockade by bupivacaine, which adds to its cardiac toxicity.

Central nervous system

- They penetrate the brain rapidly and have a biphasic effect.
- Initially, inhibitory interneurons are blocked, resulting in an excitatory phenomenon, and finally leading to depression of all central neurons.
- The dose-dependent effects include tingling of the lips, visual disturbance, tremors and dizziness, leading to convulsions, coma and apnoea.

Pharmacokinetics

Absorption

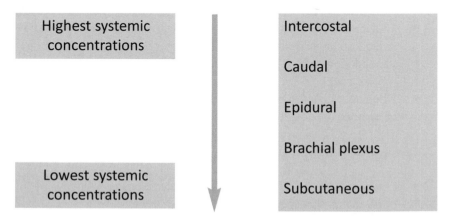

Figure 5.1. Systemic concentration of local anaesthetic and the site of injection.

- Absorption into the systemic circulation varies depending on the characteristics of the local anaesthetic agent used, additives such as vasoconstrictors and the vascularity at the site of injection.

Distribution

- Esters are minimally bound whilst amides are more extensively bound in the plasma (bupivacaine > ropivacaine > lidocaine > prilocaine).
- α-1-acid glycoprotein binds local anaesthetic with more affinity, although albumin is present in a higher abundance for binding.
- When protein binding is increased, the free fraction of drug is reduced, for instance, in the following conditions:
  - pregnancy;
  - renal failure;
  - postoperative period;
  - infancy.

Metabolism and elimination

Esters:

- Hydrolysed by plasma cholinesterases rapidly.
- Short elimination half-life due to rapid hydrolysis.
- Para-aminobenzoate (PABA) is the main metabolite and has been associated with hypersensitivity reactions.
- Cocaine is the exception, undergoing hepatic hydrolysis to water-soluble metabolite excreted in urine.
- Metabolism may be delayed when plasma cholinesterase is low (liver disease, pregnancy, atypical enzymes).

Amides:

- Undergo hepatic metabolism by amidases, which are liver microsomal enzymes.
- Initially metabolised into an amino-carboxylic acid and a cycline aniline derivative and then undergoes dealkylation and hydroxylation, respectively.

- Amidase metabolism is slower than ester hydrolysis and so amides are prone to accumulation when administered via continuous infusion.
- Metabolism is reduced by reduced hepatic blood flow or hepatic dysfunction.

Commonly used local anaesthetic agents

Amides

Lidocaine

Lidocaine is used as a local anaesthetic and also as a Class 1b anti-arrhythmic agent.

Preparations:

- Formulated as hydrochloride.
- Presented as a colourless solution (0.5-2%) and also with adrenaline 1/80,000-1/200,000.
- 2% gel, 5% ointment, spray at 10mg/dose, and 4% solution for topical use.
- 0.25-0.50% solution used for infiltration anaesthesia and intravenous regional anaesthesia.
- 1-2% solutions: nerve blocks and extradural analgesia (epidural).
- 4% solution: topical anaesthesia (mucous membranes, pharynx, larynx).
- 10% spray: topical anaesthesia via metered dose pump.
- 1-2% gel: for urethral catheterisation.

Pharmacokinetics:

- Protein binding: 64-70% protein bound (α1-acid glycoprotein).
- Percentage unionised: 25%.
- pKa: 7.9.
- Metabolism: dealkylation in the liver. Metabolites excreted in urine.
- Elimination (half-life): 100 minutes.
- Onset: fast.

- Duration: moderate.
- Relative lipid-solubility: 150.
- Relative potency: 2.0.
- Dose:
  - maximum: 3mg/kg;
  - with adrenaline: 7mg/kg;
  - airway topical anaesthesia: up to 9mg/kg.
- Toxic plasma concentration: >5µg/ml (convulsions at a level >8µg/ml).

Bupivacaine

Bupivacaine is a racemic mixture of S- and R-enantiomers.

Preparations:

- Presented as a colourless solution of 0.25% and 0.5% strengths (with/without 1/200,000 adrenaline).
- Heavy bupivacaine: 0.5% preparation containing 80mg/ml glucose 8% (specific gravity: 1.026) for use as a spinal anaesthetic.

Pharmacokinetics:

- Protein binding: 95% protein bound (α1-acid glycoprotein).
- Percentage unionised: 15%.
- pKa: 8.1.
- Metabolism: dealkylation in the liver, into pipecolic acid and pipecoloxylidide.
- Elimination (half-life): 160 minutes.
- Onset: moderate.
- Duration: long.
- Relative lipid-solubility: 1000.
- Relative potency: 8.0.
- Maximum safe dose: 2mg/kg.
- Toxic plasma concentration: >1.5ng/ml.

Levobupivacaine

Levobupivacaine is the S-enantiomer of bupivacaine.

Preparations:

- Presented as a colourless solution of 0.25% (2.5mg/ml), 0.5% (5mg/ml) and 0.75% (7.5mg/ml) strengths.

Pharmacokinetics:

- Maximum dose: 2mg/kg.
- Maximum single dose: 150mg.
- Maximum divided dose in 24 hours: 400mg.
- Toxicity:
  - in comparison to bupivacaine, levobupivacaine has a lower potential for cardiac toxicity;
  - excitatory central nervous system effects or convulsions occur at lower doses with bupivacaine than levobupivacaine.

Ropivacaine

Ropivacaine is formulated as the S-enantiomer, since the R-enantiomer is less potent and more toxic. It has a lower lipid-solubility and an improved toxic profile.

Lower lipid-solubility results in reduced penetration of the large myelinated alpha and beta motor fibres, so that initially these fibres are spared from the anaesthetic; however, they will become blocked via continuous infusion.

The motor block is slower in onset, less dense and of a shorter duration when compared to bupivacaine, and theoretically should be better for an epidural due to this sensory-motor discrimination and greater clearance.

Preparations:

- Presented in concentrations of 2mg/ml (0.2%), 7.5mg/ml (0.75%) and 10mg/ml (1%) in two volumes; 10ml or 100ml.

Pharmacokinetics:

- Protein binding: 94% protein bound (α1-acid glycoprotein).
- Percentage unionised: 15%.
- pKa: 8.1.
- Metabolism:
  - metabolised in the liver by aromatic hydroxylation mainly into 3-hydroxy-ropivacaine but also 4-hydroxy-ropivacaine, both having some local anaesthetic properties.
- Elimination (half-life): 120 minutes.
- Onset: moderate.
- Duration: long.
- Relative lipid-solubility: 300.
- Relative potency: 8.0.
- Maximum dose: 3.5mg/kg.
- Toxic plasma concentration: >4.0ng/ml.

Prilocaine

Prilocaine is usually used for intravenous regional anaesthesia (IVRA).

Preparations:

- Presented as a 0.5-2.0% colourless solution.
- 0.5-1.0% solutions for infiltration.
- 1-2% solution for nerve blocks.
- 0.5% solution for IVRA.
- Available as a 3.0% solution with felypressin for dental use.

Pharmacokinetics:

- Protein binding: 55%.
- Percentage unionised: 33%.

- pKa: 7.7-7.9.
- Metabolism:
  - rapid metabolism, occurring in the liver, kidneys and lung;
  - in large doses, one of its metabolites, o-toluidine, may precipitate methaemoglobinaemia.
- Elimination (half-life): 100 minutes.
- Onset: fast.
- Duration: moderate.
- Relative lipid-solubility: 50.
- Relative potency: 2.0.
- Dose:
  - maximum safe dose: 5mg/kg;
  - maximum single dose: 400mg;
  - maximum dose combined with adrenaline: 8mg/kg.
- Toxic plasma concentration: >5ng/ml.

Esters

Cocaine

Cocaine is mainly used for topical anaesthesia and as a local vasoconstriction agent.

Preparations:

- Alkaloid ester local derived from the leaves of *Erythroxylum coca*.
- Moffatt's solution: 2ml 8.0% cocaine, 2ml 1% $NaHCO_3$, 1ml 1/1000 adrenaline.
- 1-4% paste.

Pharmacokinetics:

- Protein binding: 95% protein bound.
- Percentage unionised: 5%.
- pKa: 8.6/8.7.

- Metabolism: hydrolysed extensively in the liver and a small amount is excreted unchanged in the urine.
- Elimination (half-life): 100 minutes.
- Onset: moderate.
- Duration: short.
- Dose: 1.5-3.0mg/kg (maximum 100mg).
- Toxic plasma concentration: 0.5ng/ml.
- Mechanism of action:
  - cocaine causes vasoconstriction by preventing uptake of noradrenaline by pre-synaptic nerve endings and blocks monoamine oxidase (MAO) whilst also stimulating the CNS;
  - CVS toxicity: hypertension, tachycardia, arrhythmias and hyperthermia;
  - CNS toxicity via stimulation: confusion, hallucinations, convulsions and apnoea;
  - chronic abuse: cardiomyopathy and sudden death.

Amethocaine, also known as tetracaine

Amethocaine is used for topical anaesthesia. As a topical cream it has a faster onset of action compared to a eutectic mixture of local anaesthetic (EMLA), producing anaesthesia in 30-45 minutes, lasting between 4-6 hours.

Preparations:

- 0.5% and 1% drops for topical use either alone or before local anaesthetic block.
- 4% cream for topical anaesthesia (Ametop®).

Pharmacokinetics:

- Protein binding: 75% protein bound.
- Percentage unionised: 7%.
- pKa: 8.5.

- Metabolism: hydrolysed completely by plasma cholinesterases to form butylaminobenzoic acid and dimethlyaminoethanol.
- Elimination (half-life): 80 minutes.
- Onset: slow.
- Duration: long.
- Relative lipid-solubility: 200.
- Relative potency: 8.0.
- Dose: 1.5mg/kg.

Eutectic mixture of local anaesthetic (EMLA)

EMLA is a mixture of two compounds producing a substance with a single set of physical characteristics.

EMLA 5% contains a mixture of crystalline bases of 2.5% lidocaine and 2.5% prilocaine in a white oil-water emulsion.

The mixture has a lower melting point, being an oil at room temperature, as opposed to crystalline.

The following are the specific characteristics of EMLA:

- Presentation: EMLA emulsion in 5g or 30g tubes.
- Duration of action: requires application to the skin for 60-90 minutes to ensure anaesthesia.
- Caution:
  - contraindicated in congenital or idiopathic methaemoglobinaemia;
  - drugs such as sulphonamides and phenytoin increase the risk of methaemoglobinaemia;
  - not to be used on mucous membranes due to rapid systemic absorption;
  - those taking Class I anti-arrhythmic drugs (tocainide, mexiletine), since toxic effects are additive and synergistic.

Case scenario 1

A 44-year-old male patient is listed for a right shoulder replacement. The patient has a past medical history of lymphoblastic leukaemia as a child and had a bone marrow transplant as a child, a right lung transplant due to pulmonary fibrosis secondary to graft versus host disease, hypothyroidism, osteoporosis and chronic kidney disease stage 3. The patient has had avascular necrosis of both hips and has had hip replacements under spinal anaesthesia. Pulmonary function tests show: VC: 1.63 (39% predicted), FVC: 1.67 (41% predicted), FEV_1: 1.43 (42% predicted), FEV_1/FVC ratio: 86%.

Medications include: co-trimoxazole, cyclosporin, prednisolone. pregabalin, lansoprazole, Adcal D3®.

Allergies include: amikacin, clarithromycin, dihydrocodeine and flucloxacillin.

A multidisciplinary team decision was made to proceed with surgery solely under awake regional anaesthesia involving an interscalene brachial plexus block, and a suprascapular and axillary nerve block.

What local anaesthetic agent would you choose to provide intra-operative anaesthesia for an interscalene block and suprascapular/axillary nerve block? And would you use more than one agent?

The chosen agent would be prilocaine 1% (20mg/ml) due to its quick onset and medium duration of action. A total of 15ml of prilocaine is used. This allows high concentration for a potent sensory and motor block with minimal volumes. This is combined with 20ml of 0.25% levobupivacaine 20ml, for the suprascapular and axillary nerve blocks, which is used to provide a longer sensory block with sparing of a motor block purely for analgesia.

Lignocaine 1% would be an alternative for intra-operative regional anaesthesia but is not chosen due to its shorter duration of action compared to prilocaine.

Case scenario 2

A 65-year-old female patient is scheduled for an elective right total knee replacement. The patient has a past medical history of hypertension, hypercholesterolaemia and suffers with anxiety. The patient has refused a spinal anaesthetic due to concerns regarding complications and a needle phobia. She also wants to be 'fully asleep and not know anything' during the operation. She has agreed to general anaesthesia with an asleep femoral nerve block.

Medications include: losartan, propranolol and sertraline.

Allergies include: Nil.

Which local anaesthetic would you use to perform a femoral nerve block?

Levobupivacaine would be the ideal agent to use in this scenario. A fast onset of action is not required for this surgery due to it being performed under general anaesthesia, and so a long-acting local anaesthetic would be best used.

What advantages does levobupivacaine have over lignocaine for this patient?

Levobupivacaine would be expected to last up to a maximum of 16 hours, whereas lignocaine may only last up to a maximum of 4 hours.

What strength of local anaesthetic would you use?

A concentration of 0.25% levobupivacaine would be ideal in this situation, as it would provide analgesia for up to 16 hours with the residual motor block lasting for much less time allowing for physiotherapy. At this concentration, a volume of between 20-30ml can be used, which would ensure an adequate spread of local anaesthetic to the femoral nerve and distal branches.

Further reading

1. Peck T, Hill S, Williams M. *Pharmacology for Anaesthesia and Intensive Care*, 4th ed. Cambridge University Press, 2014.

2. Yentis SM, Hirsch NP, Smith GB. *Anaesthesia and Intensive Care A-Z: An Encyclopedia of Principles and Practice*, 3rd ed. Elsevier, 2004.

3. Becker DE, Reed KL. Essentials of local anesthetic pharmacology. *Anesthesia Progress* 2006; 53: 98-109.

6 Peri-operative monitoring

Kavitkumar Dasari and Cyprian Mendonca

Introduction

Monitoring the anaesthetised patient is one of the key roles of an anaesthetist and is necessary not only during the induction of anaesthesia, but also during maintenance, emergence, transfer and in the recovery area. The common monitoring methods and devices used in theatre will be discussed in this chapter.

Standards of monitoring

The Association of Anaesthetists of Great Britain and Ireland (AAGBI) has recommended standards of monitoring (2015) for all patients requiring sedation and general anaesthesia. The primary aim is to anticipate and minimise any deterioration of the patient in the peri-operative period.

Minimal monitoring

Minimal monitoring refers to the presence of an electrocardiogram (ECG), a pulse oximeter and non-invasive blood pressure (NIBP) monitoring and should be attached prior to the induction of anaesthesia. These parameters should be recorded at 5-minute intervals, or more often, on the anaesthetic chart. If muscle paralysis is used, then neuromuscular monitoring via a quantitative peripheral nerve stimulator forms part of minimal monitoring. Minimal monitoring should be maintained until the patient is fully awake, responding appropriately to commands, breathing spontaneously and not requiring airway support.

Capnography is mandatory for those with infraglottic or supraglottic airway devices. For patients undergoing general anaesthesia in theatre, monitoring standards also encompass, in addition to all of the above, measurement of oxygen levels, anaesthetic vapours and airway pressure. Guidance from the National Institute for Health and Care Excellence (NICE) also states temperature monitoring is necessary for any operations longer than a 30-minute duration.

All necessary monitoring equipment should be available and checked during the sign-in process of the WHO surgical safety check list, prior to any intervention in the operating theatre.

Specific situations

Monitoring requirements for patient transfer to the recovery unit is dependent upon the size of the theatre complex, but minimal monitoring is recommended. While in recovery, the presence of NIBP, pulse oximeter, ECG and temperature monitoring is mandatory for emergence. Supplemental oxygen should be used.

For patients undergoing regional anaesthesia, with or without sedation, NIBP, pulse oximeter and ECG monitoring are recommended. Capnography should be used in patients with an airway device or in those who are deeply sedated and verbal contact must be maintained throughout.

Inter-hospital transfer and anaesthesia in remote areas such as in the emergency department, intensive care unit or labour ward requires the use of minimal monitoring as in theatre. Additional theatre monitoring is required depending on whether the patient is manually or mechanically ventilated. If infusion pumps are used, the cannula should be visible throughout the procedure and connected to the mains power. A depth of anaesthesia monitor is recommended if this includes total intravenous anaesthesia (TIVA). Handover to other anaesthetists should be recorded in the anaesthetic chart.

Clinical monitoring

The most important part of monitoring is the presence of a trained anaesthetist continuously during an anaesthetic. Human error is inevitable; however, the incidence of adverse events can be reduced by the presence of a vigilant anaesthetist. In order to provide a safe anaesthetic and prevent patient deterioration, clinical signs must be detected, alarms responded to and the use, as well as limitations, of monitoring devices must be acknowledged.

Direct observation of a patient and good basic clinical skills are crucial due to the amount of information that can be provided on cardiovascular and respiratory parameters.

For spontaneously breathing patients, the respiration rate, depth and pattern can all be observed. Observation of the reservoir bag may indicate a leak, disconnection or a hypoventilating patient. Listening to the chest can indicate pathology relating to the patient or even machine dysfunction.

Palpation of the radial or temporal artery can provide indicators on pulse rate, rhythm, volume and character. This may be coupled to measuring urine output.

Volume status can be determined by looking at skin colour, palpating for a central capillary refill time and ascertaining a patient's temperature. In addition, skin examination for rashes will be essential for those patients who have allergic reactions.

Monitoring display unit

The monitoring screen is the focal point for the anaesthetist and can display an array of observations (Figure 6.1). The display screen can be tailored to the individual anaesthetist but care must be made to not overload the screen which will be detrimental in an emergency. Important checks include that NIBP monitoring is automatically cycled, the capnograph is working properly and the alarm limits are set. Alarms provide an auditory and visual reminder in the loud and potentially stressful theatre environment.

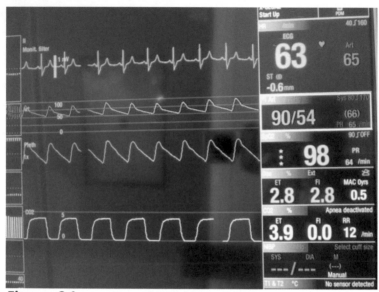

Figure 6.1. A colour-coded display unit showing the ECG, invasive arterial blood pressure, oxygen saturations, end-tidal vapour concentrations and capnography.

Monitoring standards for induction and maintenance of general anaesthesia are as follows:

- NIBP monitor, pulse oximeter and ECG are attached before induction of anaesthesia.
- Capnography.
- Inspired and expired oxygen, carbon dioxide and nitrous oxide levels.
- Anaesthetic vapour analysis.
- Airway pressure.

- Peripheral nerve stimulator (if a neuromuscular blocking agent is used).
- Temperature monitoring (if the procedure is longer than 30 minutes).

Electrocardiography

The electrocardiogram (ECG) is one of the fundamental methods of monitoring. The ECG is a surface recording that graphically displays electrical activity of the heart. It provides information regarding heart rate, rhythm and may indicate ischaemia. It doesn't provide any information regarding the cardiac output.

ECG configurations

ECG monitoring may be undertaken by standard three-lead monitoring in theatre using silver/silver chloride skin electrodes. This triangular configuration is known as Einthoven's triangle (Figure 6.2). The leads are positioned as below:

- Right shoulder (red lead).
- Left shoulder (yellow lead).
- Left leg or chest (green lead).

The potential difference between positive and negative electrodes produces the characteristic leads I, II and III seen on a standard 12-lead ECG. The signal is amplified and filters are used to prevent any unwanted noise from muscle movement, electromagnetic interference or other equipment. The signal is displayed by an oscilloscope. Differential amplifiers and filters are commonplace in modern theatre monitoring. Lead II is most commonly selected on the anaesthetic monitor as this most readily provides information regarding dysrhythmias. A standard display with a speed of 25mm/sec and sensitivity of 1mV/cm is used in the United Kingdom (UK).

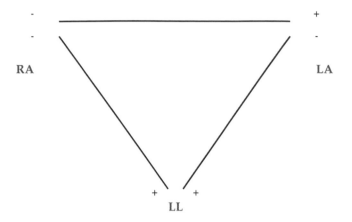

Figure 6.2. Standard lead axes forming Einthoven's triangle.

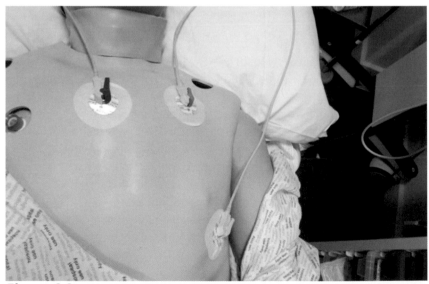

Figure 6.3. CM5 electrode positions. Note the position of the green electrode on the left clavicle or shoulder.

The 'CM5' configuration (Figure 6.3) may be used for monitoring left ventricular ischaemia and is a modified V5 lead from a standard 12-lead ECG. The configuration is:

- Manubrium of the sternum (red lead).
- 5th intercostal space, left anterior axillary line (yellow lead).
- Left clavicle (green lead).

ECG interference

Electrical interference may occur due to the mains current (50Hz in the UK) or diathermy. Checking the patient's pulse and observing the pulse oximeter waveform may be helpful in ascertaining if a true arrhythmia is present. Observing the capnography and arterial waveform is helpful in simultaneously ascertaining if there is still cardiac output.

Preventing ECG interference:

- Application of electrodes to bony prominences to prevent muscle artefact.
- Consider changing the monitoring lead or altering the amplitude.
- Correct application of the diathermy plate (and away from pacemakers).
- Appropriate alarm settings in relation to heart rate and arrhythmias.

Pulse oximetry

A pulse oximeter measures the peripheral oxygen saturation levels and displays a numerical value and pulse waveform (Figure 6.4). It provides continuous measurement and is non-invasive and portable. Alarm limits can be set for both oxygen saturation and the heart rate. Common sites include the finger, toe or ear lobe. Burns and pressure injuries may occur from prolonged use.

It is important to note that while pulse oximeters measure oxygen saturation levels, they cannot provide an indication of oxygen delivery to tissues.

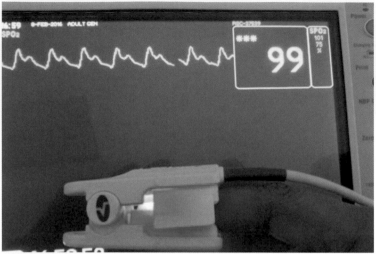

Figure 6.4. Pulse oximeter waveform and pulse oximeter probe attached to the finger.

Mechanism

A pulse oximeter probe consists of two light-emitting diodes (LED) on one side and a photodetector on the side of the probe. They measure the differential absorption of light between oxygenated and deoxygenated haemoglobin. One LED emits at a wavelength of red (660nm) and the other at infrared (910nm) and this occurs about 30 times per second. Deoxygenated haemoglobin (deoxyHb) absorbs maximum light at 660nm, and oxygenated haemoglobin (oxyHb) maximally at 910nm (Figure 6.5). The isobestic point where absorption is equal is 805nm. The greater number of haemoglobin molecules between the LED and photodetector, and the further distance the emitted light has to travel, the greater the absorbance (Beer-Lambert's law). The remaining light not absorbed is measured with a photodetector on the opposite side of the probe. A microprocessor utilises an inbuilt algorithm that subtracts the venous contribution leaving only the pulsatile arterial component. An electrical signal of the saturations is produced and then displayed in addition to the heart rate which is derived from the pulse waveform.

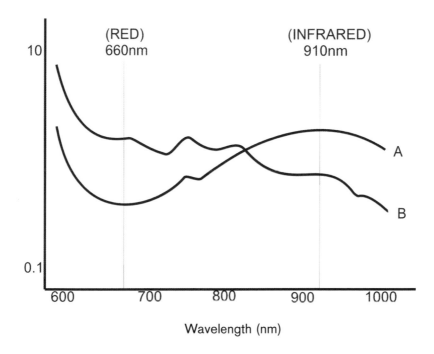

Figure 6.5. The absorbance of oxygenated and deoxygenated blood via the pulse oximeter. Oxygenated haemoglobin absorbs more infrared light (910nm) and deoxyhaemoglobin absorbs more red light (660nm).

Inaccuracies with the pulse oximeter

- Pulse oximeters are not accurate when the oxygen saturations fall below 70% due to the inability to calibrate and test at this level.
- Abnormal haemoglobins (methaemoglobinaemia — falsely low saturation; carboxyhaemoglobinaeamia — falsely high saturation).
- Reduced peripheral circulation (low cardiac output, hypothermia, vasoconstriction, peripheral vascular disease).
- Venous congestion.
- Cardiac arrhythmias.
- Extraneous interference (bright ambient light, nail varnish).
- Motion artefacts such as shivering or seizures.

In some instances, the reading may be imprecise and this may occur when the finger probe is on the same arm as the blood pressure cuff while it inflates. If frequent blood pressure readings are required then an ear probe may be advantageous. Alternatively, an arterial line may be sited.

Non-invasive blood pressure (NIBP) monitoring

NIBP measurements are a part of minimal monitoring and may be measured using manual or automated methods. Manual sphygmomanometers (aneroid) may be used but listening to Korotkoff sounds in theatre is both difficult and cumbersome; therefore, they have been superseded by automated systems.

Automated methods

The device for indirect non-invasive automated mean arterial pressure (DINAMAP) measurement using the principle of oscillometry is the mainstay of NIBP measurement in theatre. In this method, a single blood pressure cuff is used to both sense arterial pulsations and compress the brachial artery. A pneumatic cuff is inflated to a pressure greater than 160mmHg or previous systolic blood pressure by a microprocessor and slowly deflated in a stepwise manner. This is controlled by a solenoid valve. Where these reach a maximum amplitude of oscillations, the mean arterial pressure (MAP) value is generated. The diastolic blood pressure is derived from the MAP and systolic measurements. A transducer senses the changes in pressure and is fed back to the microprocessor providing information for the next inflation. The final component includes a display unit showing systolic, MAP and diastolic blood pressures, and heart rate. Lower limb NIBP measurements can be used accurately in the anaesthetised patient to represent brachial measurements when the patient is supine and the legs are at the level of the heart.

Newer methods such as finger blood pressure monitors are constantly being developed that incorporate the advantage of being non-invasive but also providing continuous NIBP measurements.

NIBP monitoring disadvantages

- Large and wide cuffs provide falsely low readings and narrow and smaller cuffs provide falsely high readings.
- Most NIBP devices only work within the normal range of blood pressures.
- Prolonged use may lead to nerve or soft tissue injury.
- Presence of dysrhythmias.
- Cycling cannot be faster than 1-minute intervals.

Invasive blood pressure monitoring

Invasive blood pressure (IBP) is measured through siting a 20 or 22G arterial cannula. These are aseptically inserted via direct or transfixation methods or via the Seldinger technique (Figure 6.6).

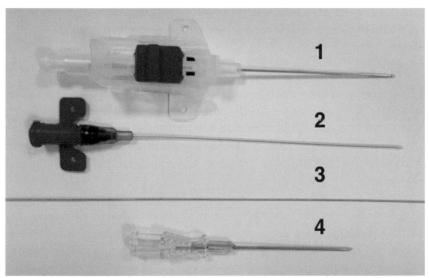

Figure 6.6. FloSwitch® 20g arterial cannula (1) with locking mechanism. In the Seldinger technique, the arterial cannula (2) is inserted over a guidewire (3) and requires an introducer needle (4).

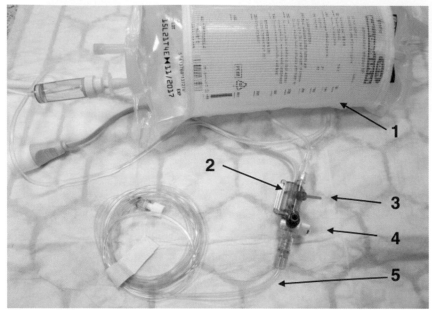

Figure 6.7. An arterial line set-up consisting of a pressured bag (1) of intravenous fluid (0.9% normal saline at 300mmHg), drip chamber (drip rate 3-4ml/hr), transducer (2), flushing device (3), three-way tap (4) and high-pressure tubing (5) ideally 120cm in length.

Commonly chosen arteries include the radial and dorsalis pedis. The ulnar artery is used less frequently as it is the dominant artery to the hand. Use of the brachial and femoral arteries predispose to distal ischaemia as they are end arteries. Additional risks include bleeding, infection and accidental injection of drugs. Figure 6.7 shows the standard arterial line set-up.

IBP monitoring can provide beat-to-beat blood pressure measurements in those patients where large pressure changes are expected, for example, septic patients with large fluid shifts, patients with pre-existing cardiac disease or patients being administered vasopressor or vasodilator drugs. Further uses include when NIBP monitoring may be inaccurate, i.e. morbidly obese patients.

Arterial line waveform

In order to generate an arterial line waveform, the arterial pulsation is transmitted up the fluid-filled column within the tubing to a diaphragm. This diaphragm is connected to four strain gauge resistors in a Wheatstone bridge configuration to amplify the signal. A transducer converts resistance to an electrical signal that is displayed on the monitor.

The normal arterial wave form, as seen in Figure 6.8, provides basic information on blood pressure and heart rate. Analysing the waveform can provide additional information such as stroke volume, myocardial contractility and peripheral vascular resistance. Problems with IBP monitoring may occur due to the cannula (ischaemia, thrombosis, bleeding, infection, nerve injury) or with the transducer (resonance, damping).

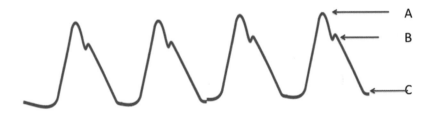

A

B

C

Figure 6.8. A normal arterial waveform. The dicrotic notch (B) represents closure of the aortic valve. A = systolic pressure; C = diastolic pressure.

Damping and resonance

- Resonance represents the tendency of the system to oscillate.
- Natural frequency is the frequency at which a system will oscillate itself.
- Damping is the tendency of the system to resist oscillation.

The measuring range frequency of an arterial system is 0.5-40Hz. An inadvertently high systolic and low diastolic blood pressure is displayed when the natural frequency is below 40Hz, as this results in amplification of the transmitted signal. This can be prevented by avoiding inappropriately stiff or short tubing.

The waveform may be inappropriately flat (overdampened) or tall (underdampened) as seen in Figure 6.9. In these situations, the MAP will

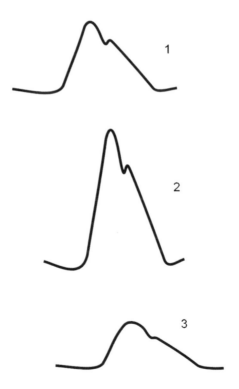

Figure 6.9. Normal (1), underdamped (2) and overdamped (3) arterial pressure waveforms.

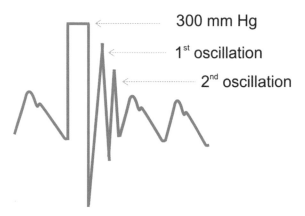

Figure 6.10. Square wave test demonstrating optimal damping.

be the same, but systolic and diastolic measurements are incorrect. An appropriate amount of damping is required and optimal damping has a coefficient of 0.64, between 0 (no damping) and 1 (critical damping). Optimal damping can be ascertained by the square wave test with an expected one to two oscillations before the true pressure reading is attained (Figure 6.10). Damping may be due to kinks, clots, air bubbles in the line or inappropriately long tubing with multiple three-way taps and results in loss of energy from the system.

Overdamping will require re-zeroing, checking the patency of the arterial cannula by attempting to aspirate blood via the three-way tap, flushing via the pressurised bag or repositioning the limb.

Practical problems with IBP monitoring

- Correctly siting an arterial cannula requires practice.
- Be vigilant to prevent disconnection, as catastrophic bleeding can occur.

- Be wary of inadvertent drug administration.
- Observe for any signs of infection or distal ischaemia.
- Recalibration is frequently required to prevent drift.
- For any change in transducer height, a 10cm change will alter blood pressure by 7.5mmHg.

Cardiac output monitoring

There are an increasing number of methods to measure cardiac output, ranging from the truly non-invasive, such as transthoracic echocardiography (TTE), to minimally invasive and, lastly, invasive techniques. Some of the commoner methods used in operating theatres are discussed here, but others such as transoesophageal echocardiography (TOE) may be used more frequently in expert hands and in specific clinical situations. Furthermore, there are many methods which employ the Fick principle and one method cannot be recommended over another.

Minimally invasive cardiac output monitoring

A minimally invasive technique for monitoring cardiac output includes the use of an oesophageal Doppler. It is a continuous method that provides information on stroke volume, heart rate, cardiac output and cardiac index and, in particular, how these change with fluid challenges.

An oesophageal Doppler consists of a flexible probe that is sited in the lower one third of the oesophagus (Figure 6.11) and contains a Doppler transducer that emits ultrasound waves at 4Hz. Caution should be taken in those with known oesophageal pathology.

The Doppler shift measures:

- Velocity of the blood flow in the descending aorta. Red blood cells in the blood that are moving away from the ultrasound beam reflect the beam back to the transducer at a lower frequency. The difference in the frequency of ultrasound is known as the frequency shift which is proportional to the velocity of flow.

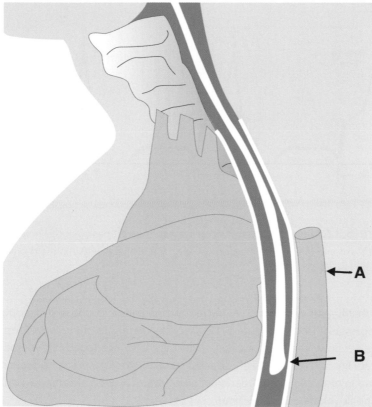

Figure 6.11. Correct position of a Doppler probe in the lower third of the oesophagus (B). A = descending aorta.

- Aortic velocity profile gives information regarding contractility and adequacy of filling.
- Aortic area is calculated using the nomogram based on patient characteristics such as age, height and weight (aortic area can be measured using an M-Mode echocardiogram).
- Stroke volume is calculated by the aortic area multiplied by this velocity.

Good lubrication and small adjustments may be needed while listening to the Doppler sound to correctly position the probe at the level of the fifth

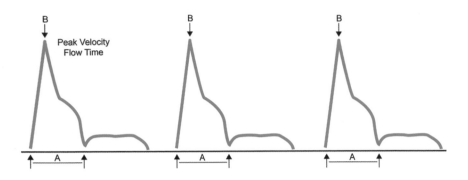

Figure 6.12. An oesophageal Doppler waveform, with peak velocity represented on the Y axis and the flow time over the X axis. The distance between the two arrows (A) is the flow time.

or sixth thoracic vertebrae. A correctly positioned probe will produce a waveform as shown in Figure 6.12. Two key elements of the waveform are corrected flow time (FTc) and peak velocity (PV). Reduced left ventricular contractility is reflected as reduced peak velocity and a reduction in preload is reflected as reduced flow time. An increased afterload will affect both peak velocity and flow time.

Invasive cardiac output monitoring

The thermodilution technique using a pulmonary artery catheter (Swan-Ganz) is the gold standard method to measure cardiac output but its use is limited due to its invasive nature and associated complications. In addition to measuring cardiac output, it is used for mixed venous oxygen sampling (pulmonary capillary sample). Pressure waveforms produced during the flotation of the pulmonary artery catheter include CVP, right atrium, right ventricle, pulmonary artery and pulmonary capillary wedge pressures (Figure 6.13). Derived indicators include cardiac index and systemic and pulmonary vascular resistance.

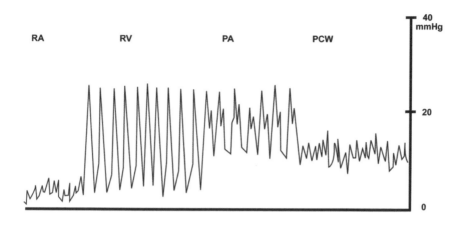

Figure 6.13. Pulmonary artery catheter trace. RA = right atrium; RV = right ventricle; PA = pulmonary artery; PCW = pulmonary artery capillary wedge pressure.

The lithium dilution (LiDCO™) technique involves injection of a known amount of lithium chloride through a peripheral or central vein and then measuring the levels via an arterial line that contains a lithium sensor.

Arterial pulse wave analysis can be used to assess the stroke volume which can be calculated based on the area under the systolic component of arterial pressure waveform. But the contour of the pressure waveform varies based on the peripheral vascular resistance and site of arterial cannulation. Therefore, it requires cannulation of either the femoral or brachial artery to obtain a good-quality pressure waveform and also requires prior calibration using either a thermodilution or lithium dilution technique.

The other less invasive techniques such as FloTrac™ and LiDCO™ rapid systems unitise advanced software which analyses the arterial wave form more than hundred times per second and compensates for the internal variation in the vascular tone. This eliminates the need for prior calibration.

The ejection of blood from the left ventricle into the aorta is associated with changes in electrical impedance of the thoracic cavity. This thoracic bioimpedance or change in electrical impedance is measured using high-frequency, low-voltage AC.

NICOM™ (totally non-invasive haemodynamic and cardiac output monitoring system) is a completely non-invasive cardiac output monitor based on bioreactance methods.

Central venous pressure monitoring

Central venous pressure (CVP) catheters are used for diagnostic, monitoring and therapeutic purposes. Commonly this includes blood sampling, drug administration, total parenteral nutrition administration and to guide fluid management. This is especially the case when large amounts of fluid are administrated or when small amounts could be potentially harmful to the patient. The CVP is more useful as a trend, and hypovolaemic patients may show a transient increase in CVP with fluid challenges, while euvolaemic patients show a sustained increase.

Sites of insertion

CVP catheters, or colloquially "central lines", are multi-lumen (although single-lumen lines do exist) and vary in length and number of ports. They are inserted via the Seldinger technique under ultrasound guidance in sterile conditions.

The internal jugular or subclavian veins are commonly chosen, though peripherally inserted central lines can be placed via the antecubital veins for patients requiring long-term access. Adequate placement requires the tip to lie in the superior vena cava (SVC) outside the right atrium. Specialised lines can be used for haemofiltration or haemodialysis and these are usually locked with heparinised saline to prevent clot formation. Subclavian lines have a higher risk of pneumothorax on insertion but are more comfortable for the patient. A central line inserted via the femoral route does not display an accurate CVP waveform due to the distance to the right atrium.

All lines should be observed for infection, kept locked when not used to reduce the risk of air embolism and correct placement should be checked using a chest X-ray prior to first use. The transducer is placed at the level of the right atrium similar to arterial lines and works via a similar mechanism.

Complications of insertion

- Bleeding, including carotid artery injury and haemothorax.
- Guide wire problems — arrhythmia on insertion, distal embolisation, loss of guide wire.
- Pneumothorax.
- Air embolism.
- Right atrial perforation.
- Infection, including endocarditis and sepsis.
- Nerve injury (brachial plexus, vagus, phrenic).

CVP waveform

The normal CVP is 0-8cmH$_2$O and if the patient is not flat or the transducer position is incorrect, then the readings, and therefore the trend, may be inaccurate.

Various characteristic waveforms have been described (Figure 6.14). Low CVP readings occur with hypovolaemia. In atrial fibrillation, the 'a' wave is generally absent. Raised right atrial pressures (in pulmonary hypertension, pulmonary stenosis) may produce giant 'a' waves. In comparison, tricuspid regurgitation produces a prominent 'v' wave. A distinctive canon pattern occurs in complete heart block that distorts the whole CVP and appreciation of the normal waves may be difficult. A prominent 'x descent' may be seen in constrictive pericarditis.

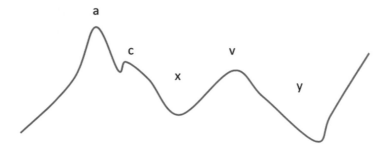

Figure 6.14. A normal CVP waveform. The a wave represents atrial contraction, c wave represents closure of the tricuspid valve (onset of ventricular systole), x descent represents atrial relaxation, v wave is due to venous filling of the atria and y descent represents early ventricular filling at the early part of diastole.

Oxygen measurement

Inspired oxygen concentration monitoring is mandatory to avoid hypoxia. The galvanic fuel cell is a safety device installed in anaesthetic machines to ensure that oxygen and not any other gas via that supply is being delivered to the patient. It utilises a chemical reaction to generate a current proportional to the partial pressure of oxygen (PO_2) in the sample. It consists of a gold or silver cathode, lead anode and potassium bicarbonate buffer solution. Oxygen molecules diffuse through the membrane and combine with the electrons and water at the cathode to give hydroxyl ions:

$$Pb + 2OH^- \rightarrow PbO + 2H_2O + 2e^-$$
$$O_2 + e^- + 2H_2O \rightarrow 4OH^-$$

The fuel cell is compact and does not require a power supply. It is not affected by nitrous oxide. It has a relatively slow response time of around 30 seconds. Hence, it cannot measure breath to breath changes in oxygen concentration. It is affected by water vapour and has a life expectancy of only 12-18 months. It is calibrated at 21% and 100% oxygen.

A paramagnetic analyser is based on the principle that oxygen unlike most anaesthetic gases or vapours is attracted to a magnetic field. Oxygen contains two unpaired electrons in the outermost orbit. Hence, it is attracted towards a magnetic field (paramagnetic). In a pulsed-field paramagnetic analyser, reference (room air) and sample gas are delivered as separate streams to a magnetic field. A differential pressure transducer measures the pressure difference across the sample and measuring chamber. When the oxygen is present, the pressure gradient between the two chambers is proportional to the partial pressure of oxygen.

A mass spectrometer can analyse oxygen from a given gas mixture. Sample gas is ionised by a beam of electrons and the charged ions are then deflected by a magnetic field. Detector plates located at various positions detect the ions according to their charge: mass ratio. It has a rapid response time, and can be used for breath to breath analysis of oxygen concentration.

PO_2 in the blood sample is measured using a polarographic (Clark) electrode and works via a chemical reaction similar to the fuel cell. It consists of a silver/silver chloride anode, a platinum cathode, electrolyte solution and a battery. A membrane permeable to oxygen separates the electrode from the blood sample.

Capnography

Capnography is the graphical representation of the measured end-tidal carbon dioxide ($EtCO_2$) level at a specific time (Figure 6.15). It also displays respiratory rate. The use of $EtCO_2$ monitoring has shown to reduce airway-related adverse events.

In healthy patients with normal physiological parameters, $EtCO_2$ approximates to the partial pressure of arterial carbon dioxide ($PaCO_2$). In normal lungs the partial pressure of $EtCO_2$ is about 0.5-0.8kPa less than the $PaCO_2$ due to the mixing of dead space gas (with no CO_2) with alveolar gas (containing CO_2).

Normal capnograph waveform

- Phase 1: inspiratory baseline (0kPa EtCO$_2$).
- Phase 2: upslope signifying onset of expiration.
- Phase 3: expiratory plateau phase due to mixing of alveolar gas in expiration.
- Phase 4: downslope signifying onset of inspiration.

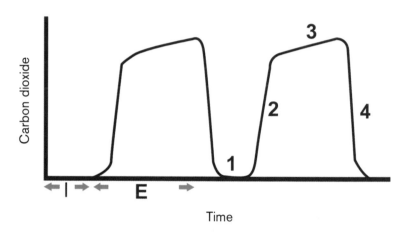

Figure 6.15. A normal capnograph waveform. Expiration results in a sudden increase in CO$_2$ and inspiration results in a sudden decrease. The EtCO$_2$ reading is taken at the end of phase 3. I = inspiratory phase; E = expiratory phase.

Uses of capnography

Capnography is increasingly essential not only for patients undergoing general anaesthesia or on intensive care but also those under sedation. Newer face masks have been developed to incorporate oxygen delivery and capnography together.

Capnography provides essential information regarding the airway, breathing, circulatory and metabolic systems.

Airway

The continuous presence of capnography is the gold standard method in confirming the correct placement of a tracheal tube. This should be used in conjunction with other markers of successful intubation such as visualisation of the tube passing through the vocal cords, misting of the tube and auscultation in the axillae for bilateral breath sounds.

Breathing

A disconnection in the breathing circuit will result in a complete loss of the capnograph waveform.

Hyperventilation will result in a lower $EtCO_2$ below normal physiological parameters and can be due to a patient with a raised respiratory rate or via mechanical ventilator settings.

Obstructive airways disease will produce a sloping phase 3 as seen in Figure 6.16B. This is more common with asthmatics and patients with chronic obstructive airway disease but may occur in those with bronchospasm due to any cause.

Rebreathing will result in a raised baseline (phase 1) and this is seen in Figure 6.16F. In this situation, the CO_2 absorber should be inspected and may necessitate changing.

Circulation

Capnography can be used as a marker of perfusion. Figure 6.16D shows a reduction in cardiac output that occurs due to a V/Q mismatch. This may occur in the settings of hypoperfusion such as hypovolaemia and pulmonary embolism.

Neuromuscular agents that are starting to wear off will show a characteristic 'M' waveform (Figure 6.16C).

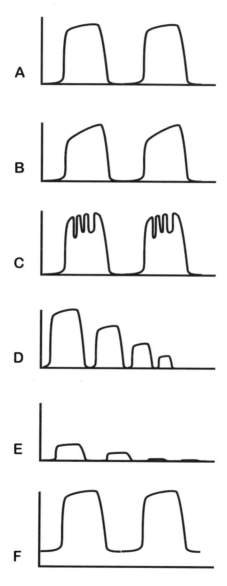

Figure 6.16. Abnormal EtCO$_2$ waveforms. A) Normal capnograph; B) Chronic obstructive airways disease; C) Neuromuscular paralysis wearing off (curare cleft); D) Reduced cardiac output; E) Oesophageal intubation; F) Rebreathing.

Metabolism

Malignant hyperthermia is an anaesthetic emergency. Classically this occurs in the setting of a raised $EtCO_2$ without any change of ventilation as the high limit alarms are set off. This is a clinical diagnosis and other markers of increased metabolism should be pursued. A similar pattern may occur in sepsis or pyrexia.

Measurement of EtCO$_2$

Mainstream and sidestream sampling

Gas can be analysed by a mainstream analyser which is contained within the breathing circuit (Figure 6.17). Sidestream sampling delivers the sampling gas externally to a separate analyser. This second mode is most commonly used in the operating theatre as it allows simultaneous analysis of the anaesthetic vapours.

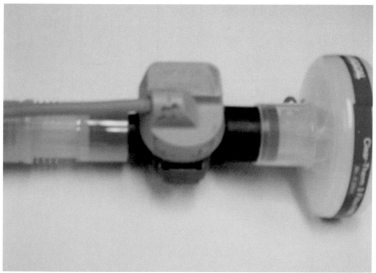

Figure 6.17. Mainstream EtCO$_2$ analyser.

Infrared spectroscopy

Infrared spectroscopy is used to measure $EtCO_2$ levels in the operating theatre. Gases or vapours with two differing molecules, such as CO_2, are absorbed by infrared radiation. Its absorbance peak is at 4.3nm.

A microprocessor-controlled infrared light is shone through an optical filter (Figure 6.18) into both a reference chamber consisting of gas with a known CO_2 concentration, and a second chamber, the sampling chamber. The amount of infrared radiation absorbed is proportional to the partial pressure of carbon dioxide (PCO_2) in that gas, as detected by a reduction in light on a photodetector.

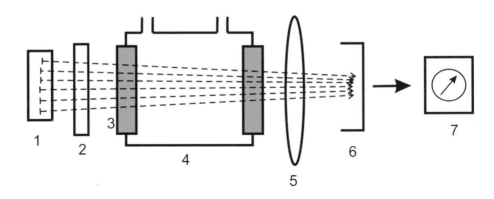

Figure 6.18. Components of an infrared carbon dioxide analyser. 1) Infrared radiation source; 2) Filter; 3) Crystal window; 4) Sample chamber; 5) Focusing optics; 6) Photodetector; 7) Display.

Errors in capnography

- Capnometers are subject to drift and require frequent calibration.
- Obstruction of the sampling line and leaks are common as is disconnection.
- Sidestream analysers are prone to damage by standing and this may lead to inaccurate results.
- Mainstream analysers increase the weight of the breathing circuit.
- There is a general lag time when sidestream analysers are used which depends on the length of the tubing and the size of the sample chamber of the analyser.
- Collision broadening occurs with nitrous oxide as it has a similar absorption spectrum to CO_2 (4.5nm). When nitrous oxide is used this may result in inaccurately high levels of measured CO_2.

Measurement of vapour concentration

While inspired levels represent delivery of a vapour, expired levels most similarly represents brain levels and therefore functional activity of the vapour, and thus this is most critically monitored. Specific end-tidal levels or the minimal alveolar concentration (MAC) value of the anaesthetic agent should be monitored. Measurement is similar to carbon dioxide (CO_2), via infrared spectroscopy, and the vapours are delivered via the same sampling lines. The absorbance pattern will be unique to each different anaesthetic vapour across a spectrum of wavelengths and optical filters are used to identify the individual vapours from each other. Other methods include Raman spectroscopy, mass spectrometry and piezo-electric absorption.

Ventilatory parameters

Mechanically ventilated patients are at risk of volutrauma and barotrauma, and therefore need to be monitored to prevent these adverse events.

The ventilator can provide information on mode of ventilation, airway pressure, gas volumes and an alternative place to visualise capnography, inspired and expired oxygen levels and vapour concentrations which are also normally displayed on the main display unit. In modern anaesthetic machines, ventilators will display rotameters where target inspired oxygen concentration (FiO_2) or end-tidal oxygen concentration (EtO_2) and flow rates can be set electronically (Figure 6.19).

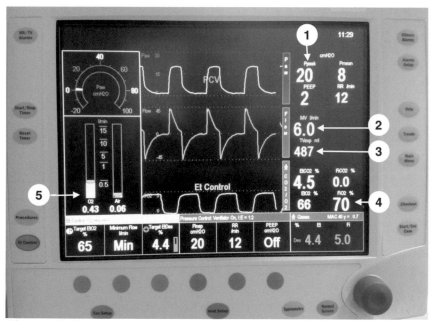

Figure 6.19. Ventilator display showing pressure-controlled ventilation. 1) Peak airway pressure; 2) Minute volume; 3) Tidal volume; 4) Inspired oxygen concentration (FiO_2); 5) Electronic rotameters.

Modes of ventilation

In pressure-controlled ventilation, a defined pressure is set and the tidal volume produced needs to be routinely checked to prevent unnecessarily large tidal volumes. A tidal volume of 6-8ml/kg is routinely used in current practice.

In volume-controlled ventilation, a defined target tidal volume is set and attentiveness is needed to maintain the peak airway pressure below $30cmH_2O$.

The addition of positive end-expiratory pressure (PEEP) may be appropriate and this can improve oxygenation.

Alternative modes of ventilation may be used depending on the ventilator manufacture and can incorporate a spontaneously breathing patient with added pressure support and apnoea back-up. In addition, the ventilator may be time-cycled in these settings.

Volume and flow measurement

A Wright's respirometer (Figure 6.20) directly measures tidal volume and minute volume when placed either on the expiratory or inspiratory limb of a breathing circuit. A rotating vane turns a set number of times in relation to the volume of gas that flows past it. This is connected to a gear mechanism and display. It is affected by water vapour and under-reads at low flows and over-reads at high flows. It only measures the volume of flow in one direction (either in inspiration or in expiration)

A pneumotachograph is used for indirect measurement of gas volume by firstly measuring the gas flow. Laminar flow is induced across a screen gauze and pressure transducers on either side of this gauze sense the alteration in pressure gradient when gas flow is present. Adding a pitot tube allows compliance to be measured and produces flow/volume and volume/pressure curves. Turbulent flow and increased resistance is created by water vapour and therefore pneumotachographs incorporate a heating element.

Rotameters, whether mechanical or electronic, are used to fine tune the delivery of oxygen, air and nitrous oxide. Mechanical rotameters consist of a conical glass tube with a floating bobbin or a ball, and gas flow is

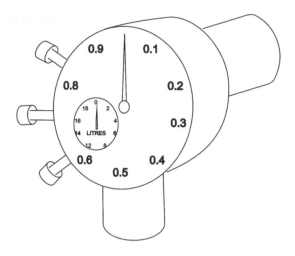

Figure 6.20. Wright's respirometer.

measured from the top of the bobbin or the middle of the ball. Checking the rotameter function should be routine practice as they are at risk of sticking or cracking.

Ventilator alarms

- Clinical observation of bellows, pulse oximeter and $EtCO_2$ all provide indicators of ventilation.
- High and low alarm limits should be set for:
  - peak airway pressure alarm (low limits for leaks and disconnection and high limit for obstruction);
  - tidal volume;
  - minute volume.

Neuromuscular monitoring

Neuromuscular monitoring is now mandatory when muscle paralysis is used. This includes prior to administrating any top-ups and prior to extubating the patient.

Peripheral nerve stimulators

These are battery-powered devices that can provide a constant current of approximately 40-60mA. Stimuli are given over 0.2-0.3ms and produce a monophasic square waveform. Common peripheral nerves used include the ulnar, facial, posterior tibial or common peroneal nerves.

To site a peripheral nerve stimulator, the negative (black or brown) electrode is placed distally over the superficial part of the nerve and the white or red positive electrode proximally (Figure 6.21).

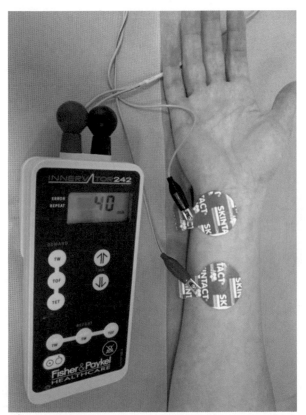

Figure 6.21. Placement of electrodes for stimulation of the ulnar nerve.

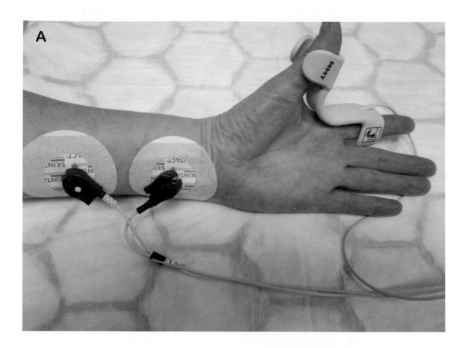

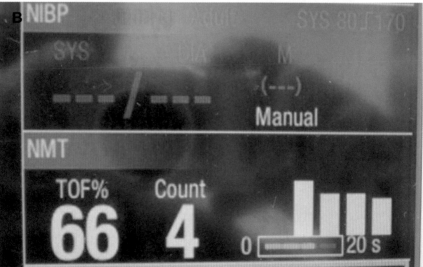

Figure 6.22. Placement of electrodes and mechanosensor of a neuromuscular transmission monitor (A) and quantitative display of the TOF ratio as a percentage, with a graphical display of the twitch amplitudes (B).

Tactile and visual evaluation is unreliable and therefore quantitative peripheral nerve stimulators are recommended. The use of kinemyography is becoming more routine in the operating theatre as they are inbuilt into some anaesthetic machines as an essential monitoring tool (Figure 6.22). They can be used for continuous monitoring and as an objective value, as the train-of-four (TOF) ratio is displayed on the monitor. Stimulation of the ulnar nerve produces contraction of the adductor pollicis resulting in adduction of the thumb. The movement of the thumb is sensed by a piezoelectric crystal and converted into an electrical signal.

Patterns of nerve stimulation

Single-twitch stimulation involves a single supramaximal stimuli of 60mA for 0.1-0.2ms with a frequency of 1Hz, repeated every 10 seconds. Twitch height is compared to before any muscle paralysis is given but it has limited use.

The TOF count is the number of responses obtained when four stimuli of 0.2ms at a frequency 2Hz are applied. The TOF ratio is a ratio of amplitude of the fourth twitch to the first twitch (T4:T1 ratio).

The degree and characteristics of the patterns produced will depend on whether depolarising or non-depolarising agents are used. Non-depolarising agents result in a fade in the response to TOF and tetanic stimulation. Fade occurs when there is a gradual reduction in twitch height after nerve stimulation, starting with a loss of the fourth twitch, then the third, second and, lastly, loss of the first twitch. Receptor occupancy by the neuromuscular agent increases as each twitch is lost from 75%, 80%, 90% and 100% receptor occupancy, respectively. On recovery, the reverse happens starting with the first twitch appearing. The return of three twitches is recommended before reversal can be given. A quantitative assessment of the response is essential to ensure adequate reversal of the neuromuscular blockade. A TOF ratio of more than 0.9 is considered as adequate reversal.

Tetanic stimulation of 50Hz for 5 seconds will produce a fade predictably. A post-tetanic count (PTC) involves stimulation with single twitches at 1Hz following a tetanic stimulus. This is used in determining deep block that usually appears as zero twitches with a standard TOF. A PTC of fewer than five twitches represents deep block and greater than 15 twitches represents sufficient return of muscle function for neuromuscular reversal to be given.

Double-burst stimulation is when two groups of three tetanic bursts are given at 750ms apart. It is more sensitive as a tactile assessment of the response as compared to TOF in determining fade.

Suxamethonium produces a phase 1 block, where there is continual depolarisation at the neuromuscular junction observed by fasciculations. Each twitch height is reduced equally and there is no fade in the response.

Objective assessment of response

- Electromyography: electrical activity in muscle measured using electrodes.
- Mechanomyography: muscle tension measured using a strain gauge and force transducer.
- Acceleromyography: acceleration of a digit produces a voltage change that is measured with a piezoelectric transducer.
- Kinemyography: movement of fingers deforms a piezoelectric mechanosensor that generates a current.

Criteria for adequate reversal

Clinical signs

- Sustained head lift for 5 seconds.
- Return of grip strength.
- Vital capacity breath of 15ml/kg.

Objective method

A TOF ratio of >0.9 is one of the most reliable indicators of returning muscle function.

Depth of anaesthesia monitoring

Although depth of anaesthesia monitoring is essential to titrate the dose of anaesthetic agents, due to various limitations it is less frequently used in current clinical practice and there is little consensus on how the depth of anaesthesia should be appropriately monitored.

Generally its use is recommended in situations where there is an increased risk of awareness during general anaesthesia. Awareness represents the conscious or unconscious memory that a patient encounters in relation to their anaesthetic or surgical procedure. Usually this represents unpleasant feelings and includes the sensation of pain. The incidence of awareness during general anaesthesia is 0.1-1.6%.

The National Audit Project 5 in the United Kingdom showed that 50% of cases of awareness occurred at induction and therefore depth of anaesthesia monitoring should be initiated prior to induction of anaesthesia, and used until the patient is fully recovered. MAC values above 1 are likely to prevent any further increase in an incidence of awareness.

Autonomic signs such as mydriasis, diaphoresis, tachycardia and sweating may all indicate a patient is aware and clinical signs should be used in conjunction with monitoring devices.

Bispectral Index

The Bispectral Index (BIS) processes cerebral electroencephalogram (EEG) activity to produce a dimensionless number from 0 to 100; 40 to 60 is said to represent an adequate depth of anaesthesia and 100 a fully awake patient.

Entropy

Entropy processes the EEG and frontal electromyography (FEMG). As anaesthesia deepens, the EEG becomes more regular and the FEMG signal become more quiet. Similar to BIS based on the irregularity of EEG and FEMG signals, an entropy monitor produces a dimensionless number from 0 to 100. A number between 40 to 60 is considered as an adequate depth of anaesthesia

Each facial electrode needs to be pressed for 5 seconds to attain proper contact with the skin (Figure 6.23). Interference may occur from diathermy or from spontaneous facial muscle activity.

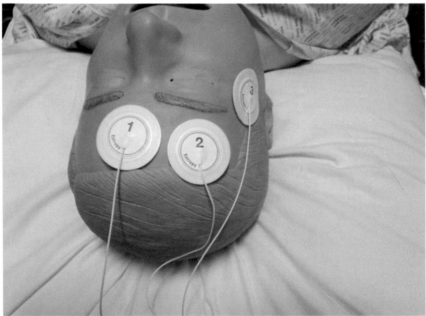

Figure 6.23. Correct placement of electrodes for entropy monitoring.

Other methods

Other less commonly used methods include measuring evoked potentials from repeated auditory or visual stimuli.

An aepEX™ monitor generates a number between 0 to 100 based on an analysis of auditory evoked potentials. Using earphones, repeated auditory stimuli are delivered to the ears and the EEG signal is detected using sensors placed at the forehead and mastoid region.

The isolated forearm technique involves inflating a tourniquet on the arm prior to the administration of any neuromuscular agent. This is thought to segregate the arm from the rest of the body and patients may spontaneously, or to command, move their arm or fingers. Caution should be taken with the prolonged use of tourniquets, including local skin, muscle and nerve damage.

There are limitations to the depth of anaesthesia monitors. In addition to anaesthesia, various other factors affecting cerebral activity such as hypotension, hypothermia, hypoxia and hypoglycaemia can affect the EEG pattern. Other drugs such as a high dose of opioids and ketamine have a variable affect on the EEG.

Patient groups at risk of awareness are:

- Previous history of awareness.
- The use of total intravenous anaesthesia (TIVA), especially when muscle paralysis is used concurrently.
- Emergency surgery, including obstetrics.
- Cardiac surgery.
- Haemodynamically compromised patients.

Monitoring temperature

Non-electrical methods

The mercury thermometer applies thermal expansion of a liquid to measure temperature. This, however, has a slow response time and poses an obvious risk of mercury spillage. Additionally, aneroid gauges also do exist. On the whole, non-electrical methods are rarely used during the peri-operative period.

Electrical methods

A tympanic infrared thermometer (Figure 6.24) measures infrared radiation at the tympanic membrane. A series of thermocouples (thermopile) is used to detect infrared radiation. Due to its proximity to the hypothalamus, tympanic measurements are considered as the equivalent

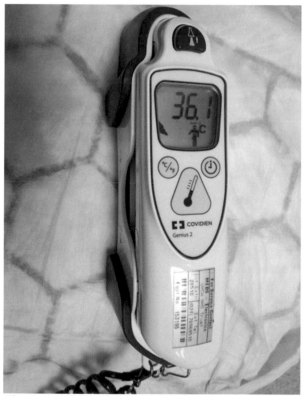

Figure 6.24. A tympanic infrared thermometer is a handheld device placed in the external auditory canal.

to core temperature. If accessible, the alternative ear should be checked if any erroneous results are displayed. This may be due to obstruction such as ear wax in the canal.

A thermistor is a semiconductor. The change in resistance is measured using a metal oxide semiconductor and this exponentially reduces with an increase in temperature. It is highly accurate and can be made very small and therefore can be used in pulmonary artery catheters and nasopharyngeal temperature probes (Figure 6.25).

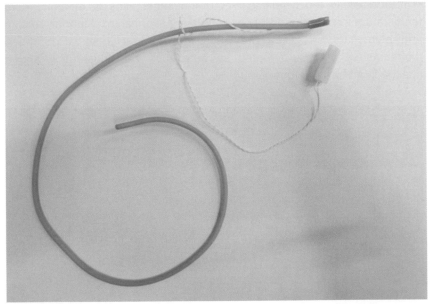

Figure 6.25. Nasopharyngeal temperature probe.

A platinum wire also measures resistance, but this increases linearly with an increase in temperature. They have a wide temperature range and do not require frequent calibration. They can be incorporated into a Wheatstone bridge as a strain gauge wire. They are also seen on flow sensors in ventilators.

Thermocouples measure temperature by exhibiting the Seebeck effect. It consists of two dissimilar metals, usually copper and constantan (copper with 40% nickel) joined together. At one end (reference end), the temperature is constant and at the other end (the measuring end), this is exposed to a different temperature. The potential difference between the two ends is directly proportional to the temperature difference between the two ends.

Sites of measurement

In addition to the tympanic membrane, other sites to measure core temperature include the distal oesophagus, nasopharynx, bladder, rectum and pulmonary artery as previously described. Chemical forehead thermometers may be affected by cutaneous vasoconstriction and a change in ambient temperature.

Case scenario 1

A 25-year-old, fit and healthy (ASA Class 1) patient is scheduled for a knee arthroscopy as a day-case procedure.

What monitoring would you consider?

Induction

- Minimum standard of monitoring — NIBP, pulse oximeter, ECG.

Intra-operative

- Minimum standard of monitoring.
- Airway pressure, tidal volume and minute volume, inspired and expired vapour concentrations, oxygen analysis.
- Capnography.
- Neuromuscular monitoring if a neuromuscular blocking agent is administered.

Postoperative

- Recovery unit — NIBP, pulse oximeter, ECG, temperature.
- Standard ward care monitoring postoperatively if uneventful.

Case scenario 2

A 65-year-old male patient with known ischaemic heart disease and hypertension presents with abdominal pain and vomiting (ASA Class 3). He has been scheduled for an emergency laparotomy with a provisional diagnosis of acute small bowel perforation.

What monitoring would you consider?

Induction

- Minimum standard of monitoring — ECG, pulse oximeter, NIBP for induction of general anaesthesia via rapid sequence intubation (RSI).
- Invasive blood pressure monitoring using an arterial line should be considered. It allows beat to beat monitoring of blood pressure during induction and titration of vasoactive drugs such as metaraminol to manage hypotension during induction.

Intra-operative

- Airway pressure, tidal volume/minute volume, inspired and expired vapour concentration, oxygen analysis.
- Capnography.
- Central venous access for fluid replacement, measurement of central venous oxygen saturations and administration of inotropes.
- Cardiac output monitoring via an oesophageal Doppler or pulse contour analysis via an arterial line.
- Hourly urine output should be monitored.

- Blood gas sampling to monitor acid-base balance, haemoglobin level and electrolytes.
- Temperature monitoring via an infrared tympanic or a continuous nasopharyngeal or oesophageal thermistor.

Postoperative

- Arrange high dependency or intensive care admission for close clinical and biochemical monitoring.
- Once the patient is awake, monitoring of pain levels and Bromage score if the epidural is sited intra-operatively.

Further reading

1. Al-Shaikh B, Stacey S, Eds. *Essentials of Anaesthetic Equipment*, 4th ed. Churchill Livingstone, 2013.

2. Davey AJ, Diba A, Eds. *Ward's Anaesthetic Equipment*, 6th ed. Saunders Elsevier, 2012.

3. Checketts MR, Alladi R, Ferguson K, *et al.* Recommendations for standards of monitoring during anaesthesia and recovery 2015: Association of Anaesthetists of Great Britain and Ireland. *Anaesthesia* 2016; 71: 85-93.

4. National Institute for Health and Care Excellence. Hypothermia: prevention and management in adults having surgery. London, UK: NICE, 2008. https://www.nice.org.uk/guidance/cg65.

5. National Institute for Health and Care Excellence. Depth of anaesthesia monitors (E-Entropy, BIS and Narcotrend). NICE Diagnostic Guideline No.6. London, UK: NICE, 2012. https://www.nice.org.uk/dg6.

6. Pandit JJ, Andrade J, Bogod DG, *et al.* 5th National Audit Project (NAP5) on accidental awareness during general anaesthesia: summary of main findings and risk factors. *Br J Anaesth* 2014; 113: 549-59.

7. Kettner S. Not too little, not too much: delivering the right amount of anaesthesia during surgery. *Cochrane Database Syst Rev* 2014; 6: 10.1002/14651858.E.

7 Anaesthetic machines

Rathinavel Shanmugam and Cyprian Mendonca

Introduction

Anaesthetic machines are used for safely delivering a mixture of oxygen, anaesthetic gases and volatile agents at a desired concentration as controlled by the operator to the patient's lungs through a breathing system. It provides a supply of anaesthetic gases, regulates the pressure of anaesthetic gases and oxygen, and allows mixing of gases and anaesthetic agents.

A basic anaesthetic machine (Figures 7.1 and 7.2) consists of the following components:

- Rigid metal framework with a compressed gas source.
- Pressure regulators: regulate the pressure of oxygen, air and nitrous oxide.
- Pressure gauges: measure the pressure of oxygen, air and nitrous oxide both in the cylinder and pipelines.
- Flow meters: reads the flow of oxygen, air and nitrous oxide.
- Back bar system: allows attachment of vapourisers.
- High-pressure release valve: protects the anaesthetic machine from high pressure due to downstream obstruction.
- Oxygen flush: enables delivery of a high flow of oxygen at a rate of 35L/min.
- Common gas outlet: a final mixture of gases and volatile agents leaves the anaesthetic machine and enters the breathing system.

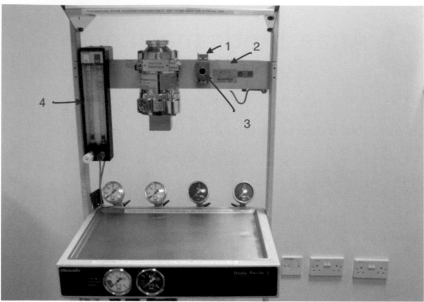

Figure 7.1. A basic anaesthetic machine. 1) Oxygen flush; 2) Back bar system; 3) Gas outlet; 4) Flow meters.

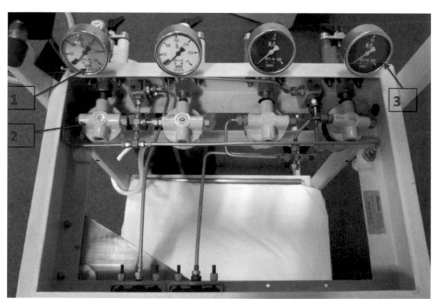

Figure 7.2. Components of a basic anaesthetic machine (top cover is removed). 1) Oxygen pressure gauge; 2) Pressure-reducing valve; 3) Nitrous oxide pressure gauge.

The anaesthetic machine performs three main functions:

- Delivers oxygen.
- Accurately mixes anaesthetic gases.
- Ventilates the patient's lungs.

The original anaesthesia machine was invented in 1917 by Henry Boyle. Prior to this, anaesthesia was delivered by anaesthetists who used to carry heavy cylinders and cumbersome airway equipment.

The modern anaesthetic machine

The moden anaesthetic machine (Figure 7.3) has the following basic subsystems:

- Gas supply via pipelines and cylinders.
- Gas flow measurement and control (flow meters).
- Vapourisers.
- Gas delivery via breathing system and ventilator.
- Scavenging.
- Monitoring.

The components of an anaesthetic machine are made up of a rigid metallic framework which is mounted on antistatic tyres with brakes.

Gas supply

Piped gas supply

Piped gases are supplied to the anaesthetic machine from a central source. Oxygen is usually supplied from a central cylinder manifold or from a vacuum-insulated evaporator. Medical air and nitrous oxide are supplied from a central cylinder manifold. The gases from the central sources are distributed via a colour-coded pipeline which terminates in the wall as a Shrader socket (Figure 7.4). Further colour-coded pipelines then connect

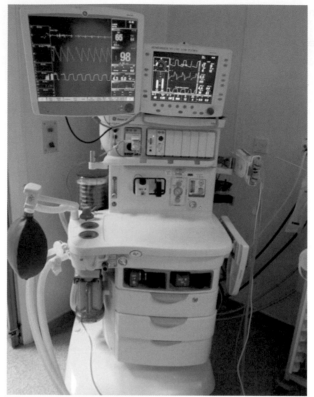

Figure 7.3. A modern anaesthetic machine.

the anaesthetic machine to the socket. There are pressure-reducing valves which ensure that the pipeline pressure is reduced to 4 bar.

The flexible pipeline has a Schrader probe (Figure 7.5) which is unique for each gas and thus prevents misconnection of gases. The pipeline is also colour-coded for each gas and they connect to the machine via a non-interchangeable screw thread (NIST) system (Figure 7.6). There is a one-way valve which ensures a unidirectional flow of gases.

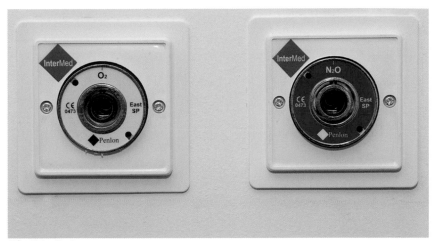

Figure 7.4. Shrader sockets.

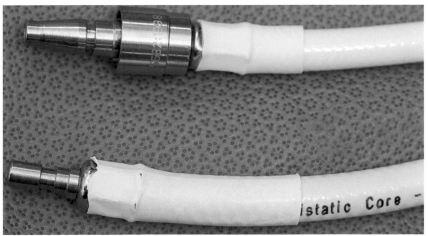

Figure 7.5. Shrader probes (standard Shrader probe and mini-Shrader probe).

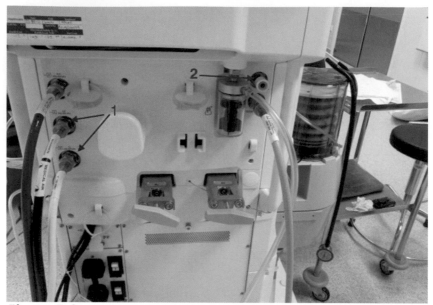

Figure 7.6. The back of an anaesthetic machine with a pipeline inlet via a non-interchangeable screw thread system (1) and mini-Shrader socket (2).

Cylinders

In addition to the central supply via the pipelines, all anaesthetic machines have cylinders present. They serve as a back-up in case there is a loss of central supply. The cylinders are made up of molybdenum steel and are strong but light. They are colour-coded for a particular gas. There is a pin index system which prevents accidental connection of a wrong cylinder to the anaesthetic machine yoke assembly (Figure 7.7) and a Bodok seal which gives a gas-tight seal. The pressures on the cylinders are measured by a Bourdon pressure gauge. There are unidirectional valves and primary pressure regulators. These pressure regulators reduce the dangerously high cylinder pressures to 4 bar.

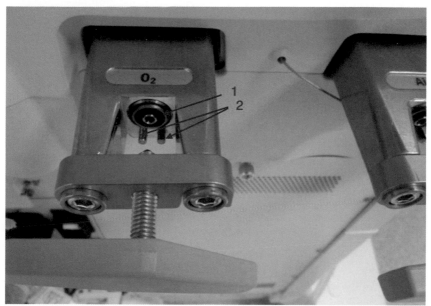

Figure 7.7. Yoke assembly. 1) Bodok seal; 2) Pins for oxygen cylinder.

Gas flow measurement

The gas pressures are further reduced from 4 bar to more manageable pressures which are just above atmospheric pressure by a flow restrictor. The gases then flow through a rotameter. The rotameters can be electronic or mechanical. The mechanical rotameter consists of calibrated tapered conical gas tubes with a bobbin. The tubes have an antistatic coating and are leak proof. In addition, the oxygen rotameter is placed downstream of other gases to add safety during any leaks. The knobs used to control flow are also differently shaped for each gas. Newer machines use microprocessors to ensure that the gas flow is controlled electronically.

Vapourisers

Anaesthetic vapourisers (Figure 7.8) deliver a given concentration of a volatile anaesthetic agent. They control the vapourisation of anaesthetic

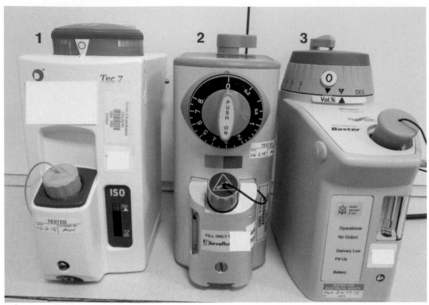

Figure 7.8. Isoflurane, sevoflurane and desflurane vapourisers.

agents from liquid, and then accurately deliver the desired concentration in the fresh gas flow. They are usually seated on the anaesthetic machine back bars and they have O-rings which help in maintaining a gas-tight seal. They have additional safety features including non-spill reservoirs and interlock systems.

The vapourisers are colour-coded and are calibrated for specific agents. Wrong-agent filling is prevented by the use of keyed filling systems. The devices are designed to consider ambient temperature, fresh gas flow and agent vapour pressure to deliver accurate anaesthetic gases.

Desflurane vapourisers differ from other vapourisers. Desflurane has a boiling point of 23.5°C; therefore, at room temperature it would not remain as liquid in the reservoir of a conventional vapouriser. In the desflurane vapouriser, the liquid desflurane is heated up to a temperature of 39°C so that it is converted into vapour.

Gas delivery: breathing systems and ventilators

Modern anaesthetic machine use a circle system to deliver the gases to the patient. The circle system (Figure 7.9) consists of a carbon dioxide (CO_2) absorber, a switch to choose between manual or mechanical ventilation mode, an adjustable pressure-limiting valve and a reservoir bag. The CO_2 absorber is soda lime which changes colour to indicate depletion.

Some machines deliver the gases via a T-piece system or a Bain circuit. These systems lack a CO_2 absorber and need higher flows to prevent rebreathing.

The ventilators are integrated with the machines. They are electronically controlled and pneumatically driven. The current machines have ventilators that support multiple modes of ventilation. In addition, most machines have spirometers which improve the efficiency of gas delivery to the patient.

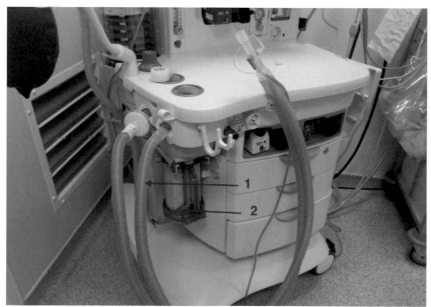

Figure 7.9. Circle breathing system (1) with a soda lime carbon dioxide absorber (2).

Scavenging

The anaesthetic gases are removed from the theatre environment by the use of a scavenging system. It is comprised of a collection system which covers the adjustable pressure-limiting (APL) valve. There is a wide-bore tube which transfers the gases to a receiving unit. The gases are then disposed of into the atmosphere. This is aided by a fan system which generates a subatmospheric pressure.

Monitoring

Most modern anaesthetic machines have integrated monitors attached. The monitors usually include ECG, SpO_2, blood pressure, temperature, end-tidal CO_2, anaesthetic agent (gas) and oxygen.

Safety features of modern machines

All anaesthetic machines incorporate features to prevent delivery of hypoxic gas mixtures:

- Oxygen failure alarm: this is an alarm that is set off if the oxygen pressure falls. In modern machines, this alarm is electronic.
- A delivery of a hypoxic gas mixture is prevented by mechanisms including chain linking of flow valves to prevent delivery of a <0.25 ratio of oxygen and nitrous oxide, as well as use of oxygen analyzers with a minimum inspired oxygen concentration (FiO_2) alarm.
- The pin index system, the NIST system and the colour coding of pipelines and cylinders prevent wrong connections of gases.
- Ventilators and monitors have alarms that can be set to identify abnormal readings.
- In the event of power failure, modern machines have a back-up battery system.
- In the event of a major fault, most modern machines switch off the delivery of gases and deliver only oxygen to the patient.

In the UK, anaesthetic machines should be regularly checked according to the guidelines published by the Association of Anaesthetists of Great Britain and Ireland or, if you are based in a different country, by the relevant association/society of that particular country.

It is essential to have an alternative source of oxygen delivery and ventilation, such as a self-inflating bag and an oxygen cylinder in the event of complete failure of the anaesthetic machine.

A breathing system delivers the mixture of anaesthetic gases from the machine to the patient. The Circle breathing system, Bain system, Magill system and modified T-piece system are commonly used. All the waste anaesthetic gases (exhaled from the patient and spilled over from the anaesthetic machine) are scavenged using a specific scavenging system. Modern anaesthetic machines also incorporate a ventilator, monitor and several safety mechanisms that enable early warning of any problems and possible critical incidents.

Case scenario 1

A 19-year-old girl is scheduled for an arthroscopy of the right knee. She has tested positive for malignant hyperthermia.

What precautions would you take In using the anaesthetic machine?

As the volatile anaesthetic is one of the triggers for malignant hyperthermia, total intravenous anaesthesia and a vapour-free anaesthetic machine should be used. In most operating theatre complexes, a dedicated vapour-free anaesthetic machine should be reserved for patients who are susceptible to malignant hyperthermia.

Another alternative option includes flushing the existing anaesthetic machine with a high fresh gas flow of 10-15L/min for 20 minutes (the manufacturer's instructions should be followed). All vapourisers should be removed from the anaesthetic machine. The carbon dioxide absorber and breathing systems should be replaced.

Malignant hyperthermia filters consisting of activated charcoal are available. These filters remove the trace levels of volatile anaesthetic by flushing the machine for 90 seconds with a high fresh gas flow.

Further reading

1.　Sinclair CM, Thadsad MK, Barker I. Modern anaesthetic machines. *Br J Anaesth CEACCP* 2006; 6: 75-8.

2.　Diba A. Anaesthetic work station. In: Davey AJ, Diba A, Eds. *Ward's Anaesthetic Equipment*, 6th ed. Saunders Elsevier; 2012: 65-106.

3.　AAGBI safety guideline. Checking anaesthetic equipment, 2012. https://www.aagbi.org/sites/default/files/checking_anaesthetic_equipment_2012.pdf.

8 Patient positioning for surgery

Vinesh Mistry and Cyprian Mendonca

Introduction

The primary aim of patient positioning is to maximise access and ease for surgery. However, various physiological systems can be influenced by various positions, increasing the potential for harm to a patient. In addition, there can be significant physical harm caused by poor positioning as an anaesthetised patient will not be able to combat anything unsafe. Inadequate attention to patient positioning is a leading cause of patient morbidity and cause for litigation.

The commonly used positions during surgery are:

- Supine.
- Lateral.
- Lithotomy/Lloyd-Davies.
- Head-up/deck chair.
- Trendelenburg/head-down.
- Prone.

For successful patient positioning, several pieces of equipment are required:

- Transfer equipment: patslide and slide sheets or hoist.
- Operating table.
- Patient supports: armboards, arm gutters, head rests, torso mattresses, vacuum mattress.
- Padding: gel pads, cotton rolls and pillows.

- Specialist equipment:
  - Mayfield® clamp — for neurological procedures;
  - stirrups — for a lithotomy position.

Supine position

The supine position is where the patient is lying flat on their back and it is the commonest position used in anaesthesia.

Physiological considerations

Respiratory

- Under general anaesthesia, lying flat will cause the tongue to fall back due to a loss of muscular tone. This causes airway obstruction and needs to be corrected immediately.
- Lying flat allows the diaphragm and abdominal contents to be pushed into the chest cavity, resulting in a reduction in the functional residual capacity (FRC). This reduces pulmonary compliance and increases ventilation-perfusion mismatching. In addition, if the closing capacity of the alveoli encroaches upon the FRC, then the alveoli are likely to collapse causing atelectasis and hypoxaemia.

Cardiovascular

- There is redistribution of blood from venous capacitance vessels within the lower limbs. This causes an increase in preload and therefore an increase in cardiac output. This does offset some of the vasodilatation caused by anaesthetic techniques.
- There is the potential for severe hypotension to occur because the inferior vena cava can be compressed against the vertebral bodies, and this is particularly an issue in obese patients and pregnant patients. Therefore, a 15° left lateral tilt is commonly used for pregnant patients to avoid supine hypotension syndrome.

Gastrointestinal

- Lying flat and relaxation of the lower oesophageal sphincter under general anaesthesia increases the potential risk of aspiration of gastric contents.

Anatomical considerations

Peripheral nervous system

- The brachial plexus is susceptible to injury from compression onto the fixed, hard structures it lies near (the clavicle, 1st rib and proximal humerus). Ideally, arms should be:
  - adducted, and crossed across the abdomen or chest; or,
  - straight and with the hands supinated by the side of the patient.
- If an armboard is to be used, this arm should only be mildly abducted, supinated and the head turned towards this abducted arm. This prevents compression of the ulnar nerve at the elbow and prevents traction on the brachial plexus.

Pressure areas

- The occiput is at risk of a pressure sore; therefore, a pillow or head ring should always be used.
- The heels are at risk too; therefore, gel heel pads should be used.
- In addition, the sacrum is also at risk and should be padded.

Eyes

- Under general anaesthesia, protective reflexes are lost as is muscular tone. This puts the eyes at risk of injury.
- There is the risk of corneal abrasion due to the lack of the corneal reflex, and from direct trauma from face masks, airway devices, airway devices ties, catheter mounts, breathing system filters.
- Corneal drying can occur if the eye is uncovered for less than 10 minutes.

- The supraorbital and facial nerves are at risk of compression injuries from the above airway devices also.

Lateral position

The lateral positon can be either a left lateral (right arm on top) or right lateral (left arm on top) position. This is commonly used for orthopaedic procedures on the hip, femur and ankle.

Physiological considerations

Respiratory

- During positive pressure ventilation, the dependent (inferior) lung is relatively under-ventilated and over-perfused, whilst the non-dependent (superior) lung is over-ventilated and under-perfused.
- Although there is a degree of ventilation perfusion mismatch, this is generally well tolerated in the majority of patients. However, patients with a lung pathology are the most likely to become compromised leading to hypoxaemia.

Cardiovascular

- Venous hypertension can occur in the dependent (lower) arm usually due to outflow obstruction. However, some of this can be prevented by flexing the arm and lying it adjacent to the head on the pillow (much the same as in the recovery position).

Anatomical considerations

Peripheral nerves and pressure areas

- A brachial plexus injury on the non-dependent (upper) side may occur if the head and neck are not supported sufficiently by a pillow or head rest.

- Padding/pillows should be placed between the legs preventing injury to the saphenous nerve and to prevent mechanical damage to the knees.
- There should be padding to the lower legs to prevent injury to the common peroneal nerve.

Eyes

- This position has the highest incidence of ocular injuries, in particular corneal abrasions which occur equally in both eyes.

Lloyd-Davies and lithotomy position

These two positions have similar physiological effects. The differences between them are the degree to which the hips and knees are flexed. The Lloyd-Davies position has less hip and knee flexion and is commonly used for urological procedures. The lithotomy position has greater hip and knee flexion and is commonly used for gynaecological and obstetric procedures.

Physiological considerations

Respiratory

- When moving the patient from the supine position into a legs up position, there will inevitably be movement of the carina cephalad. This can result in stimulation of the carina by an endotracheal tube causing bronchospasm or displacement of the tube resulting in endobronchial intubation.
- The abdominal organs are pushed into the thorax and reduce FRC, but to a lesser degree than the head-down/Trendelenburg position.

Cardiovascular

- Leg elevation causes emptying of the lower limb venous pools into the systemic circulation.

- The resultant increase in central venous pressure and right atrial pressure activates atrial stretch receptors and causes tachycardia — the 'Bainbridge Reflex'.

Gastrointestinal

- Lying flat and relaxation of the lower oesophageal sphincter under general anaesthesia increases the potential risk of aspiration of gastric contents.
- The flexed hips cause an increase in intra-abdominal pressure increasing the risk of regurgitation.

Anatomical considerations

Peripheral nerves

- Extreme flexion at the hips can cause nerve damage by stretching the sciatic and obturator nerves or by direct compression of the femoral nerve under the inguinal ligament.

Pressure areas

- Both hips and knees should be elevated simultaneously as there is a risk of hip dislocation.
- Calf compression occurs due to flexion at the knees and leg elevation above the heart which predisposes to venous thromboembolic events and compartment syndrome if surgery exceeds 4-5 hours.

Eyes

- The same issues for the supine position apply.

Head-up, deck chair and sitting position

A slight head-up tilt is used for ENT and head and neck procedures. A sitting position is commonly used for shoulder procedures and occasionally in neurosurgery as an approach to the posterior cranial fossa.

Physiological considerations

Respiratory

- The seated position maintains the normal ventilation-perfusion ratio which favours ventilation due to a maintained normal torso posture, with the apices being preferentially ventilated and the bases preferentially perfused.

Cardiovascular

- This system is the most affected, with venous pooling in the lower limbs in the presence of vasodilatation, which can lead to resistant hypotension.
- Excessive neck flexion/extension may cause obstruction to the neck veins.
- Systolic and mean arterial pressure decreases and heart rate increases.
- The feared and likely catastrophic event which may occur is a venous air embolism, more likely to be caused during a posterior fossa craniotomy. It is caused by the cranial venous plexus being below atmospheric pressure in the head-up position and the non-collapsible nature of the dural sinuses which can entrain air into the venous system.

Gastrointestinal

- Minimal effects are seen.

Anatomical considerations

Peripheral nerves

- Unsupported upper limbs can cause rotator cuff and brachial plexus injuries due to the traction caused by the weight of the limb.

Pressure areas

- A pillow or support should be placed under the knees to prevent the patient sliding down the operating table.
- This also maintains a degree of hip flexion preventing stretch of the sciatic nerve and retains the lumbar lordosis preventing back pain.

Eyes

- Eye padding and eye shields are used to prevent inadvertent pressure or injury from surgeons and surgical equipment.

Trendelenburg position

This position is used for procedures on the lower limb to reduce venous bleeding and for laparoscopic procedures on the pelvic organs. More often it is used in association with a lithotomy and Lloyd-Davies position for urology and gynaecological procedures.

Physiological considerations

Respiratory

- Cephalad movement of the diaphragm due to a pushing effect of the abdominal organs and pneumoperitoneum (in laparoscopic procedures) leads to a significant reduction in the FRC and consequent atelectasis.
- This leads to a greater ventilation-perfusion mismatch, with more lung perfused but less ventilated leading to hypoxaemia.

- There is a risk of laryngeal oedema during lengthy procedures.

Cardiovascular

- Increased systemic vascular resistance due to a significant area of the body being above the level of the heart. In addition, when pneumoperitoneum is created, venous return can be significantly reduced.

Gastrointestinal

- This position is associated with passive regurgitation due to a relaxed lower oesophageal sphincter under general anaesthesia and gravity, and the highest rate of aspiration in an unprotected airway.
- The abdominal organs are also pushed into the thorax.

Anatomical considerations

Peripheral nerves and pressure areas

For most procedures using a Trendelenburg position, the arms are abducted on the armboard. Care should be taken to avoid over-abduction of the arms, which may result in stretching of the brachial plexus. Elbows should be padded appropriately to prevent a pressure effect on the ulnar nerves. Pressure areas should be padded in a similar way to the supine position.

Eyes

- There is a raised intracranial pressure due to engorgement of the head and neck veins.
- There is also a raised intraocular pressure.

Prone position

This position is used to gain surgical access to the back, a few procedures on the lower limb, spinal surgery and for a posterior fossa

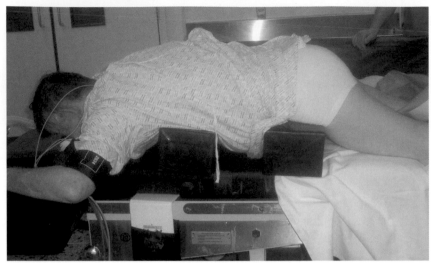

Figure 8.1. A patient positioned prone using chest and pelvic blocks. An appropriate head rest should be used to ensure the neck is neutral or slightly flexed and that there is no pressure on the eyes. Shoulders should be slightly flexed and abducted (<90° abduction).

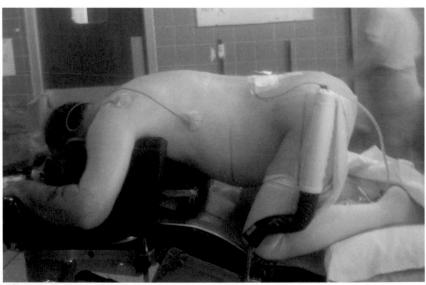

Figure 8.2. The knee chest position used for spinal surgery at the lumbar level. Note that the abdomen is free to allow easy movement of the diaphragm during ventilation.

craniotomy (Figures 8.1 and 8.2). The patient is most often anaesthetised in the supine position on a trolley and is then positioned prone on the operating table. Therefore, this involves a well-coordinated multidisciplinary theatre team involving between five to six individuals with good communication to ensure safe positioning. Special supports such as a Montreal mattress, Wilson frame, pelvic roll, chest roll or Cambridge frame are used for supporting the patient in the prone position.

Physiological considerations

Respiratory

- A beneficial ventilation-perfusion profile is achieved during positive pressure ventilation due to better matching of ventilation and perfusion.
- However, compression of the thorax will occur and dynamic chest compliance will be reduced; consequently, there is an increase in peak airway pressure.
- Adequate precautions should be taken to avoid compression of the lower thorax and abdomen so that easy movement of the diaphragm is possible during ventilation.
- Nonetheless, the breathing circuit and patient should be checked to ensure there is no compression of the circuit, kinked tubing, endotracheal tube movement causing endobronchial intubation or bronchospasm.

Cardiovascular

- Hypotension with a reflex tachycardia usually results from turning the patient into the prone position. This is due to a decrease in preload which can be caused by some or all of the following:
  - blood pooling to dependent areas in the vasodilated state;
  - compression of the IVC by the abdominal organs;
  - poor positioning of the patient causing compression of the thorax and raised intrathoracic pressure;
  - use of positive pressure ventilation and PEEP (positive end-expiratory pressure).

- Cerebral blood flow:
  - cerebral blood flow is maintained if the head and neck are kept in the neutral position during positioning and the operation;
  - turning the head to the side or having hyper-flexion of the neck can cause compression of neck vessels causing a reduction in cerebral arterial blood flow and resulting in a reduction in cerebrovenous drainage.

Anatomical considerations

Airway

- Particular attention is paid to securing the airway due to the need for stability during transfer and intra-operatively. Once the surgery is started, access to the airway in this position is very limited.
- A securely fastened, reinforced, cuffed endotracheal tube is the default airway of choice.

An appropriate plan should be in place to secure the airway in the event of accidental extubation, including help from an experienced anaesthetist and when any additional airway device is required such as a videolaryngoscope or fibreoptic scope

Pressure areas

The prone position is more likely to cause pressure injuries in various anatomical locations. From head to toe all areas should be carefully inspected soon after prone positioning to ensure appropriate padding. The anatomical areas subject to pressure injury include the forehead, supraorbital nerve, eyes, pinna of the ear, chin, tongue, ulnar nerve at the elbow, breasts, genitalia, and the femoral nerve and vessels.

Peripheral nerves

- Poor positioning or lack of padding is thought to cause peripheral nerve injury. All peripheral nerves are at risk of injury in the prone position.

- Placing the arms by the side provides the greatest protection to the brachial plexus, axillary vessels and ulnar nerve; however, this may not be feasible due to a requirement for venous and arterial access.
- The ulnar nerve is at risk if the elbow is not padded or the forearm supinated.
- The lateral cutaneous nerve of the thigh is at risk from compression injury from the support mattress.
- The supraorbital and facial nerves are at risk of compression injury if padding to the face is not sufficient or moves intra-operatively.

Eyes

- Visual loss due to direct and indirect trauma is highest in the prone position.
- Direct pressure on the globe of the eye can cause central retinal artery occlusion and cause visual loss.
- Indirect visual loss is caused by ischaemic optic neuropathy and is thought to be multifactorial, but is predicted to result from reduced venous drainage causing oedema around the optic nerve. This combination is thought to cause a form of compartment syndrome around the optic nerve.

Cardiac arrest

- In the event of cardiac arrest whilst the patient is in position, CPR should be started in the prone position.
- There are separate published guidelines for CPR in patients undergoing neurosurgical procedures.
- Cardiac compression over the posterior precordium is favoured and is identified as the angle of the scapula/level of T7 on the left of the patient.
- Defibrillation pads can be attached in an anteroposterior or anterolateral position.

Case scenario 1

A 66-year-old fit and healthy male patient (ASA Class 1) is scheduled for an incision and drainage of an abscess on his back in the lumbar region.

How would you position this patient?

This is a short surgical procedure; therefore, the airway can be secured using a supraglottic device. Anaesthesia is induced in the supine position and the airway is secured. Once the correct placement of the airway is confirmed, the patient is turned lateral for this procedure. At the minimum, four people are required to turn the patient to the lateral position. Once in the lateral position, the patient should be supported using lateral supports, one from the front at the level of the lower abdomen and the other from the back at the gluteal region. In addition, if required, safety straps should be used. The upper arm should be supported on an arm support, and care should be taken to avoid any traction on the brachial plexus.

Case scenario 2

A 62-year-old male patient is scheduled for a lumbar spinal fusion.

How would you position this patient?

This is a long surgical procedure requiring a prone position. All care should be taken to prevent accidental disconnection of infusion lines and the tracheal tube. The patient is initially anaesthetised on a trolley and then transferred to the table. Various body supports such as a Montreal mattress, Wilson frame or Allen table are used. At the minimum, six people are required to position this patient prone. Whilst the patient remains in position, a spare trolley should always be available, to transfer the patient to a supine position, in the event of a catastrophic intra-operative problem such as loss of the airway or cardiac arrest.

Further reading

1. MacDonald JJ, Washington SJ. Positioning the surgical patient. *Anaesthesia & Intensive Care Medicine* 2012; 11: 528-32.

2. Knight DJW, Mahajan RP. Patient positioning in anaesthesia. *Br J Anaesth CEACCP* 2004; 4: 160-3.

3. Feix B, Sturgess J. Anaesthesia in the prone position. *Br J Anaesth CEACCP* 2014; 14: 291-7.

4. Management of cardiac arrest during neurosurgery in adults. https://www.resus.org.uk/publications/management-of-cardiac-arrest-during-neurosurgery-in-adults.

9 Regional anaesthesia

Laith Malhas and Alastair Fairfield

Introduction

Regional anaesthesia (RA) describes the technique of causing a temporary interruption of sensory (and often motor) supply to an area in order to provide analgesia or anaesthesia, often referred to as a "nerve block" or "block". This is done by exposing nerves to local anaesthetic (LA) agents (with or without adjuncts) in order to interrupt communication with the area supplied. This can be used as a sole anaesthetic technique as an alternative to general anaesthesia (GA) or for peri-operative and postoperative analgesia in combination with a GA. They can be broadly classified as:

- Neuraxial techniques:
  - spinal anaesthesia (intrathecal/subarachnoid);
  - epidural/caudal block.
- Peripheral techniques:
  - field infiltration;
  - intravenous regional anaesthesia (IVRA);
  - peripheral nerve and plexus blocks;
  - compartment blocks.

General considerations

Advantages of regional anaesthesia

- Conscious patient — able to warn of adverse effects (during carotid surgery and transurethral resection of the prostate), less interruption of oral intake.

159

- Effects of general anaesthesia on respiratory function and mechanics can be avoided when an appropriate regional technique is chosen.
- Stable intra-operative conditions in conjunction with a GA.
- Faster recovery and improved early mobilisation.
- Better postoperative pain relief.
- Better ventilation (if pain is likely on breathing due to fractured ribs).
- Avoidance of adverse effects of GA like nausea, vomiting, sore throat and hang over.
- Avoids hazards of unconsciousness like aspiration of gastric contents, anatomical damage to skin, joints, nerves, etc.
- Avoidance/reduction of systemic opioids (reduced respiratory, gastrointestinal, urinary side effects).
- Reduced stress response to surgery.
- Reduced blood loss particularly with pelvic and hip surgery.
- Decreased incidence of pneumonia and deep vein thrombosis (DVT).

Disadvantages of regional anaesthesia

- Time-consuming.
- Adequate training and equipment are required.
- Haemodynamic instability with neuraxial techniques.
- May mask underlying conditions (e.g. compartment syndrome).
- Resumption of pain on block regression (may be sudden/at night).

Contraindications

There are few absolute contraindications to regional anaesthesia. Most are relative and the decision to continue becomes a risk to benefit balance, where it can be considered beneficial to continue when the risks of not doing so may be more severe. A careful explanation of this should be given to the patient when consent for the anaesthetic is taken. There are guidelines to aid with these decisions when considering coagulopathies and anticoagulant therapies available through The Association of Anaesthetists of Great Britain and Ireland (AAGBI).

Absolute contraindications are:

- Patient refusal.
- Severe coagulopathy.
- Active infection at the site of needle insertion.
- Inexperience of the anaesthetist with the technique.
- Allergy to local anaesthetic agents.

Relative contraindications tend to be more specific to the type of technique; some common ones are:

- Existing neurological disease.
- Systemic infection.
- Altered coagulation.
- Patient on anticoagulation therapy.
- Abnormal anatomy/previous surgery at site.

Complications of regional anaesthesia

These can arise from the procedure (needle puncture/catheter) or from the LA used and vary depending on the block area and technique used.

Procedural complications:

- Failure to perform.
- Inadequate block.
- Wrong side/wrong block.
- Infection (puncture site, epidural abscess, encephalitis, sepsis).
- Bleeding (bruising, haematoma).
- Inadvertent vascular puncture.
- Nerve damage (the majority are temporary).
- Damage to the surrounding structures (pleura, vessels).

LA complications:

- Systemic LA toxicity (immediate: direct vascular injection; delayed: systemic absorption).

- Spread to the surrounding nerves (e.g. phrenic nerve and sympathetic chain with an interscalene block).
- Anaphylactic reactions.

Safety and procedural considerations

Patients should always have the risks and benefits explained in order to gain valid consent before any technique. If part of an operative procedure, written consent is not required but verbal consent should be documented. If provided as a sole procedure, written consent may be appropriate.

Patients should have intravenous access established and secured before the procedure in case of any incident. They should be monitored continuously (SpO_2, NIBP, ECG) for the procedure and afterwards until the risk of complications dissipate.

A wrong-site or wrong-side procedure is a "never event" and safety checks should be performed in preparation for and immediately before any procedure in the form of the "Stop Before You Block" campaign and is in addition to the World Health Organisation's surgical safety checklist carried out in a theatre environment.

Performing these procedures whilst the patient is awake and non-sedated enhances safety and for neuraxial techniques they also allow the patient to be in the sitting position. An awake patient is able to report paraesthesia from the needle or catheter placement alerting the anaesthetist to immediate proximity to the nerve and the need to cease and alter the procedure. However, the need to perform all blocks on awake patients for safety reasons is still debated. Firstly, the paraesthesia elicited is not consistent with neural contact so does not preclude the occurrence of nerve damage. Secondly, it has been shown that intraneural injection does not necessarily cause nerve damage. Also, the introduction of ultrasound (US) allows real-time monitoring of the needle tip allowing the operator to avoid direct contact with the nerve theoretically reducing the risk.

Local anaesthetics

The specific pharmacology of LAs has been described in Chapter 5. The selection of a specific LA drug(s), concentrations and volumes depends on the desired effects of the technique. It is important to remember the maximum safety doses of LA when calculating how much is required.

The choice of local anaesthetic is dictated by the desired clinical effects. With the speed of onset and duration required in mind, the short-acting lignocaine and prilocaine are used when a quick onset is required and the long-acting bupivacaine, levobupivacaine and ropivacaine for a greater duration. Mixing LAs can be used to aim for a fast onset/long duration block; however, in practice, the results are unpredictable. The maximum safe dose should always be adhered to for the specific LA, otherwise there is a risk of systemic toxicity reactions.

Volume and concentration

This can affect the efficacy, density and duration of a block. A small volume of injectant may not adequately spread around a nerve or compartment to effectively block all components and will be absorbed quickly giving a shorter block. Alternatively, an excessively large volume may spread to block undesired nerves (e.g. phrenic nerve with an interscalene block or high neuraxial block), provide an excessive duration of block and increase the speed of absorption of the drug risking systemic toxicity. It may also limit the concentration of the LA that can be used in order not to exceed the maximum dose.

A weaker concentration may not provide a dense block (in some cases desirable, e.g. epidural infusions) and the smaller mass of drug molecules is cleared quicker. A high concentration provides a denser block of longer duration but limits the volume available to inject.

In practice, a balance is often sought to provide an adequate mass of drug in a solution of adequate volume and concentration for the block and its desired effects.

The type of block also affects many of these factors, with those in more vascular areas (e.g. paravertebral or epidural) having an increased rate of clearance of LA and hence a shorter duration of effect.

Calculating drug dosage

Local anaesthetic drugs are presented as percentage solutions. For example, 1% lignocaine contains 1g of lignocaine in 100ml of solution or 10mg per each millilitre of solution. The maximum safe dose is 3mg/kg, or for a patient weighing 70kg, 210mg for plain lignocaine; therefore, one can use 21ml of 1% lignocaine or 42ml of 0.5% lignocaine. For bupivacaine and levobupivacaine, the maximum safe dose is 2mg/kg.

Local anaesthetic adjuncts

Glucose is commonly added to LA solutions used with spinal techniques. This addition increases the solution's baricity (density) making it hyperbaric (or colloquially known as "heavy") compared to cerebrospinal fluid (CSF), meaning it will sink. This increases its reliability as it will spread more consistently and in the direction of gravity allowing a degree of control.

Opioids, via their direct effect on central and peripheral opioid receptors, and hence afferent pain pathways, act synergistically with LAs. Their use in neuraxial techniques is well established where they can access the spinal cord and brainstem but the evidence when used in peripheral techniques is less compelling. When used neuraxially, the resultant effects depend on the physiochemical properties. Doses and characteristics of effects differ from their epidural and intrathecal use.

Fentanyl is highly lipid-soluble producing a fast onset with little spread before fixing and a short duration. It is suitable for improving intra-operative analgesia.

Morphine is the least lipophilic so has a delayed onset of action and prolonged effect (24 hours). In the epidural space its spread is limited by binding to epidural fat but in the CSF it can spread up to the brain with possible delayed side effects, most worryingly delayed respiratory depression. It is used for postoperative analgesia.

Diamorphine is more lipid-soluble than morphine with a similar effect as it is converted to morphine within the CSF. It demonstrates less delayed side effects and has become popular where available.

The addition of adrenaline causes vasoconstriction in the area injected. Certain LAs have an intrinsic vasodilator effect (e.g. lignocaine, prilocaine). When adrenaline is added to counteract this, it reduces the blood flow to the area and hence clearance of LA. The reduced systemic absorption increases the maximum safety dose and increases the duration of the block, as the LA remains there for longer. It has little effect for longer-acting LAs as their intrinsic protein binding outlasts any effects of adrenaline and in clinical doses may have intrinsic vasoconstriction effects anyway. The addition of adrenaline is contraindicated in field blocks around end-arteries (digits, penis, nose) or around nerves with poor vascular supply (more distal nerves, sciatic nerve), as the reduction in blood supply may result in tissue necrosis and nerve damage. The adrenaline will also have an element of systemic absorption, which may be detrimental to patients with heart disease as it may trigger an ischaemic event.

Bicarbonate can be used (mainly in epidural techniques) to increase the pH of the injected solution and hence increase the non-ionised fraction of the LA resulting in a faster onset of action.

One example of using a mixed solution is for converting a lumbar epidural for labour analgesia to a sufficient block for a Caesarian section. Typically, 1ml of 8.4% bicarbonate solution and 0.1ml of 1:1000 adrenaline can be added to 19ml of 2% lignocaine and injected via the epidural catheter in 5ml boluses to effect. When used with the addition of 100µg of fentanyl, this provides a block onset of around 15 minutes capable of lasting 1½ to 2 hours.

Many other adjuncts have also been tried in an attempt to manipulate the characteristics of the block with varying evidence. Clonidine has been used, as its direct alpha-2 agonist effect can inhibit pain transmission prolonging a block. It does, however, cause vasodilatation and increased hypotension limiting its popularity. Dexamethasone, by an unknown mechanism of action, prolongs the duration of a block (from 12 to 24 hours in the case of an interscalene block). It has, however, been shown to also have this effect if given IV rather than in the LA mix, leading to most preferring the former due to an added antiemetic effect. Others that have been used include NMDA antagonists (e.g. magnesium, ketamine) and neostigmine.

Neuraxial blockade

The first subarachnoid block was performed in 1898 by August Bier using a cocaine solution; epidural anaesthesia was described 3 years later in 1901. The use of neuraxial blockade for anaesthesia has increased in recent decades. They are now used widely in clinical practice and there are several proven benefits for using these regional techniques:

- Attenuation of the stress response to surgery.
- Reduced risk of bleeding and need for a blood transfusion.
- Reduced risk of thromboembolic events (DVT or PE).
- Reduced risk of myocardial infarction and postoperative respiratory complications.

Contraindications

Additional relative contraindications for neuraxial techniques include:

- Severe stenotic cardiac disease.
- Raised intracranial pressure.
- Uncorrected hypovolaemia.
- Previous back surgery at the site of needle insertion.
- Some pre-existing neurological disorders, e.g. multiple sclerosis.

Subarachnoid (spinal) blockade

Indications

Indications for spinal anaesthesia include lower abdominal, pelvic and lower limb surgery. It is used to avoid a GA or in conjunction with a GA.

Risks of subarachnoid block

The risks of neuraxial blockade are outlined in Table 9.1.

Table 9.1. Specific risks of neuraxial blockade.

Common	Hypotension — fluid loading or vasopressors may be needed
	Technical failure — missed segments with epidural for example
	Pruritis (itching)
	Nausea
	Urinary retention — requires urinary catheters for 24-48 hours
	Confusional states — particularly elderly patients
Rare	Spinal haematoma — may cause paraplegia, needs urgent evacuation
	Spinal abscess — may cause paraplegia, needs aggressive antibiotic therapy and occasionally surgical evacuation
	Direct nerve damage — most resolve in 1-6 months
	Respiratory depression — particularly with neuraxial opioids

Relevant anatomy

The spinal cord terminates to form the cauda equina at the level of L1 in adults (L3 in children) but in 2% of adults extends to L3; therefore, attempting subarachnoid block above the L3/4 interspace is not recommended. Tuffier's line (Figure 9.1) is the line joining the superior aspects of the iliac crests posteriorly and crosses the L4 vertebra in the midline (Figure 9.1). It is an important anatomical landmark for neuraxial procedures. Ultrasound can also be used to identify the midline and lumbar interspace, which is particularly useful in the obese patient or patients with abnormal spinal anatomy.

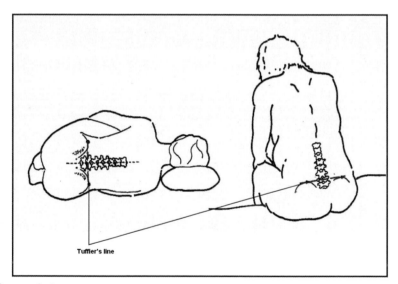

Figure 9.1. Tuffier's line.

Performing the subarachnoid block

The block is usually performed in the awake patient for safety reasons with IV access established and standard monitoring in place. Some would also advocate the use of capnography. Short-acting analgesia can be provided to aid patient positioning.

The two positions recommended are for the patient to be sat up or lying in the lateral position. The sitting up position allows for better identification of the anatomy and often a more straightforward approach to the subarachnoid space. The lateral position can be more technically challenging but may be the only position the patient can tolerate, if they have a fractured neck of the femur or perineal trauma for example. In either position, a midline or paramedian (start 1-2cm lateral from the midline) approach can be used. Flexion of the lumbar spine helps to open up the intervertebral spaces.

Full aseptic precautions should be used throughout the procedure including thorough hand washing, the wearing of sterile gloves, gown, hat and face mask, and the use of a sterile drape. The skin must be cleaned with an appropriate cleaning solution (for example, chlorhexidine 0.5% in 70% alcohol) and the equipment prepared (Figure 9.2). Lignocaine 1% or 2% is infiltrated to the dermal and subcutaneous layers at the insertion site.

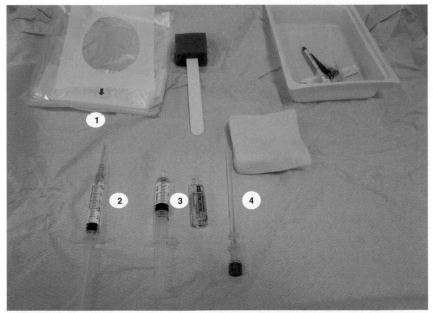

Figure 9.2. Equipment for a spinal block. 1) Clear sterile drape; 2) 1% lidocaine; 3) 0.5% heavy bupivacaine; 4) 24g Sprotte spinal needle.

The choice of spinal needle will influence the risk of post-dural puncture headache (PDPH). Pencil point needles (Sprotte or Whitacre) result in a lower incidence of PDPH than beveled needles (Quincke); therefore, a 24G or 25G pencil point needle is most commonly used in current practice. The spinal needle is inserted using the introducer needle to aid passage through the subcutaneous tissues. A slight cephalic angle may be required to negotiate the spinous processes (Figure 9.3).

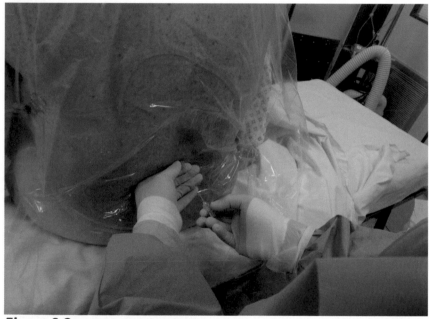

Figure 9.3. Inserting a spinal needle.

Resistance increases as the ligamentum flavum is reached and then a 'pop' can be palpated as the dura is breached and the needle tip enters the subarachnoid space. At this point the inner stylet can be removed and the position of needle placement confirmed by the flow of CSF from the needle (Figure 9.4). It should be noted that the rate of flow is reduced in the lateral position compared with the sitting up position. It is important that the needle does not move once the correct position has been confirmed.

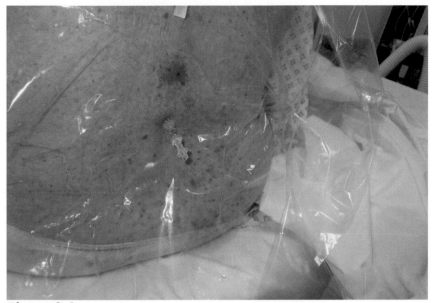

Figure 9.4. CSF demonstrated flow from a needle hub.

The local anaesthetic solution of choice can then be steadily injected through the spinal needle into the subarachnoid space. There should be minimal resistance to injection. The patient should then be aided into the supine position and time allowed for the block to be established, typically 5-10 minutes, during which time observations should be monitored and the block height assessed.

Assessment of block height

The loss of sensation to cold (using ethylene chloride spray for example) and sharp (slightly blunted needle or cocktail stick) stimuli should be tested at each relevant dermatome level. Some would recommend assessing light touch sensation but this has a heavy dependence on operator technique and can therefore be unreliable. A block from S4 to T4 would provide good analgesia for abdominal and pelvic surgery. A lower level of block would be sufficient for lower limb and prostate surgery.

Some easy to remember dermatome levels are:

- T4-5 — nipple.
- T6-8 — xiphisternum.
- T10 — umbilicus.
- L1 — groin.
- S2 — perineum

As well as the sensory block, the motor block should also be assessed using the modified Bromage score (Table 9.2).

Table 9.2. Modified Bromage score.

Grade	Patient assessment	Degree of block
I	Able to move hip, knee and ankle	None
II	Able to move knee and ankle but not hip	Partial
III	Only able to move ankle	Almost complete
IV	No movement	Complete

It is important to remember the spinal sympathetic nerves will also be blocked leading to vasodilation and hypotension. Caution should be used in patients with the inability to increase their cardiac output (e.g. fixed output states) and direct vasopressors should be prepared and readily available.

Choice of local anaesthetic for subarachnoid block

The choice and volume of local anaesthetic to be used varies greatly depending on the clinical scenario. A larger volume of local anaesthetic will result in a higher block height so that 1 or 2ml may be adequate for some lower limb surgery, whereas 2 or 3ml may be required for pelvic or abdominal surgery.

Likewise, shorter-acting agents (for example, prilocaine) may be suitable for shorter-length surgery and longer-acting agents (bupivacaine/levobupivacaine) for more lengthy surgical procedures. Bupivacaine can reliably provide operative analgesia for 1½ to 2 hours.

'Heavy' bupivacaine is the most commonly used agent as it gives a more predictable spread and a degree of manipulation using the patient's position.

Troubleshooting and tips

Patient positioning is key to successful neuraxial procedures. Having the patient relax and curl forwards to flex their lumbar spine is of key importance. Good communication with the patient and an engaged assistant can help with this. If the patient is in the sitting position, tilting the table towards you will encourage the patient to flex forwards.

Avoid the vertical centre of the space but instead aim for the upper third of the interspace. Hitting bone superficially suggests you are too high, whereas hitting bone deeply indicates you are too low.

Try to imagine a vertical line down the midline and avoid directing your needle away from this (unless performing a paramedian approach). If the patient complains of sharp pain, ask which side it is felt; this can help redirect the needle path (e.g. if pain is felt on the right side the needle needs to be directed more leftwards).

Call for assistance early if you are struggling and there is no suitable alternative to neuraxial blockade.

Check the block thoroughly using multimodal testing to ensure it is working correctly before any surgical procedure commences.

Epidural anaesthesia

Indications

In addition to providing analgesia for abdominal, pelvic and lower limb surgery, epidurals can also provide postoperative analgesia following major abdominal or thoracic surgery. Epidurals can also be used to provide analgesia in the non-operative setting, for example, rib fractures or for labour analgesia.

Contraindications

Contraindications and risks are the same as for spinal anaesthesia.

Relevant anatomy

Unlike with subarachnoid blockade, an epidural can theoretically be sited throughout the length of the spine. The epidural space is the potential space that lies between the dura and periosteum lining the inner aspect of the vertebral canal. On the posterior aspect, the ligamentum flavum completes the boundary between the lamina. The upper limit of the epidural space is the foramen magnum and its lower limit is the tip of the sacrum at the sacrococcygeal membrane. It contains lymphatics, spinal nerve roots, loose connective tissue, small arteries and a network of venous plexuses. The width of the epidural space posteriorly varies, being maximal at L2 where it is 6mm wide (4-5mm at the mid-thoracic level).

Performing an epidural

The patient position, monitoring and preparation is as mentioned in the spinal anaesthesia section. In addition, the epidural catheter should be flushed with sterile 0.9% saline using an epidural catheter bacterial filter.

The chosen inter-space is infiltrated with local anaesthetic (1% lignocaine) and a midline or paramedian approach is chosen. A Touhy needle (Figure 9.5) is inserted into the skin and then advanced to a depth of 2-3cm until a distinct sensation of increased resistance is felt as the needle enters the interspinous ligament (Figure 9.6).

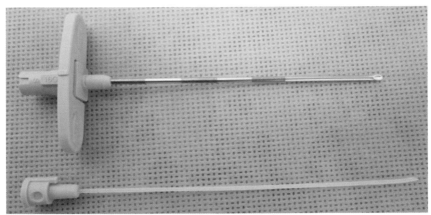

Figure 9.5. Touhy needle.

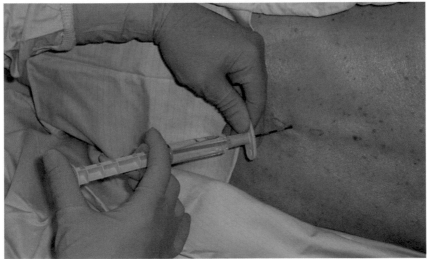

Figure 9.6. Performing an epidural; the patient is in the right lateral position.

The stylet is then removed and a saline or air-filled 'loss of resistance' syringe is attached. The needle and syringe are slowly advanced, constantly checking for the loss of resistance, which will be felt as the needle exits through the ligamentum flavum and enters into the epidural space (saline or air is injected). At this stage, the syringe is removed and the catheter is inserted (Figure 9.7) for about 15-18cm at the hub. The depth of the needle into the epidural space is noted and the needle is gradually withdrawn. About 3-5cm of catheter should be left inside the space.

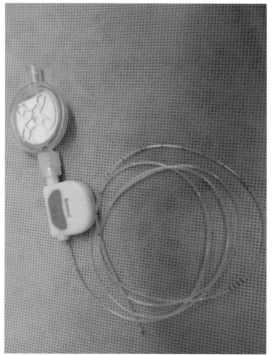

Figure 9.7. Epidural catheter, showing the blue tip, centimetre markings, connector and filter.

A drop in the meniscus level in the epidural catheter suggests correct placement within the epidural space.

A 'test dose' should then be administered to ensure that the catheter is not intrathecal. A typical regime would be 3ml of 2% lignocaine which would produce profound and fast-onset motor and sensory block if injected intrathecally rather than into the epidural space.

The epidural infusion can then be started. A typical infusion solution would be 0.1% bupivacaine with 2µg/ml fentanyl. Depending on the indication for the epidural, a 'loading dose' may be required which could be 10-20ml of the above infusion solution or 0.25% bupivacaine (with or without fentanyl) as examples.

The block height can be assessed, as discussed above for spinal anaesthesia.

Troubleshooting and tips

The same tips for a spinal technique also apply. Once in the interspinous ligament, resistance to saline can help direct the path: if there is full resistance, the needle tip is likely to still be in the ligament; if there is a slight give (but not easy injection), the path may have diverted laterally and the needle tip may be in the muscle; once in the epidural space there is no resistance.

On removing the stylet some fluid may como back if saline is used. If a full 10ml was instilled, this may seem alarming but will slow and stop, as opposed to a dural tap, which would continue. If a dural tap is recognised, replace the stylet to prevent further loss. The options are then to remove the needle and re-attempt the procedure at a different level, or place a catheter and label it clearly to be used as an intrathecal catheter. This decision should be guided by local policies, senior advice and the patient should be kept informed at all times.

Threading the epidural catheter requires constant pressure. Some resistance may be felt when passing the Huber tip (at the 10cm mark) but then it should pass freely. If there is a lot of resistance the tip may be placed incorrectly. The needle should not be rotated to try and overcome this, as it is highly likely to rupture the dura. If there is further resistance beyond this point, the catheter should not be forced as it may be against vulnerable structures (dura or blood vessels).

The catheter should never be withdrawn from the needle as this may shear off the catheter tip. If it is to be withdrawn, either the needle should be withdrawn first or both removed together.

By threading the catheter to the 15cm mark at the hub, this leaves 5cm in the space. Any more increases the risk of curling or diverting laterally.

Once the needle is removed, the depth to skin should be checked to ensure the catheter has not migrated significantly. If blood is aspirated from the catheter it should be withdrawn 1cm, flushed with saline and aspirated again; if no aspirate is present a test dose can be given if the drop test is satisfactory. If less than 3cm is left in the space the epidural may not be reliable and 2cm or less requires removal and replacement.

The catheter should then be secured to prevent it being dislodged. There are many devices available and local policies should be followed.

Benefits after epidural analgesia

A number of studies have shown that epidural analgesia reduces postoperative complications; however, an overall reduction in mortality has not been reliably demonstrated. The MASTER study investigated the effects of epidural analgesia versus systemic opioids in high-risk patients undergoing major surgery. Those patients with epidural analgesia had fewer thromboembolic events and respiratory complications. They also had better analgesia. However, there was no reduction in overall mortality, perhaps because despite being high risk, overall mortality rates for major surgery are small.

Combined spinal/epidural (CSE)

A combined spinal/epidural (CSE) technique can sometimes be used where a spinal anaesthetic is given for intra-operative analgesia followed by placement of an epidural catheter so that further analgesia can be given for prolonged surgical procedures (that will outlast the effects of a spinal anaesthetic) or for postoperative analgesia. It also allows the spread of the intrathecal drug to be manipulated; by filling the epidural space the dural sack is compressed increasing cephalad spread and block height.

Although CSE techniques give a clinical advantage they can be technically more difficult and the combined risks are higher.

The technique involves finding the epidural space with a Touhy needle as described above but then inserting a spinal needle through the Touhy needle (generally included in CSE kit packs) into the subarachnoid space to give a spinal dose of local anaesthetic. The spinal needle is then removed and an epidural catheter threaded into the epidural space.

Peripheral techniques

Peripheral nerve blocks (PNBs) allow more targeted analgesia and anaesthesia if the pain or operation is confined to their distribution. They can be used for the upper body (as opposed to neuraxial blocks) and although each varies slightly in their associated risks, they are generally less than neuraxial techniques. A variety of choices with LAs, single shot or catheter techniques, boluses or infusions, allow a variety of options available to tailor for individual case requirements. A summary of the different types are given below. A detailed description and discussion of each individual technique is beyond the remit of this book; however, tabulated brief summaries are provided and further information can be found in the further reading resources.

Traditionally, PNBs are performed using anatomical surface landmarks to target the area where there is little inter-patient anatomical variability. Counting fascial planes transferred (as 'pops') can be used to identify compartments. The precise identification of a nerve was originally by eliciting paraesthesia in its distribution by contact with the needle. In order to minimise the risk of damaging the nerve with the needle, the use of a peripheral nerve stimulator can be used to elicit a motor response when the needle tip is in close proximity. With the advent of powerful portable ultrasound (US) machines their use allows direct visualisation of the target, surrounding anatomy, needle as it is guided into position and spread of the injectant. Ultrasound regional anaesthesia (USRA) is now becoming standard practice with many advantages and few disadvantages (see Table 9.3 below). It is important to note that attempts to quantify advantages such as risk reduction are mainly theoretical as research has not always been able to prove statistical differences.

Table 9.3. Use of ultrasound in regional anaesthesia.

Advantages	Disadvantages
Visualisation of the nerve, allowing identification of the optimal level to block	Equipment cost
Visualisation of anatomy, including any variations and abnormalities, allowing the choice of needle entry and path	Availability of machine
Identification of the surrounding sensitive structures, allowing their avoidance, e.g. vessels	Extra skills required
Visualisation of needle advancement and course corrections	Steeper learning curve
Visualisation and confirmation of LA spread and correct catheter placement	
Increased safety in asleep patients	
Able to perform in a paralysed patient	
Increased patient satisfaction allows blocks to be done without the use of a peripheral nerve stimulator and with fewer needle passes	
Lower volumes of LA can be used with confidence, with a reduction of side effects	

Equipment and procedure

Needles used for peripheral techniques tend to have a short bevel tip as opposed to a cutting tip present on most hypodermic needles (Figure 9.8). This creates greater resistance when traversing tissue planes allowing for feedback of a 'pop' to indicate piercing a fascia. The short bevel tip also gives a safety advantage if contact were to be made with a nerve. By being blunter it is more likely that a nerve in its path is pushed aside rather than transfixed or cut as would happen more readily with a cutting tip. However, it is still possible to damage a nerve and in this instance a short bevel will create more damage compared to a clean cut from a cutting tip which will tend to heal quicker.

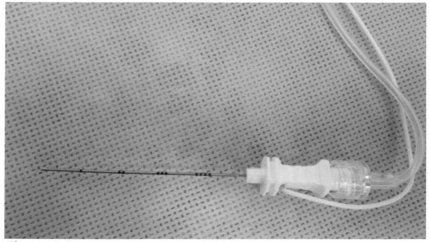

Figure 9.8. Peripheral nerve block needle.

A peripheral nerve stimulator (PNS) can be used to identify nerves by electrically stimulating it causing a motor twitch (in a non-paralysed patient) and paraesthesia (in an awake patient) in its distribution.

Ultrasound techniques require a suitable machine and transducer (Figure 9.9). Most techniques require a linear transducer using 10-12MHz, while in those with deeper structures, a curvilinear probe of 2-5MHz may be more suitable. Sterility of the procedure should still be maintained either as an aseptic non-touch technique for single-shot procedures or maintaining a full sterile field for catheter techniques.

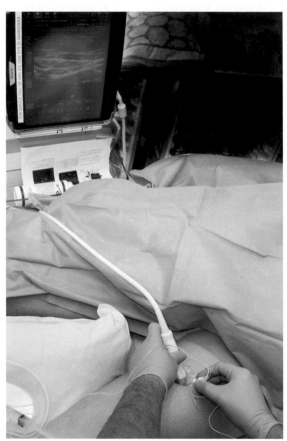

Figure 9.9. Sub-sartorial saphenous nerve block using ultrasound. The needle is inserted in the ultrasound plane and the tip should be visualised throughout the procedure.

Field infiltration

This describes the technique of injecting LA subcutaneously with the aim of blocking small nerves supplying the immediate area or more distal area known to be supplied by those nerves. These include simple subcutaneous infiltration for needle puncture, blocks for carpal tunnel release, analgesia for inguinal hernia operations and a ring block for digital anaesthesia

Intravenous regional anaesthesia

A simple and once popular technique involving isolating the vascular tree of a limb and injecting LA intravenously resulted in anaesthesia of the limb by reaching local nerves via their venous vascular supply. It has fallen out of fashion due to the risk of the LA reaching the remaining circulation (mostly by technical errors) causing systemic toxicity. A full description of the technique can be found in the further reading section. Prilocaine has been the LA of choice as it has less systemic toxicity with partial clearance by the lungs, but can cause methaemoglobinaemia.

Peripheral plexus blocks

By injecting LA directly around the nerve or plexus supplying the desired area, anaesthesia or analgesia can be reliably provided. PNBs can be performed as single-shot techniques with desired characteristics depending on the solution used (as described above) or combined with catheter placement for continuous LA infusion for prolonged analgesia. As the needle is directed towards the nerve there is the additional risk of damaging it. In general, they therefore require more caution.

Compartment blocks

Where nerves are difficult to identify individually, but are known to traverse an anatomical compartment, they can be blocked by instilling LA into that compartment. Examples include a fascia iliaca block, paravertebral block and the ophthalmic blocks (sub-tenon, peribulbar). The increasing use of US has made compartment blocks more reliable (e.g. transversus abdominal plane block) and has allowed further compartment blocks to be possible (e.g. adductor canal, serratus anterior and pectoralis blocks). These blocks tend to rely on higher volumes of initial injectant in order to reliably fill the compartment and block all the desired nerves but are amenable to subsequent catheter placement for continuous infusions.

The various types of block are outlined in Tables 9.4 to 9.7.

Table 9.4. Upper limb blocks.

	Nerves targeted	Area blocked	Examples of uses	Typical volumes	Notes
Interscalene	Brachial plexus at trunks (C5/6/7)	Shoulder and upper limb surgery to elbow	Shoulder and humeral surgery	10-20ml	Side effects of phrenic nerve palsy and Horner's syndrome occur more with larger volumes (>20ml).
Supraclavicular	Brachial plexus at divisions	Upper limb distal to shoulder	Elbow, forearm and hand surgery	10-20ml	Pleural damage can be prevented by blocking the plexus when above the 1st rib. Can spare the ulnar nerve, ensure full spread to 'corner pocket'.

Continued

Table 9.4 *continued*. Upper limb blocks.

	Nerves targeted	Area blocked	Examples of uses	Typical volumes	Notes
Infraclavicular	Brachial plexus at cords	Distal humerus and below	Elbow, forearm and hand surgery	10-20ml	Variable location of cords around artery, abducting the arm useful to bring them together. Deep structures increase difficulty.
Axillary	Terminal branches of brachial plexus	Elbow, forearm and hand	Forearm and hand surgery	5-10ml per nerve	Useful also to block the musculocutaneous nerve. T1 (thoracobrachial nerve) can be blocked by subcutaneous field infiltration at this level and this helps to prevent tourniquet pain.
Distal upper limb blocks	Ulna, medial, radial nerves	Dermatome of each nerve	Forearm and hand surgery Useful when long-acting LA in individual nerves for postop analgesia, and can be done in combination with a short-acting brachial plexus block for awake surgery	5-10ml per nerve	Each nerve can be traced with ultrasound to find the optimal position or desired block. Injecting next to the ulnar nerve in the cubital tunnel can cause compression damage. The radial nerve can be traced proximally above the elbow with US until superficial and deep branches merge for a more effective block. Dermatome distribution may be variable or overlap. Advise blocking nerve supplying the adjacent dermatome to minimise failure if selective blocks are used.

Table 9.5. Lower limb blocks.

	Nerves targeted	Area blocked	Examples of uses	Typical volumes	Notes
Lumbar plexus	Femoral, obturator and lateral cutaneous nerve of thigh	Hip, anterior and medial upper leg	Total hip replacement	20-30ml	Deep block which has been associated with a high complication rate.
Obturator	Anterior and posterior obturator nerve	Medial and posterior aspect of thigh and knee	Adjunct for knee surgery. Adductor muscle surgery	10ml	Used in conjunction with femoral and sciatic block for complete anaesthesia of the leg. Communication with the area of the femoral nerve is disproven and hence the "3 in 1" block is refuted.
Sciatic	Proximal sciatic nerve	Posterior thigh, knee and lower leg apart form saphenous distribution	Lower leg surgery. Knee surgery in combination with femoral ± obturator blocks	20ml	May be suboptimal for lower leg surgery unless the saphenous branch of the femoral nerve is blocked separately. Large nerve requires enough volume to encircle nerve and ensure all components blocked.
Popliteal	Distal sciatic nerve dividing into the common peroneal and common tibial nerves	Lower leg apart form saphenous distribution	Lower leg surgery. Knee surgery in combination with femoral ± obturator blocks	10-20ml	US use allows tracing the divisions proximally until they merge into the sciatic nerve.

Continued

Table 9.5 *continued*. Lower limb blocks.

	Nerves targeted	Area blocked	Examples of uses	Typical volumes	Notes
Ankle	Deep and superficial peroneal, saphenous, sural and tibial	Mid foot distally	Mid foot and toe surgery	~5ml per nerve	Not all five nerves require blocking depending on surgery planned. Beware of dermatome variability. Some simply consist of subcutaneous infiltration using landmark techniques.
Femoral	Femoral nerve as it passes under the inguinal ligament	Femur and anterior thigh	Femoral surgery, hip surgery excluding acetabulum	10-20ml	Divides into the anterior and posterior divisions soon after entering the upper leg. Ensure blocked as proximally as feasible.
Fascia iliaca	Iliac muscle compartment for the femoral and lateral cutaneous nerve of the thigh	Anterior and lateral thigh, femur	Fractured neck of femur surgery	30-40ml	Compartment block with generally less efficacy than femoral nerve block but fewer complication rates. Block of the lateral cutaneous nerve of the thigh is useful for dynamic hip screw procedures.
Adductor canal	Branches of femoral (including saphenous) and obturator nerves	Sensory to anterior aspect of the knee (quadriceps sparing)	Knee surgery	20-30ml	May be suboptimal as does not block sciatic component to the knee.

Table 9.6. Truncal blocks.

	Nerves targeted	Area blocked	Examples of uses	Typical volumes	Notes
Cervical plexus	Deep or superficial cervical plexus C2-4	Anterolateral neck, ante- and retro-auricular areas, skin over and just inferior to clavicle	Carotid endart-erectomy, clavicular fracture	10-15ml	US has made superficial cervical plexus block a simple procedure. Many advocate its use in simple procedures such as central line insertion for awake patients.
Paravertebral	Ventral rami of spinal nerves as they leave the vertebral canal	Hemi-thorax in dermatomes above and below level injected	Thoracotomy, breast surgery, fractured rib pain, upper abdominal surgery	20-40ml for single shot, 5-10ml per injection for multiple levels	5ml adequately blocks dermatome. 20ml reliably blocks five adjoining dermatomes (more caudal than cephalad due to gravity). Catheter techniques are directed cephalad so entry should be below the main target level. Many recipes have been described.
Intercostal	Ventral ramus of spinal nerve	Thoraco-abdominal wall of dermatome	Thoracotomy, fractured rib pain	3-5ml	Requires repeating for each level of required dermatomes to block. Simple, but still risks pneumothorax and systemic absorption of LA is high.
Transversus abdominal plane	Ventral ramus of spinal nerves while in abdominal wall	T10-L1 dermatomes by single shot	Lower abdominal surgery, bilateral blocks often required	20-30ml	May be suboptimal for incisions above the umbilicus and for visceral pain. Subcostal 'top-up' of cephalic rectus sheet blocks may be required for larger incisions.

Continued

Table 9.6 *continued*. Truncal blocks.

	Nerves targeted	Area blocked	Examples of uses	Typical volumes	Notes
Rectus sheath	Anterior cutaneous branches of spinal nerves	Paramedian abdominal wall	Midline abdominal incision	10-20ml	Variable spread, may need repeating at different levels.
Ilioinguinal/ Iliohypogastric	Ilioinguinal and Iliohypogastric nerves	Inguinal area	Inguinal hernia repair	20ml total	Requires 5ml in each anatomical layer and a fan-like field injection to ensure adequate block. A midline field block from the pubic symphysis ensures blocking any cross-innervation.
Penile	Terminal branch pudendal nerve, dorsal nerves of penis	Skin of penis	Circumcision	Children 1ml + 0.1ml/kg	Bilateral injections required (avoid midline due to artery). Used in conjunction with a subcutaneous injection around the base of the penis for greater effect.

Table 9.7. Ophthalmic blocks.

	Nerves targeted	Area blocked	Examples of uses	Typical volumes	Notes
Retrobulbar	CN — III, IV, Va, VI within muscle cone	Anaesthesia and akinesia of the globe Does not block VII for lid function (may require separate block)	Ophthalmic surgery	3-5ml	Produces comparatively superior akinesia and reduced ocular pressures but carries highest risk of injury to the globe or surrounding structures. Near the apex, these structures are packed in a very small space and are fixed by the tendon of Zinn, which prevents them from moving away from a needle.
Peribulbar	Spreads outside cone for CN — III, IV, Va, VI, also anterior spread for orbicularis	Blocks lid function but less akinesia	Ophthalmic surgery	6-8ml	Requires larger volume for spread into the cone. May require top-up injections in alternate area if block is inadequate. Superseded retrobulbar techniques due to increased safety.
Subtenon	Spreads in episcleral space blocking ciliary nerves and motor nerves to muscle sheaths	Causes ptosis and provides analgesia to the anterior compartment alongside akinesia	Ophthalmic surgery	5-6ml	Surgical approach with a curved blunt cannula may be technically difficult. There is a possibility of suboptimal akinesia but it is adequate for anterior compartment surgery. Post-block pressure may aid spread and reduce subconjunctival protrusion.

Case scenario 1

A 72-year-old man is referred to the acute pain team for pain from fractured ribs. He was admitted the previous day after falling off a ladder and sustaining fractures to his right radius, right ankle and anterior-lateral aspects of ribs 4-7 on the right side. He is a long-term smoker with moderate COPD on inhalers with a previous admission a year ago for an infective exacerbation. His current analgesia includes paracetamol and intravenous morphine patient-controlled analgesia (PCA). With this he only has mild pain at rest but severe pain in his chest on movement. He is due to go to theatre later in the day but the respiratory physiotherapist has referred him to the acute pain team as he is unable to breathe deeply or cough, is drowsy from his PCA, used to try and manage the pain, and is now requiring continuous supplemental oxygen.

What further options would be available to manage his pain?

Further options include one of the following regional techniques:

- Thoracic epidural.
- Paravertebral block.
- Serratus anterior block.

On review by the pain team he is referred to the anaesthetic team and a right-sided paravertebral block and catheter placement are performed with a local anaesthetic pump attached, which has a good effect allowing him to cough comfortably.

Pain from fractured ribs can be difficult to manage and can lead to delayed respiratory compromise 24-48 hours after. A cycle forms; reluctance to deep breathe and cough leads to atelectasis and pneumonia. Opioid analgesia tends to be ineffective as the pain is mainly on movement and side effects from opioids can worsen respiratory function further. If medical pain management is ineffective, regional techniques include a thoracic epidural, paravertebral block, intercostal blocks and now serratus anterior blocks can also be used to good effect.

An epidural has the best effect and covers bilateral fractures but carries higher risks and has more contraindications (e.g. coagulopathies, associated spinal fractures).

Case scenario 2

A 54-year-old woman is listed on the emergency list for debridement of her left foot. She is a smoker with a BMI of 52. Her past medical history includes insulin-dependent diabetes, peripheral vascular disease, lumbar disc prolapse and a previous MI 2 years ago. Her regular medications include oxycontin for her back pain. She has presented to hospital feeling unwell with necrotic 4th and 5th toes on the left side with cellulitis tracking to her mid-calf. She is being treated with IV antibiotics after she spiked a temperature with raised inflammatory markers and a white cell count. Anaesthetic pre-assessment reveals symptoms suggestive of obstructive sleep apnoea.

What would be the best anaesthetic option for this patient?

Conscious sedation with a popliteal sciatic nerve block with an adductor canal block can be used.

Patients requiring lower limb debridement or amputations are challenging due to associated comorbidities. This case is potentially at high risk of complications from a GA due to a high BMI and obstructive sleep apnoea. A spinal anaesthetic is also contraindicated, due to signs of systemic sepsis.

A good functioning popliteal sciatic nerve block can provide intra-operative anaesthesia and continue on to provide postoperative analgesia which is useful in this case due to her previous opioid use and possible tolerance.

Further reading

1. Regional Anaesthesia and Patients with Abnormalities of Coagulation. http://www.aagbi.org/sites/default/files/rapac_2013_web.pdf.

2. New York School Of Regional Anaesthesia. http://www.nysora.com.

3. Ultrasound Regional Anaesthesia, Canada. http://www.usra.ca.

4. Kettner SC, Willschke H, Marhofer P. Does regional anaesthesia really improve outcome? *Br J Anaesth* 2011; 107(1): i90-i5.

5. Neal JM. Ultrasound-guided regional anesthesia and patient safety: an evidence-based analysis. *Reg Anesth Pain Med* 2010; 35: S59-S67.

6. Curatolo M. Adding regional analgesia to general anaesthesia: increase of risk or improved outcome? *Eur J Anaesthesiol* 2010; 27: 586-91.

7. Johnson RL, Kopp SL, Burkle CM, *et al.* Neuraxial vs. general anaesthesia for total hip and total knee arthroplasty: a systematic review of comparative-effectiveness research. *Br J Anaesth* 2016; 116: 163-76.

10 Pre-operative anaesthetic assessment

Chandrashekhar Vaidyanath and Meghna Sharma

Introduction

An individual's physiological status changes over a period of time from birth until death. The human body compensates for the changes in lifestyle choices or physical disabilities during this process. If at any point a medical intervention is needed for which the individual requires either sedation or any form of anaesthetic, then understanding of compensatory mechanisms becomes essential. A pre-operative anaesthetic assessment is a systematic and essential part of preparing the anaesthetist to deal with these situations and aid in decision-making.

The aim of doing a pre-operative anaesthetic assessment is to identify and assess coexisting medical conditions and ensure that the appropriate pre-op investigations have been done. It helps to assess the risk versus benefit of undergoing both anaesthesia and surgery. It may help allay any fears and anxiety, and provide the opportunity for explanation and discussion, and also explain in detail the anaesthetic procedure and risks to the patient. It gives us the time to institute pre-operative optimisation and management. It helps the anaesthetist to choose the most appropriate type of anaesthesia for the patient, e.g. local, regional, general anaesthesia. It also identifies any special requirements for the surgical procedure, e.g. bariatric surgery. It also gives an opportunity for the patients to clarify any concerns that they have with regard to the process of anaesthesia and surgery.

ASA Physical Status grading

The American Society of Anesthesiologists' Physical Status (ASA PS) grading (Table 10.1) that has recently been updated in 2014 gives us an

Table 10.1. The ASA Physical Status grading.

ASA PS grading	Definition	Examples, including, but not limited to:
ASA I	A normal healthy patient	Healthy, non-smoking, no or minimal alcohol use.
ASA II	A patient with mild systemic disease	Mild diseases only without substantive functional limitations. Examples include (but not limited to): current smoker, social alcohol drinker, pregnancy, obesity (BMI <40), well-controlled diabetes, hypertension and mild lung disease.
ASA III	A patient with severe systemic disease	Substantive functional limitations; one or more moderate to severe diseases. Examples include (but not limited to): poorly controlled diabetes or hypertension, COPD, morbid obesity (BMI ≥40), active hepatitis, alcohol dependence or abuse, implanted pacemaker, moderate reduction of ejection fraction, end-stage renal disease undergoing regularly scheduled dialysis, history of MI (>3 months ago), CVA, TIA, or coronary artery disease/stents.
ASA IV	A patient with severe systemic disease that is a constant threat to life	Examples include (but not limited to): recent history of MI (<3 months), CVA, TIA, coronary artery disease, ongoing cardiac ischaemia, severe valve dysfunction, severe reduction of ejection fraction, sepsis, DIC, end-stage renal disease not undergoing regularly scheduled dialysis.
ASA V	A moribund patient who is not expected to survive without the operation	Examples include (but not limited to): ruptured abdominal or thoracic aortic aneurysm, massive polytrauma, intracranial bleed with mass effect, ischaemic bowel in the face of significant cardiac pathology or multiple organ/system dysfunction.
ASA VI	A declared brain-dead patient whose organs are being removed for donor purposes	

** The addition of 'E' denotes emergency surgery.

insight into the pre-operative state of the patient. It does not take into consideration the age of the patient despite the fact that neither the newborn nor the geriatric population even in the absence of any systemic disease when exposed to anesthetics respond poorly in comparison to young adults. It also has nothing to do with the type of surgery or other factors that can affect surgical outcome. Despite this, the ASA Physical Status grading is the most commonly used classification across the globe.

History taking

A system approach to history taking is a more complete and structured method of obtaining the information required in order to proceed to the next step of clinical examination.

Respiratory system

It is vital to understand if the patient is suffering from any medical condition such as asthma, COPD, obstructive sleep apnoea, cystic fibrosis, pulmonary tuberculosis or asbestosis.

This is important, as peri-operative pulmonary complications are higher in patients with existing disease, especially following prolonged surgeries lasting more than 4 hours or if they are graded ASA III and above.

Cardiovascular system

If patients have a history of coronary artery disease, then symptoms of angina, exertional dyspnoea, orthopnoea and paroxysmal nocturnal dyspnoea need to be addressed. Based on the New York Heart Association (NYHA) classification, they need to be graded (see Chapter 25 for more details). We also need to know if there is a presence of congenital heart disease, heart failure, hypertension and valvular heart disease.

The incidence of peri-operative arrhythmias and myocardial ischaemic events are higher in this cohort and, hence, pre-optimisation is essential following specific cardiac investigations.

Gastrointestinal system

It is important to find out if patients suffer from gastro-oesophageal reflux disease, as the incidence of aspiration pneumonitis is higher in this population. Associated factors such as obesity or diabetes make patients more prone to gastro-oesophageal reflux disease.

Genitourinary system

Patients with renal failure need to be asked about dialysis, existing arteriovenous fistulas and associated medical conditions. It is vital to know the background because an electrolyte imbalance is most common in this group of patients.

Endocrine system

Patients with a history of diabetes need to be identified, as control of blood glucose prior to surgical intervention is known to improve post-surgical outcome. Other endocrine diseases such as Cushing's disease or thyroid disorders need to be treated accordingly in the pre-operative period.

Central nervous system

If patients mention episodes of headache, vomiting and double vision, they need to be investigated soon. One should also ask for a history of transient ischaemic attacks (TIAs), amaurosis fugax, facial drops or slurred speech. Constant episodes of migraine or visual disturbances should not be ignored.

Otorhinolaryngeal system

In patients with a history of dysphagia or hoarseness of voice, it is important to elicit more information because special equipment may be required for airway management in this group of patients. In patients for middle ear surgery, the use of nitrous oxide should be avoided.

Musculoskeletal system

Obese patients are an anaesthetic challenge as they have associated medical conditions such as obstructive sleep apnoea, high blood pressure and diabetes that need to be controlled before anaesthesia and surgical intervention. We also need to find out about conditions such as myasthenia gravis, myotonic dystrophy and Lambert-Eaton syndrome if they complain of tiredness or drooping eyelids. Maxillofacial abnormalities could be difficult for airway management.

Anticoagulants

Advances in medicine have led to the introduction of anticoagulants, the complexity of which need to be understood. Patients could be on warfarin if they have mechanical heart valves, or for conditions such as atrial fibrillation, pulmonary embolus or a previous history of deep vein thrombosis. Bridging therapy is essential in high-risk patients. The cases of patients with coronary artery disease on dual antiplatelet therapy need to be discussed with multidisciplinary teams including a cardiologist and haematologist prior to operative interventions. Regional anaesthesia is a highly debatable topic, especially for patients on anticoagulants; hence, the choice of anaesthetic needs to be considered based on the risk versus benefit on an individual case basis taking advice from guidelines.

Family history and previous anaesthetic experience

We should take a family history in order to identify conditions such as porphyria, malignant hyperthermia and haemophilia. Also, it is vital to find out if the patient has experienced any previous anaesthetic difficulties and complications, or a presence of drug allergies and sensitivities. We should also ask about a previous history of postoperative nausea and vomiting (PONV), deep vein thrombosis and pulmonary embolus.

Social history

A history of alcohol consumption is essential since regular alcohol intake leads to the induction of liver enzymes and tolerance to anaesthetic drugs. Excessive alcohol intake causes both hepatic and cardiac damage. Delirium tremens may occur in alcoholics during the postoperative recovery phase as a result of alcohol withdrawal.

A history of smoking is associated with five to six times more postoperative complications. It is associated with vascular diseases, ischaemic heart disease, COPD and lung cancer. The half-life of carbon monoxide is short and so abstinence from smoking even for 12 hours leads to an increased arterial oxygen content.

It is also essential to find out if patients suffer from existing infectious diseases such as HIV, Hepatitis B and C or methicillin-resistant *Staphylococcus aureus* (MRSA). Universal precautions will need to be adhered to in the presence of these conditions.

Lastly, pregnancy should be ruled out in female patients, as in early pregnancy anaesthetic drugs are theoretically teratogenic. Also, general anaesthesia may induce abortion and hence it is best avoided in the first and third trimester.

In an emergency setting it may not be possible to elicit as much history, but still any available information should be noted.

Clinical examination

Examination of the airway is very important as it helps in planning the airway management strategy to avoid any potential difficulties that may be faced following an anaesthetic induction. It includes grading the airway based on Mallampati scoring, identification of the thyromental and sternomental distance, and the inter-incisor gap, as well as identification of flexion deformities of the cervical spine and the presence of loose teeth or dentures (see Chapter 20 for more details).

Physical examination of the cardiorespiratory system is equally important, especially in the paediatric and geriatric population. It is not advisable to go ahead with administration of a general anaesthetic in the presence of audible wheeze or bronchial breath sounds. In the event of audible murmurs, such as undiagnosed valvular heart disease, it is wise to postpone the procedure and investigate.

Laboratory investigations

The National Institute for Health and Care Excellence (NICE) guidance (NG45), published in April 2016, covers routine pre-operative tests for people aged over 16 who are having elective surgery. It aims to reduce unnecessary testing by advising which tests to offer people before minor, intermediate and major or complex surgery (Tables 10.2, 10.3 and 10.4), taking into account specific comorbidities (cardiovascular, renal, respiratory conditions, diabetes and obesity).

Table 10.2. Laboratory investigations to conduct before minor surgery.

Test	ASA 1	ASA 2	ASA 3 or ASA 4
Full blood count	Not routinely	Not routinely	Not routinely
Haemostasis	Not routinely	Not routinely	Not routinely
Kidney function	Not routinely	Not routinely	Consider in people at risk of AKI
ECG	Not routinely	Not routinely	Consider if no ECG results available from the past 12 months
Lung function tests/ arterial blood gas	Not routinely	Not routinely	Not routinely

AKI = acute kidney injury.

Table 10.3. Laboratory investigations to conduct before intermediate surgery.

Test	ASA 1	ASA 2	ASA 3 or ASA 4
Full blood count	Not routinely	Not routinely	Consider for people with cardiac or renal disease if any symptoms not recently investigated.
Haemostasis	Not routinely	Not routinely	Consider in people with chronic liver disease. If people taking anticoagulants need modification of their treatment regimen; make an individualised plan in line with local guidance. If clotting status needs to be tested before surgery (depending on local guidance), use point-of-care testing.
Kidney function	Not routinely	Consider in people at risk of AKI	Yes
ECG	Not routinely	Consider for people with cardiac, renal disease or diabetes	Yes
Lung function tests /arterial blood gas	Not routinely	Not routinely	Consider seeking advice from a senior anaesthetist as soon as possible after assessment for people who are ASA Grade 3 or 4 due to known or suspected respiratory disease.

AKI = acute kidney injury.

Table 10.4. Laboratory investigations to conduct before major or complex surgery.

Test	ASA 1	ASA 2	ASA 3 or ASA 4
Full blood count	Yes	Yes	Yes
Haemostasis	Not routinely	Not routinely	Consider in people with chronic liver disease. If people taking anticoagulants need modification of their treatment regimen, make an individualised plan in line with local guidance. If clotting status needs to be tested before surgery (depending on local guidance), use point-of-care testing.
Kidney function	Consider in people at risk of AKI	Yes	Yes
ECG	Consider for people aged over 65 if no ECG results are available from the past 12 months	Yes	Yes
Lung function tests /arterial blood gas	Not routinely	Not routinely	Consider seeking advice from a senior anaesthetist as soon as possible after assessment for people who are ASA Grade 3 or 4 due to known or suspected respiratory disease.

AKI = acute kidney injury.

Specialist investigations

Based on the system involved, specialist investigations need to be carried out if there is any doubt regarding the patient's physiological ability to tolerate the surgical procedure based on information available from the history and clinical examination. The following is a list that may be required.

Respiratory system

- Flow volume loops.
- Cardiopulmonary exercise testing (CPET).
- Ventilation-perfusion scan.
- Bronchoscopy.
- CT/MRI scan.

Cardiovascular system

- Echocardiogram.
- CPET.
- Myocardial perfusion scans.
- Electrophysiological studies.
- B-type natriuretic peptide.

Endocrine system

- HbA1c for diabetics.
- Thyroid function tests.
- Tests for pheochromocytoma, etc.

Central nervous system

- Carotid Doppler ultrasound.
- CT/MRI scan.

Otorhinolaryngeal system

- Nasoendoscopy.
- CT/MRI scan.
- Musculoskeletal system.
- Cholinesterase levels.

Miscellaneous

- Sickle cell test for all patients of African descent.
- Pregnancy test for all females of childbearing age.

Risk stratification for surgery

Pre-operative assessment helps to identify potential anaesthetic difficulties, existing medical conditions and tries to improve safety by assessing and quantifying risks. Thus, risk stratification before surgery helps in planning for the peri-operative care of the surgical patient.

There are various methods and risk index systems that have been developed. These include the Goldman Multifactorial Cardiac Risk Index, Eagle's Cardiac Risk Index, Detsky's Cardiac Risk Index, Lee's Revised Cardiac Risk Index and the American College of Cardiology (ACC) and the American Heart Association (AHA) Cardiac Risk Stratification for Non-Cardiac Surgery. The latter two are the most commonly used.

Lee's Revised Cardiac Risk Index

This estimates the risk of cardiac complications after non-cardiac surgery. The factors included in determining the risk are:

- High-risk surgery (intrathoracic, intra-abdominal or suprainguinal vascular).
- History of ischaemic heart disease (defined as a history of MI, pathologic Q waves on an ECG, use of nitrates, abnormal stress test or chest pain secondary to ischaemic causes).

- History of congestive heart failure.
- History of cerebrovascular disease.
- Pre-operative treatment with insulin.
- Pre-operative creatinine >2mg/dL (176.8μmol/L).

Each of the six risk factors is assigned one point. Patients with none, one, or two risk factor(s) are assigned to RCRI (Revised Cardiac Risk Index) Classes I, II and III, respectively, and patients with three or more risk factors are considered Class IV.

The risk associated with each class is 0.4%, 1%, 7% and 11% for patients in Classes I, II, III and IV, respectively.

ACC/AHA Cardiac Risk Stratification for Non-cardiac Surgical Procedures

The ACC and AHA have jointly classified surgeries into various categories of risk such as high risk, intermediate risk and low risk.

High risk (reported cardiac risk often >5%)

- Emergent major operations, particularly in older patients.
- Aortic and other major vascular surgeries.
- Peripheral vascular surgery.
- Anticipated prolonged surgical procedures associated with large fluid shifts, blood loss, or both.

Intermediate risk (reported cardiac risk >1% but <5%)

- Carotid endarterectomy.
- Head and neck surgery.
- Intraperitoneal and intrathoracic surgery.
- Orthopaedic surgery.
- Prostate surgery.

Low risk (reported cardiac risk generally <1%)

- Endoscopic procedures.

- Superficial procedure.
- Cataract surgery.
- Breast surgery.

Surgical Outcome Risk Tool (www.sortsurgery.com)

More recently in practice, the Surgical Outcome Risk Tool (SORT) is a pre-operative risk prediction tool for death within 30 days of surgery. It has been developed and validated for use in inpatient non-neurological, non-cardiac surgery in adults (aged 16 or over).

It divides the operative procedure based on system and subgroups. The severity of the procedure is determined. It also takes into consideration the ASA physical status as well as the NCEPOD (National Confidential Enquiry into Patient Outcome and Death) urgent nature of the operation. Further to this, it also factors in age, the presence of cancer and type of surgery, in particular thoracic, gastrointestinal or vascular.

Pre-operative fasting

Adults

Pre-operative fasting in adults undergoing elective surgery is outlined below:

- '2' — intake of water up to 2 hours before induction of anaesthesia.
- '6' — a minimum pre-operative fasting time of 6 hours for food (solids, milk and milk-containing drinks).

The anaesthetic team should consider further interventions for patients at higher risk of regurgitation and aspiration.

Postoperatively, patients should be encouraged to drink when ready, providing there are no contraindications.

Children

Pre-operative fasting in children undergoing elective surgery is outlined below:

- '2' — intake of water and other clear fluids up to 2 hours before induction of anaesthesia.
- '4' — breast milk up to 4 hours before.
- '6' — formula milk, cow's milk or solids up to 6 hours before.

Postoperatively, oral fluids can be offered to healthy children when they are fully awake following anaesthesia, providing there are no contraindications. There is no requirement to drink as part of the discharge criteria.

Chewing gum

Chewing gum may be allowed up to 2 hours before induction of anaesthesia.

Case scenario 1

A 75-year-old female patient with a history of atrial fibrillation, hypertension and gastro-oesophageal reflux is scheduled for a total hip replacement surgery. She has been on warfarin for her atrial fibrillation. She has agreed to have a spinal anaesthetic.

What investigations would you like her to have?

Based on NICE guidance, for intermediate-risk surgery in a ASA 3 patient who is on anticoagulants, this patient should have a full blood count, coagulation profile, renal function tests and an ECG.

How would you risk stratify this patient?

Based on Lee's Revised Cardiac Risk Index, this patient would be in RCRI Class I, but based on the ACC/AHA classification, as she is having an orthopaedic operation, she is having an intermediate-risk surgery with a reported cardiac risk of >1% but <5%.

What is the chance of her death in the first 30 days after the operation?

Based on the Surgical Outcome Risk Tool calculation, it is 0.56%. We need to note that this is only a pre-operative tool. There may be lots of confounding factors that may increase this, based on intra-operative and postoperative care.

The procedure is planned under spinal anaesthetic. Would you still want her to be fasted as per the AAGBI guidance?

Yes, it is better to prepare the patient as per the AAGBI fasting guidance, because in the event of a regional anaesthesia failure, at least the option of administering a general anaesthetic can be offered to the patient.

Further reading

1. Minto G, Biccard B. Assessment of the high-risk perioperative patient. *Br J Anaesthesia CEACCP* 2014; 14: 12-7.

2. Fleisher LA, Fleischmann KE, Auerbach AD. 2014 ACC/AHA Guideline on perioperative cardiovascular evaluation and management of patients undergoing noncardiac surgery. A report of the American College of Cardiology/American Heart Association Task Force on Practice Guidelines. http://content.onlinejacc.org/article.aspx?articleid=1893784.

3. The National Institute for Health and Care Excellence. Routine preoperative tests for elective surgery. NICE guidance, NG45. London, UK: NICE, 2016. https://www.nice.org.uk/guidance/ng45.

4. Surgical Outcome Research Centre (SOuRCe). A source of expert advice on risk adjustment and outcomes analysis for the surgical specialities. www.sortsurgery.com.

5. The Association of Anaesthetists of Great Britain and Ireland. AAGBI safety guideline of preoperative assessment and patient preparation the role of an anaesthetist, January 2010. https://www.aagbi.org/sites/default/files/preop2010.pdf.

Peri-operative pharmacology

Mark Pais

Introduction

Stopping and restarting medications in the peri-operative period is an essential component to peri-operative care. Appropriate management helps to maintain stability of chronic conditions, prevent medication withdrawal and avoid interactions with anaesthetic agents. The principles of peri-operative pharmacology are:

- Medications with significant withdrawal potential that do not affect anaesthesia should be continued in the peri-operative period.
- Medications that increase surgical risk and are not essential to the prognosis of the chronic condition should be withdrawn.
- If a medication does not meet these two concerns, clinical judgement on the part of the physician should be used based upon the stability of the condition and the surgical/anaesthetic risk.

Respiratory pharmacology

Patients suffering from respiratory conditions have a greater than normal risk of postoperative respiratory compromise due to the effects of pain, surgery, general anaesthesia, bronchospasm and peri-operative drugs. It is important to optimise these conditions prior to surgery by controlling chronic disease and addressing any acute deterioration.

Inhaled beta-agonists and anticholinergic drugs

Bronchodilators relax bronchial smooth muscle and have a maximal effect by 30 minutes with a duration of action that lasts up to 4-6 hours. Inhaled beta-agonists (e.g. salbutamol, salmeterol) and anticholinergics (e.g. ipratropium and tiotropium) have been found to reduce the risk of postoperative respiratory complications in patients with asthma and chronic obstructive pulmonary disease (COPD). They should be continued in the peri-operative period, including the day of surgery and immediately postoperatively. They can be administered via a metered dose inhaler, nebulised or, in the case of beta-agonists, intravenously. Caution should be exercised with beta-agonists as cardiac side effects (increase in heart rate, reduction in serum potassium) may be significant for patients with cardiac comorbidities.

Steroids

Steroids are used for preventing and reducing pulmonary inflammation. Most steroids are administered via the inhaled route (e.g. beclomethasone, fluticasone) that limits their side effect profile. Oral steroids, however, are usually used in acute deterioration, where their optimal effect can take up to 6 hours. Adrenal suppression, hyperglycaemia, infection, delayed healing, electrolyte abnormalities and fluid retention are common complications of long-term treatment. Steroids, both inhaled and systemic, should be continued in the peri-operative period. Patients who have been taking systemic corticosteroids for >2 weeks during the prior 6 months should be considered at risk for adrenal suppression in the setting of severe acute disease, trauma or major surgery and may need steroid supplementation (Table 11.1).

Theophylline

Theophylline inhibits phosphodiesterase and increases the level of cyclic adenosine monophosphate (cAMP) in bronchial smooth muscles resulting in bronchodilation. There is no evidence that continuing theophylline in the peri-operative period reduces pulmonary complications. Furthermore, it has a narrow therapeutic index with the potential to cause cardiac arrhythmias and neurotoxicity.

Table 11.1. Steroid dose supplementation.

<10mg/day	Normal hypothalamic pituitary adrenal axis	No additional steroids
>10mg/day	Minor surgery	Add hydrocortisone 25mg IV at induction
	Intermediate surgery	Add hydrocortisone 25mg IV at induction and 6-hourly for 24 hours
	Major surgery	Add hydrocortisone 25mg IV then 6-hourly for 48-72 hours
Stopped taking steroids	>3 months	No additional steroids
	<3 months	Treat as if on steroids

Leukotriene inhibitors

These agents (montelukast, zafirlukast) inhibit the leukotriene pathway, a mediator for bronchoconstriction. They are not useful in the acute treatment of bronchospasm and are second-line after steroids in the management of asthma. They can be stopped safely prior to surgery as their effect on asthma symptoms and pulmonary function persists 3 weeks after stopping treatment.

Endocrine pharmacology

Glucocorticoids

Steroids should be continued in the peri-operative period; however, whether it is necessary to supplement the dose depends on the usual dose of steroids, the duration of therapy and the extent of the surgery. Adrenal suppression, hyperglycaemia, infection, delayed healing, electrolyte abnormalities and fluid retention are common complications of long-term treatment. It is possible that if the dose is not supplemented there will be an impaired stress response to surgery due to hypothalamic pituitary adrenal axis (HPA axis) suppression from long-term steroids manifesting as an Addisonian crisis (hypotension/hyponatraemia/hyperkalaemia and hypoglycaemia).

In general, patients who have taken steroids for less than 3 weeks are unlikely to have a suppressed HPA axis and no supplementation is required. Patients taking prednisolone at a dose greater than 10mg/day for 3 months or more should receive increased doses pre-operatively and postoperatively.

For postoperative steroids an intravenous infusion is useful as it avoids swings in the plasma steroid levels.

Hypoglycaemic drugs

Diabetes can be managed by diet control, tablets or insulin therapy. While insulin stimulates the body to take up and store glucose, oral hypoglycaemic drug actions can broadly be defined as:

- Increasing the cell's sensitivity to absorb glucose (e.g. pioglitazone, rosiglitazone, metformin).
- Increasing the secretion of endogenous insulin (e.g. gliclazide, glibenclamide).
- Reducing absorption of glucose from the gut (e.g. acarbose).

The aim in peri-operative management is to maintain normoglycaemia and minimise lipolysis and proteolysis by the provision of exogenous glucose and insulin. It has been recommended that blood glucose levels of between 6-10mmol/L strike this balance well. All patients on regular insulin should be managed with a variable rate intravenous insulin infusion (VRIII) regimen with supplementary potassium/fluids (typically 0.9% saline, 5% glucose and 0.3 or 0.15% potassium). The infusion is started as soon as possible after admission on the morning of surgery and is continued for at least 1 hour after the first meal. It can then be stopped and replaced with a SC QDS regime before meals and sleep.

Type 2 diabetics on oral hypoglycaemic drugs should have these omitted on the day of surgery. Exceptions to this include metformin and glitazones, which can be continued as they increase the body's sensitivity to insulin during the surgical stress response. For type 2 diabetics a VRIII should be started in those with poor diabetic control (>10mmol/L) and those undergoing major surgery to contend with the large insulin requirements. The glucose/insulin infusion should be administered though the same cannula to avoid giving insulin without glucose and should be regulated with volumetric pumps with antireflux/siphon valves. Blood glucose measurement should be performed hourly and the rate of insulin should be adjusted according to local policy.

Thyroid medication

The mainstay of treatment for thyroid disorders includes drugs that reduce the level of thyroid hormones (e.g. carbimazole, propylthiouracil and iodine) in hyperthyroidism and increase levels (e.g. thyroxine) in hypothyroidism. Beta-blockers can supplement carbimazole in improving symptoms and reducing the heart rate in hyperthyroidism but do not affect hormone production or reduce the risk of a thyroid storm. Prior to theatre the patient should be euthyroid, as failure to achieve a normal hormonal balance can lead to over-administration of anaesthetic agents as well as a potential high risk of cardiovascular complications.

For patients with hypothyroidism they should take thyroxine in the peri-operative period and postoperatively, as soon they are able to drink. One can withhold this medication safely for as long as a week because of its long half-life. In patients with severe hypothyroidism or those that need rapid preparation for theatre, L-thyroxine can be given intravenously.

In hyperthyroidism, patients should receive their antithyroid drug with propranolol on the day of surgery. They should resume the drug postoperatively within 24 hours after surgery. It should be noted that carbimazole and propylthiouracil can take up to 4 months to render a patient euthyroid. In the case of emergency surgery, a euthyroid state can be achieved with a combination of beta-blockers, steroids and iodine.

Oral contraception/hormonal therapy

Patients taking an oral contraceptive pill (OCP) have an increased risk of postoperative venous thromboembolism (VTE) because of the combined effects of hormones and the hypercoagulable state, which accompanies surgery and postoperative immobility. The risk of thrombosis increases within 4 months of starting and decreases to previous levels after 4 months of stopping treatment.

The recommendation by the BNF is that for those at high risk of VTE, they should switch to alternative contraception, 4-6 weeks prior to surgery and then restart at 2 weeks after regaining full mobility. During this period, it would be sensible to exclude pregnancy before the operation.

Hormone replacement therapy (HRT) may increase the risk of postoperative VTE despite having a lower oestrogen content. The risks of discontinuing HRT are minimal but the discomfort of postmenopausal symptoms might be unacceptable to the patient. Treatment should be stopped 4-6 weeks prior to surgery and can be resumed when the risk of VTE has diminished.

If the OCP/HRT is continued, adequate thromboprophylaxis is required.

Pain pharmacology

Multimodal analgesia

Many drugs have been used as part of multimodal analgesia with the aim of improving pain management and decreasing opioid consumption and side effects. Of these, the benefits of paracetamol and non-steroidal anti-inflammatory agents have been well documented.

Poorly controlled pain at the time of surgery predisposes to chronic post-surgical pain. Because of this, drugs used for chronic neuropathic pain are now finding a place in the peri-operative period. Only ketamine and the gabapentinoids (pregabalin and gabapentin) have firm evidence for peri-operative use. Ketamine has been shown to be a useful adjuvant in patient-controlled analgesia (PCA) and is useful for painful procedures, e.g. abdominal, thoracic and orthopaedic operations. For those patients on high-dose opioid therapy, ketamine can reduce opioid consumption in the peri-operative and postoperative period. Drawbacks to ketamine relate to its side effect profile, which include feelings of dissociation and delirium, nausea and an increased sympathetic drive.

Peri-operative gabapentin and pregabalin are useful in procedures causing acute neuropathic pain requiring high opioid doses (e.g. cardiothoracic surgery, arthroplasty). Both also have a useful analgesic effect that prevents post-op pain but are no better than other analgesics in established neuropathic pain.

Chronic opioid medication

It is essential to continue chronic pain medications in the peri-operative period, as evidence suggests that it attenuates the stress response to surgery, reduces postoperative pain and avoids precipitating a post-op withdrawal syndrome of a hyperadrenergic state and hyperalgesia. Patients taking long-term opioids for management of chronic pain need to continue these agents up till the time of surgery. If unable to take the oral dose of morphine postoperatively, a continuous IV morphine infusion should be set up which corresponds with the patient's regular 24-hour opioid requirements. Breakthrough pain can be managed with a PCA or boluses of IV morphine.

For patients on methadone for drug dependency, this can be continued immediately postoperatively and PCA/IV rescue boluses to cover additional opioid needs. All patients on chronic opioid therapy should receive opioid-sparing analgesics (paracetamol, NSAIDs) to reduce their opioid requirement in the immediate postoperative period. The regime should be tailored to the patient's pain requirements and advice from a pain physician should be sought to guide therapy.

Cardiac pharmacology

Common conditions encountered in the peri-operative setting include ischaemic heart disease, hypertension, congestive cardiac failure and arrhythmias. In general, it is important to avoid acute changes in chronic medications peri-operatively, as these can lead to decompensation of the disease.

Beta-blockers

Beta-blockers are primarily used to reduce ischaemia by decreasing oxygen demand due to catecholamine release and for managing arrhythmias. Other common uses include therapy for hypertension, migraines and anxiety. Patients who chronically take beta-blockers should continue taking them pre-operatively as abrupt cessation can lead to withdrawal resulting in cardiac ischaemia.

There is controversy regarding whether to start beta-blockers in the peri-operative period. Mangano *et al* showed that for patients who are at high risk for coronary artery disease and undergo non-cardiac surgery, treatment with atenolol during hospitalisation could reduce mortality and the incidence of cardiac complications for at least 2 years after the surgery. However, the POISE trial cast doubt upon these benefits having shown increased mortality with peri-operative beta-blockers from strokes, bradycardia and hypotension. It did, however, find a reduction in the incidence of fatal and non-fatal myocardial infarction.

Current guidance states that for high-risk surgery, peri-operative beta-blockade may be useful, providing the benefits outweigh the risks (e.g. the patient does not have an underlying stroke). Suitable patients should be commenced on treatment a month prior to surgery and cardioselective, long-acting agents (e.g. atenolol) could be used to avoid rebound effects if treatment is interrupted.

Calcium channel blockers

These medications are safe to continue in the peri-operative period and do not cause withdrawal symptoms if stopped abruptly. One meta-analysis has shown that calcium channel blockers are associated with reduced ischaemia and arrhythmias undergoing non-cardiac surgery.

Diuretics

Diuretics are usually administered for the treatment of hypertension and heart failure. In general, diuretics should be withheld on the day of surgery because of the potential adverse effects of diuretic-induced volume depletion, potassium derangement, and interactions with anaesthetic agents. If a rapid diuresis is required intra-operatively, IV frusemide can be used reliably. The diuretics can be resumed in the postoperative period once the patient is able to drink sips. In patients receiving diuretics for heart failure, volume status should ideally be optimised pre-operatively.

ACE inhibitors/angiotensin-2 receptor blockers

These drugs (e.g. ramipril, captopril, losartan) are renin-angiotensin modifiers and are used in hypertension, ischaemic heart disease, congestive cardiac failure and renal protection in diabetics.

Continuing these drugs in the peri-operative period can lead to profound intra-operative hypotension especially in the presence of a regional blockade or large fluid shifts. The benefits of continuing ACE inhibitors peri-operatively are conflicting as they do not confer any immediate protective effects against surgery; however, interrupting this drug can lead to worsening of congestive heart failure and hypertension. Therefore, it would be sensible to consider continuing ACE inhibitors in congestive cardiac failure and if it is the sole drug used to control hypertension.

Statins

Evidence has been emerging that statins may prevent vascular events through mechanisms other than lowering cholesterol. These pleiotropic effects include plaque stabilisation and endothelial stabilisation. The Decrease III trial found a statistically significant reduction in MI and cardiac death in high-risk surgery (e.g vascular surgery) compared with placebo. However, the Decrease IV trial could not find a statistically significant reduction in mortality for patients undergoing intermediate-low-risk non-cardiac surgery. Furthermore, the evidence suggests a benefit of peri-operative statin therapy in patients at increased peri-operative cardiac risk. Therefore, any patient on statins should continue these in the peri-operative period. The clinician should also consider starting statins for those at high peri-operative cardiac risk starting at least 1 week prior to surgery.

Psychotropic pharmacology

Management of patients taking psychotropic drugs is influenced by the class of drug, their interaction with other agents and the severity of the psychiatric condition. Decisions to stop these medications should take into account the psychiatric and physiological consequences of withdrawal. Furthermore, many agents do not have parenteral alternatives for patients whom the oral route is unavailable, so other drugs from different classes may be needed to maintain mood and behaviour.

Antidepressants

These can be classified into tricyclic antidepressants (TCAs), selective serotonin reuptake inhibitors (SSRIs) and monoamine oxidase inhibitors (MAOIs).

TCAs are used in the treatment of depression and chronic pain. Common examples include amitriptyline, nortriptyline, and dosulepin. They exert their effects by inhibiting presynaptic uptake of serotonin and noradrenaline but also have antimuscarinic, antihistaminergic and anti-adrenergic effects. Important side effects include prolongation of the cardiac QTc interval, a reduction in the seizure threshold and sedation. They can be potentiated by indirect sympathomimetic agents (e.g. ephedrine and metaraminol) and can lead to seizures if co-prescribed with tramadol. Abrupt withdrawal should be avoided as this can precipitate cholinergic symptoms (sweating, anxiety, nausea) and can lead to a relapse of the condition.

SSRIs are the most common drug used for depression and work by inhibiting pre-synaptic serotonin reuptake. Side effects include multiple drug interactions and an increased risk of bleeding due to its interference with platelet aggregation. Tramadol in particular should be avoided for fear of precipitating a serotonin syndrome (hyperreflexia, seizures, hyperthermia and agitation). Stopping SSRIs can also lead to withdrawal symptoms and difficulty in reinstituting the drug in the post-op period. On balance, SSRIs should be continued in the peri-operative period but may be discontinued where the risks of bleeding can lead to morbidity or in patients on antiplatelet therapy undergoing surgery.

MAOIs are rarely used and are only prescribed for patients with refractory mood disorders. They work by either irreversibly (e.g phenelzine) or reversibly (e.g. moclobemide) blocking the enzyme monoamine oxidase, which is responsible for breaking down amine neurotransmitters (e.g. serotonin, noradrenaline).

For patients taking MAOIs, coadministration of indirect sympathomimetics, such as ephedrine or metaraminol, can cause a massive release of stored noradrenaline causing a hypertensive crisis. Furthermore, administration of anticholinergic drugs can lead to serotonin syndrome. It is recommended that discontinuation of MAOI requires close collaboration with a psychiatrist and if done should be stopped 2 weeks before elective surgery and an alternative antidepressant regime put in its place.

Mood stabilisers

Lithium is used in the treatment of mania, bipolar disorders and in refractory depression. It is believed to mimic sodium and causes a reduction of neurotransmitters in the central nervous system.

Lithium has a number of physiological effects that may be important peri-operatively. It has a narrow therapeutic index, which is highly dependent on renal clearance. It is subject to a number of drug interactions with NSAIDs, ACE inhibitors, serotonergic drugs (tramadol, methylene blue) and can prolong the effects of neuromuscular blockers. It is usually recommended to omit lithium 24 hours prior to surgery. If, however, a decision to continue lithium is made, attention should be paid to checking electrolyte abnormalities and thyroid status. Plasma lithium levels should also be measured pre-operatively.

Antipsychotics

Antipsychotics are conventionally classed as being typical or atypical. Typical antipsychotics include prochlorperazine and chlorpromazine. In addition to blocking dopamine receptors, these drugs also block histamine, adrenergic, and cholinergic receptors. As a result of the large number of receptors blocked, these drugs have a large side effect profile.

Atypical antipsychotics include drugs such as quetiapine and risperidone. These drugs, however, have a significantly lower propensity to produce side effects and are thus better tolerated. As a result, atypical antipsychotics have become the first-line drugs in the treatment of schizophrenia.

Important side effects again include the neuroleptic malignant syndrome and postural hypotension. Importantly, these patients have a high relapse rate when their medication is discontinued and ideally should be continued in the peri-operative period

Antithrombotic pharmacology

Uses for anticoagulation include prophylaxis against thrombosis (e.g. in prosthetic heart valves, arrhythmias, stent insertion, patients with high-risk factors for clots) and treatment of established thrombosis (e.g. pulmonary embolism, ischaemic and cerebral vascular disease).

Common types of anticoagulation include antiplatelet agents, warfarin and heparin. With all antithrombotics, a balance must be struck whereby the coagulation system must be functional enough to minimise surgical blood loss but at the same time be able to prevent excessive clot formation.

Antiplatelet agents

The main antiplatelet agents used are salicylates (e.g. aspirin), thienopyridines (e.g. clopidogrel) and glycoprotein IIb/IIIa inhibitors (e.g. tirofiban, abciximab).

The antiplatelet activity of aspirin relates to its ability to irreversibly block the activity of the COX-1 enzyme on the platelet. Inhibiting COX-1 reduces platelet aggregation and vasoconstriction. Platelet function will return to normal after 7-10 days, whereby new platelet stores are replenished. Aspirin is used alone as monotherapy (e.g. cerebrovascular accidents/stable angina ischaemic heart disease) or as dual antiplatelet therapy with a thienopyridine (e.g. post-stent insertion/after a recent acute coronary syndrome).

Thienopyridines reduce platelet aggregation by irreversibly binding to the P2Y ADP receptor on the platelet. Like aspirin, platelet function will return to normal after 7-10 days and can only be overcome with a platelet transfusion before this time. Clopidogrel has a more potent antiplatelet activity than aspirin and is associated with a greater incidence of peri-operative bleeding.

GP IIb/IIIa receptor antagonists are used primarily in the management of acute coronary syndrome (ACS) and percutaneous coronary intervention (PCI). They act to block the final common pathway of platelet activation. In contrast to salicylates and thienopyridines, they offer reversible platelet inhibition in a dose-dependent manner. Tirofiban and eptifibatide are the shortest-acting of these agents, with half-lives of around 2-5 hours. Both are cleared by the kidney unchanged, with normal platelet function usually returning within 6-8 hours of stopping an infusion.

It is recommended to continue aspirin pre-operatively as cardiovascular risk is increased by its removal. The only exceptions are when bleeding can be catastrophic or heavy (e.g. intracranial surgery/vitreous surgery/radical prostatectomy and hip surgery). Aspirin does not contraindicate regional anaesthesia. Clopidogrel should be stopped 7 days prior to most surgery unless the risk of bleeding is low. Regional anaesthesia is contraindicated if the patient has been on clopidogrel within 7 days due to the possibility of neuraxial haematoma.

Dual antiplatelet therapy (DAPT) is used to reduce the risk of stent thrombosis and for additional cover after an acute coronary syndrome. Those with stents represent a high-risk group, whereby the risk of thrombosis is related to the type of stent inserted. For bare metal stents, a minimum of 6 weeks is recommended before clopidogrel can be omitted. However, for patients with drug-eluting stents, this period is extended to 12 months due to the inhibition of re-endothelialisation of the vessel from the antiproliferative drugs within the stent.

If surgery cannot be delayed beyond a stent's high-risk period, a balance must be struck between thromboprophylaxis and surgical bleeding. In situations of catastrophic haemorrhage requiring emergency surgery, only a platelet transfusion will reverse the actions of aspirin and clopidogrel.

In general, if there is a low risk of operative bleeding, DAPT can be continued. If there is a moderate risk of operative bleeding, one should maintain DAPT where possible unless the bleeding risk outweighs the risk of thrombosis, whereby clopidogrel should be stopped. If there is a high risk of bleeding, stop clopidogrel and maintain aspirin. If surgery involves the intracranial/posterior compartment of the eye (where bleeding would be catastrophic), both antiplatelet agents should be stopped.

Note that in situations where the risk of thrombosis is high and clopidogrel is stopped, bridging therapy with GP IIb/IIIa inhibitors can be used prior to surgery as they are reversible and short-acting. Clopidogrel can be restarted when the bleeding risk has subsided. Most of these cases require consultation with a cardiologist prior to omitting treatment.

Warfarin

Warfarin is an anticoagulant whose effect cannot be controlled easily. It takes 3-4 days to clear and is only available as an oral preparation. Warfarin acts by inhibiting vitamin K synthesis and thereby limiting the coagulation factors that are dependent on vitamin K (II, VII, IX, X and proteins C and S).

The anticoagulant effects can best be measured using the prothrombin time (PT), a measure of the extrinsic coagulation pathway. This is usually documented as the International Normalised Ratio (INR), a ratio of the patient's PT over the control for the normal population. Warfarin is indicated for the prevention of intravascular thrombosis in patients with a history of deep vein thrombosis (DVT), pulmonary embolism (PE), prosthetic heart valves or patients with chronic atrial fibrillation. The recommendations by the British Society for Haematology suggest an INR of 2.0-2.5 for DVT prophylaxis; an INR of 2.5-3.0 for patients with a history of PE, atrial fibrillation, cardioversion, dilated cardiomyopathy, mural thrombus and rheumatic mitral valve disease; an INR of 3.5 for recurrent deep vein thrombosis and PE, and patients with mechanical heart valves.

Unfortunately, most surgery cannot take place within these INR ranges and can only be performed when the INR is <1.5. Only minor surgery can take place with an INR of <2. Therefore, once a decision has been made to stop warfarin, an alternative anticoagulant would be required.

General guidance for patients on warfarin requiring surgery is as follows:

- Evaluate the extent of surgery:
  - minor surgery: ensure the INR is <2.0 on the day of surgery by reducing the dose and monitoring the INR. One can recommence the standard dose the following day;
  - major surgery: stop warfarin 3 days pre-operatively and monitor the INR. Proceed with surgery after ensuring an INR of <1.5.
- Evaluate the risk of thrombosis (if heparin cover is needed once the warfarin is stopped):
  - high risk: heparin infusion is started once the INR is <2.0, usually 48 hours after stopping warfarin. Stop heparin 4 hours pre-operatively. Restart warfarin as soon as the risk of surgical haemorrhage has passed, using heparin to bridge the time until the INR is therapeutic;
  - moderate risk: anticoagulation is decided on a case-by-case basis;
  - low risk: no alternative anticoagulation is required.

Note that if the INR is high despite stopping warfarin, vitamin-K/fresh frozen plasma/prothrombin complex concentrate can be given to replenish clotting factor stores.

Heparin

Heparin can be classified into low molecular weight and unfractionated. They are used as prophylaxis against venous thrombosis, treatment for established thrombosis and priming extracorporeal circuits for haemodialysis or cardiac bypass to prevent clot formation.

Unfractionated heparin acts by binding reversibly to antithrombin III (AT III), accelerating its action on coagulation factors XII, XI, X, IX, plasmin and thrombin. It inhibits platelet activation by fibrin. It is administered intravenously and its effect can be reversed quickly with protamine; however, merely stopping the infusion is enough to reverse anticoagulation, as its half-life is 1-2 hours. It does have side effects, which include thrombocytopenia and osteoporosis.

Low-molecular-weight heparins (LMWH) inhibit factor Xa and because they interact less with platelets, have a lower tendency to cause bleeding. They have become a standard in the management of patients at risk of DVT because of their longer half-life and therefore can be given as a daily maintenance dose for prophylaxis without the need for monitoring; however, if titration of the dose is necessary, factor Xa assays can be measured.

In general, LMWH should be stopped 12 hours (prophylactic dose) and 24 hours (treatment dose) prior to surgery. Unfractionated heparin can be stopped 4-6 hours prior to surgery. Ensure the activated partial thromboplastin time (APTT) is satisfactory before commencing surgery. Following the procedure, the acceptable time for LMWH to be restarted after central neuraxial block or epidural catheter removal is 4 hours.

Other agents

Fondaparinux is a new thromboprophylaxis drug that achieves its effect by indirectly inhibiting antithrombin through factor Xa inhibition. The onset of anticoagulation is 2 hours and the plasma half-life is 21 hours in adults. It is licensed for thromboprophylaxis in major joint replacement surgery, the treatment of DVT and PE, and the management of ACS. It is administered postoperatively and is useful if there is a contraindication to heparin.

Dabigatran is an oral reversible thrombin inhibitor whose onset of anticoagulation is 2 hours. It has received the National Institute for Health and Care Excellence (NICE) approval for the prevention of stroke and systemic embolism in a select group of patients with non-valvular atrial fibrillation.

Prior to major surgery dabigatran should be stopped 4 days prior, shortened to 2 days if there is a standard operative bleeding risk. The acceptable time to recommence the drug after central neuraxial blockade (CNB) or epidural catheter removal is 6 hours.

Rivaroxaban is an oral selective factor Xa inhibitor whose onset of anticoagulation is 2-4 hours. It is approved for stroke prevention in atrial fibrillation and for VTE prophylaxis following orthopaedic surgery. Prior to major surgery, rivaroxaban should be stopped 2 days prior, shortened to 1 day if there is a standard operative bleeding risk. Precautions for restarting this drug post-procedure are identical to dabigatran.

For patients awaiting central neuraxial blockade (CNB), guidance is outlined in Table 11.2.

Table 11.2. Guidance for timing of central neuraxial blockade for patients on antithrombotic drugs.

Drug	Acceptable time after drug for block performance	Acceptable time after block or catheter removal to (re)commence drug
Aspirin and NSAIDs	No additional precautions	No additional precautions
Clopidogrel	7 days	6 hours
Prasugrel	7 days	6 hours
Unfractionated heparin prophylaxis (subcutaneous)	4 hours or normal APTTR	1 hour
Unfractionated heparin treatment (IV)	4 hours or normal APTTR	4 hours
LMWH (prophylactic dose)	12 hours	4 hours
LMWH (therapeutic dose)	24 hours	4 hours
Warfarin	INR ≤1.4	After catheter removal
Fondaparinux (for prophylaxis)	36-42 hours	6 hours after surgery/CNB; 12 hours after catheter removal
Abciximab	48 hours	6 hours

Continued

Table 11.2 *continued*. Guidance for timing of central neuraxial blockade for patients on antithrombotic drugs.

Drug	Acceptable time after drug for block performance	Acceptable time after block or catheter removal to (re)commence drug
Rivaroxaban (prophylaxis) Creatinine clearance >30ml/min	18 hours	6 hours
Rivaroxaban (treatment) Creatinine clearance >30ml/min	48 hours	6 hours
Dabigatran (prophylaxis or treatment) Creatinine clearance >80ml/min	48 hours	6 hours
Creatinine clearance 50-80ml/min	72 hours	6 hours
Creatinine clearance 30-50ml/min	96 hours	6 hours

Case scenario 1

A 53-year-old man with a history of type 2 diabetes, congestive heart failure, COPD and chronic stable angina is scheduled for an umbilical hernia repair.

His medications include simvastatin, atenolol, ramipril, frusemide, metformin, digoxin and PRN inhalers for his COPD.

How would you manage his medication peri-operatively?

The anaesthetic options include a general anaesthetic or regional anaesthetic with a GA being preferred by most anaesthetists.

Cardiovascular medication

Continue up to and including the day of surgery — atenolol, digoxin, simvastatin. Withhold on the morning of surgery — frusemide.

Consider holding on the morning of surgery — ramipril (ACE inhibitor). However, this can lead to decompensation of heart failure, so it is reasonable to continue this drug, as regional blockade is unlikely, as are large fluid shifts intra-operatively.

Endocrine medication

Recent guidance has advised to continue metformin in the peri-operative period. The patient should be triaged to be the first patient on the operating list so that diabetic medication can resume early after surgery.

Respiratory medication

His inhalers should be used on the morning of surgery to avoid intra-operative bronchospasm and postoperative respiratory complications.

Case scenario 2

A 69-year-old patient with chronic angina underwent a revascularisation procedure 4 weeks ago with a drug-eluting stent. He is booked for an elective rotator cuff repair. His drug list includes aspirin, clopidogrel, atenolol and simvastatin.

How would you manage his medication peri-operatively?

The operation is elective. The options for anaesthesia include a general anaesthetic (+/- regional block) or sole regional block.

Antithrombotic medication

The risk for thrombosis is high if dual antiplatelet therapy is discontinued. A period of 12 months is recommended before DAPT can be stopped. It would be prudent to delay surgery until the risk of thrombosis has decreased. A sole regional anaesthetic block for a patient on DAPT is not a contraindication.

Cardiovascular medication

Atenolol and a statin can be safely continued in the peri-operative period.

Further reading

1.   BNF: British National Formulary, 2015.
2.   Huyse FJ, Touw FJ, van Schijindel RS, *et al*. Psychoactive drugs and the perioperative period: a proposal for a guideline in elective surgery. *Psychosomatics* 2006; 47; 8-22.
3.   Management of adult patients with diabetes undergoing surgery and elective procedures. NHS England, 2011.
4.   Lee AF, Kirsten AF, Andrew DA, *et al*. Perioperative beta blockade in noncardiac surgery: a systematic review for the 2014 ACC/AHA guideline on perioperative cardiovascular evaluation and management of patients undergoing noncardiac surgery. *J Am Coll Cardiol* 2014; 64(22): e77-e137.
5.   Association of Anaesthetists of Great Britain and Ireland. AAGBI guidelines: regional anaesthesia and patients with abnormalities of coagulation. AAGBI, Nov 2013.

12 Peri-operative fluid therapy

Gemma Dignam and Ahmed Mesbah

Introduction

Intravenous fluids are drugs. They have a dose, indications and contraindications. Not all patients need intravenous fluids peri-operatively. This chapter will address four questions relevant to the peri-operative period:

- Why should I give intravenous fluids?
- When should I give intravenous fluids?
- Which intravenous fluids should I use?
- How much volume should I give?

The goal of peri-operative fluid therapy is to optimise (although not necessarily maximise) cardiac output in order to maintain oxygen delivery to injured tissues. Both too little and too much fluid administration is associated with poor outcomes.

Why should I give intravenous fluids?

In a healthy adult, 60% of total body mass is water. Two-thirds of this water lies within the body's cells, whereas the remaining one-third lies outside the cell and is shared amongst the following:

- The interstitial space where the fluid bathes the cells and fills the lymphatic system.
- The intravascular space, which incidentally, consists of both extracellular fluid (plasma volume) and intracellular fluid (fluid within blood cells).

- The transcellular fluids such as cerebrospinal, intestinal and joint fluid.

Water and electrolytes move across all the compartments via diffusion, osmosis and active transport in order to maintain an electrochemical equilibrium. Total body water is then regulated by a system of cardiovascular, neuroendocrine and renal sensors and effectors such as the hypothalamic osmoreceptors, high- and low-pressure baroreceptors in the carotid sinus and right atrium, respectively, which respond to changes in plasma volume by controlling the release of angiotensin II, antidiuretic hormone (ADH) and the sensation of thirst. The goal of these mechanisms is to maintain adequate plasma volume and thus cardiac preload, ensuring adequate oxygen delivery (DO_2) to the tissues. However, note that DO_2 is dependent on several other factors, of which preload and haemoglobin concentration are the most commonly manipulated in peri-operative fluid therapy (Figure 12.1).

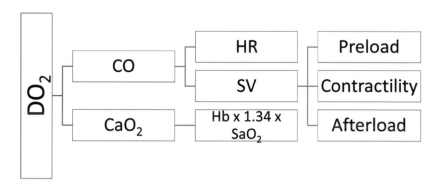

Figure 12.1. The components of global oxygen delivery (DO_2). Peri-operative fluid administration will specifically manipulate preload and haemoglobin concentration.

This equilibrium is disrupted during surgery in two main ways. First, a fluid deficit occurs which can be absolute, due to blood or gastrointestinal loss or relative due to the vasodilation that accompanies anaesthesia and the inflammatory effects of surgical trauma. Secondly, the neuroendocrine stress response to surgery results in the retention of sodium and, consequently, water, thus reducing replacement requirements. The goal of peri-operative fluid management is thus the same as that of the cardiovascular system in health; to assess and replace fluid losses in order to maintain an adequate blood flow to organs and tissues so as to not compromise the former and to enable effective wound healing in the latter. Collateral damage such as interstitial oedema, acidosis and coagulopathies should be avoided when attempting to achieve this.

When should I give intravenous fluids?

Currently, our standard practice is to administer intravenous fluids to maintain blood pressure and to replace presumed losses. We do so based on several assumptions: the patient has been fasted and therefore must be hypovolaemic; insensible evaporative losses continue throughout the peri-operative period; fluid shifts due to 'third space losses' are significant and must be replaced; hypervolaemia due to excessive fluid administration will be excreted by the kidneys; blood loss must be replaced to three or four times its volume in crystalloids; hypotension due to vasodilatation following induction produces a relative hypovolaemia that must be corrected.

Many of these assumptions have now been found to be flawed; however, they continue to lead to the replacement of unsubstantiated losses leading to an excessive positive fluid balance and complications. We will examine them in turn.

Pre-operative fasting

Extended pre-operative fasting with no bowel preparation for 8-10 hours has been shown to have a negligible effect on intravascular volume. Very few of us actually require a litre of tea following a good night's sleep to rehydrate, so why do we give our patients a litre of crystalloid?

Furthermore, current guidelines restrict fluids to only 2 hours pre-operatively. The utility of bowel preparation, considered a significant source of pre-operative hypovolaemia, is being questioned and is now used less often. Current anaesthetic, analgesic and antiemetic agents now enable patients to resume oral intake much sooner.

Insensible evaporative losses

In 1977, Lamke *et al* performed direct measurements of evaporative losses in a specially designed humidity chamber and found that basal evaporation in an awake adult at rest to be approximately 0.5ml/kg/hr. This may increase to 1ml/kg/hr in open abdominal operations with extensive bowel exposure. However, much of surgery today is minimally invasive or laparoscopic, with constant irrigation if performed open, and is carried out in operating theatres where temperature and humidity are controlled.

The third space

The concept of the 'third space' was developed 60 years ago by Shires *et al* following a study measuring plasma volume, red blood cell mass and extracellular volume in two groups of patients, five undergoing minor operations and 13 undergoing major colorectal procedures. A reduction of up to 28% of the extracellular fluid was found in the second group. This was attributed to the peri-operative loss of extracellular fluid to spaces, which normally contain little or no fluid such as the peritoneal and bowel cavities as well as other non-localised compartments. However, since this initial study, the third space has never been localised. It was only quantified in experiments with considerable weaknesses using a sulphate tracer with a relatively short equilibration time. Subsequent experiments with various other tracers and longer equilibration times refute the existence of this fluid-consuming third space. The mysterious fluid deficit that the third space is intended to account for is most likely a shift from the intravascular to the interstitial space.

Hypervolaemia and renal excretion

The generous administration of intravenous fluids with the assumption that the kidneys will excrete excessive volume overlooks that urinary output is frequently low peri-operatively due to ADH secretion, pre-existing renal disease or impaired function secondary to the use of nephrotoxic drugs peri-operatively. Excess fluid is thus more likely to cause hypervolaemia and interstitial oedema rather than a diuresis, possibly due to damage to the endothelial glycocalyx.

The endothelial glycocalyx

The luminal side of the endothelium is coated by a 1µm layer of membrane-bound proteoglycans and glycoproteins called the endothelial glycocalyx. When intact, this layer covers the fenestrations and intercellular clefts of the endothelium, forming a barrier, and prevents platelet and leukocyte adhesion. Water and electrolytes pass freely from the intravascular space to the interstitium through the glycocalyx and endothelium; however, proteins are filtered at the level of the glycocalyx. This results in a subglycoceal layer (between the glycocalyx and endothelium) that contains up to 700-1000ml of protein-poor plasma that forms part of the intravascular space. Damage to this layer results in protein-rich plasma shifting towards the interstitial space.

The glycocalyx can be damaged peri-operatively both by the surgeon and anaesthetist. Surgically, inflammation, mechanical trauma, endotoxin exposure and ischaemia-reperfusion injury all have deleterious effects on the integrity of the glycocalyx. Anaesthetically, hypervolaemia seems to have a similar effect. Irrespective of the mechanism, the result is a compromise in the gateway to the interstitial space with resultant oedema. The glycocalyx also influences the volume effect of infused fluids as discussed below.

Replacing blood with crystalloids

The practice of replacing blood loss with three or four times its volume in crystalloid solution stems from tracer studies consistently finding that approximately 20% of the infused volume remained intravascularly, the remainder being lost to the interstitium. However, clinical studies comparing crystalloids with hydroxyethyl starches (HES), which one would expect to expand plasma volume by the infused amount, challenge this. Recent clinical trials such as 6S, VISEP and CHEST, found that only 15-32% more crystalloid than colloid was used. Furthermore, in a volunteer study in which 900ml of blood was withdrawn and replaced by 900ml of lactated Ringer's solution, pulmonary artery and central venous pressures were maintained while cardiac output was only 4% less than baseline.

These observations can be partly explained by the glycocalyx. Infused colloids are excluded from the subglycocalyceal layer, therefore producing a volume effect by remaining within the plasma with a concomitant reduction in haematocrit. Crystalloids, however, leave the intravascular space and distribute throughout all compartments thus producing a lesser drop in haematocrit. These findings are interpreted in tracer studies as only 20% of crystalloids remaining intravascularly. However, crystalloids, unlike colloids, also distribute to the subglycocalyceal layer, which forms parts of the intravascular compartment, thus exhibiting a volume effect that exceeds what the tracer studies suggest.

Therefore, we can draw two conclusions: (1) the volume effect of crystalloids is larger than expected; meanwhile, colloids may not, in some pathologies, actually remain intravascularly; and (2) excessive fluid crystalloid infusion in the context of massive haemorrhage will lead to interstitial oedema that impairs lung and gut function. Massive haemorrhage should therefore be replaced with blood and blood products.

Vasodilatation following induction

Using intravenous fluids to treat vasodilation and the resultant relative hypovolaemia that accompanies the reduction in sympathetic tone caused by anaesthesia ignores the fact that the vascular tone will be restored at the conclusion of the anaesthetic, resulting conversely in a relative hypervolaemia and/or interstitial oedema at the conclusion of surgery. This relative hypovolaemia should be treated with vasopressors.

Fluid therapy indications

The National Institute for Health and Care Excellence (NICE) created a set of guidelines to aid the non-expert clinician in the general principles of intravascular fluid therapy in adults. They specifically acknowledge that the intra-operative and critical care patient populations are outside the scope of the recommendations. However, the guidance describes a useful aide-memoire for all clinicians to consider before prescribing parental fluids — the 5 Rs: Resuscitation, Routine maintenance, Replacement, Redistribution and Reassessment. The first four are concerned with the prescriber having a clear indication and are discussed below. The fifth, Reassessment, is a reminder that whatever the original indication, the ongoing requirement and the patient's fluid status should be evaluated regularly. This ensures timely de-escalation of therapy and avoids the morbidity associated with poor fluid management.

Resuscitation

Fluid boluses (set volumes of fluid) are administered rapidly (500ml in under 15 minutes) to correct dangerous physiological values suggestive of impending cardiovascular collapse. It should be noted that measurements to guide the response to the fluid boluses should be simple and rapid to perform, for example, central capillary refill, allowing ongoing management without delay.

Routine maintenance

Intravenous therapy should not be considered routine. When prescribing 'maintenance' ask the fundamental question: can any of this fluid be administered via the oral/enteral route and if not, how can I expedite this patient's return to enteral intake? This may involve optimising analgesia and antiemetic therapy, in addition to promoting early mobilisation, which can aid the return of normal gut function. Enteral feeding tubes can supplement insufficient oral intake. Of course, some cannot receive enteral feeding peri-operatively and this is when maintenance fluid is indicated. However, it is important to understand maintenance fluids do not provide nutritional benefit and patients who remain unable to tolerate the enteral route should be considered for parental nutrition.

The normal daily requirement of water is 25-30ml/kg/day with approximately 1mmol/kg/day of potassium, sodium and chloride. Starvation ketosis may be limited by the administration of 50-100g/day of glucose. The volume of intravenous maintenance should take into account fluid administered orally, parentally or via drugs.

Replacement

Two components will usually require replacement: (1) existing fluid and electrolyte imbalance (excess or deficit), and (2) fluid loss from perspiration, and the renal or gastrointestinal tract. Currently, it is believed that the basal fluid loss via insensible perspiration is approximately 0.5ml/kg/hr, extending up to 1ml/kg/hr during major abdominal surgery. Accurate recording of measurable body fluid output (for example, stoma output or indeed urine in high-output renal failure) is important. The NICE guidelines provide a good summary of the composition of some body fluids and this can be used with volume lost to guide rational replacement.

Redistribution

Redistribution describes the movement of fluid across compartments, for example, from the intravascular compartment to the interstitium. This indication is perhaps the most difficult to assess. It requires careful clinical assessment combined with a good understanding of the pathophysiology of the potential fluid shifts that occur peri-operatively. Indeed, these shifts are further complicated by comorbid disease states such as sepsis, trauma and organ failure that lead to electrolyte and protein imbalance. Fluid management in these cases is complex and requires regular (at least daily) clinical and biochemical monitoring, remembering that excess peri-operative fluid is retained for around 3 weeks.

Which intravenous fluids should I use?

Having a clear indication will guide the clinician in choosing the appropriate fluid. An accurate clinical assessment of the volume and electrolyte status including ongoing fluid losses is vital. Knowledge of the electrolyte content of body fluids can then be used to predict ongoing electrolyte deficits. Thus, the identified existing and predicted deficits can then be compared to the physiochemical properties of available fluids (Table 12.1) and the solution that provides the best match should be chosen.

Crystalloids

Crystalloid solutions consist of crystalline solids dissolved in water. They diffuse easily across semipermeable membranes and are classified according to their tonicity in relation to plasma as hypotonic, isotonic or hypertonic. Isotonic solutions (normal saline and Hartmann's solution) distribute freely in the extracellular space and therefore limit the movement of water between the extracellular fluid compartment and intracellular fluid compartment. Hypotonic solutions, such as dextrose 5%, allow the free movement of water between the compartments once the glucose is metabolised and therefore are used for rehydration. Hypertonic solutions, such as 3% saline, raise the osmolality of the extracellular fluid and therefore shift water from the intracellular fluid compartment to the extracellular fluid compartment. This can be indicated in the management of cerebral oedema.

Normal (0.9%) saline

Normal (0.9%) saline is not actually 'normal'. It contains 154mmol/L of both sodium and chloride and is slightly hypertonic (osmolality 308mOsm/kg). Excessive administration may cause hyperchloraemic acidosis and sodium overload.

Table 12.1. The physiochemical properties of some commonly available fluids.

Fluid	Na mmol /L	K mmol /L	Cl mmol /L	Ca mmol /L	Mg mmol /L	HCO$_3$ mmol /L	Lac mmol/ L	Ace mmol/ L	Gluc mmol/ L	Gluc g/L	Osm mOsm /L	pH
Plasma	140	4.5	100	2.5	1.2	24	1				285	7.4
0.9% NaCl	154		154								308	6.0
5% dextrose										50	252	4.5
5% dextrose/ 0.45% NaCl	77		77							50	406	4.0
4% dextrose/ 0.18% NaCl	31		31							40	271	
Compound sodium lactate	131	5	111	4			29				275	6.5
Plasma-Lyte® 148	140	5	98		1.5			27	23		294	4-6.5
5% albumin	150		150								300	
20% albumin	145		145								310	
Gelofusine® 4%	154		125								290	
Isoplex® 4%	145	4	105		0.9		25				284	7.4
Gelaspan® 4%	151	4	103	1	1			24			284	7.4
Voluven® 6% HES	154		154								308	4-5.5
Volulyte® 6% HES	137	4	110		1.5			34			286	5.7-6.5

Lac = lactate; Ace = acetate; Gluc = glucose; Osm = osmolarity; NaCl = normal saline; HES = hydroxyethyl starch.

Compound sodium lactate solution (Hartmann's solution)

Hartmann's solution is very slightly hypotonic. It contains less sodium and chloride than 0.9% saline but also contains potassium and calcium, and as such is usually considered more 'physiological' than 0.9% saline.

Colloids

Colloids contain macromolecules such as gelatin, starches or protein. Examples include the gelatins (Gelofusine®), hydroxyethyl starches (Volulyte® and Voluven®) and albumin. In theory, these large particles should confine the fluids to the intravascular space, as opposed to crystalloids, and are therefore referred to as plasma expanders. However, as alluded to earlier, this does not seem to be the case. Substantial volumes of colloids diffuse out of the intravascular space depending on the clinical state of the patient and the integrity of the vascular endothelium and glycocalyx. All semi-synthetic colloids have an effect on the blood coagulation.

A number of studies comparing crystalloids and colloids have demonstrated either similar outcomes or harm associated with colloid administration. The Saline versus Albumin (SAFE) study compared albumin and normal saline in an intensive care population and demonstrated that albumin was not inferior to saline. It also showed that to achieve the equivalent goal-directed targets, the ratio of normal saline to albumin was 1.4:1 as opposed to the 3:1 as previously thought. Furthermore, the Volume Substitution and Insulin Therapy in Severe Sepsis (VISEP) study found that resuscitation with hydroxyethyl starches was associated with an increased risk of renal failure and mortality. This was echoed by the findings of the 6S study in 2011, which led the UK's Medicines and Healthcare products Regulatory Agency (MHRA) in 2013 to suspend their use in critically ill patients and peri-operatively.

How much volume should I give?

The volume of fluid should be individualised to the patient and surgery, with continuous reassessment.

Striking the balance between avoiding morbidity from excessive fluid and maintaining perfusion is arguably the most important element of peri-operative fluid management. However, evaluating the optimal volume of fluid to be administered can be challenging. Two main approaches have been suggested:

- A traditional approach whereby a calculation of pre- and intra-operative loss is made based upon the patient's weight and the surgical insult; or
- Goal-directed therapy (GDT), the targeted administration of fluid challenges based upon the measurement of physiological variables with reassessment to maintain these values within a desirable optimum range (goals).

Currently, evidence supports the use of goal-directed therapy (GDT) to practically guide the clinician in their goal of using fluid to optimise the tissue oxygen delivery. GDT should be encouraged peri-operatively and is strongly recommended for intra-operative use, especially for high-risk surgical procedures.

Volume estimation by calculation

Although administering a calculated volume of fluid is more individualised than a recipe type approach (administration of a set volume for a particular operation), calculations may still fail to accommodate for individual variations in fluid handling. See the example below.

Case example

John (65kg) is a 68-year-old who had a 3-hour right hemicolectomy with 300ml blood loss. He consumed water up to 2 hours pre-operatively.

Pre-operative deficit: maintenance (using the 4-2-1 rule) was calculated and multiplied by the starvation period. 4(10)+2(10)+1(45) = 105ml/hr. 105 (2) = 210ml. However, we now estimate the pre-operative starvation deficit to be 0.5ml/kg/hr = 65ml.

Intra-operative maintenance: 3(105) = 315ml. However, we now estimate the daily water requirement as 25-30ml/kg (25 x 65 x 3/24) to (30 x 65 x 3/24) = 203ml-244 ml.

Insensible losses: the requirement was estimated to be as large as 0-2ml/kg/h for minimal, 2-4ml/kg/h for modest and 4-8 ml/kg/hr in severe tissue trauma or large surface area exposure. Insensible losses for 3 hours: 3(4 x 65) to 3(8 x 65) = 780 to 1560ml. This is now actually thought to be 0.5ml/kg/h extending to 1.0ml/kg/hr for major surgery. 3(65 x 1) = 195ml.

Blood loss: replace on a 1:1 basis for colloid/blood or 1:3 ratio for crystalloid administration. These ratios are based upon the myth that crystalloids redistribute across the entire extravascular compartment and that colloids will remain in the entirely intravascular compartment. 3(300) = 900ml of crystalloid or 300ml of colloid/blood. However, observational data suggest a 1:1.5 colloid to crystalloid ratio is actually used to achieve the desired effect clinically. Using this 1:1.5 ratio, his crystalloid requirement would be reduced to 1.5(300) = 450ml.

Traditional calculations were based upon many of the fluid myths we discussed above and may lead to the administration of significant volumes of excess fluid. Indeed, 2205-2985ml would be estimated for the scenario. However, if we apply our current understanding of fluid handling, the estimated volume would reduce to 918-959ml. These traditional calculations therefore do not have a place in current practice.

Goal-directed therapy (GDT)

Goal-directed therapy (GDT) can be described as a dynamic process in which the user targets a specific objective endpoint (see Figure 12.2). In its modest form, the goal could be a simple capillary refill time or blood pressure. The fundamental part of the process is the reassessment: following an intervention the current status is reassessed and action to achieve the goal decided using the previous response. Once the goal is reached, regular reassessment is performed to direct the actions to keep that parameter within the goal range.

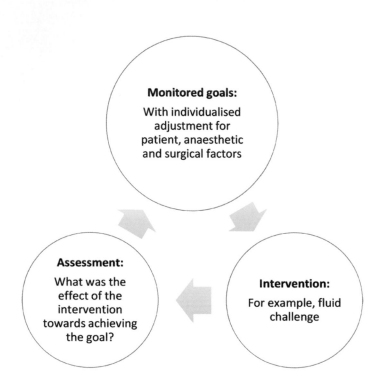

Figure 12.2. A basic schematic of goal-directed therapy (GDT) emphasizing it is a dynamic process. Monitoring of desired goals prompts intervention when there is a deviation from the desired range. This intervention is always reassessed; if it partially or fully returns the parameter towards the desired range, it may be repeated as necessary. If unsuccessful, another intervention should be selected.

Enthusiasm for GDT occurred following the observation by Shoemaker, that surgical mortality could be reduced if a patient's cardiac indices were manipulated to replicate the values observed in the survivors of high-risk surgery from a previous study. This approach uses fluids and inotropes to produce these supra-normal predetermined values on a population basis.

The modern approach to peri-operative GDT includes maintaining normal values (for example, targeting the corrected flow time [FTc] between 330-360 milliseconds) or individualised targets (for example, a 10% improvement in stroke volume following the administration of a fluid challenge, may indicate that individual is on the upstroke of the Starling curve).

Few would agree with a fluid management approach that administered fluid without reassessment (which as discussed above is GDT at its basic level). However, the uptake of GDT using cardiac output monitors has met resistance — perhaps, because of the lack of strongly positive large randomised controlled trials and concerns about the invasiveness and technical skills required with some monitoring techniques. A 2012 Cochrane systematic review concluded that peri-operative GDT was associated with reduced peri-operative 28-day mortality and morbidity including renal impairment, respiratory complications, postoperative wound infection and reduced hospital length of stay.

NICE has endorsed the use of goal-directed peri-operative fluid management for a wide variety of surgical populations. The NICE Technology Adoption Centre specifically evaluated the oesophageal Doppler monitor (ODM). However, it is likely that the potential benefits relate to the process of fluid administration and crucially re-evaluation is based upon objective endpoints rather than the measurement device (assuming a degree of device accuracy).

Individual considerations

There are numerous circumstances where fluid management needs to be adjusted to avoid excess morbidity and mortality (Figure 12.3).

Cardiac disease	• May have salt and fluid retention from activation of the renin, angiotensin, and aldosterone (RAA) system. • Diuretics may lead to chronic electrolyte and volume depletion. • Failing ventricles are poorly compliant. Intravascular hypovolaemia and short diastolic times are poorly tolerated. • Invasive monitoring is often required to guide optimal fluid therapy.
Renal disease	• Perform surgery when euvolaemic to avoid the adverse features of hypervolaemia or hypovolaemia. • Post-dialysis there is ongoing fluid and electrolyte equilibration between compartments and the dialysis anticoagulants may still be functioning, so usually plan surgery for the following day.
Neonates	• Dextrose replacement required for starvation. • Monitor blood glucose during starvation. • Eliminate air from infusion tubing. • Care not to unintentionally infuse excessive volumes.
Neurosurgery & neurotrauma	• Avoid hypotonic fluids and albumin.
Thoracic surgery or ARDS	• Avoid over-hydration.
Trauma	• Replace blood loss with blood products. • Avoid hypothermia by warming fluids administered. • Avoid acidosis and coagulopathy but ensuring euvolaemia and remembering to administer plasma and platelets with packed red cells.
Transurethral resections	• Large volumes of hypotonic irrigation fluid may potentially be absorbed. Therefore, consider limiting additional intravenous fluid.
Burns	• Large evaporative and blood loss intra-operatively. • Initially crystalloid therapy, primarily guided by urine output, followed by administration of albumin-containing fluids.

Figure 12.3. A brief summary of some circumstances where adjustments may need to be made.

Case scenario 1

A 78-year-old male is booked for an urgent laparotomy for a suspected perforation. He had presented to hospital after experiencing sudden onset colicky upper abdominal pain and his chest X-ray revealed free air under the diaphragm; however, computed tomography failed to reveal the source of the perforation.

He tells you that he suffers from high blood pressure and 'wear and tear' arthritis of his knees, going on to report that he had suffered a heart attack 6 years ago. He then had coronary artery stenting of two vessels and now only suffers infrequent attacks of angina (less than once or twice a year). Prior to this admission today he reports being able to complete a single flight of stairs in one go.

He has no allergies and he takes the following medications regularly: aspirin 75mg OD, atenolol 25mg OD, ramipril 2.5mg OD, simvastatin 40mg nocte and furosemide 40mg OD. Additionally, he takes paracetamol 1g QDS, codeine phosphate 15mg QDS and some ibuprofen gel 5% applied topically TDS when required for his painful knees.

On examination, he is peripherally cold to his mid-calves with reduced skin turgor. His central capillary refill is 4s and heart rate is 93 beats per minute. His blood pressure is 91/47mmHg. You are unable to visualise the jugular venous pulse and he has dry mucous membranes. There is 5ml of concentrated urine in the urometer for the last 45 minutes (documented residual volume of 50ml). He has received a litre of 0.9% sodium chloride in the last hour.

The lactate is recorded as 3.8mmol/L on a venous blood gas. On reviewing his laboratory results, you note his urea is elevated at 16.2mmol/L and creatinine is 141µmol/L (baseline creatinine appeared to be 98µmol/L). He has raised inflammatory markers and his haemoglobin was 149g/L with a haematocrit of 52%.

What is your clinical assessment of this patient's fluid balance?

The patient has severe hypovolaemia; indeed, he is shocked and requires resuscitation fluid management. Physiological compensation usually maintains blood pressure until the blood volume is reduced by more than 30% and this usually hypertensive gentleman is hypotensive. Note he is not particularly tachycardic due to his beta-blockade. He remains alert — it should be noted that a deteriorating conscious level is a very late sign in shock and is a worrying pre-terminal sign.

What immediate steps would you take to address this situation?

Administer 500ml of Hartmann's solution rapidly using a pressure bag, via a 16-gauge cannula. His capillary refill remains prolonged. You therefore give a further 500ml, which improves his capillary refill time to 2 seconds. You then take his blood pressure — it is now 106/54mmHg.

What would you do now?

You contact critical care and they accept him for postoperative care but are unable to provide immediate pre-operative optimisation. You therefore arrange to take him to the operating department, for ongoing fluid optimisation. Invasive monitoring (radial arterial and jugular central venous pressure) is inserted. He receives two 250ml warmed Hartmann's solution challenges in response to a lactate of 3.4mmol/L and central venous saturation of 62%. These both improve. His capillary refill and blood pressure remain stable. You decide to aim for an intra-operative mean arterial blood pressure of 65mmHg. Anaesthesia is then induced; following intubation and mechanical ventilation, the patient then becomes hypotensive and the administration of an α-agonist successfully restores the blood pressure. You choose to use an oesophageal Doppler monitor (ODM) to guide further fluid management. The Doppler probe is inserted and you record the corrected flow time (FTc) and stroke volume (SV). The surgeons confirm and undertake the repair of a perforated duodenal ulcer. The monitor guides you to administer three further 250ml boluses. After the third bolus the SV remains static, with an FTc of 410ms. The CVP increases by 3cmH$_2$0. However, the MAP is only 58mmHg; you therefore decide to administer vasopressors at this point to target the desired mean arterial pressure. You transfer him to critical care ventilated, as he remains acidotic.

What would be your postoperative fluid management instructions?

You calculate his daily requirements for maintenance fluid therapy. He weighs 70kg, so requires 1750ml (25 x 70) to 2100ml (30 x 70) per day. His electrolyte needs are: 70mmol of potassium, sodium and chloride. You decide the best match would be 1L of 4% dextrose/0.18% NaCl + 20mmol KCl and 1L of 4% dextrose/0.18% NaCl + 40mmol KCl at 83ml/h (12-hourly), providing 62mmol of both sodium and chloride, with 60mmol of potassium and 80g of glucose in 24 hours. You prescribe each bag to be infused over 12 hours.

You leave the ODM monitor *in situ* and you direct that additional fluid boluses should be considered in response to a falling SV (aiming for a 10% improvement following the fluid challenge) or FTc <350ms.

The patient is successfully extubated the following day and the ODM monitor removed. (There are awake probes available; however, patients often cannot tolerate these, most likely due to the regular signal manipulation.) Reviews of his electrolytes reveal normal potassium, chloride and sodium levels so the current maintenance regimen is continued. However, the surgical team agree to establish enteral feed via the nasogastric tube. Therefore, the maintenance fluid prescription is altered to direct a reduction in rate as the enteral feed is built up so that the total volume given is 83ml/h. Once the patient is providing his own maintenance requirements enterally, the intravenous fluids are discontinued.

Case scenario 2

A 20-year-old male is scheduled to undergo a complex tympanoplasty (estimated to take 3-4 hours) to repair damage to the middle ear sustained following a cholesteatoma. He is fit and well with no other comorbid disease and weighs 70kg. You review him at 08:00 and find he last ate and drink at 22:00 the previous evening. There are several other small paediatric cases on the list. At the theatre team briefing, the list order is decided and it is estimated that this gentleman's surgery will commence at around 13:00, allowing the children to be operated on in the morning. The admissions nurse therefore asks you to prescribe some pre-operative intravenous fluid for him.

What would you prescribe pre-operatively?

The patient is not going to be operated on before the afternoon. He only needs 2 hours abstinence from clear oral fluids. You therefore advise her that he can take free clear fluids orally until 11:00.

He eventually arrives in theatre at 13:30. He tells you he drank a jug of water over the course of the morning, having his last oral intake at 10:30.

How much fluid would you anticipate administering during this case?

Much of the pre-operative deficit has been addressed by allowing him to drink orally during the morning until 2 hours before the predicted surgical start time. He has been nil by mouth for only 3 hours. You calculate his pre-operative deficit using the 0.5ml/kg/hr formula: 0.5 x 70 x 3 = 105ml.

You calculate his maintenance rate using 30ml/kg/day: 30 x 70 = 2100ml per 24 hours. A rate of 87.5ml/hr. This is 350ml for 4 hours.

There is minimal surgical trauma, blood loss and evaporative losses during this procedure. You therefore only anticipate administering 350 + 105 = 455ml and ask your anaesthetic assistant to prepare a 500ml bag of Hartmann's solution.

The anaesthesia and surgery proceed uneventfully; you use a total intravenous anaesthesia technique and administer intravenous dexamethasone 3.3mg and cyclizine 50mg as prophylactic antiemetics. You hand over his care to the recovery nurse — she asks if you have prescribed another bag of fluid.

What would be your postoperative fluid instructions?

The patient is awake, pain- and nausea-free. You instruct her that he can drink oral fluids immediately and does not require any further intravenous fluid.

Further reading

1. National Institute for Health and Care Excellence (NICE). Intravenous fluid therapy in adults in hospital. NICE clinical practice guideline 174. London, UK: NICE, 2013. https://www.nice.org.uk/guidance/cg174.

2. Chappell D, Jacob M, Hofmann-Kiefer K, et al. A rational approach to perioperative fluid management. Anesthesiology 2008; 109: 723-40.

3. Powell-tuck J, Gosling P, Dileep N, et al. British consensus guidelines on intravenous fluid therapy for adult surgical patients, 2011: 1-50. http://www.bapen.org.uk/pdfs/bapen_pubs/giftasup.pdf.

4. Corcoran T, Rhodes JEJ, Clarke S, et al. Perioperative fluid management strategies in major surgery: a stratified meta-analysis. Anesth Analg 2012; 114: 640-51.

5. Grocott MPW, Dushianthan A, Hamilton MA, et al. Perioperative increase in global blood flow to explicit defined goals and outcomes following surgery. Cochrane Database Syst Rev 2012; 11: CD004082.

13 Peri-operative blood transfusion

Anuja Patil and Cyprian Mendonca

Introduction

Anaesthetists play an important role in the decision of peri-operative blood transfusion. Thorough pre-operative assessment and planning are essential. This includes a history, clinical examination, investigations and type of surgery. Attention should be paid to a personal or family history of bleeding disorders, and the use of medications affecting coagulation (e.g. salicylates, NSAIDs, antiplatelet drugs and anticoagulants). Wherever possible, pre-operative anaemia should be corrected with the use of iron, folate supplements and recombinant human erythropoietin. Strategies to minimise blood loss during surgery and alternatives to allogeneic blood transfusion should be considered when appropriate.

Pre-operative assessment and preparation should include:

- A thorough history and clinical examination for symptoms and signs of anaemia.
- Appropriate laboratory investigations.
- Measures to optimise pre-operative haemoglobin.
- Correction of coagulopathies.
- Discontinuing any medications that affect coagulation.
- Strategies to minimise intra-operative blood loss.
- A plan for autologous blood transfusion and intra-operative cell salvage.
- Confirmation of blood group and availability of blood products.
- Discussion with the patient and consent for blood transfusion.
- Discussion with surgical colleagues with regard to steps to minimise blood loss.

Physiology of blood loss

Acute blood loss results in a decrease in circulating blood volume. This triggers the body's acute compensatory response to maintain perfusion of vital organs, i.e. brain, heart and kidney. This is achieved by increasing cardiac output by various neurohumoral mechanisms which lead to increased pre-load, cardiac contractility and afterload. Activation of the sympathetic nervous system stimulates the adrenal medulla to secrete catecholamines. This in turn causes peripheral and splanchnic vasoconstriction directing blood from the skin and gut back to the heart. The resulting increase in the venous return increases cardiac output.

Direct stimulation of the sino-atrial node causes an increase in heart rate and increased levels of circulating adrenaline has a positive inotropic effect on the heart which further increases cardiac output.

Reduced firing from the baroreceptors leads to increased sympathetic output from the vasomotor centre resulting in vasoconstriction and increased cardiac output. This helps to maintain the perfusion of vital organs.

Decreased blood flow to the kidneys causes activation of the renin-angiotensin-aldosterone system (Figure 13.1), which leads to retention of water and sodium in the kidneys helping to restore intravascular volume.

Lost haemoglobin is replaced over a period of 6-8 weeks. Kidneys secrete more erythropoietin which increases the production of red blood cells by the bone marrow.

Clinical presentation of blood loss

Patients with acute blood loss can present with the following signs and symptoms:

- Pale, sweaty, anxious and confused.
- Cold peripheries.
- Tachypnoea.
- Tachycardia.

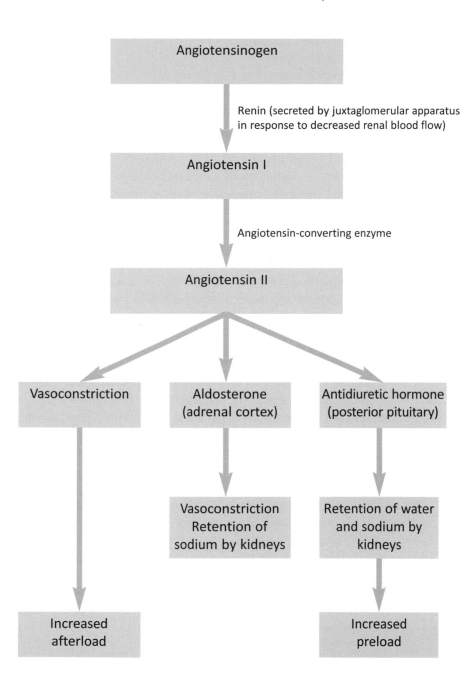

Figure 13.1. Renin-angiotensin system.

- Low systolic blood pressure.
- Narrow pulse pressure.
- Decreased urine output.

Indications and haemoglobin triggers for transfusion

The main aim of blood transfusion is to increase the oxygen-carrying capacity of the blood. A neurohumoral stress response to surgery leads to an increased basal metabolic rate. This leads to an increased oxygen demand. Blood transfusion helps to balance the oxygen demand and supply:

- A haemoglobin concentration below 70g/L is a strong indication for blood transfusion.
- A haemoglobin concentration of 80-100g/L is a safe level even for those patients with significant cardiorespiratory disease.

Contraindications to blood transfusion

Although blood transfusion can be lifesaving, a patient's wish not to receive blood transfusion should be respected (e.g. Jehovah's Witness). This is the absolute contraindication for blood transfusion. Other relative contraindications are a previous severe reaction to blood transfusion, non-urgent surgery in a patient with anaemia, severe congestive cardiac failure and massive haemorrhage.

Anaesthetists encounter patients with massive haemorrhage in a variety of situations. These include major trauma, obstetric patients, intra-operative blood loss and patients with a known coagulation disorder. Awareness of the situation, knowledge and understanding of the management of massive haemorrhage and effective teamwork are of paramount importance.

Massive haemorrhage

Massive haemorrhage can be defined as a situation where 1 to 1.5 times the total blood volume may need to be replaced acutely or in 24 hours. A major haemorrhage protocol should be in place in hospitals. This ensures that blood and blood products can be rapidly obtained and team members perform their tasks according to the pre-designated roles.

The principles of managing a massive haemorrhage include:

- Rapid control of bleeding.
- Maintenance of perfusion to vital organs.
- Management of coagulopathy.

Immediate actions include activation of a major haemorrhage protocol, communicating with other theatre team members and control of obvious bleeding by direct pressure, tourniquets, and surgical or radiological techniques.

Management of massive haemorrhage

- Administer high-flow oxygen.
- Monitor vital signs and peripheral oxygen saturation.
- Establish wide-bore IV access.
- Obtain blood samples for a full blood count, blood group and cross-match, urea & electrolytes, clotting profile, fibrinogen levels, thromboelastography and arterial blood gas.
- Replace blood loss with blood products. Use blood group O Rhesus negative blood (O negative) until group-specific and cross-matched blood is available. Major haemorrhage packs (Table 13.1) are issued by blood banks according to local policy.
- Administer 1g tranexamic acid.
- Keep the patient warm using a forced air warmer and administer warm blood products.
- Transfuse fresh frozen plasma (FFP), platelets and other blood products as indicated.
- Radiological investigations as indicated, e.g whole body CT scan or FAST (focused assessment with sonography for trauma) in major trauma.
- Treatment of hypocalcaemia and hyperkalemia.
- Ongoing assessment of the response to treatment.
- Normalise blood pressure, coagulation abnormalities, temperature.

- Admit to the high dependency unit or intensive care unit for continuous monitoring.

Table 13.1. Components of major haemorrhage packs. Initially, transfuse pack 1; with ongoing blood loss transfuse pack 2; and finally pack 3.

Pack 1	4 units red cells + 4 units FFP
Pack 2	4 units red cells + 4 units FFP + 1 unit of platelets
Pack 3	4 units red cells + 4 units FFP + unit of platelet + 1 unit of cryoprecipitate

---

Practical procedure of blood transfusion

All hospitals should have a local policy for the transfusion of blood and blood products. All the members of staff must be trained and qualified to administer blood. Strict adherence to the recommendations should minimise the risk of transfusion of an incorrect blood. Complete traceability of the administered blood is a legal requirement.

The steps involved in blood transfusion

At the bedside:

- A decision is made by the clinicians to give a blood transfusion to the patient.
- Discussion with the patient and obtaining informed consent as per the local protocol before the surgery.
- Confirming the identity of the patient. Patient identification labels should be checked. Removed labels should be immediately replaced.
- Obtaining the sample and labelling it correctly at the bedside.

In the laboratory:

- Safe transfer of the sample to the laboratory.
- Blood group determination and compatibility testing at the laboratory.
- Issuing of the blood. Most hospitals now issue blood electronically.

In the anaesthetic room/theatre:

- Positive patient identification (confirm their identity against the patient identification label before induction of anaesthesia) by two qualified personnel.
- Check the unit and tags.
- Check prescription.
- Check special requirements, e.g. irradiated, *Cytomegalovirus* (CMV)-negative.
- Record the details (number, volume, etc.) of the blood unit administered on the anaesthetic chart.
- Use the products within the appropriate time after they have been left out of the fridge.
- Return unused blood to the blood bank.

In recovery:

- Complete handover of the transfused blood products.
- Advice on monitoring the patient for blood transfusion reactions.

Blood products

In the UK, blood is donated by volunteers who have undergone health screening. Donated blood is tested for HIV 1, HIV 2, hepatitis B, hepatitis C and syphilis. White cells are commonly removed from the blood, thus reducing the risk of transmission of Creutzfeldt-Jacob disease and CMV. Whole blood is collected into an anticoagulant solution (citrate-based) and is further processed to obtain the blood products (CMV-negative blood is available for immunosuppressed patients and neonates). Whole blood is rarely used for blood transfusion; packed red cells tend to be used instead.

Whole blood is centrifuged to remove plasma and then filtered to remove platelets and leucocytes. The red cells are then suspended in additive solutions — saline, adenine, glucose and mannitol (SAG-M) or citrate phosphate dextrose adenine (CPDA).

A bag of packed cells has an approximate volume of 200-400ml with a haematocrit of 60-70%. It has a shelf-life of 35 days and is stored at 2-6°C.

Platelets

Two types of platelets are available: pooled or apheretic. A pool is derived from four donations of whole blood by the buffy coat method of preparation. During apheresis, platelets are derived from a single donor. Approximate volume is up to 300ml, with a shelf-life of 5 days. They are stored at 20-24°C on an agitator rack

Fresh frozen plasma

Fresh frozen plasma (FFP) is obtained by centrifugation of whole blood or apheresis and then rapidly frozen. It contains both labile and stable clotting factors including albumin, gamma globulin, fibrinogen and factor VIII. There are currently two types of viral-inactivated FFP available in the UK: methylene blue treated and solvent detergent treated. Approximate volume is about 300ml, with a shelf-life of 1 year (frozen). It is stored at -30°C.

Cryoprecipitate

Cryoprecipitate is obtained by slowly thawing fresh frozen plasma at 2-6°C. The precipitate is separated from the supernatant and refrozen. Cryoprecipitate has a higher concentration of factor VIII, fibrinogen, von Willebrand factor, factor XIII and fibronectin as compared to FFP. It is indicated in situations where fibrinogen levels are critically low (<1g/L). Approximate volume is about 300ml, with a shelf-life of 1 year (frozen). It is stored at -30°C.

Factor VIII and IX concentrates

These factors are the treatment of choice in patients with haemophilia A who do not respond to desmopressin. Only recombinant preparations are available in the UK to eliminate the risk of viral-borne infection. They are available as freeze-dried powders and need to be reconstituted before intravenous use. A shorter half-life of factor VIII (8-12 hours) necessitates twice-daily injection, whereas factor IX has a longer half-life (12-18 hours) and once-a-day administration is adequate for a sustained effect.

Prothrombin complex concentrates

The main indication for the use of prothrombin complex concentrates is urgent reversal of over-anticoagulation or bleeding due to coumarin anticoagulants, e.g. warfarin. These are derived from plasma and contain vitamin K-dependent coagulation factors (II, VII, IX, X), thus increasing their levels.

Immunoglobulins

Specific immunoglobulins are obtained from donor plasma. These immunoglobulins are used for passive prophylaxis of certain infections, e.g. tetanus, *Varicella zoster*. They can also be used in the prevention of haemolytic disease of the newborn and idiopathic thrombocytopenic purpura.

Non-specific immunoglobulins are obtained from pooled plasma of multiple donors. These are used in passive prophylaxis of commonly prevalent conditions like hepatitis A.

Jehovah's Witnesses

A Jehovah's Witness is part of a Christian movement. They believe that God views blood as sacred and holy, and its purity is lost when it is removed from the body. It should, therefore, not be used for transfusion

263

regardless of the consequences. So, the procedures involving removal and storage of their own or a donor's blood are unacceptable. All Jehovah's Witnesses refuse whole blood transfusion, plasma, red blood cells and autologous predonation. Recombinant factors, cardiopulmonary bypass, renal dialysis and acute hypervolaemic haemodilution are acceptable. Individuals need to make their own decision about accepting derived products like platelets, albumin, clotting factors, immunoglobulins and procedures like cell salvage and epidural blood patches. Transfusion-free medical and surgical treatment is a challenge faced by healthcare professionals. At the same time, respecting a patient's beliefs is an important aspect of good medical practice. Thus, a familiarity of the various techniques available for the management of these patients is important.

Legal and ethical issues

By law, every competent adult has the right to refuse any medical or surgical treatment (including lifesaving treatments). Administering treatment against a patient's wishes is unlawful and may lead to a legal action against the doctor. Most Jehovah's Witnesses carry an advanced directive signed and witnessed outlining acceptable and unacceptable products. A copy of this must be filed in the patient's clinical notes. Anaesthetists have the right to refuse treating a Jehovah's Witness for elective surgery but are obliged to provide care for emergency procedures. This should involve respecting a patient's wishes for not receiving a blood transfusion.

In emergency situations, when the patient's Jehovah's Witness status is not known, a doctor is expected to act in the patient's best interest which may include blood transfusion. A patient's general practitioner can be contacted for evidence of the advanced directive if required.

The care of children (less than 16 years of age) of Jehovah's Witnesses may present as a difficult situation. For an elective procedure, pre-operative assessment should involve a detailed discussion by the anaesthetist and surgeon with the parents. A "Specific Issue Order" can be applied by the court if the parents refuse the blood transfusion and this puts the child at risk. It is essential that two consultants document the necessity of blood transfusion before this step is undertaken. In the case of an emergency, a doctor should give blood if the child is likely to develop serious harm or die without immediate blood transfusion. All hospitals should have a policy outlining the management of Jehovah's Witness patients. A Jehovah's Witness Hospital Liaison Officer should be contacted for advice if required.

Pre-operative management

Pre-operative management should include:

- Early communication with the anaesthetic team.
- Pre-operative assessment by a senior member of the team willing to anaesthetise the patient in elective situations.
- Outlining the acceptable and unacceptable products.
- Signing the Advanced Directive if not already done.
- Investigate and treat anaemia (iron supplements or recombinant erythropoietin).
- Discuss and document intra-operative strategies (acute normovolaemic haemodilution and cell salvage).
- Review medications, especially antiplatelet agents and anticoagulants.
- A plan to stage a major surgery.
- Involve other speciality teams such as haematology.

Intra-operative management

- Reduce venous oozing by avoiding venous congestion, high intrathoracic pressure and hypercarbia.
- Prevent hypothermia (use a fluid warmer and forced air body warmer), thus preventing coagulopathy.
- Hypotensive anaesthesia.
- Acute hypervolaemic haemodilution or cell salvage (needs to be discussed pre-operatively).
- Antifibrinolytic agents such as tranexamic acid.
- Red cell substitute, e.g. perfluorocarbons and haemoglobin solutions.

Surgical management

- Use a staged or laparoscopic procedure where appropriate.
- Meticulous haemostasis.
- Use of tourniquets.

Postoperative management

- ICU care.
- Close monitoring of bleeding and immediate treatment.
- Avoid hypothermia.
- Hyperbaric oxygen in the case of severe blood loss.

Cell salvage

Cell salvage is a procedure where lost blood from the operating site is collected. It is then processed and transfused back to the patient. This reduces the need for allogeneic blood transfusion and thus eliminates the risks associated with it. It is also more cost effective as compared to allogeneic blood transfusion.

Indications for cell salvage include:

- Anticipated blood loss of >1000ml or >20% estimated blood volume.
- Patients with a low haemoglobin or increased risk factors for bleeding.
- Patients with multiple antibodies or rare blood types.
- Patients with objections to receiving allogeneic (donor) blood.

Contraindications for cell salvage are patient refusal and blood contaminated with bowel contents.

The procedure of cell salvage includes collection of blood from the surgical site, separation of blood components and retransfusion.

Collection

Blood from the surgical site is collected by a double-lumen suction tube. It is immediately mixed with anticoagulants to prevent clotting. Blood is then filtered to remove large clots and collected in a reservoir.

Separation and washing

Collected blood is centrifuged to separate its components. Red blood cells are then washed with normal saline and passed through a semi-permeable membrane. This removes white blood cells, platelets, plasma and free haemoglobin which are collected in a separate bag and then removed.

Retransfusion

Red blood cells are resuspended in normal saline and transfused back to the patient. The salvaged blood has a haematocrit of about 50-80%. This can be done as a continuous circuit if requested by the patient. Otherwise, blood can be transfused within 6 hours.

Benefits of cell salvage

- Reduced need for allogeneic blood transfusion.
- More cost effective.
- Accepted by some Jehovah's Witnesses.
- Increased 2,3 diphosphoglycerate (2,3 DPG) and adenosine triphosphate (ATP) as compared to stored blood.

Risks of cell salvage

- Haemolysis.
- Contamination with surgical-site cleaning solutions, amniotic fluid.
- Coagulopathy due to removal of clotting factors, platelets and use of anticoagulants.

- Incomplete removal of leucocytes, plasma and platelets.
- Febrile non-haemolytic reactions.

Case scenario 1

A 60-year-old lady is scheduled for an elective total hip replacement. Her past medical history includes hypertension, previous deep vein thrombosis and hypercholesterolaemia. Her exercise tolerance is limited by arthritis. Her medications include enalapril, warfarin and simvastatin.

Her blood investigations are shown in Table 13.2.

What measures would you take to minimise the need for peri-operative blood transfusion?

This is an elective procedure that can lead to significant blood loss considering the patient is on oral anticoagulants. The patient's pre-operative haemoglobin does not warrant blood transfusion. Measures include the following:

- A further history and investigation may be necessary to find out the cause of her anaemia. Pre-operative oral iron therapy should be initiated to increase the haemoglobin concentration. Consider delaying the procedure until the haemoglobin is within normal limits. This should be discussed with the patient and surgeons.
- Warfarin should be stopped at least 5 days before the procedure and the INR normalised. Discuss this with the haematologist.
- Consider intra-operative cell salvage.
- Strategies to minimise intra-operative blood loss by the anaesthetist and surgeons as discussed earlier in the chapter.
- Monitor blood loss postoperatively. Restart oral anticoagulants as advised by the haematologist.

Table 13.2. Blood investigations.

		Normal values
Hb	9.1g/dL	11-16g/dL
Haematocrit	0.23	0.4-0.5 males, 0.37-0.47 females
RBC	2.75×10^{12}/L	$3.8-4.8 \times 10^{12}$/L
WBC	9.5×10^9/L	$4-11 \times 10^9$/L
Platelets	296×10^9/L	$150-450 \times 10^9$/L
INR	4.0	0.9-1.2

Case scenario 2

A 35-year-old female patient is undergoing an emergency Caesarean section under general anaesthesia. The indication for a Caesarean section was the previous two Caesarean sections. Her pre-operative blood investigations were normal. Following delivery of the baby, the surgeon informs the team that there is a significant amount of scar tissue and her uterus is not contracting well. Her heart rate is 120 beats per minute, blood pressure is 90/50mmHg and SpO_2 is 98%. Estimated blood loss is 1.5L.

What would be your management plan?

The management of this scenario includes:

- Call for more help and activate the major haemorrhage protocol.
- Establish another wide-bore intravenous access.
- Send bloods for a full blood count, cross-match and coagulation screen if not already done.

269

- Do not use excessive amounts of crystalloids.
- Use O-negative blood if required.
- Maintain temperature by using fluid warmers and forced air body warmers.
- Use vasopressors such as metaraminol to maintain mean arterial pressure above 60-70mmHg.
- Administer agents which will help the uterus to contract, such as Syntocinon®, ergometrine, carboprost.
- Administer tranexamic acid.
- Secure an arterial line and check the arterial blood gas.
- Administer blood and blood products as appropriate. Repeat the clotting profile to assess the response to transfusion.
- Admit the patient into a critical care setting postoperatively. Monitor for further blood loss and uterine tone, coagulation abnormalities, hourly urine output and inflammatory response.

Further reading

1. Contreras M, Ed. *ABC of Transfusion*, 4th ed. Blackwell Publishing Ltd, 2009.
2. Jabbour N, Ed. *Transfusion-Free Medicine and Surgery*. Blackwell Publishing Ltd, 2005.
3. The Association of Anaesthetists of Great Britain and Ireland (AAGBI). Blood transfusion and the anaesthetist, red cell transfusion 2, 2008. https://www.aagbi.org/sites/default/files/red_cell_08.pdf.
4. The Association of Anaesthetists of Great Britain and Ireland (AAGBI). Management of anaesthesia for Jehovah's Witnesses, 2nd ed, 2005. https://www.aagbi.org/sites/default/files/Jehovah's%20Witnesses_0.pdf.
5. The Association of Anaesthetists of Great Britain and Ireland (AAGBI). AAGBI safety guideline: blood transfusion and the anaesthetist, intra-operative cell salvage, 2009. https://www.aagbi.org/sites/default/files/cell%20_salvage_2009_amended.pdf.
6. Milligan L, Bellamy M. Anaesthesia and critical care of Jehovah's Witnesses. *Br J Anaesth CEACCP* 2004; 4: 35-9.
7. Ashworth A, Klien AA. Cell salvage as part of a blood conservation strategy in anaesthesia. *Br J Anaesth* 2010; 105: 401-16.
8. Klein AA, Arnold P, Bingham RM, et al. AAGBI guidelines: the use of blood components and their alternatives. *Anaesthesia* 2016; 71: 829-42.
9. Clevenger B, Richards T. Pre-operative anaemia. *Anaesthesia* 2015; 70 (Suppl. 1): 20-8.

14 Peri-operative temperature regulation

Anuji Amarasekara and Cyprian Mendonca

Introduction

Surgery and general anaesthesia impair the normal balance between heat production and heat loss, leaving patients essentially poikilothermic. The normal core temperature in adults is maintained between 36.5°C and 37.5°C.

Hypothermia is defined as a core body temperature of less than 36°C (96.8°F).

General or neuroaxial anaesthesia eliminates the natural behavioural modification to maintain body temperature effectively. Anaesthetised patients alter their thermoregulatory mechanisms, allowing unwarmed patients to be hypothermic.

Peri-operative hypothermia is associated with postoperative instability, an increased risk of myocardial infarction and prolonged recovery. Hypothermia also causes an increase in surgical blood loss, an increase in allogeneic blood transfusion and a three-fold increase in surgical-site infection. Increased shivering occurring as a result of hypothermia causes patients to increase oxygen utilisation.

Hyperthermia is a term used to indicate that the core body temperature has exceeded the normal values. This can be:

- Passive hyperthermia.
- Excessive heat production.

Passive hyperthermia does not result from thermoregulatory intervention and can simply be treated by discontinuing active warming and removing excess insulation.

Excessive heat production occurs in malignant hyperthermia where there is an enormous production of heat from internal organs and skeletal muscles. The thermoregulatory centre is intact in this condition; however, the heat loss mechanism may be compromised by intense vasoconstriction that occurs due to an almost 20 times increase in concentration of catecholamines.

Physiology

Core temperature is maintained at a very tight range of preset values. The reason for this is because the speed of chemical reactions varies with temperature. Normal enzymatic function and normal body functions occur optimally at a narrow therapeutic range of core temperature.

Thermoregulation can be considered in a two-compartmental model:

- Core compartment. This contributes to two-thirds of the body heat content and the temperature varies from 36.5-37.5°C. This helps to facilitate the cellular enzyme function. Core temperature is composed of well-perfused tissues and is generally higher and more uniform than the rest of the body.
- Peripheral compartment. This consists of skin and subcutaneous tissue. It is used to maintain the core temperature by absorbing and releasing thermal energy. This contributes to one-third of the total body heat content. The temperature in this compartment varies widely.

Temperature is regulated by three components (Figure 14.1):

- Afferent input.
- Central integrating system.
- Efferent response.

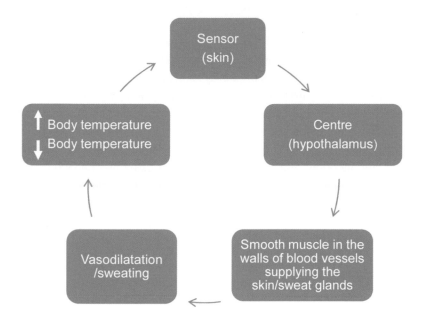

Figure 14.1. Normal temperature regulating system.

Afferent input

Afferent input is triggered by receptors found in the skin and all over the body. Receptors for cold are distinct from those for heat. Cold receptors get excited below a set threshold and generate impulses that are carried via A-delta fibres. Temperature above a certain threshold will stimulate the heat receptors, which would generate impulses via unmyelinated C fibres, which also carry pain sensation. Cell bodies of these nerve fibres are at the dorsal root ganglion. These connect the skin to the spinal column and brain. This information is then conducted at various levels to the brain and the spinal cord, finally arriving at the hypothalamus.

Central integrating system

Vertebrate species have the ability to maintain core body temperature by heat production and heat loss, which is primarily integrated by the hypothalamus. This gives us the ability to maintain core temperature within a narrow range regardless of the environmental temperature. The primary centre for thermoregulatory control is in the hypothalamus. Although some integration and temperature control may occur at the spinal cord, most afferent inputs coordinating various efferent outputs required to maintain normothermia occur at the hypothalamus. The exact mechanism by which the body maintains temperature control is unclear. However, it involves a number of neurotransmitters such as noradrenaline, dopamine, serotonin, acetylcholine and prostaglandin E1.

Efferent response

The efferent response is broadly divided into an autonomic and behavioural response.

About 80% of the autonomic response (sweating and shivering) is dependent on core temperature and is regulated by the anterior hypothalamus.

The behavioural response (seeking warm/cold environment or clothing) is 50% governed by skin temperature and controlled by the posterior hypothalamus.

Efferent output from the hypothalamus regulates body temperature by altering the subcutaneous blood flow, skeletal muscle tone and overall metabolic activity. This includes: sweating, pre-capillary vasodilatation, arteriovenous shunt, vasoconstriction, non-shivering thermogenesis and shivering.

Neural reflex control of cutaneous blood flow is by means of the adrenergic vasoconstrictive system and sympathetic vasodilator system, which is responsible for the majority of cutaneous vasodilatation during heat stress.

Maintenance of body temperature occurs as a form of negative feedback. Biochemical processes will not function adequately if the body temperature is too high or too low. At very high temperatures, enzymes lose their activity, and at very low temperatures, there is insufficient energy to maintain metabolic processes. The metabolic rate is reduced by up to 10% for every 1°C fall in body temperature.

Anaesthesia and temperature regulation

Peri-operative heat loss occurs mainly by radiation (60%), convection (25%) and evaporation (10%). Hypothermia during general anaesthesia occurs in the following three phases — outlined below (Figure 14.2).

Phase 1

Phase 1 is characterised by a rapid reduction in core temperature of 1-1.5°C, occurring within the first 30-45 minutes, mainly due to radiation. Vasodilatation induced by general anaesthesia inhibits normal tonic vasoconstriction causing a redistribution of heat from the core to peripheral tissues. This creates a temperature gradient between the core and peripheral tissues. Volatile anaesthetics, propofol and opioids promote heat loss through vasodilatation. In addition, opioids also depress overall sympathetic outflow, which further impairs any attempt on maintaining temperature.

Phase 2

Phase 2 is characterised by a more linear and gradual reduction in core temperature at a rate of 1°C over 2-3 hours of anaesthesia, occurring due to heat loss by radiation, convection and evaporation. Heat loss exceeds heat gain by metabolism.

Phase 3

Phase 3 is a plateau phase where heat loss is matched by heat production. When the core temperature is below a certain thermoregulatory threshold, peripheral vasoconstriction limits the heat loss from the core. When a balance is reached between the core heat production and the heat loss from the peripheries, the core temperature plateaus. The temperature does not plateau in diabetics, in those with impaired vasoconstriction or in those having combined regional and general anaesthesia

Regional anaesthesia also produces hypothermia, especially seen in epidural and spinal anaesthesia. Local anaesthetics do not have a direct action on the hypothalamus; however, the thermoregulatory centre can

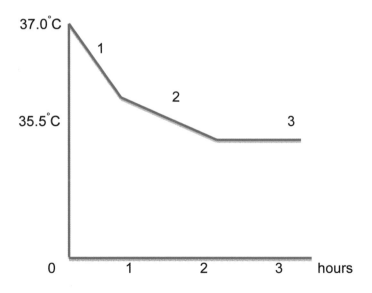

Figure 14.2. Three phases of heat loss during general anaesthesia.

become impaired. The thermoregulatory centre judges the skin temperature in the blocked region to be abnormally elevated. As a result, even though the core temperature has dropped, the patient will feel warm because the hypothalamus misinterprets the skin temperature. This can lead to patients becoming so hypothermic that they commence shivering despite having a subjective feeling of warmth. The use of sedation along with regional anaesthesia can worsen the depression of the thermoregulatory centre.

Consequences of peri-operative hypothermia

The consequences of peri-operative hypothermia are as follows:

- Cardiovascular effects. During the intra-operative period hypothermia decreases cardiac output and heart rate. Impairment of thermal comfort in the postoperative period causes shivering. This increase in stress could lead to a rise in heart rate and blood pressure, and an increase in oxygen consumption causing cardiac arrhythmias and ischaemia.
- Left shift of the oxygen dissociation curve results in decreased oxygen delivery to the tissues.
- Increased risk of surgical-site infection due to impaired immune function and thermoregulatory vasoconstriction as a result of decreased oxygen delivery.
- Coagulopathy due to decreased activity of enzymes that control the coagulation cascade and cold-induced inhibition of platelets.
- Altered mental status.
- Impaired renal function.
- Poor wound healing.
- Decreased drug metabolism: minimum alveolar concentration (MAC) of volatiles are reduced by 5% for each 1°C reduction in temperature.
- Increased intra-operative blood loss.
- Increased allogeneic blood transfusion requirement.

Prevention and management of hypothermia

Pre-operative

Pre-operative warming of peripheral tissue reduces the core to peripheral temperature gradient, thereby preventing the sudden drop of core temperature seen in Phase 1. For this to be effective, the patients need to be exposed to radiant heat for about 1 hour before anaesthesia. Advice can be given to patients to dress appropriately. This is an inexpensive way to minimise heat loss.

Intra-operative

Passive insulation with space blankets reduces the cutaneous heat loss by 30% due to entrapment of air between the blanket and the skin.

Active warming is more effective than passive insulation. Active warming involves a forced-air warmer such as a Bair Hugger™ (Figure 14.3), which

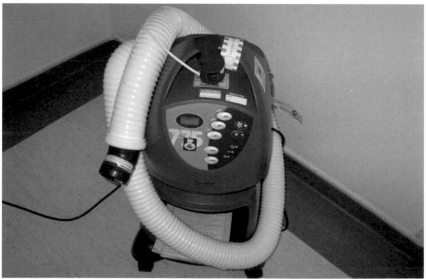

Figure 14.3. Bair Hugger™ warming device.

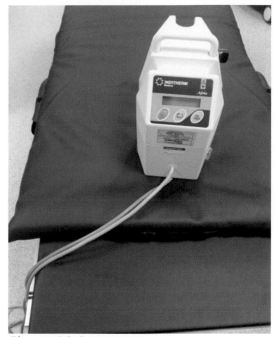

Figure 14.4. Warming mattress.

blows hot air into a blanket, thereby reducing heat loss by convection and radiation. It also increases the heat gain when the forced air is warmer than the skin. Active warming can also be provided using an electrical mattress (Figure 14.4), which can be placed on the operating table underneath the patient.

Fluid warming by administering fluid at room temperature reduces body temperature by 0.25°C; therefore, fluid should be warmed to body temperature before transfusing. A dry heat warmer (Figure 14.5) consists of two plates between which a PVC bag connected to the fluid giving set can be inserted.

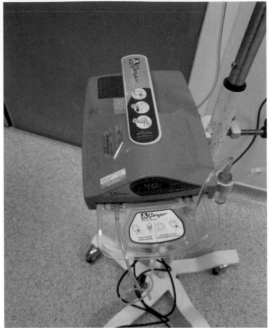

Figure 14.5. A fluid warming device — a dry heat warmer.

Airway humidification with a heat and moisture exchanging filter and low-flow breathing system prevents heat loss from respiration. As only <10% of body heat is lost via the respiratory tract, this does not contribute significantly to the prevention of hypothermia.

The room temperature of the operating theatre should be warmed to greater than 24°C during induction and whilst the patient is being prepared and draped.

The National Institute for Health and Care Excellence (NICE) guidelines

NICE guidelines published in 2008 provides the following key priorities for the prevention of peri-operative hypothermia.

Pre-operative phase

- Information should be given to the patient and their family with regard to the importance of staying warm before surgery which helps to reduce the risk of postoperative complications.
- Inform the patient that the hospital environment may be colder than their home.
- Advise the patient to bring additional clothing.
- Ask the patient to inform the hospital staff if they are feeling cold during their hospital stay.

On admission to the hospital

- Each patient should be assessed for the risk of inadvertent peri-operative hypothermia and the potential adverse consequences before transfer to the theatre suite.
- If a patient's temperature is <36°C, a forced-air warmer should be started unless there is a need to expedite surgery due to clinical urgency.

Intra-operative phase

- Temperature should be measured and documented every 30 minutes.
- Induction of anaesthesia should not commence until the temperature is 36°C or above.
- Intravenous fluids (>500ml) and blood should be warmed to 37°C using a fluid warming device.
- All patients having anaesthesia for more than 30 minutes should be warmed intra-operatively from induction using a forced-air warming device.
- All patients who are at high risk for inadvertent hypothermia should be warmed using a forced-air warming device intra-operatively from induction of anaesthesia.

Postoperative phase

- The patient's temperature should be measured and documented on admission to the recovery room and then every 15 minutes.
- Ward transfer should not be arranged until the patient's temperature is 36°C or above.
- If the patient's temperature is <36°C, they should be actively warmed using a forced-air warming device.

Case scenario 1

An 83-year-old male patient with intestinal obstruction secondary to possible malignancy is scheduled for a hemi-colectomy. His medical history includes ischaemic heart disease, moderate aortic stenosis and insulin-dependent diabetes mellitus.

Vital signs from the ward shows that his HR is 120/min, BP is 90/70mmHg, SaO_2 is 96% and temperature is 35.4°C.

How would you manage this patient?

Pre-operative management

His temperature should be checked on the ward. However, as this is an emergency, it would be unsuitable to delay the operation until his temperature is optimised. The patient should be given warm blankets on the ward and be transferred to theatre.

Intra-operative management

The patient's temperature drops quite steeply within the first 2 hours of induction.

In patients having a laparotomy, there is a continuous loss of temperature due to a loss of fluids via evaporation and due to third space loss. Intra-operative temperature monitoring is essential to maintain normothermia. A forced-air warmer should be used throughout the intra-operative period. Intra-operative fluids and blood should be warmed prior to transfusion. Temperature should be measured and recorded every 15 minutes due to heat loss by radiation, convection and evaporation.

Postoperative management

Continuous monitoring and maintenance of temperature is important to prevent hypothermia. The continuous use of a forced-air warmer may be necessary to prevent complications. The patient should ideally be managed in the intensive care unit or high dependency unit.

Further reading

1. Insler SR, Sessler DI. Perioperative thermoregulation and temperature monitoring. *Anaesthesiology Clinics* 2006; 24: 823-37.

2. Diaz M, Becker DE. Thermoregulation: physiological and clinical consideration during sedation and general anaesthesia. *Anaesth Prog* 2010; 57: 25-33.

3. Sessler DI. Temperature monitoring. In: Miller RD, ed. *Miller's Anaesthesia*, 6th ed. Elsevier Churchill Livingstone, 2005: 1571-97.

4. The National Institute for Health and Care Excellence. Inadvertent hypothermia guidelines. London, UK: NICE, 2008. www.nice.org.uk/nicemedia/pdf/CG65 Guidance.pdf.

15 Anaesthesia and endocrine disease

Kate Bosworth

Introduction

There are several important endocrine diseases that the anaesthetist needs to be aware of. This is because they can affect many areas of anaesthetic management including airway difficulties, drug interactions and acute changes in patient physiology. This chapter will explain the anaesthetic considerations for patients with a thyroid abnormality, adrenocortical disorder, diabetes mellitus, pituitary disease and porphyria.

Thyroid abnormality

Anaesthesia for thyroid surgery requires the anaesthetist to think about several important considerations. Firstly, the systemic manifestations of thyroid disease need to be determined and, secondly, the impact of goitres on the airway. There are many indications for thyroid surgery, which can range, depending on the cause (Table 15.1), from excision of a single nodule to removal of a complex, retrosternal goitre. The indication for surgery may be to remove malignancy, relieve airway obstruction or as part of the management of the systemic effects of hyperthyroidism.

Pre-operative assessment

The aim of pre-operative assessment is to assess for systemic complications of thyroid disease and to ensure that the patient is euthyroid. This is determined through taking a full history, examination and investigations.

Table 15.1. Causes of thyroid disease.

Hyperthyroidism	Hypothyroidism	Malignancy
Graves' disease - autoimmune condition	Hashimoto's thyroiditis	Papillary carcinoma
	Iodine deficiency	Follicular carcinoma
Toxic multinodular goitre		
		Medullary carcinomas
Solitary nodule/adenoma		- multiple endocrine neoplasia II (MEN II)
Others		
- exogenous		Lymphomas
- iodine		
- irradiation		
- amiodarone		

History

Symptoms such as dysphagia, orthopnoea, stridor and change in voice can indicate potential airway problems during induction of anaesthesia. The duration of any goitre is also important as this can determine the risk of postoperative complications such as tracheomalacia.

Examination

Patients should be examined for any systemic features of thyroid disease (Table 15.2). A thorough airway examination should be performed to determine whether there is any compromise or risk of a difficult intubation. The neck should be examined to assess the size of the goitre and whether there is any tracheal deviation.

Table 15.2. Clinical features of thyroid disease.

System	Hyperthyroidism	Hypothyroidism
General	Weight loss, increased appetite, malaise, heat intolerance	Weight gain, poor appetite, cold intolerance
Central nervous system (CNS)	Anxiety, tremor, irritable	Depression, psychosis, mental slowness, slow relaxing reflexes
Cardiovascular system (CVS)	Palpitations, tachy-arrhythmias, atrial fibrillation (AF), angina, hypertension, heart failure	Bradycardia, heart failure, anaemia
Gastrointestinal system (GI)	Diarrhoea, vomiting	Constipation
Genito-urinary system (GU)	Loss of libido, oligomenorrhoea	Loss of libido, menorrhagia
Eye	Blurred vision, exophthalmus, lid lag, conjunctival oedema	
Musculoskeletal system	Proximal muscle weakness and wasting	Myalgia
Skin	Palmar erythema, pretibial myxoedema (Graves' disease only)	Dry, coarse, 'peaches and cream' complexion

Investigations

The following investigations should be performed:

- Blood tests: full blood count (FBC), urea & electrolytes (U&Es), thyroid function tests (TFTs) and corrected calcium.
- Chest X-ray (CXR): to assess for tracheal deviation and retrosternal extension of goitres.
- CT scan: to assess for tracheal invasion or narrowing.
- Nasendoscopy: to determine any vocal cord palsy.
- Flow-volume loops: to check for fixed upper airway obstruction.

Intra-operative management

Premedication

The patient should take their usual antithyroid drugs on the day of surgery except carbimazole as this increases vascularity of the thyroid. Benzodiazepines can be given for anxiolysis but should not be used if there are any airway concerns. If an awake fibreoptic intubation is planned, anticholinergic drugs (e.g. glycopyrrolate 200µg) can be given to dry secretions.

In emergency surgery, symptoms of hyperthyroidism can be controlled using beta-blockers, intravenous hydration and cooling. Intravenous T3 and T4 can be given to severely hypothyroid patients.

Choice of anaesthetic technique

Thyroid surgery in the UK is mainly performed under a general anaesthetic. However, regional techniques have been used safely in other countries. Regional anaesthesia is achieved using deep and superficial cervical plexus blocks combined with or without sedation.

General anaesthesia

There are a variety of techniques used. After establishing standard monitoring (electrocardiogram [ECG], non-invasive blood pressure

[NIBP], pulse oximetry), intravenous (IV) access and pre-oxygenation, the following techniques can be used:

- Intravenous induction followed by a non-depolarising muscle relaxant and intubation with a reinforced endotracheal (ET) tube.
- Inhalational induction, using sevoflurane, can also be used if there are concerns regarding airway patency and abnormal anatomy.
- Awake fibreoptic intubation may be used if there is distorted anatomy or concern that the airway may be lost on induction.
- A tracheostomy under local anaesthetic can be performed by the surgeons prior to surgery if appropriate.
- Rigid bronchoscopy may be used to ventilate the patient if there is a failure to pass an ET tube due to mid-tracheal obstruction.

Anaesthesia is maintained using either IV or inhalational agents. Good muscle relaxation is important and this needs to be monitored. Remifentanil infusions are popular as they provide intra-operative analgesia and contribute to hypotensive anaesthesia. Remifentanil also reduces the need for muscle relaxants, thereby allowing intra-operative testing of the recurrent laryngeal nerve. During the procedure, there will be limited access to the airway so the ET tube should be taped securely. A head-up tilt is useful to allow venous drainage and eyes should be adequately padded. Intravenous dexamethasone is useful to reduce postoperative oedema and as an antiemetic. At the end of the procedure, the surgeon may request a Valsalva manoeuvre to check for haemostasis. Extubation is performed after full reversal of muscle relaxant, with the patient fully awake, breathing spontaneously and sat up. The ET tube cuff should be deflated to ensure a leak prior to extubation. Analgesia includes local anaesthetic infiltration by the surgeon, regular paracetamol, NSAIDs and weak opioids. Morphine may be required. Antiemetics such as ondansetron, cyclizine and dexamethasone should also be prescribed.

Postoperative complications

- Bleeding — haematoma formation can lead to neck swelling and airway obstruction. Therefore, stitch cutters must be kept by the patient's bedside just in case there is not enough time to take the patient to theatre.

- Laryngeal oedema — causing respiratory obstruction. Treatment is humidified oxygen and steroids.
- Recurrent laryngeal nerve palsy — unilateral palsy results in respiratory difficulty, a hoarse voice and difficulty in phonation. Bilateral palsy causes stridor and requires reintubation.
- Hypocalcaemia — due to parathyroid glands being damaged or removed. Features include perioral tingling, confusion, twitching and tetany. Treatment is with IV calcium replacement as hypocalcaemia can cause laryngospasm, cardiac irritability, arrhythmias and seizures.
- Tracheomalacia — due to tracheal compression by large tumours; this usually requires reintubation.
- Thyroid storm — this is a medical emergency characterised by hyperpyrexia, tachycardia, altered conscious level and hypotension. Treatment is with active cooling, hydration, beta-blockers and antithyroid drugs.
- Pneumothorax — very rare due to retrosternal dissection.

Adrenocortical disorders

The adrenal glands lie superior to each kidney and consist of an outer cortex and inner medulla. The cortex secretes glucocorticoids, mineralocorticoids and androgens. These steroid hormones have roles in metabolism, the stress response and fluid and electrolyte balance. The medulla secretes adrenaline and noradrenaline.

Hyperaldosteronism

This can be primary (Conn's syndrome) or secondary. In primary hyperaldosteronism, there is excess secretion of aldosterone from an adrenal adenoma, bilateral adrenal hyperplasia or carcinoma. Secondary hyperaldosteronism is due to high renin and aldosterone levels in plasma.

Clinical features include hypertension, hypokalaemia and a metabolic alkalosis, which should all be corrected pre-operatively. Treatment is with spironolactone (an aldosterone antagonist), ACE inhibitors and surgical removal of the adenoma.

Manipulation of the adrenal gland during removal can cause cardiovascular instability due to catecholamine secretion. This can be treated with a short-acting alpha-blocker, e.g. phentolamine. Patients may require replacement corticosteroids and mineralocorticoids with IV hydrocortisone (Table 15.3). Intra-operative hypokalaemia can prolong the duration of non-depolarising muscle relaxants.

Cushing's syndrome

This is due to excessive levels of glucocorticoids. This may be due to excess adrenocorticotropic hormone (ACTH) secretion from a pituitary adenoma (Cushing's disease) or from an adrenal adenoma or carcinoma. Patients may present with central obesity, a moon face, buffalo hump and thin skin. They may also have impaired glucose tolerance or diabetes mellitus, hypertension and obstructive sleep apnoea. There may be evidence of end-organ damage and an ECG may show evidence of ischaemic heart disease. A dose of steroids may be required pre-operatively (Table 15.3) if the cause of Cushing's syndrome is iatrogenic.

Adrenocortical insufficiency (Addison's disease)

Addison's disease is due to reduced or absent secretion of glucocorticoids and mineralocorticoids. It may be due to destruction of the adrenal cortex by autoantibodies, tuberculosis (TB), carcinoma or haemorrhage. Secondary hypoadrenalism results from prolonged steroid use and hypopituitarism. Clinical features include fatigue, weight loss, postural hypotension and increased pigmentation. They may be hypoglycaemic, hyponatraemic and hyperkalaemic. Diagnosis is with a short Synacthen test. Treatment is by replacement of steroids and mineralocorticoids.

Prior to surgery, these patients should have their regular medications. Serum potassium and glucose should be checked pre-operatively and regularly in the postoperative period. Steroid replacement may be necessary (Table 15.3) in patients who have been taking 10mg prednisolone daily or more in the past 3 months.

Table 15.3. Guidelines for peri-operative steroid replacement.

Type of surgery	Recommendation
Minor	25mg hydrocortisone at induction
Moderate	Usual pre-operative steroids + 25mg hydrocortisone at induction + 25mg hydrocortisone 6-hourly for 24 hours
Major	Usual pre-operative steroids + 25mg hydrocortisone at induction + 25mg hydrocortisone 6-hourly or 48-72 hours

Diabetes mellitus

Diabetes is the most common metabolic disorder and patients who present for surgery often have coexisting comorbidities and complications of diabetes. Microvascular complications include: diabetic nephropathy leading to renal failure; retinopathy leading to retinal detachment and vitreous haemorrhage; and neuropathy leading to sensory, motor and autonomic polyneuropathies. Macrovascular complications include cardiovascular disease, hypertension, peripheral vascular disease and cerebrovascular disease. The presence of these complications and glycaemic control need to be assessed and optimised at the pre-operative assessment.

Pre-operative assessment

As well as the complications of diabetes, the type, duration and current treatment need to be ascertained. Glycaemic control over the previous 3 months can be determined using haemoglobin A1c (HbA1c) and this should be optimised. The degree of peripheral neuropathy should be assessed and documented prior to performing any regional technique. Symptoms of autonomic neuropathy such as orthostatic hypotension, gustatory sweating and impotence need to be considered. These patients are at increased risk of regurgitation and aspiration. Patients may also suffer from stiff joint syndrome, which may affect cervical spine movement. Investigations performed should include blood glucose, HbA1c, urinalysis for albumin and ketones, FBC, U&Es and an ECG.

Intra-operative management

- Maintenance of normoglycaemia peri-operatively (blood glucose between 6-10mmol/L). Hyperglycaemia can occur due to catabolic hormones increasing blood glucose levels. This can be reduced by the use of regional anaesthetic techniques and opioids. Hypoglycaemia may occur due to prolonged starvation. Patients taking oral hypoglycaemics should omit these on the morning of surgery. Patients who have an anticipated short starvation period and who are taking insulin should be managed according to local policies. Patients who are likely to have prolonged periods of starvation, however, will most likely require a variable rate intravenous insulin infusion (VRIII).
- Minimise pre-operative starvation and early resumption of oral intake and usual medication — patients should be first or early on in the operating list order.
- Prevention of postoperative nausea and vomiting.

Choice of anaesthetic technique

There is no evidence that regional anaesthesia improves morbidity and mortality after major surgery in diabetics compared with general anaesthesia. Advantages of regional techniques include: an awake patient, no need for airway intervention, a decreased catabolic hormone response and good postoperative care. Disadvantages of neuraxial techniques include increased cardiovascular instability with diabetic autonomic neuropathy and increased risk of infection. Disadvantages of peripheral nerve blocks include worsening of neuropathy by direct damage and increased risk of local anaesthetic toxicity. Whichever techniques are used, blood glucose levels should be regularly measured intra-operatively and postoperatively. Insulin infusions may need to be adjusted and glucose may need to be given. Potassium levels should also be measured regularly.

Postoperative care

Patients should be prescribed appropriate analgesia, antiemetics and intravenous fluids for the postoperative period. Good analgesia will decrease catabolic hormone secretion, which helps with glucose control. NSAIDs should be avoided as they may impair renal function.

Pituitary disease

The pituitary gland has a central role in the neuroendocrine axis and controls the secretion of many hormones. Pituitary tumours can present in different ways. They may present as hormone hyper-secretion, e.g. Cushing's disease (excess adrenocorticotrophic hormone [ACTH]) and acromegaly (excess growth hormone [GH]) or hypo-secretion, e.g. adrenocortical insufficiency, hypothyroidism and diabetes insipidus. They may also present with mass effects, e.g. headache, visual field defects and cranial nerve palsies or as an incidental finding. Management of pituitary tumours can either be medical or surgical. The majority of surgical resections are via the trans-sphenoidal approach. The extent of pituitary dysfunction needs to be determined and a full endocrine review should be sought. Hormonal and antihypertensive medications should be continued.

Acromegaly

A careful airway assessment is required in patients with acromegaly. These patients may be difficult to intubate due to macrognathia, macroglossia and upper airway tissue hypertrophy. Awake fibreoptic intubation may be required in these patients. Patients with acromegaly may also have obstructive sleep apnoea due to enlarged upper airway soft tissue and symptoms of these patients need to be assessed, as this may lead to postoperative airway difficulty and cardiorespiratory instability. Patients with acromegaly may also have hypertension and left ventricular hypertrophy, ischaemic heart disease, arrhythmias and ventricular dysfunction. A pre-operative echocardiogram may be required.

Central diabetes insipidus

This is due to failure of antidiuretic hormone (ADH) secretion. It is treated with desmopressin orally or intranasally. It may be given intramuscularly or subcutaneously in the peri-operative period.

Intra-operative management

Aims of anaesthesia:

- Optimise cerebral oxygenation.
- Maintain haemodynamic stability.
- Facilitate surgical exposure.
- Smooth, rapid emergence.
- Invasive monitoring including invasive arterial blood pressure and central venous pressure if required.

Choice of anaesthetic technique

This depends on the patient's comorbidities. During induction, patients should be given antibiotics and IV hydrocortisone. Induction can either be via the intravenous or inhalational route. Remifentanil is useful for stimulating parts of the surgery and it maintains good haemodynamic control and rapid recovery. This allows early postoperative neurological assessment and reduces postoperative airway problems. Analgesia includes paracetamol and opioids. NSAIDs are generally avoided due to the risk of haematomas. Routine antiemetic prophylaxis should also be given. Intra-operative complications during pituitary surgery include haemorrhage and venous air embolism due to the semi-sitting position, although these are both rare.

Postoperative care

Patients should be nursed on a high dependency area due to the risk of airway obstruction. The level of consciousness, eye movements, visual fields and acuity should all be regularly tested postoperatively. Postoperative complications after transsphenoidal surgery include CSF rhinorrhoea, meningitis, vascular damage, cranial nerve injury, cerebral ischaemia and stroke. Patients can also develop postoperative neuroendocrine abnormalities such as diabetes insipidus. This usually develops within the first 24 hours and can be treated with oral or intranasal desmopressin. Hyponatraemia due to the syndrome of inappropriate ADH secretion (SIADH) may also occur. This is treated with fluid restriction of 500-1000ml daily. Patients require hormone replacement such as steroids and other hormones depending on the patient's hormone function.

Porphyria

The porphyrias are a heterogeneous group of inherited disorders involving the biosynthesis of haem. They are classified into acute and chronic but only the acute porphyrias are relevant to anaesthesia as these are the ones that can deteriorate into an acute crisis. The acute porphyrias include: acute intermittent porphyria (AIP), variegate porphyria (VP), hereditary coproporphyria (HCP) and 5-aminolevulinic acid (ALA) dehydratase deficiency.

Pre-operative assessment

A full medical and family history needs to be taken as well as a systemic examination, with particular attention to the neurological system. Any peripheral or autonomic neuropathy needs to be noted as this may indicate active disease. All staff involved in the care of the patient in the peri-operative period need to be aware. Patients may be admitted on the day of surgery and may be administered an anxiolytic, e.g. a benzodiazepine. Fasting should be minimised and they should receive IV dextrose saline. Patients are not suitable for day-case surgery.

Intra-operative management

There are many drugs that are safe to give to these patients for general anaesthesia (Table 15.4). There is no absolute contraindication for the use of regional anaesthesia in porphyria but a full neurological and cardiovascular examination should be performed prior to this. There is no evidence to suggest that one technique is superior to the other in these patients.

Implications for anaesthesia

The acute porphyrias can develop into life-threatening neurovisceral crises that may be triggered by certain factors and drugs. Signs and symptoms of an acute crisis may include abdominal pain, tachycardia, arrhythmias, hypertension, muscle weakness, confusion, mood disturbance, pain and sensory disturbance, seizures and a vesicular rash. The patient's urine may also darken on standing. They may also present with hyponatraemia and hypomagnesaemia. Crises are more common in females and usually occur in their early 30s. It is therefore important to avoid any precipitating triggers. Triggers include: fasting, dehydration, infections, drugs, endogenous hormones, physical or emotional stress, smoking and alcohol. The management of an acute crisis is to remove all precipitants, avoid a catabolic state by administering carbohydrate supplements and IV haem arginate. Haem arginate will suppress hepatic production of ALA and other precursors by replenishing haem. The dose is 3mg/kg once a day for 4 days. Supportive care is also necessary, such as analgesia, antiemetics and anxiolytics. Seizures may be treated with benzodiazepines whilst hypertension and tachycardia can be treated safely with beta-blockers. Ventilatory support may be required if there is respiratory failure.

Table 15.4. Drug safety in porphyria.

Drug class	Unsafe	Undetermined	Safe
IV anaesthetic agents	Thiopentone Ketamine	Etomidate	Propofol
Inhalational anaesthetic agents	Sevoflurane		Isoflurane Desflurane Nitrous oxide
Local anaesthetics		Levobupivacaine Ropivacaine	Bupivacaine Prilocaine Lignocaine
Muscle relaxants and reversal			Suxamethonium NDMRs Neostigmine
Analgesia	Oxycodone Diclofenac	Mefenamic acid	Fentanyl Alfentanil Remifentanil Morphine Tramadol Ibuprofen Aspirin Paracetamol
Sedatives			Lorazepam Phenothiazines Temazepam

Continued

Table 15.4 *continued.* Drug safety in porphyria.

Drug class	Unsafe	Undetermined	Safe
Antibiotics	Rifampicin Erythromycin		Gentamicin Co-amoxiclav Penicillins Vancomycin Tazocin
Cardiovascular drugs	Vasopressin Metaraminol	Ephedrine	Adrenaline Noradrenaline Atropine Glycopyrrolate Beta-blockers Phenylephrine Magnesium Milrinone
Others		Dexamethasone Hydrocortisone Clopidogrel	Fibrinolytics Syntocinon Carboprost Tranexamic acid Aprotinin

NDMR = non-depolarising muscle relaxant.

Postoperative care

Avoidance of precipitating factors and drugs is also important in the postoperative period. Effective analgesia is important in the postoperative period and patients may require a patient-controlled analgesia (PCA) system. Diclofenac should be avoided as it may precipitate a crisis. Nausea can be safely managed with ondansetron and prochlorperazine.

Case scenario 1

A 65-year-old non-insulin-dependent diabetic patient presents for a knee arthroscopy. His diabetes is well controlled on metformin alone.

Can he be listed for a day-case procedure?

If his diabetes is well controlled and he has no major comorbidities, then he can have this as a day-case procedure.

What advice do you need to give him in the pre-operative assessment clinic?

He does not need to take his metformin on the day of his operation.

Does he require an insulin infusion during his period of starvation?

No, as long as there is not a prolonged period of fasting and his blood sugars are checked regularly in the peri-operative period.

Are there any other considerations that need to be taken into account for this patient in the peri-operative period?

He should be put first on the operating list. It should be mentioned at the WHO team brief that he is a diabetic patient. His blood sugars need to be regularly measured.

When can he restart his metformin?

As soon as he is eating and drinking normally.

Case scenario 2

A 78-year-old non-insulin-dependent diabetic lady presents with acute small bowel obstruction. She is vomiting and is booked for an emergency laparotomy.

What is important for you to know from the pre-operative assessment?

We need to know how well her diabetes is controlled and what her blood sugars have been since admission; during an acute illness, blood sugars can increase due to the release of stress hormones. Also, we need to know if she has any complications of diabetes including ischaemic heart disease, renal disease, peripheral or autonomic neuropathy.

What should be done regarding her usual medications?

Any oral hypoglycaemic agents should be stopped during the time in which she is 'nil by mouth'. She should be started on a variable rate intravenous insulin infusion (VRIII)(Table 15.5).

Should she be started on an insulin infusion?

Yes. She should be started on a VRIII at the standard rate initially. Capillary blood glucose should be checked every hour and VRIII adjusted accordingly. The blood glucose level should ideally be between 6-10mmol/L.

Which IV fluid should be prescribed alongside the VRIII?

- Always check the patient's U&Es before prescribing IV fluids.
- If blood glucose is ≥14.0mmol/L, use 0.9% sodium chloride with 20-40mmol potassium at 125ml/hr.

- If blood glucose is <14.0mmol/L, use 5% glucose with 40mmol potassium at 125ml/hr.
- The rate of fluid replacement must be set to deliver the hourly fluid requirements of the individual patient.
- Aim to keep potassium levels between 4.5-5.5mmol/L.

How should her diabetes be managed in the postoperative period?

- Her blood sugars need to be regularly measured.
- She will need to continue the VRIII until she is eating and drinking normally.
- She may need a referral to the diabetes nurse or team to adjust her medications.

Table 15.5. Example of a variable rate insulin infusion (49.5ml 0.9% sodium chloride + 50 units Actrapid® in a 50ml syringe).

Glucose mmol/L	Insulin rates (ml/hr) Commence on standard rate unless otherwise indicated		
	Reduced rate	Standard rate	Increased rate
<4.0	0	0	0
4.1-8.0	0.5	1	2
8.1-12.0	1	2	4
12.1-16.0	2	4	6
16.1-20.0	3	5	7
20.1-24.0	4	6	8
>24.1	6	8	10

Further reading

1. Menon R, Murphy P, Lindley A. Anaesthesia and pituitary disease. *Br J Anaesth CEACCP* 2011; 11: 133-7.

2. Adams L, Davies S. Anaesthesia for thyroid surgery. Anaesthesia tutorial of the week: 162, 2009.

3. Malhotra, Sodhi V. Anaesthesia for thyroid and parathyroid surgery. *Br J Anaesth CEACCP* 2007; 7: 55-8.

4. Davies M, Hardman J. Anaesthesia and adrenocortical disease. *Br J Anaesth CEACCP* 2005; 5: 122-6.

5. Findley H, Philips A, Cole D, Nair A. Porphyrias: implications for anaesthesia, critical care, and pain medicine. *Br J Anaesth CEACCP* 2012; 12: 128-33.

6. Nicholson G, Hall G. Diabetes and adult surgical inpatients. *Br J Anaesth CEACCP* 2011; 11: 234-8.

16 Anaesthesia and cardiovascular disease

Narcis Ungureanu and Cyprian Mendonca

Introduction

One in 30 patients suffer cardiac complications following surgery and anaesthesia. Most of these cardiac complications are due to ischaemic heart disease, as 60% of patients who die within 30 days of their surgery have coronary artery disease.

Significant coronary artery stenosis and unstable coronary artery plaques are the main pathophysiological mechanisms behind ischaemic heart disease. Peri-operative tachycardia, hypertension and inflammatory markers disrupt these unstable plaques which can lead to temporary or permanent occlusion.

The imbalance between oxygen demand and oxygen supply caused by hypotension, hypertension, tachycardia, hypoxia, anaemia or left ventricular distension in the presence of coronary artery stenosis causes myocardial ischaemia and subsequent structural damage to the cardiac muscle.

The prevention of cardiovascular peri-operative complications of ischaemic heart disease include:

- Identification of high-risk patients.
- Coronary revascularisation in selected patients.
- Prophylactic pharmacological protection.
- Monitoring and management of peri-operative haemodynamic abnormalities.

Similar principles to prevent peri-operative complications apply to other cardiovascular conditions which are relevant to anaesthetists and surgeons. The peri-operative safe management of patients with pacemakers as well as that of patients with hypertension, cardiomyopathy and valvular diseases will be addressed in this chapter.

The emphasis will be on the fact that vigilance should be exercised at all times in order to provide safe peri-operative care, especially because patients with some of these conditions could present for an emergency or elective surgery with very few clues in the history or even undiagnosed.

The new evidence-based modalities such as plasma brain natriuretic peptide (BNP) concentration and cardiopulmonary exercise testing (CPET) have the potential to contribute significantly to the evaluation of peri-operative cardiac risk.

The new guidelines from the National Institute for Health and Care Excellence (NICE) for the diagnosis and management of essential hypertension and for antibiotic prophylaxis for patients with valvular disease who undergo other non-cardiac procedures will be presented in their respective sections.

The peri-operative management of patients on dual-antiplatelet therapy, who are in the high-risk period following a percutaneous coronary intervention, will be discussed. The emphasis will be on the use of novel therapies like the oral reversible platelet aggregation blocking agent (the non-thienopyridine P2Y12 receptor antagonist ticagrelor) or the intravenous version of the same class of drug (cangrelor) and their potential combination with a bridging therapy like a GPIIb/IIIa inhibitor (e.g. tirofiban).

Hypertension

Hypertension is defined by NICE as a measurement of 140/90mmHg or higher in clinic, with subsequent ambulatory or home measurement of 135/85mmHg or higher.

NICE guidelines define three stages of hypertension after the measured clinic blood pressure: Stage 1 (140/90mmHg or higher), Stage 2 (160/100mmHg or higher) and Stage 3 — severe hypertension (180/110mmHg or higher).

The link between hypertension and cardiovascular disease is well established, the greatest risk being associated with the highest pressures. A significant percentage of adult patients undergoing anaesthesia are hypertensive. Patients with hypertension-induced end-organ damage like heart failure, ischaemic heart disease, cerebrovascular disease or renal failure have an increased risk of peri-operative cardiovascular complications.

Antihypertensive medication

The NICE guidelines on the treatment of hypertension were updated in 2011. They describe and advise a four-step approach to treatment:

- Step 1 can include an angiotensin-converting enzyme inhibitor (ACEI), an angiotensin-II receptor blocker (ARB) or a calcium channel blocker (CCB) if the patient is over 55 years of age or of Afro-Caribbean descent. Thiazide-like diuretics can replace any of the above in the case of intolerance.
- Step 2 includes a calcium channel blocker (CCB) in combination with an ACEI or an ARB (preferred for African or Caribbean patients). A thiazide-like diuretic can replace the CCB in the case of intolerance.
- Step 3 includes triple therapy — an ACEI (or ARB) in combination with a CCB and a thiazide-like diuretic.
- Step 4 introduces a forth antihypertensive to the triple therapy. This could be another diuretic like spironolactone, an increase in the thiazide diuretic therapy or an alpha- or beta-blocker in the case of failure or intolerance with the above mentioned drugs.

The patient can present for anaesthesia on single therapy or with a combination of the above drugs which could suggest the hypertension stage and point towards a particular end-organ damage.

Patients who are an elective surgical case are usually given their regular antihypertensive medications on the morning of surgery.

The use of drugs that block the renin-angiotensin system in the peri-operative period

It is generally recommend that ACEIs and ARBs be withheld on the day of surgery in order to reduce the risk of hypotension under anaesthesia. However, in patients with heart failure or resistant hypertension, continuing to take ACEIs peri-operatively may be beneficial provided the episodes of hypotension are managed with intravenous fluids and vasopressors. Other benefits provided by these agents are renal protection, neuroprotection in cerebrovascular surgery and reduced rates of peri-operative atrial fibrillation.

Pre-operative evaluation and investigations

The first step is to try and establish if it is primary (also called essential) or secondary hypertension. Secondary hypertension due to phaeochromocytoma, hyperaldosteronism, renal vascular or parenchymal diseases or pre-eclampsia have particular anaesthetic implications.

The second step is to ascertain the stage of the hypertension. Patients with Stage 3 hypertension (systolic >180mmHg, diastolic >110mmHg) or above should have this treated prior to elective surgery. Emergency and urgent surgery can be performed in these patients after careful consideration of the risks and benefits, with regional techniques playing an important role if the decision was taken to proceed with anaesthesia.

The third step is to establish if there is any end-organ damage. The presence of coronary or cerebrovascular disease, renal impairment, ventricular hypertrophy and cardiac failure will require not only the control of the elevated blood pressure but also further investigations and possibly other treatments prior to surgery.

Investigations

ECG changes may include left ventricular hypertrophy, bundle branch block and evidence of an old myocardial infarction such as Q waves. If significant cardiac disease is suspected, an exercise tolerance test should be performed.

Peri-operative management

The cardiovascular risk of patients with systolic blood pressure of less than 180mmHg and diastolic pressure of less than 110mmHg is not significant and surgery should not be deferred based on a single hospital reading or even after several readings done on the day of surgery. The patient's primary care doctor should have records which could help decision making on the day. Proven 'white coat' hypertension does not represent an increased peri-operative risk and surgery should not be delayed unnecessarily.

Patients with Stage 1 and Stage 2 hypertension are not at an increased risk of cardiovascular complications. Surgery should go ahead as scheduled and they should continue their antihypertensive medication peri-operatively.

Patients with Stage 3 hypertension and no evidence of end-organ involvement should not be deferred only on the basis of elevated blood pressure. The aim during surgery is to maintain cardiovascular stability by using invasive monitoring and correcting deviations of greater than 20% from the baseline. Postoperative monitoring in the high dependency unit is advised if these patients are cardiovascularly unstable during surgery or have undergone major procedures.

An elective surgical procedure in a patient with Stage 3 hypertension and evidence of end-organ damage should be postponed for 4 weeks to have his/her blood pressure controlled and the cause investigated.

Conduct of anaesthesia

Cardiovascular stability and pre-optimisation of blood pressure through investigations and treatment allow a better manipulation of physiology and pharmacology, making anaesthesia safer.

In addition to standard monitoring, invasive blood pressure monitoring in high-risk patients allows early detection and pharmacological intervention during anaesthesia.

Hypertensive patients require higher than normal levels of blood pressure in keeping with their existing day-to-day readings for adequate organ perfusion (especially the elderly). Avoiding apparent normotension and hypotension in these cases prevents complications of underperfusion. This approach is also relevant in managing patients in the postoperative period on the ward or in the HDU/ICU setting.

Induction of anaesthesia

Significant hypotension may occur on induction of anaesthesia and a significant hypertension may occur during stimulating procedures such as laryngoscopy, intubation and surgical interventions.

Short-acting opioids such as fentanyl 1µg/kg or alfentanil 10µg/kg and a target-controlled infusion of remifentanil in conjunction with the induction agent of choice will provide more haemodynamic stability at induction. Ketamine should be avoided due to its cardiovascular stimulatory effects.

Maintenance

In order to minimise the hypertensive episodes during surgery, one should avoid hypoxia, hypercarbia, light anaesthesia and provide adequate pain management by using opioids and regional techniques when suitable.

Vasopressor drugs and intravenous fluids may be required and could be used if cardiac depression causes hypotension or when this happens following spinal or epidural anaesthesia, especially in dehydrated patients on vasodilator drugs.

Management of intra-operative hypertensive crisis

The aim is to prevent a hypertensive stroke and/or subendocardial ischaemia of the myocardium. The surgeon should be informed and requested to stop the surgery until the blood pressure is under control.

The depth of anaesthesia and analgesia (a target-controlled remifentanil infusion is useful here) should be increased.

Pharmacological methods to decrease blood pressure include the use of vasodilators (hydralazine 5mg every 15 minutes or a GTN infusion 50mg diluted in 50ml of 0.9% NaCl started at 3mg/hour or magnesium sulphate 2-4g IV over 10 minutes), beta-blockers (especially if an arrhythmia or tachycardia are present) (labetalol 5-10mg IV or esmolol 25-100mg bolus followed by an IV infusion of 50-200µg/kg/min) or alpha-blockers such as phentolamine 10mg diluted in 10ml of 0.9% NaCl, administered as 1mg IV boluses until the desired effect is seen (especially if bradycardia or a normal heart rate is present).

If the increase in blood pressure was unexpected, prolonged, and difficult to control or the patients have symptoms in recovery, they should be investigated with serial ECGs, cardiac enzymes, thyroid function tests and a 24-hour urinary catecholamine excretion assessment.

Recovery

Standard monitoring and a calm recovery room with suitable trained staff are important, especially for confused anxious patients.

Emergence cough hypertension can be prevented by anaesthetising the vocal cords pre-operatively or by performing deep extubation.

Hypertension can have many reversible causes in recovery (pain, anxiety, uterine retention, hypercarbia) and once these are treated or excluded, it is reasonable to treat persistent systolic blood pressure readings of 200mmHg or above.

Ischaemic heart disease

Ischaemic heart disease is a significant risk factor for peri-operative morbidity. A significant number of patients who die within 30 days of surgery have evidence of ischaemic heart disease. In the presence of coronary artery stenosis, peri-operative hypotension, tachycardia and hypertension causes an imbalance between oxygen supply and demand to the myocardium resulting in myocardial ischaemia. In addition, peri-operative release of inflammatory mediators as well as hypertension and tachycardia promote plaque disruption in the presence of unstable plaques. This will result in temporary or permanent occlusion of the respective coronary artery.

Peri-operative risks associated with ischaemic heart disease

Ischaemic heart disease may lead to myocardial infarction, which can be non-fatal or extensive enough to cause death.

The risk is determined by patient factors, including their functional capacity (Tables 16.1, 16.2 and 16.3), and the nature of surgery.

The surgery can be regarded as high-risk (>5% death/non-fatal MI), intermediate-risk (<5% death/non-fatal MI) and low-risk (<1% death/non-fatal MI).

The functional capacity can be assessed by using the Duke Activity Status Index and is expressed in metabolic equivalents of task (METs).

Patients who are unable to sustain 4 METs of physical activity (that is eating, dressing, walking around the house) and undergo high-risk surgery, have adverse outcomes.

Table 16.1. Major risk predictors (suggesting unstable coronary disease).

- Recent MI (<1 month before surgery).
- Unstable/severe angina.
- Significant arrhythmia.
- Severe valvular disease.
- Ongoing ischaemia.
- Decompensated heart failure.
- Bare-metal stent (BMS) <6 weeks before.
- Drug-eluting stent (DES) <1 year before.

Table 16.2. Intermediate risk predictors (suggesting stable coronary disease).

- MI >1 month before.
- Stable angina.
- Abnormal renal function.
- Diabetes.
- Compensated heart failure.

Table 16.3. Minor risk predictors (suggesting a high probability of cardiac pathology).

- Abnormal ECG (especially other rhythms).
- Previous CVA.
- Uncontrolled hypertension.
- Low functional capacity.
- Decreased physiological reserve.

Pre-operative evaluation and investigations of patients with suspected ischaemic heart disease

The aim is to confirm the diagnosis (starting with a thorough history and clinical examination) and to identify high-risk patients.

An electrocardiogram (ECG) may reveal arrhythmias or conduction abnormalities, but it can be normal in many patients.

A dynamic investigation like dobutamine echocardiography, radionuclide angiography or myocardial dipyridamole thallium scintigraphy under physical- or pharmacological-induced stress will reveal reversible myocardial ischaemia.

Cardiopulmonary exercise testing (CPET) can be performed as part of a protocol for major intra-cavity or vascular surgery. An anaerobic threshold of less than 11ml/min/kg associated with evidence of ischaemia on the pre-operative ECG is indicative of high mortality in these patients.

B-type natriuretic peptide (BNP) estimation is a biochemical marker used in the diagnosis and prognosis of left ventricular dysfunction, but recent studies have indicated it to be an independent predictor for postoperative cardiac mortality in non-cardiac surgery.

Coronary artery bypass surgery (CABG) before non-cardiac surgery

Indications for CABG include patients with poorly controlled angina, significant main stem stenosis, severe coronary artery disease involving two or three vessels including the proximal left anterior descending artery and coronary lesions associated with significant left ventricular dysfunction. Some patients with less important coronary lesions might benefit from undergoing prophylactic revascularisation before high-risk surgery (major thoracic, vascular, major head and neck or other procedures with significant fluid shifts and haemodynamic changes).

Percutaneous coronary interventions (PCIs) involve balloon angioplasty and the insertion of bare-metal (BMS) or drug-eluting stents (DES) followed by dual-antiplatelet therapy (aspirin plus a thienopyridine (e.g. clopidogrel) or a P2Y12 reversible receptor blocker (e.g. ticagrelor) for 12 months or more (for complicated lesions).

Surgery after coronary revascularisation procedures

Following CABG, subsequent elective surgery should be delayed for at least 3 months.

Aspirin is normally continued for life by these patients.

The second antiplatelet agent is recommended for a minimum of 6 weeks for bare-metal stents (BMS) and a minimum of 12 months for drug-eluting stents (DES). Stopping this second antiplatelet agent during this high-risk period carries an increased risk of stent thrombosis.

Peri-operative management of patients who underwent percutaneous coronary intervention and stent insertion within the high-risk period

There is conflicting evidence between large studies regarding the risk of a severe haemorrhage in most types of elective surgery when dual antiplatelet therapy is continued. Most of the elective surgeries can be postponed until agents like clopidogrel can be safely stopped. In the situation where a surgery cannot be postponed, the benefits of stopping antiplatelet agents should be balanced against the risk of stent thrombosis and possible death. Therefore, in some situations, surgery can be carried out without stopping antiplatelet agents. The exceptions are spinal and neurosurgery, posterior eye surgery and transurethral prostatectomy procedures when the haemorrhage could be catastrophic and antiplatelets like clopidogrel should be stopped. Spinal and epidural anaesthesia cannot be performed if the patient is on dual-antiplatelet therapy. The newer reversible antiplatelet agents (e.g. ticagrelor — an oral non-thienopyridine P2Y12 receptor antagonist), are recently recommended by NICE for the management of patients who undergo PCI for acute coronary syndromes, as they may have some benefit over clopidogrel.

Clinical studies show that the bleeding risk of stopping ticagrelor for 24 to 72 hours is comparable to that of stopping clopidogrel for 5 days. This rapid 'off-set' of its action can be used in combination with the so-called bridging therapy infusion (a GPIIb/IIIa inhibitor, e.g. tirofiban) that could continue until 4 hours before the scheduled surgery. The ticagrelor can be reloaded after the surgical intervention if the decision to stop it before surgery was taken by a multidisciplinary team which includes the surgeon, the anaesthetist and the cardiologist.

Peri-operative medical therapy

Chronic beta-blockade therapy should be continued due to its anti-inflammatory properties which stabilise the plaques. Acute peri-operative beta-blockade, although beneficial in reducing the risk of non-fatal MI, increases the risk of stroke and overall mortality and should be avoided.

Alpha 2 agonists like clonidine (up to 300µg a day) are beneficial and represent an alternative to beta-blockers.

Nitrates and calcium channel blockers should be continued during the peri-operative period.

ACE inhibitors improve survival in patients with left ventricular dysfunction and offer benefits to patients with diabetes or vascular disease with normal ventricular function. If continued, they increase the risk of peri-operative hypotension and more invasive monitoring is required.

Statins are likely to offer cardiac protection through their anti-inflammatory effects and their chronic use should continue as there is a significantly increased risk of cardiovascular events if statins are stopped during the peri-operative period.

Conduct of anaesthesia

No particular anaesthetic technique is superior for patients with ischaemic heart disease.

Intra-operative attention to blood pressure and heart rate are mandatory and this can be achieved for most patients and procedures by using the standard monitoring as per The Association of Anaesthetists of Great Britain and Ireland (AAGBI) recommendations. High and intermediate-risk patients undergoing major surgery are likely to benefit from invasive arterial pressure and cardiac output monitoring. In addition, central venous access is useful for administering inotropic drugs. Blood pressure and heart rate should be maintained within 20% of their initial values.

Regional anaesthesia offers the benefit of preventing pain-induced tachycardia and should be used if indicated and possible. Intra-operative hypertension and tachycardia can be treated using short-acting beta-blockers.

Postoperatively, tachycardia and hypertension are best avoided by adequate pain management which should include the use of regional anaesthesia. Haemoglobin levels should be maintained above 9g/dL. High- and intermediate-risk patients undergoing major surgery should be monitored in HDU postoperatively and should receive supplemental oxygen for 72 hours.

Cardiomyopathy

Cardiomyopathy is a disease of the heart muscle. Classically it has been described as being idiopathic or secondary to other disease processes.

There are three main types of cardiomyopathy:

- Hypertrophic obstructive cardiomyopathy (HOCM).
- Dilated cardiomyopathy.
- Restrictive cardiomyopathy.

Most patients suffering with cardiomyopathy have arrhythmias or heart failure and have little reserve for surgery and anaesthesia. All patients with a history of cardiomyopathy require careful anaesthetic management.

Hypertrophic obstructive cardiomyopathy (HOCM)

HOCM is an autosomal dominant cardiovascular disease that causes inappropriate and asymmetrical changes in the myocardium in the absence of a stimulus which normally causes hypertrophy. It is a diagnosis of exclusion, as 60% of these unexplained left ventricular hypertrophies are caused by HOCM.

HOCM can be completely asymptomatic, but can present with arrhythmias, angina (due to hypertrophy, increased diastolic pressures and oxygen demand), heart failure or sudden death.

Sudden death is more likely in patients with a family history of such deaths (first-degree relatives), significant ventricular ectopics, unexplained syncope, massive left ventricular hypertrophy and the presence of the malignant genotype.

The pathophysiology involves diastolic dysfunction with ventricular hypertrophy, poor ventricular compliance and preserved systolic function. Twenty percent of patients have septal involvement with outflow tract obstruction. This is often dynamic and is affected by the patient's volume status.

Ventricular systole is associated with the abnormal movement of the anterior mitral valve leaflet towards the septum (SAM — systolic anterior motion) and further obstruction of the outflow tract. This is followed by development of mitral regurgitation in some patients.

Dilated cardiomyopathy

Dilated cardiomyopathy has a poor prognosis with a 5-year survival of 40-50% once heart failure has been diagnosed. It is familial in 25% of cases. Other causes are alcohol consumption, Coxsackie or HIV infections, high cardiac output states (found in pregnancy, thyrotoxicosis or anaemia), drugs (cocaine, heavy metals), thiamine deficiency and phaeochromocytoma.

The pathophysiology involves systolic dysfunction and ventricular chamber enlargement with normal ventricular wall thickness. There is a progressive decrease in ventricular contractile function of the myocardium and subsequent heart failure.

The main complications of dilated cardiomyopathy are ventricular and supraventricular arrhythmias, conduction system problems, mitral and tricuspid incompetence and thromboembolism. The low cardiac output state activates the renin-angiotensin system with consequences like heart failure and/or sudden cardiac death.

Restrictive cardiomyopathy

Restrictive cardiomyopathy is a progressive condition that leads to a low cardiac output heart failure, liver cirrhosis, thromboembolism and eventually death.

The commonest cause is endomyocardial fibrosis affecting adults in tropical and subtropical Africa. Outside these regions, the causes can be idiopathic (associated with increasing age) or secondary to infiltrative diseases (sarcoidosis, amyloidosis), storage diseases (haemachromatosis), eosinophilic endocarditis, myocarditis, metastatic cancer or cardiac transplant.

The pathophysiology involves diastolic dysfunction with stiff ventricles, often prominent right heart failure with impaired diastolic filling which causes pulmonary venous congestion and dilated atria. The systolic function is normal.

Anaesthesia in restrictive cardiomyopathy is hazardous as catastrophic events can be triggered by vasodilatation, myocardial depression and reduced venous return.

Peri-operative risks associated with cardiomyopathy include arrhythmias (common and require intervention), exacerbation of cardiac failure and cardiac arrest.

Patients with HOCM are usually treated with beta-blockers with or without verapamil or disopyramide as negative inotropes. An electrocardiogram (ECG) is likely to show ventricular hypertrophy. A transthoracic echocardiogram (TTE) gives an estimate of the degree of dynamic obstruction and ventricular hypertrophy.

Most patients with HOCM will have dual-chamber pacing and/or an automatic implantable cardioverter defibrillator (AICD).

Treatment for patients with restrictive cardiomyopathy includes ACE inhibitors, beta-blockers and diuretics. Supraventricular or ventricular arrhythmias are treated with amiodarone or digoxin. These patients are frequently anticoagulated due to the risk of malignant arrhythmias. Arrhythmias may warrant the use of a permanent pacemaker and an AICD.

Patients with dilated cardiomyopathy are normally on diuretics, ACE inhibitors and vasodilators. Amiodarone is the drug of choice for arrhythmias as it has the least myocardial depressant effect. These patients are frequently anticoagulated and some will have synchronised biventricular pacers/defibrillators in place.

Pre-operative investigations and management should include an ECG, a transthoracic echocardiogram, electrolytes and a pacemaker/ICD check.

Conduct of anaesthesia

Invasive cardiovascular monitoring is required during anaesthesia in the form of an arterial line. Non-invasive cardiac output monitors such as oesophageal Doppler, PiCCO or LiDCO should be used. Transoesophageal echocardiography (TOE) is useful in assessing the dynamic changes during surgery, but is not always available and has not been shown to change the outcome.

In general, the haemodynamic goals are to maintain the sinus rhythm and an adequate volume status. The specific haemodynamic goals for HOCM are to maintain a low to normal heart rate, a high normal systemic vascular resistance (similar to the management of aortic stenosis patients) and a low ventricular contractility by avoiding increases in sympathetic activity (as increased contractility will exacerbate the outflow obstruction).

The haemodynamic goals for dilated cardiomyopathy are a normal systemic vascular resistance and to avoid myocardial depression (frequently by using inotropes or inodilators like phosphodiesterase inhibitors).

The haemodynamic goals for restrictive cardiomyopathy are a high normal systemic vascular resistance and to avoid myocardial depression.

The main aims of intra-operative management of the three types of cardiomyopathy are highlighted in Table 16.4.

Table 16.4. Intra-operative management of the three types of cardiomyopathy.

	Main aims	Avoid	Contraindicated	In case of instability, use	Postop
HOCM	• Prevent/treat LVOT obstruction and arrhythmia	• Tachycardia • ↑ sympathetic drive • ↓ vascular resistance • ↓ venous return	• Inotropes (they increase LVOT obstruction)	• Alpha agonists • IV fluids • Correct arrhythmia	• Avoid sympathetic stimulation by providing good pain relief and avoiding hypothermia
Dilated CM	• ↓ in afterload is beneficial and the use of regional anaesthesia encouraged	• Tachycardia • ↑ in SVR	• N/A	• Inotropes	• ICU fluid management
Restrictive CM	• Maintain filling pressures • Maintain SVR	• Vasodilatation • Myocardial depression • ↓ venous return	• Regional anaesthesia		• CO monitoring • Maintain right ventricular filling

HCOM = hypertrophic obstructive cardiomyopathy; LVOT= left ventricular outflow tract obstruction; CM = cardiomyopathy; SVR = systemic vascular resistance.

Pacemakers

The indications for permanent pacemaker insertion continue to expand and now include the prevention of atrial fibrillation and the management of congestive cardiac failure.

There are three types of cardiac permanent pacemakers in use:

- Single-chamber pacemaker — one pacing lead is implanted in the right atrium or ventricle.
- Dual-chamber pacemaker — two pacing leads are implanted (one in the right ventricle and one in the right atrium).
- Biventricular pacemaker (known as cardiac resynchronisation therapy [CRT]) — in addition to single- or dual-chamber right heart pacing leads, a lead is advanced to the coronary sinus for left ventricular pericardial pacing.

Published guidelines on the indications for cardiac pacing are available from both the American Heart Association (AHA) and the European Society of Cardiology (ESC).

The indications for permanent pacemaker insertion are:

- Sinus node. Sick sinus syndrome, recurrent Stoke-Adams syndrome and sinus node dysfunction.
- Conduction system. Complete heart block, symptomatic second-degree heart block, symptomatic bifascicular and trifascicular heart block.
- Chronic atrial fibrillation.
- Persistent and symptomatic second- or third-degree atrioventricular block associated with myocardial infarction.
- Atriobiventricular pacing in moderate to severe heart failure.

The pacemaker type and function is described using a five-letter code (Table 16.5) are:

- The first letter describes the chamber paced.
- The second letter describes the chamber sensed.

- The third letter describes the response for sensing.
- The fourth letter describes the rate modulation or programmability.
- The fifth letter describes the anti-tachycardia function.

Table 16.5. Five-letter pacemaker codes.

Chamber paced	Chamber sensed	Response to sensing	Rate modulation	Anti-tachycardia function
Atria (A)	Atria (A)	Triggered (T)	Rate modulated (R)	Pacing (P)
Ventricle (V)	Ventricle (V)	Inhibited (I)	No action (O)	Shocking (S)
Dual (D)	Dual (D)	Dual (D)		Dual (D)
No action (O)	No action (O)	No action (O)		No action (O)

Peri-operative management

Most patients have a card that has details of the pacemaker as well as information about the last time it was checked.

All modern pacemakers can be remotely programmed. The pacing rate, energy output, sensitivity, mode of operation and other functions can be amended. They can also be interrogated regarding rhythm and critical events.

Despite inbuilt protection, radiofrequency and microwave electromagnetic interference can cause inappropriate inhibition or triggering of impulses, asynchronous pacing, reprogramming to a back-up mode (VOO) or damage to the pacemaker. Magnetic resonance imaging (MRI) is a contraindication for patients with pacemakers. Recently, advances in cardiac device technology have led to the first generation of MRI-conditional devices.

For emergency surgery where pacing is indicated but there is insufficient time for temporary or permanent pacing wires, the patient should have external transcutaneous pacing pads attached before surgery.

The potential intra-operative interference and their consequences are presented in Table 16.6.

Table 16.6. Pacemaker response to various interference during anaesthesia and surgery.

Interference	Response
Monopolar diathermy	• Inhibition (if sensed as cardiac activity) • Back-up mode (if too much noise sensed)
Shivering/fasciculations	• Back-up mode (if rate modulator gets confused)
Nerve stimulators or TENS machines	• Potential interference; generally safe if well away
Defibrillation	• Potential damage or reprogramming; generally safe if paddles are well away

Pre-operative evaluation

It is good practice to establish the location of the pacemaker and the reason for its insertion, avoiding making assumptions about the device without taking a history or without written evidence.

A detailed history (dizziness, syncope) and review of all available records should be made. This will establish the most recent pacemaker check and its mode of action. Pacemakers without a rate modulator should be deactivated prior to anaesthesia.

The history should include questions about dizziness, syncope or worsening symptoms of heart failure as these suggest recent pacemaker malfunction and/or are signs of a deteriorating cardiac function which should be managed before surgery.

The physical examination should include an examination for scars over the chest or upper abdomen. A chest X-ray will confirm the integrity of the leads, the location and the type of device.

The 12-lead ECG will reveal the underlying rhythm, evidence of pacing activity and electrical capture.

Electrolyte levels should always be checked prior to surgery.

There are two important aspects of managing patients with a pacemaker during the peri-operative period:

- Ensuring that the pacemaker is functioning optimally.
- Ensuring that external electrical devices such as diathermy do not interfere with pacemaker function.

Conduct of anaesthesia

Standard AAGBI monitoring should be employed. Invasive arterial blood pressure monitoring, although not mandatory, should be given consideration because it provides real-time evidence of mechanical capture.

The ECG should be monitored carefully when changing patient position or starting mechanical ventilation as lead displacement can cause loss of mechanical capture or an increase in the pacing threshold.

The ECG monitor should be kept in diagnostic mode because it has a wider frequency response range (0.05-100Hz) which enables accurate assessment of QRS morphology and ST segment analysis.

Suxamethonium should be avoided if possible as fasciculations can produce pacemaker over-sensing.

Bipolar diathermy should be used whenever possible. If unipolar diathermy must be used, then the diathermy and the ground plate need to be as far away as possible from the pacemaker and a back-up pacing method should be immediately available.

In the case of intra-operative pacemaker dysfunction, an external transthoracic pacemaker is the best back-up plan.

An isoprenaline infusion could be used to improve the rate or rhythm and buy time. Invasive temporary pacing methods (such as transoesophageal or transvenous) take longer to set up and might be impractical in the case of device malfunction during surgery.

Defibrillation during surgery

For implantable cardioverter defibrillators, the shocking mode should be disabled, and defibrillator pads should be attached and connected to the defibrillator. The heart rhythm should be continuously monitored and if the rhythm changes to ventricular fibrillation, the heart should be manually defibrillated using an external defibrillator. The pads should be placed in an anteroposterior position and as far away from the pacemaker as possible.

Postoperative management

The technician should be asked to recheck the pacemaker after surgery and reinstitute the rate modulation and any deactivated specific pacing modes.

Valvular heart diseases

Patients might present for non-cardiac surgery, knowing about their valvular disease, being symptomatic and already on treatment or they could be asymptomatic and diagnosed on the same admission as the planned anaesthetic and surgery.

A murmur in asymptomatic fit and well individuals with good functional capacity and normal ECGs does not signify cardiac disease but more often a physiological increase in blood flow. They can undergo anaesthesia safely.

In general, stenotic lesions are more challenging to manage in the peri-operative period than regurgitant lesions. The American College of Cardiology/American Heart Association (ACC/AHA) 2014 recommendation was that a pre-operative transthoracic echocardiography should be performed for all patients with clinically suspected moderate or severe valvular stenosis or regurgitation.

The echocardiography should also be performed if a year has passed since the most recent one or there is significant change in the clinical status since the most recent review.

Aortic stenosis

The most common causes include degenerative calcification (especially over 70 years of age) and a bicuspid aortic valve (2% of population).

Pathophysiology

The normal aortic valve area (AVA) is 2.6-3.5cm^2. Significant obstruction occurs when the AVA approaches 1cm^2. The initial response is left ventricle hypertrophy which maintains the gradient across the valve, followed by left ventricle stiffness and diastolic dysfunction. Eventually the left ventricle filling becomes dependent on atrial contraction and sinus rhythm is essential for maintaining cardiac output. All these changes produce a mismatch between oxygen supply and demand leading to angina despite normal coronary circulation. The ventricle becomes sensitive to changes in preload and susceptible to ischaemia especially with decreases in diastolic blood pressure. In the final stages, the cardiac output, stroke volume and the pressure gradient across the valve fall. Dilatation of the left ventricle occurs at a late stage.

The three cardinal symptoms are angina, syncope and dyspnoea. Clinical examination may reveal a slow rising pulse with a narrow pulse pressure. The ejection systolic murmur radiating to the neck is heard at the aortic area.

Investigations

- ECG: left ventricular hypertrophy and ST-T wave abnormalities.
- Echocardiography: reveals the anatomy of the aortic valve, calculates the valve gradient and assesses the left ventricular function.
- Angiography: recommended in patients over 50 years of age to detect concurrent coronary artery disease, as bypass grafting could be performed at the same time with the valve replacement.

Conduct of anaesthesia

Pre-operative care includes the important multidisciplinary decision on whether to replace the valve or not before elective surgery. Symptomatic patients and asymptomatic patients undergoing major surgery with a marked fluid shift and patients with a gradient across the valve >50mmHg may require valve replacement.

The haemodynamic goals during anaesthesia and surgery are presented in Table 16.7.

These are best achieved through invasive monitoring (CVP, oesophageal Doppler or TOE) to guide fluid management and intra-arterial pressure monitoring (except for very short procedures) and the use of direct-acting alpha-agonists to maintain the blood pressure.

The selected technique should maintain afterload and avoid tachycardia.

Central neuraxial blocks should be used with caution because of the danger of afterload reduction.

Peripheral nerve blocks are useful in preventing tachycardia.

Table 16.7. Intra-operative haemodynamic goals during aortic valve surgery for aortic stenosis.

Goal	Reason
Sinus rhythm	Prevents haemodynamic collapse
(Low) normal heart rate	Tachycardia disrupts the balance between myocardial oxygen supply and demand
Adequate fluid volume	Prevents hypotension, myocardial ischaemia and reduced contractility
(High) normal systemic vascular resistance	Prevents hypotension, myocardial ischaemia and reduced contractility

Postoperative management includes consideration for HDU/ITU admission, attention to pain management, fluid balance and sometimes the use of vasoconstrictors.

Aortic regurgitation

Rheumatic heart disease and endocarditis are causes of primary aortic regurgitation.

Secondary aortic regurgitation is caused by aortic dissection, Marfan syndrome and ankylosing spondylitis.

Pathophysiology

The left ventricle gradually becomes eccentrically hypertrophic and dilates, as it has to maintain a supra-normal stroke volume. A massively enlarged left ventricle is less compliant, and small changes in filling pressures can cause important changes in preload and cardiac output. The incompetent valve lowers the diastolic blood pressure, which can reduce coronary flow even in the absence of coronary artery disease.

At end stage, as ventricular function deteriorates, the ejection fraction declines and left end-diastolic pressure (LEDP) increases and leads eventually to mitral regurgitation (MR).

Afterload reduction (ACE inhibitors), diuretics, and digoxin are typically used for medical management. The aortic valve should be replaced before irreversible ventricular changes occur.

Investigations

- ECG: shows left ventricular hypertrophy.
- Chest X-ray: enlarged 'boot-shaped' heart.
- Echocardiography: shows the degree of regurgitation and the cardiac anatomy.

Conduct of anaesthesia

Asymptomatic patients tolerate surgery well. Symptomatic patients with poor functional capacity should be referred for valve replacement before elective surgery.

The intra-operative haemodynamic goals are presented in Table 16.8.

Invasive intra-arterial pressure monitoring is required for major surgery. Non-invasive cardiac output monitors are inaccurate.

The selected technique should avoid bradycardia (which needs urgent treatment with beta-agonists or anticholinergic agents) and maintain the afterload in the low to normal range. Arrhythmias like supraventricular tachycardia and atrial fibrillation (especially if associated with low blood pressure) need prompt DC cardioversion.

Ephedrine is the preferred first-line vasopressor, but small doses of phenylephrine (25-50µg) can be considered.

Table 16.8. Intra-operative haemodynamic goals during aortic valve surgery for aortic regurgitation.

Goal	Reason
(High) normal heart rate (around 90 bpm)	Maintains forward flow/decreases degree of regurgitation
(Low) normal systemic vascular resistance	Maintains forward flow and diastolic pressure and decreases the degree of regurgitation
Adequate fluid volume	Maintains diastolic pressure/cardiac output
Maintain contractility	Maintains forward flow/diastolic pressure

Central neuraxial blocks are well tolerated provided intravascular volume is maintained.

Mitral stenosis

Rheumatic fever is the commonest cause. Rarer causes include malignant carcinoid disease, systemic lupus erythematosus, rheumatoid arthritis and mucopolysaccharidosis. It could also be congenital in origin.

Very few patients have isolated stenosis and the majority have mixed mitral valve disease.

Pathophysiology

The stenosis prevents the ventricle from filling and the pressure and volume upstream to the valve are increased. The left ventricle has normal function but it is small and under-filled.

Initially the left atrium dilates and the pulmonary pressure is low, but as the disease progresses, chronic reactive pulmonary hypertension develops, the right heart hypertrophies, then fails, and secondary pulmonary and tricuspid regurgitation develops.

Atrial fibrillation decreases the diastolic filling time and it is not tolerated well.

A slow heart rate is desirable as it optimises left ventricular filling.

Dyspnoea, haemoptysis, fatigue and palpitations are the most common symptoms.

Hoarseness can develop from compression of the left recurrent laryngeal nerve against the pulmonary artery by the enlarged left atrium.

Clinical examination may reveal signs of right heart failure (raised JVP, peripheral oedema, ascites, hepatomegaly) and a diastolic low pitch rumble murmur at the apex. The first heart sound is usually loud and may be palpable (tapping apex beat) because of increased force in closing the mitral valve.

Investigations

- ECG: will reveal atrial fibrillation in most patients or signs of atrial enlargement if the sinus rhythm is present.
- Chest X-ray: could show a large left atrium on a lateral film and a double shadow behind the heart on a PA film; splaying of the carina and Kerley B pulmonary congestion lines could also be features.
- Echocardiography: is used to ascertain the valve area and the gradient.

Conduct of anaesthesia

Asymptomatic patients tolerate non-cardiac surgery well. Symptomatic patients with poor functional capacity should be referred for valve replacement before elective surgery.

The intra-operative haemodynamic goals are presented in Table 16.9.

Table 16.9. Intra-operative haemodynamic goals during mitral valve surgery for mitral stenosis.

Goal	Reason
(Low) normal heart rate (around 50-70 bpm) and maintain sinus rhythm	Prevent decreases in diastolic filling time
Adequate preload	Prevents a decrease in cardiac output
(High) normal systemic vascular resistance	Prevents a decrease in cardiac output
Avoid hypercarbia, hypoxia and acidosis	Prevent exacerbation of pulmonary hypertension

Invasive intra-arterial pressure monitoring is required for major surgery.

The anaesthetic technique is similar to that for aortic stenosis as there is a relatively fixed cardiac output state and aims to provide a slow heart rate, adequate preload (measure CVP or PAOP if needed) and afterload.

Central neuraxial blocks should be avoided as they pose significant risks.

Mitral regurgitation

The most common causes for mitral regurgitation (MR) include mitral valve prolapse (MVP), rheumatic heart disease, infective endocarditis, annular calcification, cardiomyopathy and ischaemic heart disease.

Pathophysiology

Regurgitation from the ventricle produces a massively dilated left atrium and is then followed in evolution by pulmonary congestion and secondary pulmonary hypertension. The left ventricular ejection fraction is supra-normal. Patients might remain asymptomatic for years until left ventricular dysfunction develops, when symptoms of fatigue, weakness, palpitations (most will have AF) and dyspnoea occur. They may also present with pulmonary oedema on the initial assessment.

Clinical examination may reveal atrial fibrillation, an apical pansystolic murmur radiating to the axilla with a soft first heart sound and a loud third heart sound on auscultation.

Investigations

- ECG: normally shows atrial fibrillation and left atrial enlargement.
- Chest X-ray: shows left atrial and ventricular enlargement.
- Echocardiography: shows cardiac anatomy and the degree of regurgitation.

Brain natriuretic peptide (BNP) assessment is used for prognostic purposes.

Conduct of anaesthesia

Asymptomatic patients tolerate non-cardiac surgery well. Symptomatic patients with poor functional capacity should be referred for valve replacement before elective surgery.

The intra-operative haemodynamic goals are presented in Table 16.10.

The chosen anaesthetic technique aims are similar to those for aortic regurgitation. Because the preload is difficult to estimate, a pulmonary artery catheter might be useful in major non-cardiac surgery.

Table 16.10. Intra-operative haemodynamic goals during mitral valve surgery for mitral regurgitation.

Goal	Reason
(High) normal heart rate (>90 bpm)	Decreases time for regurgitation in systole and the time for diastolic filling, reducing the LV overload
Adequate preload	Prevents a decrease in cardiac output
Low systemic vascular resistance	Stimulates forward flow
Avoid hypercarbia, hypoxia and acidosis	Prevent exacerbation of pulmonary hypertension

Patients with prosthetic valves

Most of these patients are under surveillance and take life-long anticoagulation if their valve is mechanical. Tissue valves do not need anticoagulation.

Modern aortic valves have a low risk of thromboembolisation, so warfarin can be stopped 5 days before surgery and cover provided peri-operatively with prophylactic low-molecular-weight heparin.

Old aortic and mitral mechanical valves have a much higher risk of thromboembolisation (>4%/year) and are best managed with stopping warfarin 5 days before surgery and instituting a bridging therapy with either an infusion of unfractionated heparin (to be stopped 6 hours before surgery) or a daily subcutaneous therapeutic dose of low-molecular-weight heparin (to be stopped 12 hours before surgery).

Peri-operative antibiotic prophylaxis for patients with valvular heart diseases

Peri-operative antibiotic prophylaxis is no longer recommended by NICE guidelines for patients with valvular heart disease undergoing dental, gastrointestinal, genitourinary tract or respiratory tract procedures unless the procedure involves a site where there is suspected infection.

Case scenario 1

A 49-year-old Afro-Caribbean lady known to have hypertension presents on the morning theatre list for a laparoscopic cholecystectomy under general anaesthesia. Her regular medication includes losartan 50mg once daily and amlodipine 5mg OD. Her blood pressure is normally well controlled according to her GP and she does not have symptoms, signs or investigations to suggest any end-organ damage. She was seen in the pre-operative clinic and advised not to take losartan on the morning of surgery.

She is anxious and the blood pressure readings on the day of surgery are 200/110mmHg, 197/107mmHg and 185/95mmHg.

What would be the management plan for this patient?

This patient was advised correctly to stop the losartan (angiotensin-II receptor blocker on the day). The surgery proceeds as scheduled without any adverse events.

Drugs that block the renin-angiotensin system should be continued for patients with persistent elevated blood pressures or hypertensive patients with signs of cardiac failure.

Case scenario 2

A 46-year-old gentleman is admitted to the emergency department with a reduced GCS. Four weeks prior to his admission he had a myocardial infarction for which he underwent an emergency PCI, balloon angioplasty and a drug-eluting stent insertion in the LAD artery. He has been on dual-antiplatelet therapy for 12 months (aspirin and ticagrelor). A CT scan of the head shows a large subdural haematoma, which the neurosurgical team would like to evacuate in theatre.

What would be the best way to manage his antiplatelet therapy during the peri-operative period?

As the surgery is an emergency, the patient needs to go to theatre in a timely manner. A possible solution would be to stop his ticagrelor, continue the aspirin and provide 2 units of platelets (guided by TEG platelet mapping) during surgery with a view to starting bridging therapy with a GPIIb/IIIa inhibitor (e.g. tirofiban) infusion postoperatively in case he needs to return to theatre at a later stage. This plan should be formulated following a discussion with the cardiologist.

This patient is managed as above. The surgical procedure is uneventful. The patient makes a good recovery over the next few days, the tirofiban infusion is stopped and the ticagrelor is restarted.

Case scenario 3

A 48-year-old obese (BMI 34) male patient with a history of hypertension presents for an emergency laparotomy for small bowel obstruction. His exercise tolerance is between 4-10 METs, as he claims he could manage 1 flight of stairs normally. His current medication includes ramipril 10mg OD and bisoprolol 5mg OD.

He states that he had "problems with his heart" 5 years ago when he was a heavy drinker. He had an echocardiogram at the time which showed dilated cardiomyopathy with a left ventricle ejection fraction of 25%. The ECG recorded on the day of surgery is unremarkable.

He feels well in himself, he still has mild abdominal pain and his MEWS score is zero.

What would be the management plan for this patient?

This patient needs an emergency operation. In view of his history and previous echocardiography findings, he has a high risk of cardiovascular morbidity. The fact that he is relatively asymptomatic does not predict the exact individual risk in this case.

It is unlikely that any other last-minute investigations will alter the anaesthetic management of this patient, but a repeat bedside echocardiogram and cardiology opinion would be useful. His regular medication including the ACE inhibitors and the beta-blocker should be continued.

The anaesthetic technique should include invasive blood pressure monitoring and non-invasive cardiac output monitoring.

The haemodynamic goals should be maintenance of an adequate fluid status and sinus rhythm as well as avoidance of tachycardia and of increases in systemic vascular resistance and myocardial depression (use inotropes/inodilators if this happens).

Case scenario 4

An 89-year-old lady is booked to have an open reduction and internal fixation of a humeral fracture under a general anaesthetic after sustaining a mechanical fall.

She is keeping well for her age, but she states that she had "cardiac problems and collapses" in the past for which she was fitted with a pacemaker 10 years before. This was inserted in a different district general hospital. She only knows "her heart was slow" before that. She is now asymptomatic from that point of view. She does not have a pacemaker card with her, but she mentioned the device was checked at that hospital within the last year.

What would be the management plan for this patient?

Obtain as much information as possible from the clinical records, previous clinical letters and from the patient.

The patient should be asked about any symptoms of dizziness, syncope or worsening symptoms of heart failure as these suggest recent pacemaker malfunction and there are signs of deteriorating cardiac function which should be managed before anaesthesia. The ECG may show valuable information about the rhythm and patient's dependency on the device.

As no exact information could be ascertained from any of the above mentioned in-hospital available sources, the hospital where the pacemaker was fitted is contacted and the required information is obtained relatively easily from the electrophysiology department. It was a DDD pacemaker inserted for symptomatic bradycardia and sick sinus syndrome. It was checked within the year and found to be in perfect condition. As the patient did not describe any deterioration in her symptoms, it is safe to proceed with the surgery.

In the case of intra-operative pacemaker dysfunction, a non-invasive transthoracic pacemaker is the best contingency plan. An isoprenaline infusion can also be used to improve the rate or rhythm and buy time until definitive treatment is instituted.

Case scenario 5

A 58-year-old gentleman is on the trauma list for an open reduction and internal fixation of a mid-shaft tibial fracture.

He states that he suffers with mitral stenosis and that he gets short of breath on exertion.

What would be the best way to anaesthetise him?

Find out as much information as possible about the mitral stenosis from the patient and clinical records. If the echocardiography is older than 1 year or if he has developed worsening symptoms since his assessment, a new one should be requested.

A carefully titrated opioid-based general anaesthetic with invasive arterial blood pressure monitoring before induction is probably the best option in this case.

Further reading

1. NCEPOD. Then and Now: The 2000 Report of the National Confidential Enquiry into Postoperative Deaths. The National Confidential Enquiry into Postoperative Deaths, 2001.

2. Sear JW, Howard-Alpe G. Preoperative plasma BNP concentrations: do they improve our care of high-risk non-cardiac surgical patients? *Br J Anaesthesia* 2007; 99: 151-4.

3. National Institute for Health and Care Excellence guideline 127. Hypertension: clinical Management of Hypertension in Adults. Manchester, UK: NICE, 2011.

4. Howell SJ, Sear JW, Foex P. Hypertension, hypertensive heart disease and perioperative cardiac risk. *Br J Anaesthesia* 2004; 92: 570-83.

5. Hartle A, McCormack T, Carlisle J, *et al*. The measurement of adult blood pressure and management of hypertension before elective surgery. *Anaesthesia* 2016; 71: 326-37.

6. Auron M, Harte B, Kumar A, *et al*. Renin-angiotensin system antagonists in the perioperative setting: clinical consequences and recommendations for practice. *Postgrad Med J* 2011; 87: 472- 81.

7. Townsend N, Wickramasinghe K, Bhatnagar O, *et al.* Coronary Heart Disease Statistics. London, UK: British Heart Foundation, 2012.

8. Biccard BM, Devereaux PJ, Rodseth RN. Cardiac biomarkers in the prediction of risk in the non-cardiac setting. *Anaesthesia* 2014; 69: 484-93.

9. DeVile MPJ, Foex P. Antiplatelet drugs, coronary stents, and non-cardiac surgery. *Br J Anaesth CEACCP* 2010; 10: 187-91.

10. POISE Study Group. Effects of extended release metoprolol in patients undergoing non-cardiac surgery (POISE Trial): a randomized controlled trial. *Lancet* 2008; 371: 1839-47.

11. Biccard BM, Sear JW, Foex P. Statin therapy: a potentially useful perioperative intervention in patients with cardiovascular disease. *Anaesthesia* 2005; 60: 1106-14.

12. Davies MR, Cousins J. Cardiomyopathy and anaesthesia *Br J Anaesth CEACCP* 2009: 9: 189-93.

13. Spirito P, Autore C. Management of hypertrophic cardiomyopathy. *Br Med J* 2006; 332: 1251-5.

14. Tracey CM, Epstein AE. 2012 ACCF/AHA/HRS Focused update of the 2008 guidelines for device-based therapy of cardiac rhythm abnormalities. *Circulation* 2012; 126: 1784-800.

15. Shinbane JS, Colletti PM, Shellock FG. Magnetic resonance imaging in patients with cardiac pacemakers: era of "MR Conditional" designs. *J Cardiovasc Magn Res* 2011; 13: 63.

16. Brown J, Morgan-Hughes NJ. Aortic stenosis and non-cardiac surgery. *Br J Anaesth CEACCP* 2005; 5: 1-4.

17. Otto CM. Valvular stenosis: diagnosis, quantitation, and clinical approach. In: Otto CM. *Textbook of Clinical Echocardiography*, 2nd ed. WB Saunders Company, 2000; 229-64.

18. Vahanian A, Alfieri O, Andreotti F, *et al.* Guidelines on the management of valvular heart disease (version 2012): The Joint Task Force on the Management of Valvular Heart Disease of the European Society of Cardiology (ESC) and the European Association for Cardio-Thoracic Surgery (EACTS). *Eur Heart J* 2012; 33: 2451-96.

19. National Institute for Health and Care Excellence guideline CG64. Prophylaxis against infective endocarditis: antimicrobial prophylaxis against infective endocarditis in adults and children undergoing interventional procedures. London, UK: NICE, 2008.

20. Pervez R. Pacemakers and implantable cardioverter-defibrillators (ICDs). World Federation of Societies of Anaesthesiologists. Anaesthesia Tutorial of the Week 2013: 299 and 300.

17 Anaesthesia and respiratory disease

Ranjna Basra, Chandrashekhar Vaidyanath and Melanie Sahni

Introduction

Patients suffering from respiratory diseases are at increased risk of peri-operative complications. This can have a significant effect on their morbidity and mortality. Common problems that arise are due to basal atelectasis, hypoventilation, poor lung compliance and superseding infection. Respiratory physiology can be dramatically altered in patients relying on compensatory processes resulting in complications. By identifying these patients in the pre-operative period, pulmonary function can be optimised and a carefully planned approach towards their anaesthetic management undertaken, which will lead to a reduction in risks such as reintubation, unplanned admission to the intensive care unit (ICU) and prolonged hospital stay. This chapter will briefly describe the pathophysiology of common respiratory diseases with their implications on the anaesthetic technique and intra-operative management.

General principles

Although the effects of general anaesthesia (GA) are usually mild and dissipate within 24 hours, it can instigate respiratory failure in those known to have limited respiratory reserve by a variety of mechanisms:

- Manipulation of the airway and surgical stimuli can precipitate laryngospasm or bronchospasm.
- Bypassing pharyngeal humidification and filtering functions with endotracheal intubation permits entry of pathogens and dries secretions; therefore, the use of a heat and moisture exchange (HME) filter is advised.

- The respiratory response to hypoxia, hypercapnia and clearing secretions is depressed by the use of volatile agents. An associated reduction in functional residual capacity (FRC) and increase in pulmonary shunt leads to hypoxia. This can be further exaggerated by patient positioning (e.g. lithotomy and Trendelenburg) and patient factors such as obesity.
- Intermittent positive pressure ventilation (IPPV) may cause a ventilation/perfusion (VQ) mismatch requiring an increased inspired oxygen concentration.
- Despite adequate reversal from neuromuscular blockade, residual anaesthesia effects may depress upper airway muscular tone and cause airway obstruction.
- Patients can easily be tipped into pulmonary oedema with excessive fluid therapy or on extubation (negative pressure pulmonary oedema).

Drugs affecting the respiratory system

A number of drugs used as part of a general and/or regional anaesthetic can effect respiratory function and need to be dealt with carefully:

- A transient apnoea can follow intravenous induction agent use (thiopentone, propofol and etomidate). On the contrary, ketamine maintains both airway patency and respiratory drive, although it increases the secretions.
- Thiopentone increases airway reactivity.
- Volatile anaesthetics depress respiratory drive — in decreasing order: enflurane > desflurane > isoflurane > sevoflurane > halothane.
- Certain agents are known to cause bronchospasm, partly due to histamine release, e.g. atracurium, morphine.
- Opiates and benzodiazepines depress respiratory drive and response to hypoxia and hypercapnia.

Surgical effects on the respiratory system

Surgical insult can also contribute greatly to the development of pulmonary complications, with thoracic and upper abdominal procedures associated with the highest risk. This is not only due to the functional respiratory muscle impediment from the surgical incision or from reflex inhibition of the phrenic nerve (due to visceral stimulation by mechanical traction), but it can also be due to hypoventilation secondary to poorly controlled postoperative pain.

Large volumes of gas insufflation, e.g. during hand bag-mask ventilation, CO_2 insufflation during laparoscopy and/or fluid sequestration within the bowel and peritoneal cavity can also externally impede ventilation.

It is widely known that pulmonary complications increase dramatically if surgical time exceeds 3 hours. It can take up to 2 weeks for postoperative lung function to return to baseline and therefore the benefits of the proposed surgery must outweigh any risks, even in healthy individuals.

Asthma

Pathophysiology

Asthma is defined as a disease of intermittent reversible airflow obstruction. Increased resistance to airflow is caused by the occlusion of the airway lumen (e.g. bronchial wall inflammation resulting in mucus hypersecretion) and pathology within the airway wall (e.g. smooth muscle bronchoconstriction). The incidence of an asthmatic patient suffering bronchospasm whilst having elective surgery is less than 2%, especially if they have well-controlled disease. Nevertheless, care should be taken to schedule elective surgery during a period of optimum disease control. Factors increasing complication rates include patient age over 50 years, major surgery and patients suffering from brittle asthma.

Asthma classically presents with symptoms such as shortness of breath, wheeze, cough and sputum production, which develop after antigen is exposed to the dendritic cells of the airway. This process activates T-lymphocytes resulting in the release of cytokines and an influx of mast cells, basophils, eosinophils, neutrophils, macrophages and subsequently by a release in mediators such as histamine, prostaglandins and leukotrienes.

Specific trigger factors (exercise or allergy) can often be identified, which precipitate symptoms. Poor control often results in persistent

Table 17.1. Medications to control asthma.

Class of drug	Examples	Intra-operative use	Key notes
Beta two agonists	Salbutamol	Nebulised via ET tube	Be aware of tachycardia (sympathetic stimulation) and tremor, $\downarrow K^+$
Anticholinergic drugs	Ipratropium	Nebulised via ET tube	Minimum 4-hourly
Inhaled steroids	Beclomethasone Fluticasone	Nil	Beware of adrenal suppression in high doses
Oral steroids	Prednisolone	IV hydrocortisone	Beware of adrenal suppression in high doses
Leukotriene inhibitors	Montelukast	Nil	
PDE inhibitors	Aminophylline	Can be used intravenously	Sparse clinical evidence. Consider infusion for severe cases

ET = endotracheal; PDE = phosphodiesterase.

diurnal symptom patterns; however, impairment of ventilatory capacity can often still be demonstrated between attacks.

Several different types of medications can be employed to control asthma, and they are summarised in Table 17.1.

Anaesthetic management

Elective surgery should whenever possible be performed when the disease is well controlled. Figure 17.1 displays the stepwise management of acute severe asthma occurring outside of theatre. Additionally, for abdominal or thoracic surgery, pre-operative optimisation should include regular chest physiotherapy, reducing the risk of postoperative infectious complications.

Patients suffering from wheeze should be pre-medicated with inhaled/ nebulised salbutamol. Certain commonly used agents are known to exacerbate asthma in poorly controlled individuals, by means of histamine release and these include morphine, atracurium, etc. Intubation in a lightly sedated patient may provoke bronchospasm and particular care needs to be taken to avoid this. Topical application of local anaesthetic to the vocal cords may help in reducing their incidence.

Regional anaesthetic techniques provide an excellent alternative to a general anaesthetic for brittle asthmatics. Invasive monitoring may be required for severe asthmatics undergoing major surgery.

Postoperatively, the patient's regular medication and oxygen therapy should be prescribed as appropriate. Alternative analgesia should be considered, if bronchospasm has occurred with previous exposure to morphine. Corticosteroid doses should be prescribed daily and if symptoms persist despite optimal therapy, other causes (e.g. pulmonary oedema, pulmonary emboli, pneumothorax) should be ruled out.

When faced with a patient suffering from severe bronchospasm under an anaesthetic, it is advised to increase the inspired fraction of oxygen to 100% and minimise the surgical stimulus or cease surgery until the patient's condition is stable. Potential precipitants should be reviewed.

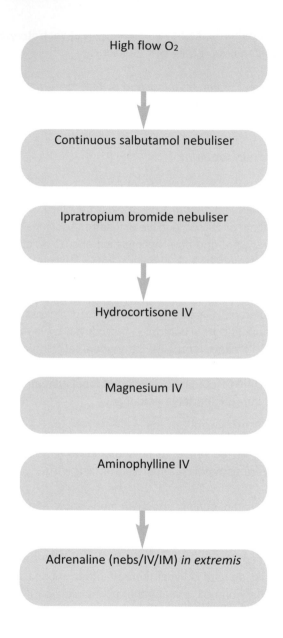

Figure 17.1. Management of acute severe asthma occurring outside of theatre.

Inhalational anaesthetic agents act as potent bronchodilators and can be employed to break the spasm. Certain IV induction agents such as ketamine also have bronchodilatory effects and can be used.

High inspiratory pressures may be required to achieve adequate tidal volumes. Raised airway resistance will obstruct expiration leading to gas trapping in the alveoli, ultimately resulting in 'auto-PEEP'. Barotrauma and pneumothorax are therefore common complications.

High pressures can also impede venous return resulting in a reduced cardiac output. To counteract these issues a longer expiratory time is needed. Permissive hypercarbia is relatively well tolerated. Metered doses of a salbutamol inhaler can also be delivered inside the ET tube by placing the canister in a 50ml syringe connected to appropriate tubing or a catheter.

Chronic obstructive pulmonary disease

Pathophysiology

Chronic obstructive pulmonary disease (COPD) is a commonly encountered respiratory disease. The risk of peri-operative complications is substantially higher in this category of patients, the length of hospital stay is often longer and the general mortality is increased. It has been estimated that 3 million people in the UK suffer from COPD, with almost two-thirds not being formally diagnosed. Long-term survival in patients with COPD while undergoing major operations is generally poor and postoperative pulmonary complications are commonly encountered.

COPD constitutes chronic and progressive inflammatory disease characterised by poorly reversible airway narrowing, remodelling of pulmonary smooth muscle, raised numbers of goblet cells, mucus hypersecretion and vasculature changes ultimately leading to pulmonary hypertension. Smoking is widely considered the main culprit; however, other causes have been identified, with genetic predisposition recently being implicated. Characteristically, COPD is associated with expiratory airflow limitation due to small airway inflammation (obstructive bronchiolitis) and destruction of lung tissue architecture (emphysema).

Obstructive bronchiolitis leads to air trapping causing hyperinflation, affecting V/Q mismatch as well as the mechanics of breathing. Emphysema on the other hand leads to the breakdown of elastin due to inflammation leading to loss of alveoli structure and thereby causing decreased gas transfer and further worsening of V/Q matching.

In advanced COPD it is the V/Q mismatch, reduced gas transfer and alveolar hypoventilation that ultimately leads to respiratory failure. To complicate matters even further, COPD is often present in a number of other conditions associated with smoking, such as lung cancer and pulmonary hypertension. Several guidelines for the diagnosis and management of COPD are available. Smokers older than 35 presenting with shortness of breath on exertion, chronic cough, regular sputum production, winter bronchitis and/or wheeze should be tested for COPD. Spirometry is the cornerstone to diagnosis. Airflow obstruction is defined by a ratio of forced expired volume in the first second to forced vital capacity (FEV_1/FVC) of 0.7, at which point COPD is formally diagnosed. The severity of COPD depends on the level of airflow obstruction and ranges from mild, moderate, severe to very severe.

The main therapy consists of inhaled agents, with short-acting beta-agonists being initially employed to provide symptomatic relief. For ongoing symptoms long-acting beta-agonists (LABA) as well as long-acting muscarinic agents (LAMA) may be employed in combination with inhaled corticosteroids. Smoking cessation, however, remains vital, at any stage in the disease as it can contribute to slowing down the disease progress before disability or death occurs.

Although regular oral therapy is rarely recommended, in severe cases oral corticosteroids are recommended. Occasionally, oral theophyllines are also used, mainly for patients who are unable to use inhaled therapy, or suffer from severe disease. Patients with chronic productive cough will often benefit from oral mucolytic therapy (for example, carbocysteine). These agents can lead to a reduction in the number of excerbations in certain individuals.

In severe cases of COPD, long-term oxygen therapy (LTOT) is advised. LTOT reduces pulmonary arterial pressure and prolongs life with oxygen saturations >90%. To have a beneficial effect on mortality, supplemental oxygen needs to be breathed in for at least 15 hours a day.

Non-invasive positive pressure ventilaton (NPPV) is now also widely used for patients suffering from respiratory failure secondary to COPD. It can reduce mortality if tried early in the course of respiratory failure. Exacerbations of COPD lead to accelerated loss of lung function, poorer quality of life and increased mortality. It is therefore of utmost importance to adhere to treatment, avoid excerbations, recognise them early and treat promptly.

Anaesthetic management

COPD patients requrire an extensive pre-operative review early enough to allow appropriate interventions to be implemented. A clinical history should be taken in order to ascertain the severity of COPD, with special focus on exercise tolerance. Often, questions will yield more reliable answers when relatives are questioned, as well as being specific in asking about the maximal level of exertion possible, e.g. do you get breathless when dressing yourself/climbing the stairs? The number of previous excerbations, last course of antibiotics and any hospital admissions requiring invasive and/or non-invasive ventilation should be identified. Smoking history and current status are also important.

In addition to routine blood tests, evidence of right-sided heart disease (cor pulmonale) should also be sought out. A chest X-ray itself is not mandated, unless there is clinical suspicion of an infective process. Extensive bullae can highlight the risk of a pneumothorax. A baseline arterial blood gas can provide a lot of information regarding the severity of the disease. Nutritional status is also an important determinant in postoperative pulmonary complications and nutritional supplements should be considered in malnourished patients. A pre-operative examination can help to predict complications and in the presence of active infection surgery should be postponed when possible.

It has been widely shown that general anaesthesia, especially tracheal intubation and intermittent positive pressure ventilation, is associated with a higher rate of adverse events in COPD patients. These patients are prone to laryngospasm, bronchospasm, cardiovascular compromise, barotrauma, hypoxaemia and a higher rate of postoperative complications. Regional anaesthesia should therefore be chosen, if feasible. Many patients will struggle to lie flat, which can complicate regional anaesthetic technique. If a general anaesthetic is required, COPD patients are often at risk of haemodynamic compromise on induction and appropriate precautions should be taken. Preoxygenation should be used in any hypoxic patients. In patients with severe COPD and hypoxia, continuous positive airway pressure (CPAP) might be used. Ventilating these patients can be very challenging, mainly due to the raised intrathoracic pressure when using intermittent positive pressure ventilation (IPPV). Limited expiratory flow rate due to airway narrowing leads to the next inhalational breath to start before expiration has finished. This is called breath stacking or air trapping and leads to the development of intrinsic/auto positive end-expiratory pressure (PEEP) leading to a number of undesirable pulmonary and cardiovascular side effects.

One of the first signs of air trapping is seen on manually ventilating the patient. The reservoir bag fills very slowly at induction. Upon initiation of mechanical ventilation, a capnography trace which does not reach plateau will indicate auto-PEEP. When attempting to reduce air trapping, several methods can be employed, namely allowing more time for expiration by reducing respiratory rate or increasing expiratory time via the I:E ratio. However, this will lead to a build up of carbon dioxide, which can lead to hypercarbia and acidosis. External PEEP can keep small airways open during late exhalation and thereby reducing internal PEEP.

Ventilating COPD patients is therefore often a compromise between oxygenation, normocapnia and cardiovascular stability and some derangments will have to be accepted in certain cases. Prior to extubation it is important to optimise the patient's condition. A peri-extubation bronchodilator can be useful and sometimes extubation directly to non-invasive ventilation (NIV) can reduce the work of breathing and air trapping. Postoperatively, patients should be closely monitored. Patients with significant disease or comorbidities are often monitored in high dependency units. Provision of effective analgesia is vital to ensure a speedy recovery.

Restrictive lung disease

Pathophysiology

Restrictive lung disease is a category that comprises a large number of respiratory conditions, which can affect either the lung parenchyma, pleura or may be due to an extrapulmonary cause resulting in restriction of lung expansion. This leads to increased work of breathing and V/Q mismatch. They can be primarily divided into two categories: intrinsic and extrinsic. The causes of intrinsic restrictive lung disease include pulmonary fibrosis due to pneumoconiosis, tuberculosis, acute respiratory distress syndrome (ARDS), drug-induced fibrosis due to bleomycin, radiation, sarcoidosis and interstitial lung disease. The causes of extrinsic restrictive lung disease include pleural thickening, obesity, ascites, diaphragmatic hernia and kyphoscoliosis.

The physiological effects of diffuse parenchymal disorders reduce all the lung volumes. Expiratory airflow is reduced in proportion to lung volume due to pulmonary fibrosis. There is ventilation-perfusion mismatching with an intrapulmonary shunt leading to arterial hypoxaemia. The reflexes arising from the lungs and the need to maintain minute ventilation by reducing tidal volume and increasing respiratory frequency cause hyperventilation at rest and exercise. The total compliance by the respiratory system is reduced in cases of disorders of the pleura and thoracic cage, leading to lung volume reduction. In kyphoscoliosis, a Cobb angle greater than 100° is associated with severe respiratory failure. Neuromuscular disorders affect the respiratory pattern at the level of the central nervous system (CNS), spinal cord, neuromuscular junction (NMJ) or respiratory muscles. The type of ventilatory impairment is dependent on the nature of the specific neuromuscular disorder. Obesity is also a cause of restrictive lung disease. BMI and lung volumes share an inverse relationship where FRC and expiratory reserve volume (ERV) are the parameters most dramatically reduced by increasing body mass index (BMI).

Anaesthetic management

Patients with restrictive lung disease need to be investigated thoroughly to allow appropriate interventions to be implemented. A clinical history should be taken in order to ascertain the degree of severity and also to focus on exercise tolerance. Questions regarding occupational history, exposures to certain drugs as well as a previous history of surgical intervention are helpful. This is more so in patients with kyphoscoliotic disorders. Smoking history and current status are equally important. Preoptimisation of the existing condition is important before going ahead with lung reduction surgery. Corticosteroids, immunosuppressive agents and cytotoxic agents are the mainstay of therapy for many of these diseases. Routine blood tests, respiratory function tests, chest X-rays, CT scans and an arterial blood gas can provide a lot of information regarding the severity of disease. Nutritional status as with any chronic condition is important in postoperative pulmonary rehabilitation and nutritional supplements should be considered. A history of significant exercise intolerance or evidence of a raised JVP, hepatic congestion or peripheral oedema should prompt a cardiac function evaluation with an echo. In the presence of active infection, surgery should be postponed when possible and antibiotic therapy should be commenced immediately.

Patients with restrictive lung disease are a real challenge to anaesthetists. Some of them come with coexisting lung disease to be operated on for a different procedure while some come for scoliosis corrective surgery. General anaesthesia with IPPV can be associated with adverse events like bronchospasm, cardiovascular collapse, hypoxaemia and a higher rate of postoperative complications. Regional anaesthesia may be beneficial occasionally. Patients who struggle to lie flat should be positioned accordingly to avoid further respiratory compromise.

Patients undergoing scoliosis corrective surgery can be challenging for several reasons, including body positioning, advanced disease and the large area of exposure required for a posterior approach to the spine. Endotracheal tube placement and intravenous lines should be secured and pressure points should be padded. The abdomen should be free to prevent an increase in abdominal pressure that can compromise venous return via the inferior vena cava. This in turn may raise pressure in the epidural veins, which would be responsible for increased blood loss during surgery. Hypothermia can be avoided by warmed intravenous fluids and forced-air warmers, as these patients often have a large surface area exposed for a prolonged period of time. In patients with restrictive lung disease, especially due to neuromuscular disease, the lung volumes and capacities can very easily be compromised in the postoperative period due to prolonged procedure time or due to positioning. Hence, it is better to have a HDU or ITU bed available as back-up when managing such patients. To avoid haemodynamic compromise on induction and to prevent intra-operative hypoxaemia, appropriate precautions should be taken. CPAP might be useful.

Ventilating patients with interstitial lung disease can be a compromise between oxygenation and cardiovascular stability, as these patients tend to have a certain degree of pre-existing pulmonary hypertension. This will be discussed later in the chapter. Postoperatively, patients should be closely monitored. Pain relief in the form of regional anaesthesia is essential to help with recovery especially in these patients.

Pulmonary hypertension

Pathophysiology

Pulmonary hypertension is a rare condition, having received more interest in the past 10 years as specifically targeted therapies have been devised, improving the survival rate of patients from previously less than 30% to over 50%.

Pulmonary hypertension is defined as a mean pulmonary artery pressure (MPAP) >25mmHg at rest or 30mmHg upon exercise. Five distinct types of pulmonary hypertension have been described (Table 17.2). The underlying cause is of crucial importance as it ultimately defines treatment.

Idiopathic pulmonary hypertension has an annual incidence of 1-2 cases/million and is more common in women. Without targeted therapy, median survival after diagnosis is less than 3 years. It has now been recognised that it is associated with other systemic diseases, such as systemic sclerosis, sickle cell disease or congenital heart disease. The more common forms and also of more interest to the anaesthetist are, however, cases caused by left-sided heart disease and lung disease.

Table 17.2. Types of pulmonary hypertension.

Pulmonary arterial hypertension	Idiopathic pulmonary hypertension or Persistent pulmonary hypertension of the newborn or pulmonary artery hypertension with venous/capillary involvement
Pulmonary hypertension with left heart disease	
Pulmonary hypertension associated with lung diseases and/or hypoxaemia	
Chronic thromboembolic pulmonary hypertension (CTEPH)	
Unclear multifactorial mechanism	

Pulmonary hypertension leads to increased pulmonary vascular resistance (PVR), with increased work and strain being placed on the right side of the heart, ultimately leading to a fall in cardiac output and right ventricular failure in severe cases. The correct diagnosis and treatment can be a difficult undertaking, with many diagnostic tests requiring invasive and dangerous procedures. Symptoms are often non-specific, with the cardinal symptom being breathlessness, which can later be associated with chest pain and syncope. Syncope usually stems from a low cardiac output indicating severe disease.

Pulmonary function tests are often normal, although a reduced gas transfer coefficient may be noted. ECGs and a chest X-ray, albeit helpful, often only exhibit non-specific signs of disease and are therefore not useful in disease diagnosis. The most common non-invasive investigation is the transthoracic echocardiogram, where the systolic pulmonary pressure can be estimated and indicate disease. In order to confirm the disease, right-sided heart catherisation is required.

Anaesthetic management

Giving a safe anaesthetic to patients suffering from pulmonary arterial hypertension (PAH) requires a good knowledge of underlying cardiovascular physiology and poses many challenges. Right ventricular output is dependent on preload, afterload, contractility and heart rate, which all need to be optimised pre-operatively. In order to maintain coronary perfusion pressure to the right side of the heart, particular care needs to be given to the systemic vascular pressure, ensuring adequate perfusion of the aortic root.

Additional pressure is added on the right ventricle by raised pulmonary vascular resistance (PVR), which the heart is not designed to withstand. This increase in afterload will ultimately result in right-sided failure, leading on to left-sided failure due to reduced volume and septal disturbances. Factors that will increase PVR are hypoxia, hypercarbia, low temperature and acidosis. Hence, any anaesthetic should therefore aim to prevent these complications. Anaesthetising patients with PAH therefore relies on extensive monitoring, e.g. invasive blood pressure monitoring, pulmonary artery catheter, useful in monitoring trends in PAP, and cardiac output monitoring.

A number of different induction agents have been used in PAH patients, with etomidate being described as the ideal agent, but thiopentone and propofol being employed much more commonly due to a more favourable side-effect profile. Ketamine has been used cautiously due to concerns it may raise PVR.

Most agents used regularly, such as muscle relaxants, volatile agents and analgesic agents can be used safely. Nitrous oxide however should be used cautiously as it is also implicated in a rise in PVR. A systemic vasoconstrictor may often be employed during induction to ensure a well-controlled SVR. Right-sided failure and a high PVR can be specifically treated with inhaled selective pulmonary vasodilators and agents such as nitric oxide and prostacyclin are therefore nowadays often in use peri-operatively.

Regional techniques such as neuraxial anaesthesia and analgesia are safe in this patient group. The resulting sympathetic blockade and cardiovascular consequences, however, must be monitored. As there are no alpha-1 adrenoreceptors in the pulmonary circulation, neuraxial blockade does not have a direct effect on PVR. Nevertheless, systemic hypotension will reduce aortic coronary perfusion pressure and venous return to the right heart, leading to a reflex bradycardia. Sympathetic blockade can also lead to a loss of the cardio-accelerator fibres at T1-T4, augmenting the bradycardia and loss of inotropy. This cardiovascular compromise can precipitate right-sided failure.

Case scenario 1

A 20-year-old poorly controlled asthmatic patient on oral steroids presents for open reduction and internal fixation (ORIF) of a fractured radius. He is slightly breathless and wheezy at rest.

Describe your peri-operative anaesthetic management for this case

This case is not an emergency life- or limb-saving operative procedure. There is time to treat his asthma. Nebulised salbutamol and high-flow oxygen should be prescribed initially. If there is no response, then in a stepwise manner as outlined in Figure 17.1, treatment should be escalated. Pre-operative optimisation should also include regular chest physiotherapy. This may help in reducing the risk of postoperative infectious complications.

Regional anaesthetic techniques like a brachial plexus block may be an excellent alternative to a general anaesthetic for brittle asthmatics. Invasive monitoring may be required for severe asthmatics. In the event that the patient does not wish to have a regional anaesthetic block, then certain precautions need to be in place for a general anaesthetic.

Certain commonly used agents known to exacerbate asthma in poorly controlled individuals by means of histamine release, such as morphine and atracurium, should be avoided. Intubation in a lightly sedated patient may provoke bronchospasm and particular care needs to be taken to avoid this. Topical application of local anaesthetic to the vocal cords may help in reducing the incidence.

Postoperatively, the patient's regular medication and oxygen therapy should be prescribed as appropriate. Alternative analgesia should be considered if bronchospasm has occurred with previous exposure to morphine.

Case scenario 2

A 72-year-old patient with a history of COPD is scheduled to have a right hemicolectomy. He also gives a recent history of dyspnoea on mild exertion.

Outline your peri-op anaesthetic management for this patient

This patient not only has COPD but is also beginning to show signs of cor pulmonale. Besides standard monitoring as per The Association of Anaesthetists of Great Britain and Ireland (AAGBI) requirement, we also need invasive monitoring in the form of an arterial line and a central venous line to help in the anaesthetic management of this patient. An epidural may be used to help in controlling the pain associated with this procedure. It will help in the reduction of intravenous opioids that have their own side effects.

Induction of anaesthesia should be with either ketamine or propofol, followed by vecuronium or rocuronium. The patient will need to be ventilated throughout surgery. Try to avoid breath stacking or air trapping. This leads to the development of intrinsic/auto-PEEP that can cause a number of undesirable pulmonary and cardiovascular side effects. Analgesia in theatre can be with intravenous opioids and these should be prescribed postoperatively as well. In the event of bronchospasm worsening during surgery, it may be treated with a combination of a volatile agent, salbutamol (inhaler/nebuliser/intravenous), or in severe cases an intravenous adrenaline infusion through a CVC line.

If ventilation has been easy throughout surgery then plan for extubation in the sitting position postoperatively. Postoperatively, bronchodilators and steroids should be given regularly and patients should be closely monitored. Patients with significant disease or comorbidities are often monitored in high dependency units. The provision of effective analgesia is vital to ensure a speedy recovery.

Further reading

1. Canet J, Mazo V. Postoperative pulmonary complications. *Miverva Anesthesiol* 2010; 76: 138-43.

2. Stanley D, Tunnicliffe W. Management of life threatening asthma in adults. *Br J Anaesth CEACCP* 2008; 8: 95-9.

3. Hong CM, Galvagno Jr SM. Patients with chronic pulmonary disease. *Med Clin North Am* 2013; 97(6): 1095-107.

4. Scarlata S, Costanzo L, Giua R, *et al.* Diagnosis and prognostic value of restrictive ventilatory disorders in the elderly: a systematic review of the literature. *Exp Gerontol* 2012; 47(4): 281-9.

5. Elliot CA, Kiely DG. Pulmonary hypertension. *Br J Anaesth CEACCP* 2006; 6: 17-22.

18 Anaesthesia and obesity

Mahul Gorecha and Cyprian Mendonca

Introduction

Obesity is a multisystemic disorder affecting all the body systems but the area particularly affected is the cardiorespiratory system. Anaesthesia and surgery in the obese can be challenging and can present considerable risk.

The most widely used method of classifying obesity is according to the Body Mass Index (BMI)(Table 18.1) and can be calculated by dividing the patient's weight in kilograms by their height in metres squared.

$$BMI = \frac{\text{weight in kg}}{(\text{height in metre})^2}$$

Table 18.1. Classification of obesity.

BMI (kg/m^2)	
<18	Underweight
18-25	Normal
25-30	Overweight
>30	Obese
>35	Morbid obese
>55	Super morbid obese

Another important factor is the actual distribution of the fat and this can form an android or gynaecoid distribution (apple or pear). Pear distribution involves fat distributed to peripheral sites like arms, legs and buttocks. Apple distribution involves more central fat which can involve the liver and spleen. Classifications have been suggested based on the waist-to-hip ratio with values of >0.8 in women and 1.0 in men which is typical of apple distribution. Interestingly, it is this regional distribution of fat that is more predictive than BMI for morbidity and mortality, and central fat is more predictive of diabetes, hypertension and cardiovascular diseases. An obese individual has a 1 in 7 chance of reaching normal life expectancy, and mortality from surgery is twice that of the non-obese population.

Anaesthetic implications of obesity

Since obesity is a multisystemic disorder affecting all organs, there are a number of anaesthetic implications.

Respiratory system

Obstructive sleep apnoea (OSA) is defined as apnoeic episodes secondary to pharyngeal collapse occurring during sleep and present in at least 5% of morbidly obese patients. Patients with OSA often have increased adipose tissue in the pharyngeal wall resulting in increased pharyngeal wall compliance and a tendency for airway collapse when exposed to negative pressure. The diagnosis of OSA can often be made on clinical history and examination alone but the most suitable diagnostic aid for surgical patients is the STOP-BANG questionnaire (Table 18.2).

In the long term, OSA affects the control of breathing by respiratory centre desensitisation and eventually Type two respiratory failure. Obesity hypoventilation syndrome, which is different from OSA, can often be found in the same individuals and affects the control of breathing.

Chest wall compliance is also reduced due to the extra weight of adipose tissue surrounding the thoracic cage. Functional residual capacity

Table 18.2. STOP BANG questionnaire as a screening tool for obstructive sleep apnoea. *From: Chung F, Subramanyam R, Liao P, et al. High STOP-BANG score indicates a high probability of obstructive sleep apnoea. Br J Anaesth 2012; 108: 768-75. This is an open access article under the terms of the Creative Commons Attribution Non-Commercial License (http://creativecommons.org/licenses/by-nc/2.5/uk/).*

Snoring — Do you snore loudly? (louder than talking or loud enough to be heard through doors)	Yes/No
Tired — do you often feel tired, fatigued or sleepy during daytime?	Yes/No
Observed — Has anyone observed you stop breathing during your sleep?	Yes/No
Blood **P**ressure — Do you have or are you being treated for high blood pressure?	Yes/No
BMI — more than 35kg/m^2?	Yes/No
Age — Age more than 50 years old?	Yes/No
Neck circumference — greater than 40cm?	Yes/No
Gender — Male?	Yes/No

One point scored for each positive feature. There is a high risk of OSA if the score is >3 and a low risk of OSA if the score is <3.

(FRC) is also reduced by small airway collapse, displacement of the diaphragm by abdominal contents and increased thoracic blood volume. As BMI increases then FRC declines steeply and closing volume can encroach on FRC during normal breathing causing airway closure. The increase in adipose tissue of the neck and upper chest can make intubation and ventilation with a face mask difficult.

A combination of the above effects on the respiratory system, combined with supine position and anaesthesia, result in hypoxia and rapid desaturation during induction of general anaesthesia.

Cardiovascular system

All cardiac indices are increased including cardiac output, ventricular workload, oxygen consumption, carbon dioxide production and blood volume due to the increased metabolic demands of excess adipose tissue.

Blood volume relative to body mass is low and there is increased activation of the renin-angiotensin system. Systemic hypertension is common in the obese and can be found in about 50% of subjects. This increased left ventricular wall stress and subsequent dilatation can lead to diastolic dysfunction.

Obese patients are also more at risk of arrhythmias, sudden cardiac death, a prolonged QT interval and ischaemic heart disease.

Gastrointestinal system

In obese patients, there is an increased incidence of hiatus hernia, gastro-oesophageal reflux and an increased volume and acidity of gastric contents and increased intra-abdominal pressure increasing the risk of aspiration.

Endocrine system

The risk of developing diabetes is increased five-fold due to a relative insulin resistance and inadequate production. Obese patients also develop a macrovesicular fatty liver which can progress to steatohepatitis and cirrhosis.

Metabolic syndrome is a cluster of conditions including diabetes, hypertension, excess fat around the waist and abnormal cholesterol levels that occur together and increase the risk of developing heart disease and stroke.

Practical considerations

Obese patients can be very challenging to move, lift and nurse. All practical procedures including venepuncture, and local and regional blocks can be technically demanding. Accurate drug dosing can be difficult and non-invasive arterial pressure monitoring can be inaccurate.

Drug handling

The mass of adipose tissue makes pharmacokinetics and pharmacodynamics unpredictable in obese patients. Therefore, close attention to clinical endpoints such as loss of verbal contact is paramount. Obese patients have reduced total body water, a higher fat mass, a higher glomerular filtration rate (GFR), increased renal clearance and normal hepatic clearance. The volume of distribution of fat-soluble drugs is increased. Some drugs are cleared more rapidly in obese patients due to a higher cardiac output and splanchnic blood flow. Calculating the drug dosage in obese patients is a complex issue. Table 18.3 describes what weight can be used for calculating the drug dosage.

Table 18.3. Body weight used for the initial dosing of commonly used anaesthetic drugs for healthy obese adults. *Reproduced from The Association of Anaesthetists of Great Britain and Ireland. Peri-operative management of the obese surgical patient 2015. Anaesthesia 2015; 70: 859-76.*

Lean body weight	Adjusted body weight
Propofol (induction)	Propofol (infusion for maintenance)
Thiopentone	Antibiotics
Fentanyl	Low-molecular-weight heparin
Rocuronium	Alfentanil
Atracurium	Neostigmine
Vecuronium	Sugammadex
Morphine	
Paracetamol	
Bupivacaine	
Lidocaine	

Adjusted body weight = 0.25x (ABW-IBW) + IBW
ABW = actual body weight
IBW = ideal body weight
IBW for males is height in cm - 100; for females is height in cm - 105

Lean body weight (LBW) = actual body weight - body fat. It is calculated using complex mathematical formulae. In general, lean body weight rarely exceeds 100kg for men and 70kg for women.

Pre-operative assessment

The peri-operative management of obese patients presents significant organisational and practical issues. A detailed anaesthetic assessment must be performed and symptoms and signs of cardiac failure and OSA should be actively sought. It is also important to assess the ability to tolerate the supine position. Mouth opening, Mallampati score, neck movements and collar size should all be noted.

Investigations should be tailored to patient comorbidities and type of surgery. A full blood count, urea and serum electrolytes, coagulation profile and blood glucose are useful pre-operative investigations. An arterial blood gas (ABG) should be done in those suspected of respiratory disease and will be useful in deciding if postoperative respiratory support is likely. A pre-operative ECG should be requested to evaluate cardiac rhythm, ischaemic changes and left ventricular hypertrophy. Also, patients with right heart failure, cor pulmonale, day-time somnolence or pulmonary hypertension may benefit from a period of elective non-invasive ventilation before surgery.

Echocardiography is useful in estimating ventricular function but it is technically difficult to obtain good quality transthoracic images due to body habitus.

Prophylaxis with histamine H_2 receptor antagonists or proton pump inhibitors is advisable and can be administered at the time of premedication. Obese patients are also at risk of venous thromboembolism and adequately sized compression stockings and low-molecular-weight heparin should be used until full postoperative mobilisation.

Patient optimisation should include weight loss advice, treating cardiovascular disease and managing glycaemic control.

Regional anaesthesia

Good regional anaesthesia may reduce opioid requirement in the postoperative period; however, regional anaesthesia is technically harder due to the loss of landmarks, increased movement of the skin and the need for long needles. Due to the extra fat constricting the potential space and engorgement of the extradural veins, less local anaesthetic is needed for epidural analgesia.

Conduct of anaesthesia

To reduce moving and handling, many anaesthetists choose to induce anaesthesia in theatre on an appropriately sized operating table (Figure 18.1) with enough trained and experienced staff. Standard monitoring

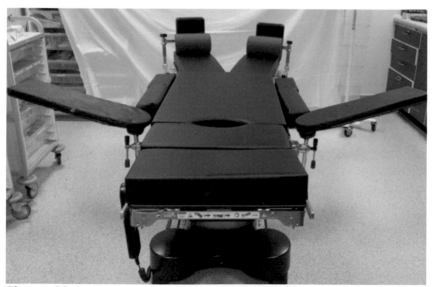

Figure 18.1. Bariatric table with arm attachments, side extensions and foot pads with support.

must include a correct-sized blood pressure cuff and if measurement is difficult then an arterial line should be considered. Venous cannulation can be difficult and central venous cannulation may be necessary. It is important to appropriately position the patient before induction of anaesthesia.

Positioning and pre-oxygenation

About 20-25° of head-up tilt position ensures better functional residual capacity of the lungs and improves oxygen reserve. Pre-oxygenation should be carried out using a tight fitting face mask and expired oxygen concentration should be monitored. An expired oxygen concentration above 0.8 ensures an adequate pre-oxygenation. In addition, oxygen can also be administered using nasal cannulae. High-flow nasal oxygen administration prior to induction of anaesthesia, continued during the apnoeic period, prolongs the duration of apnoea without desaturation.

A 'sniffing in the morning air' position may be difficult to achieve in obese patients and a wedge or blanket beneath the shoulders can aid positioning. An elevated head position with ramping improves the laryngoscopic view and success of tracheal intubation. A ramped position is achieved either using a purpose made mattress (Figure 18.2) or using blankets under the shoulder so that the external auditory meatus is aligned with the suprasternal notch.

Bag and mask ventilation can be difficult in obese patients and can be overcome by either a two-handed technique or by the use of a mechanical ventilator. Laryngoscopy can be difficult; therefore, plans should be in place for managing difficult intubation. Effective temperature maintenance is important as it reduces postoperative wound infection. Care must be taken over pressure areas, arm over abduction to avoid brachial plexus injuries and calf compression devices should be used.

Using short-acting anaesthetic agents such as remifentanil, sevoflurane or desflurane will help to aid rapid recovery from anaesthesia and reduce postoperative hypoventilation and hypoxaemia. Monitoring neuromuscular blockade is also important as inadequate reversal is poorly tolerated in obesity.

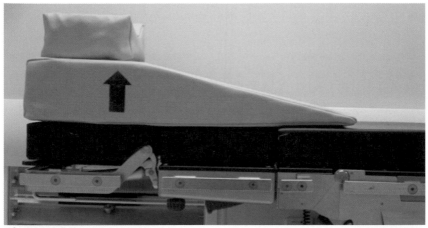

Figure 18.2. Additional mattress and pillow used to achieve a ramping position for obese patients.

Postoperative management

Obese patients should be extubated wide-awake in the sitting position. Patients who have obesity-related comorbidities have a high risk of perioperative complications and these patients should be nursed in a high dependency unit. Many obese patients who suffer from significant sleep apnoea or arterial desaturation will benefit from postoperative CPAP. The analgesic plan should consist of a multimodal approach involving paracetamol, NSAIDs, patient-controlled opioid analgesia and regional anaesthesia. All precautions should be taken to minimise the effects on the respiratory system. NSAIDs should be used with caution as they can cause postoperative renal dysfunction.

Early mobilisation is encouraged as it reduces postoperative atelectasis and venothromboembolism. Finally, the stress response of surgery can cause hyperglycaemia, so an insulin infusion may be required in some patients.

Case scenario 1

A 50-year-old male patient with a BMI of 58 is scheduled for an emergency repair of an incarcerated epigastric hernia. He has a past medical history of type 2 diabetes mellitus treated with insulin, hypertension and obstructive sleep apnoea for which he is on home CPAP.

How would you manage this patient?

Pre-operative management

Pre-operative assessment should include a detailed history to evaluate ischaemic heart disease, cardiovascular and renal complications of diabetes and hypertension. Investigations should include a full blood count, urea and electrolytes, an ECG and a coagulation profile. The patient should be kept NBM and an insulin sliding scale should be started. A nasogastric tube should be inserted to drain the stomach contents.

Intra-operative management

The patient should be positioned 20° head up on the bariatric operating table and ramped up using a HELP® mattress. An arterial line should be inserted to monitor his blood pressure. Following optimum pre-oxygenation (by monitoring end-tidal oxygen concentration), a modified rapid sequence induction using propofol and rocuronium can be performed. Following induction of anaesthesia, an ultrasound-guided bilateral posterior rectus sheath block (20ml 0.375% levobupivacaine injected on either side) should be performed. This provides postoperative analgesia and reduces the dose of opioids. The use of a target-controlled remifentanil infusion facilitates smooth and controlled extubation. It is useful to use non-invasive cardiac output monitoring such as LiDCOrapid™ to ensure optimum fluid balance.

Postoperative management

After the operation, neuromuscular blockade should be reversed. In this case, sugammadex is preferable. The patient should be extubated in a 45° sitting-up position. Regional analgesia allows the patient to wake up faster due to low opiate usage. Postoperatively, he should be transferred to the HDU for CPAP and monitoring. DVT prophylaxis should be commenced and glycaemic control should be monitored. Urine output and fluid balance should also be monitored.

Case scenario 2

A 65-year-old male patient with a BMI of 50 is scheduled for an elective left total knee replacement. He has no other significant past medical history.

How would you manage this patient?

Pre-operative management

This patient should be seen in the anaesthetic pre-operative assessment clinic and routine blood tests carried out. As this is an elective scenario, the patient should be referred to the obesity clinic in order to reduce his weight.

Intra-operative management

A regional anaesthetic technique is preferred. It may be difficult to locate the intervertebral space; an ultrasound can be used to locate the midline and depth of the space. Either a single injection of spinal anaesthetic or a combined spinal epidural can be chosen as a preferred regional technique. A long spinal needle of 120mm length (24G pencil-point spinal needle) may be required. In addition, an adductor canal block can be performed using 20ml of 0.25% levobupivacaine to provide postoperative analgesia. Peri-articular infiltration of a local anaesthetic solution also provides postoperative analgesia.

Postoperative management

In the postoperative period, the patient should be encouraged to eat and drink straightaway. Regular paracetamol and non-steroidal analgesics (if not contraindicated), and gabapentin are used for postoperative analgesia. The patient should be mobilised on the first postoperative day. Mechanical prophyalxis against deep vein thrombosis should be commenced during the intra-operative period and pharmacological prophylaxis in the postoperative period.

Further reading

1. The Society for Obesity and Bariatric Anaesthesia uk. http://www.sobauk.co.uk.
2. Cortínez LI, Anderson BJ, Penna A, *et al.* Influence of obesity on propofol pharmacokinetics: derivation of a pharmacokinetic model. *Br J Anaesth* 2010; 105: 448-56.
3. Lotia S, Bellamy MC. Anaesthesia and morbid obesity. *Br J Anaesth CEACCP* 2008; 8: 151-6.
4. Ingrande J, Lemmens HJM. Dose adjustment of anaesthetics in the morbidly obese. *Br J Anaesth* 2010; 105: i16-i23.
5. Members of working party; Nightingale CE, Margarson MP, Shearer E, *et al.* Peri-operative management of the obese surgical patient 2015 AAGBI. *Anaesthesia* 2015; 70: 859-76.
6. Chung F, Yegneswaran B, Liao P, *et al.* STOP questionnaire: a tool to screen patients for obstructive sleep apnea. *Anesthesiology* 2008; 108: 812-21.
7. Chung F, Subramanyam R, Liao P, *et al.* High STOP-BANG score indicates a high probability of obstructive sleep apnoea. *Br J Anaesth* 2012; 108: 768-75.
8. Chung F, Yang Y, Liao P. Predictive performance of the STOP-BANG score for identifying obstructive sleep apnea in obese patients. *Obes Surg* 2013; 23: 2050-7.

19 Postoperative recovery and care

George Madden

Introduction

Postoperative complications have a negative impact on patient recovery, efficiency of service provision and healthcare costs. The past 30 years has seen a gradually increasing focus on the causes of complications, and attempts to prevent them.

Postoperative complications can broadly be classified into those related to the operative procedure, those related to the anaesthetic and those related to the patient's physiology. Complications due to the surgical procedure itself may be reduced by refinements of surgical techniques and the development of minimally-invasive procedures. Complications related to anaesthesia are rare because of improvements in patient monitoring and modern anaesthetic agents. The patient's own physiology is the major contributing factor for postoperative complications following surgery.

Any tissue trauma, including surgery, prompts a cascade of physiological changes that alter oxygen requirements, cardiopulmonary stress and induces endocrine and metabolic changes. As these effects are related to surgery they are termed the surgical stress response. Many attempts have been made over the years to modify this response, though no single intervention has been demonstrated to be effective.

Common postoperative problems

The common problems during recovery and the postoperative period include pain, gut dysfunction, postoperative hypoxaemia, catabolism and complications associated with immobilisation. A multimodal approach, which is now known as enhanced recovery after surgery (ERAS) has been developed to address the common recovery and postoperative problems.

Pain

Pain is an unpleasant sensory and emotional experience associated with actual or potential tissue trauma. Aside from its obvious unpleasant nature, it has a number of important adverse effects. Firstly, it encourages the sufferer to become immobile, which then delays postoperative recovery. Secondly, it contributes to the magnitude of the stress response, with its negative cardiorespiratory and metabolic effects. Thirdly, severe pain can increase the likelihood of subsequent chronic pain syndromes, which is pain that persists beyond the tissue injury and which may represent a primary dysfunction of the nervous system. In addition, traditional analgesia is opioid-based, which generally have side effects including nausea, sedation and delayed gastric emptying.

Gut dysfunction

Delayed gastric emptying and gut motility may be the consequences of the original insult (e.g. intra-abdominal sepsis), pain, opioids, postoperative complications (e.g. collections, anastomotic leak, infection) or simply a response to gut handling during surgery. Clearly, the shortest possible time between surgery and restoration of gut function is an important factor in postoperative rehabilitation.

Postoperative hypoxaemia

It has been well established that hypoxaemia occurs after surgery due to a combination of pain, restricted movements, positioning and hypoventilation related to anaesthesia. These problems are classically worsened by the pattern of sleep disturbance over the first 72 hours. Initially, the patient's sleep will be disturbed, returning to a normal pattern on the second or third postoperative night. At this point, the patient will enter REM sleep with associated hypoventilation. Susceptible patients may then experience hypoxaemia sufficient to cause myocardial or cerebral ischaemia. Even those who are at low risk for such complications may suffer an increased risk of wound complications if they are hypoxaemic postoperatively.

Catabolism

The stress response to surgery results in mobilisation of amino acids, fatty acids and other metabolic substrates. This, in extreme circumstances, may cause overall loss of muscle mass, which if prolonged will delay mobilisation. This situation is worsened by excessive pre-operative fasting. There has been much interest in reducing this response, by either reducing the stress response itself, emphasising early mobilisation to prevent muscle loss, electrical stimulation of muscles and minimising fasting times.

Immobilisation

Reduced mobility is a major contributor to delayed recovery and discharge. It also contributes to loss of muscle mass and hypoxaemia. Minimising immobilisation is therefore an important part of enhanced recovery. To achieve this, there are two important considerations: firstly, factors that restrain the patient from mobilising must be minimised. These include postoperative drains, urinary catheters and unnecessary infusions. Efforts must be made to avoid using these routinely. Secondly, pain must be well controlled and in this instance, regional anaesthetic techniques may be superior to opioid-based regimes.

Principles of enhanced recovery

The aims of enhanced recovery after surgery (ERAS) are to reduce surgical stress, maintain physiological function and facilitate mobilisation after surgery. The ultimate aim is to reduce morbidity and the length of stay in hospital. Added to this is the benefit of a protocol-based care system.

Pre-operative management

Preadmission counselling

The aims of counselling are to reduce fear and anxiety related to surgery and to give the patient information regarding their expected postoperative recovery. This can help to reduce time to feeding, mobilisation, pain control, and aid in postoperative physiotherapy, and as a consequence reduce complication rates. It can also give patients a sense of empowerment as they can play a more active role in their own recovery.

Pre-operative optimisation

Medical optimisation of comorbidities has been advocated for many years. Abstinence of alcohol or tobacco has been shown to reduce postoperative morbidity.

It used to be a longstanding tradition that patients should be "nil by mouth from midnight" prior to surgery. Though the importance of an empty stomach prior to induction of anaesthesia is well established, the optimum fasting times should be 6 hours for foods and particulate fluids (e.g. milk), and 2 hours for clear fluids. This balances the reduced aspiration risk associated with fasting along with the benefits of reduced catabolism and hydration. Complex carbohydrate drinks, containing 12.5% maltodextrins, drunk up to 2 hours pre-operatively have been found to reduce pre-operative thirst, hunger, anxiety and insulin resistance, without increasing aspiration risk. Furthermore, carbohydrate drinks have been found to better maintain body mass and muscle strength and accelerate recovery. Carbohydrate drinks are thus a recommended part of enhanced recovery.

Premedication

Pharmacological sedation and anxiolysis have previously been part of common pre-operative practice. Anxiolytics have been shown to have an adverse effect on immediate postoperative recovery, impairing the ability to mobilise, eat and drink. As such, these agents are no longer routinely advocated.

Antimicrobial prophylaxis

Antimicrobial agents are indicated where contamination into a sterile area may occur. The optimum time for administration is 30-60 minutes prior to skin incision and the choice of antibiotics should be made in conjunction with local guidelines. Hair removal in the surgical field reduces the risk of wound infection and is best achieved with clipping rather than razors. Chlorhexidine-alcohol solutions are superior to povidone-iodine as skin preparation, though care must be taken with the use of alcohol-based solutions in the presence of diathermy, as ignition and burns have been reported.

Standardised anaesthetic technique

ERAS aims to introduce certain evidence-based anaesthetic techniques into practice.

The newer and short-acting anaesthetic agents with more rapid clearance and minimal hangover effects are deemed preferable. Agents such as propofol for induction along with opioid adjuncts such as fentanyl, alfentanil or remifentanil are recommended during induction. Amongst the inhalational anaesthetic agents used for maintenance, sevoflurane and desflurane have the most desirable properties.

Depth of anaesthesia monitoring should be used in cases where titration of anaesthesia may be compromised by the patient's physiological state and where excessively 'deep' anaesthesia may be detrimental.

Fluid management

Goal-directed fluid therapy has been shown to reduce morbidity. The National Institute for Health and Care Excellence (NICE) now recommends their use in non-invasive cardiac output monitoring (such as oesophageal Dopplers) to guide fluid and vasopressor administration with the intention of achieving normovolaemia and maintaining adequate cardiac output. In some studies this has led to a reduction in overall fluid administration, which in turn reduces bowel oedema and thus improves a return to function along with good outcome. Invasive monitoring utilising cardiac output monitoring may also be of benefit. Central venous pressure monitoring, which has traditionally been used to guide fluid administration is a poor measure of fluid balance and should no longer be used for this purpose.

Postoperative nausea and vomiting

Postoperative nausea and vomiting (PONV) is a major cause of patient dissatisfaction and delayed discharge. It affects one in three to four patients. There are many factors that cause PONV, including patient-related risk factors, particular types of surgery and also anaesthetic techniques. There is good evidence that risk stratification followed by a multimodal approach to prophylaxis is effective.

Surgical technique

It has become clear that the stress response to surgery is directly related to the extent of tissue trauma. Thus, it follows that the least invasive technique will minimise stress and thus expedite recovery. Added to that, minimising tissue trauma may also reduce the inflammatory response. It is of little surprise, therefore, that laparoscopic and robot-assisted procedures have been demonstrated to reduce the length of stay while achieving comparable results to open surgery.

Since the CRASH-2 trial demonstrated the effectiveness of tranexamic acid in traumatic major haemorrhage, there has been increasing interest in using it in elective surgery. It is now a routine component of most enhanced recovery hip and knee arthroplasties.

Nasogastric tubes

There is no evidence to support the use of nasogastric intubation in routine colorectal surgery and it has been demonstrated to increase the incidence of fever, atelectasis and pneumonia.

In pancreaticoduodenal surgery, however, there is justification for occasional use when delayed gastric emptying is a problem; in this instance, nasojejunal intubation may be utilised so the patient can receive enteral nutrition. It is not, however, advised as a routine measure and attempts to resume a normal enteral diet should still be encouraged in the first instance.

Maintenance of normothermia

Peri-operative hypothermia increases the incidence of wound infection, cardiac events, haemorrhage and worsens postoperative pain scores. Shivering dramatically increases total body oxygen consumption at a time when oxygen consumption is already raised by tissue trauma.

Maintenance of normothermia is superior to restoration of normothermia after a period of hypothermia. It is therefore important to ensure patients arrive into theatre normothermic, and are kept around normal temperature (>36°C) via a range of techniques until discharge from the post-anaesthetic care unit. Techniques commonly utilised include forced air warming devices, underbody warming mattresses and warmed fluids, while also limiting heat loss through evaporation by increasing theatre humidity and applying hydrophobic filters to breathing circuits to retain respiratory humidity. Underpinning this is close monitoring of the patient's temperature to ensure normothermia is maintained.

Postoperative management

Analgesia

Epidural analgesia has been widely acknowledged to improve pain control, reduce postoperative nausea and vomiting (PONV) and reduce complications, compared to opioids in colorectal surgery. Other regional techniques have also been shown to reduce opiod use and in doing so, facilitate rapid awakening from anaesthesia and reduce the time to mobilisation and enteral feeding. In addition, it may also attenuate the surgical stress response. The type of regional anaesthetic depends upon the surgical procedure and different blocks have different advantages and disadvantages. In the setting of lower limb arthroplasties, the benefits in analgesia gained by nerve blocks are negated by the duration of limb paralysis and thus the delay in mobilising. This is particularly relevant to lower limb arthroplasties as early mobilisation and physiotherapy reduces the length of hospital stay.

In addition to the above measures, there has been interest in using adjunctive analgesic agents such as gabapentin, magnesium sulphate and in some settings, intravenous lidocaine.

Surgical drains

In colorectal surgery, drains were thought to remove unwanted intraperitoneal fluid and to provide an early warning of anastomotic dehiscence. In both counts the evidence to support their use is lacking and drains probably only serve to delay mobilisation.

Venous thromboembolism (VTE) prophylaxis

Venous thromboembolism (deep vein thrombosis and pulmonary embolism) is a recognised complication following major surgery and carries a significant morbidity and mortality. A triad of measures has been shown to significantly reduce the incidence of VTE: intermittent pneumatic calf compression intra-operatively, compression stockings and low-molecular-weight heparin (LMWH) administration. The duration of use of LMWHs is debatable and currently extended courses of 28 days are advocated for major cancer surgery in the abdomen or pelvis and in some centres for lower limb arthroplasty. Other patients receive LMWHs while in hospital, and low-risk patients may only require LMWHs until mobile.

Prevention of postoperative ileus

Postoperative ileus is a big challenge in major abdominal surgery. Prolonged ileus appears to be associated with open surgery, intravenous opioids and fluid overload. The mainstay of management is to avoid these where possible, thus laparoscopic surgery, neuraxial analgesia, and restrictive, goal-directed fluid management are the main measures to be recommended.

Additionally, some novel interventions have been tested with varying outcomes: prokinetic agents do not appear to be effective, whereas oral magnesium oxide, bisacodyl and chewing gum have been shown to be effective. In patients receiving opioid analgesia, the μ-opioid agonist, alvimopan, has been shown to be effective.

Postoperative analgesia regimens

The ideal analgesic regimen varies according to the surgery performed. Midline laparotomies are best managed with epidural analgesia; however, for laparoscopic surgery, epidurals probably provide little benefit and may actually increase length of stay. Spinal opioids may be a better solution as, though shorter lasting, the pain from laparoscopy is lower and improves faster. An alternative technique is local infiltration and transversus abdominis plane block. Though providing effective local anaesthesia to the abdominal wall, it does not reduce the visceral pain from surgery and is primarily an adjunct.

Postoperative nutrition

Pre-operatively, it is important to maintain normal nutrition and avoid excessive fasting. In all but the most malnourished patients, a normal diet is sufficient, supplemented with a carbohydrate drink 2 hours before surgery to compensate for pre-operative fasting. Postoperatively, the patient should be allowed to drink immediately after surgery and eat as soon as possible. Though this is associated with higher rates of vomiting due to ileus, it does reduce length of hospital stay and infection, and is not associated with anastomotic dehiscence.

Glucose control

It has been recognised in critical care patients that hyperglycaemia is associated with worse outcomes, particularly infection-related. Insulin resistance is a known consequence of the stress response to surgery, and thus the measures taken in the enhanced recovery programme to reduce the surgical stress response should also reduce insulin resistance. Nonetheless, in some patients, hyperglycaemia may still occur and here insulin infusions to maintain blood glucose below 10mmol/L can help reduce the incidence of complications and also prevent glycosuria, which has osmotic effects which may ultimately cause excessive diuresis.

Early mobilisation

Early mobilisation is associated with a reduced incidence of chest complications and in combination with good nutrition, can improve muscle strength in the early postoperative phase. It may also reduce insulin resistance. It is also a good marker of ERAS success. Failure to mobilise is often related to impaired pain control, a requirement of intravenous fluids or continued urinary catheterisation, although it may also be due to patient comorbidities or motivation. It is strongly associated with increased length of hospital stay, and thus day one mobilisation may be used as an early marker of whether ERAS interventions have been successful.

Benefits and limitations of enhanced recovery

ERAS has been demonstrated to reduce postoperative morbidity and length of stay, and has showed no difference in readmission rates compared with traditional care. It does not, however, appear to affect mortality.

ERAS was designed for an elective population and original studies excluded those who had coexisting problems which may have impaired mobilisation or compliance. It did, however, include patients of all ASA grades (American Society of Anesthesiologists Physical Status). Subsequent recommendations have suggested that though the ERAS programme itself may not be feasible in especially complex, high-risk or emergency cases, the general principles should be adhered to.

Case scenario 1

A 68-year-old woman with a history of hypertension, rheumatoid arthritis and gastro-oesophageal reflux disease has to undergo a hip replacement surgery.

How would you manage this patient?

Pre-operative management

This patient should be assessed in the pre-operative assessment clinic and it should be ensured that her blood pressure is well controlled and, if anaemic, anaemia is corrected.

Pre-medication mainly consists of analgesics administered about an hour prior to the surgery:

- Gabapentin 300mg PO.
- Paracetamol 1g.
- Ibuprofen 400mg.

A carbohydrate drink should be given 2 hours prior to the surgery.

Intra-operative management

Anaesthetic technique:

- Spinal anaesthesia using 3ml of isobaric levobupivacaine 0.25% is preferred.

Analgesia:

- Local infiltration analgesia.

150mg levobupivacaine with 0.75mg adrenaline and 30mg ketorolac made up to 150ml total volume and infiltrated during the intra-operative period by the surgeon.

Circulatory support:

- Tranexamic acid 1g on induction.
- 1000ml of crystalloid.

Drains/catheters:

- Avoid drains or urinary catheters if possible.

Antimicrobial prophylaxis:

- 2% chlorhexidine gluconate skin preparation.
- Single-dose antibiotics 30-60 minutes prior to the skin incision.

Thromboprophylaxis:

- Thromboembolic deterrent (TED) and pneumatic compression stockings applied to the non-operated lower limb.

Postoperative management

Regular prescription:

- Paracetamol 1g QDS.
- Diclofenac 50mg/ibuprofen 400mg TDS (if there are no contraindications).
- Gabapentin 300mg TDS (reduce to 100mg if over 70 years or known chronic kidney disease).
- Morphine sulphate (MST) 20mg BD for 5 days.
- Omeprazole 20mg OD.
- Ondansetron 4mg TDS.
- Lactulose 15ml or senna 15mg OD.

As needed prescription:

- Oramorph 10-20mg 2-hourly.
- Naloxone 40-400µg if there is respiratory depression.
- Cyclizine 50mg.

Nutrition:

- Resume normal oral intake immediately.

Fluids:

- 500ml crystalloid boluses prior to mobilisation to offset orthostatic hypotension.

Thromboprophylaxis:

- Enoxaparin 40mg OD SC for 30 days.

Rehabilitation:

- Exercises in bed in the evening (for morning surgery) or the next morning (for afternoon surgery).
- Weight-bearing exercises on the first postoperative day (including mobilising).

The patient can be discharged once it is deemed safe by the physiotherapists.

Case scenario 2

A 72-year-old man who has no other systemic illness is scheduled for a right hemicolectomy

How would you manage this patient?

Pre-operative management

He should be seen in the pre-operative assessment clinic and the following measures should be taken in preparation for his surgery:

- Optimise comorbidities.
- Optimise anaemia.
- An instruction leaflet and verbal advice on the peri-operative course should be given.

Premedication:

- A phosphate enema on the day of surgery to the empty rectum (when required).

A carbohydrate drink should be given 2 hours prior to the surgery.

Intra-operative management

Anaesthetic technique:

- General anaesthetic with modern anaesthetic agents (sevoflurane, desflurane or total intravenous anaesthesia).

Antiemesis:

- Dexamethasone 8mg.
- Ondansetron 4mg.

Analgesia:

- Thoracic epidural with a low-dose infusion (e.g. 0.1% levobupivacaine and 2µg/ml fentanyl) for open surgery.
- Spinal opioid (e.g. 500µg diamorphine, 200µg morphine) for laparoscopic surgery.

Circulatory support:

- Goal-directed fluid therapy guided by a non-invasive cardiac output monitor.

Drains/catheters:

- Avoid drains or urinary catheters if possible.
- No nasogastric tubes.

Antimicrobial prophylaxis:

- 2% chlorhexidine gluconate skin preparation.
- Single-dose antibiotics 30-60 minutes prior to the skin incision.

Thromboprophylaxis:

- TED and pneumatic compression stockings.

Postoperative management

Regular prescription:

- Paracetamol 1g QDS.
- Regular ibuprofen (if not contraindicated).
- Epidural infusion (as commenced intra-operatively) for 3 days postoperatively.
- Prophylactic low-molecular-weight heparin.

As needed prescription:

- Naloxone 40-400µg if there is respiratory depression.
- Ondansetron 4mg 8-hourly.
- Cyclizine 50mg 8-hourly.
- Oramorph 10-20mg hourly (to be commenced when the epidural is removed).

Day 0:

- Maintenance crystalloid (1-1.5ml/kg/h until taking adequate oral fluids).
- Encouraged to eat and drink normally.
- Target oral fluid intake >1000ml, including carbohydrate drinks.
- Mobilsation begins ~6 hours after surgery.

Day 1:

- Urinary catheter removed (if present).
- Eating and drinking normally.
- Target oral fluid intake >200ml, including carbohydrate drinks.
- Mobilise during the day, sitting out when not mobilising.
- Plan for discharge.

Day 2:

- Remove the epidural catheter and convert to oral analgesia.
- Normal diet and fluids.
- Full mobilisation.
- Aim to discharge that day.

Further reading

1. Place K, Scott NB. Enhanced recovery for lower limb arthroplasty. *Br J Anaesth CEACCP* 2014; 14: 95-9.
2. Gustafsson UO, Scott MJ, Schwenk W, *et al.* Guidelines for perioperative care in elective colonic surgery: enhanced recovery after surgery (ERAS®); Society recommendations. *World J Surg* 2013; 37: 259-84.
3. Khan SK, Malviya A, Muller SD, *et al.* Reduced short-term complications and mortality following enhanced recovery primary hip and knee arthroplasty: results from 6000 consecutive procedures. *Acta Orthopaedica* 2014; 85: 26-31.
4. Lassen K, Coolsen MME, Slim K, *et al.* Guidelines for perioerative care for pancreaticoduodenectomy: enhanced recovery after surgery (ERAS®); Society recommendations. *World J Surg* 2013; 37: 240-58.
5. Nygren J, Thacker J, Carli F, Fearon KCH, *et al.* Guidelines for perioperative care in elective rectal/pelvic surgery: enhanced recovery after surgery (ERAS®); Society recommendations. *World J Surg* 2013; 37: 285-305.
6. Basse L, Jakobsen DH, Billesbolle P, *et al.* A clinical pathway to accelerate recovery after colonic resection. *Ann Surg* 2000; 232: 51-7.

20 Airway management

Vassilis Athanassoglou and Cyprian Mendonca

Introduction

The key aim of airway management is to maintain a clear air passage from the exterior to the trachea or to bypass the obstructed airway. In addition, it should facilitate assisted or controlled ventilation and should protect the lungs from aspiration.

In a critically ill patient, rapid assessment and institution of a patent airway, ventilation and oxygenation of the lungs are essential in preventing secondary damage to the brain and other organs due to hypoxia.

The unconscious patient and the airway

In an unconscious patient, airway obstruction can occur anywhere from the nose and mouth down to the bronchial level and can be partial or total. The commonest site of airway obstruction in the unconscious patient is at the level of the pharynx due to the tongue and surrounding soft tissue falling back onto the pharyngeal wall due to loss of muscle tone. Regurgitation of food, a foreign body or blood clots may cause airway obstruction. In a semi-conscious patient, laryngeal obstruction can occur as a result of spasm of the laryngeal muscles (occurring as a result of stimulation of the upper airway) or laryngeal oedema (as a result of burns, inflammation or anaphylaxis). Infraglottic airway obstruction can occur as a result of excessive secretions, mucosal oedema, bronchospasm or aspiration of gastric contents.

Airway obstruction can be recognised by a *look, listen and feel* approach:

- *Look* for chest and abdominal movements.
- *Listen and feel* for airflow at the mouth and nose.

In the presence of airway obstruction, in a spontaneously breathing patient, the accessory muscles of respiration come into play. The neck and shoulder muscles will be contracting to assist the expansion of the thoracic cage. In a patient with complete airway obstruction, the spontaneous respiratory effort produces paradoxical chest and abdominal movement. During normal breathing, the chest and abdomen move synchronously; during inspiration, the chest expands and the diaphragm is pushed down, with the opposite happening during expiration. In complete airway obstruction during inspiration the chest expands and the abdomen is drawn in, with the opposite happening during expiration; this is called 'see-saw' breathing. In complete airway obstruction, the breath sounds can be absent.

Airway obstruction can also be partial, in which case air entry is diminished and usually noisy. Different types of noisy breathing can be observed depending on the site of airway obstruction:

- Inspiratory stridor — caused by obstruction at or above the glottic level.
- Expiratory wheeze — obstruction of the lower airways.
- Gurgling — due to the presence of liquid or semisolid material in the major airways.
- Snoring — due to a partially occluded pharynx by the tongue or palate.

It is important to remember that normal breathing is quiet, partially obstructed breathing is noisy, and complete airway obstruction is silent. Airway obstruction should be relieved promptly to facilitate adequate oxygen delivery to the lungs.

Basic airway management

The airway should be cleared by removing any visible foreign body and suctioning the secretions in the oral cavity. This should be done before attempting to open the obstructed airway due to tongue or other upper airway structures. There are three manoeuvres that can be used to relieve the obstruction caused by the tongue:

- Head tilt — this can be attained by placing one hand on the patient's forehead and tilting the head backwards gently (Figure 20.1A). This

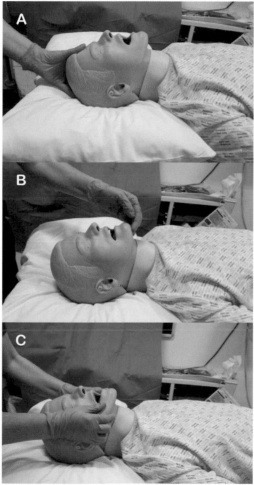

Figure 20.1. Basic airway opening manoeuvres. A) Head tilt; B) Chin lift; C) Jaw thrust.

manoeuvre is contraindicated in the presence of suspected cervical spine disease or injury.

- Chin lift — the patient's chin is lifted to open the airway using the fingertips of the other hand (Figure 20.1B).
- Jaw thrust — after identifying the angle of the mandible, the ring and little fingers are placed behind the angle, the index and middle fingers are placed over the body of the mandible to apply a steady upward and forward pressure to lift the mandible. The thumbs are used to open the mouth slightly by downward displacement of the chin (Figure 20.1C). This is the technique of choice to open the airway in order to facilitate face mask ventilation.

Basic airway adjuncts

In addition to the above manoeuvres, airway adjuncts, such as oropharyngeal or nasopharyngeal airways, may also be required to maintain the airway patency. These separate the tongue and other soft tissues from the posterior pharyngeal wall.

Oropharyngeal airway (Guedel airway)

The oropharyngeal airway follows the curvature of the tongue, pulling it and the epiglottis away from the posterior pharyngeal wall and providing a channel for air passage. It is a curved tube made of plastic, flanged and reinforced at the oral end with a flattened shape to ensure that it fits correctly between the tongue and the hard palate. It is available in various sizes to suit a newborn to large adults.

A rough estimate of the size required may be obtained by selecting an airway with a length corresponding to the vertical distance between the patient's incisors and the angle of the mandible (Figures 20.2 and 20.3).

Technique of inserting an oropharyngeal airway

The patient's mouth is opened and the airway is introduced so that the curvature (concavity) faces towards the palate until the tip of the airway reaches the junction between the hard and soft palate and then the airway

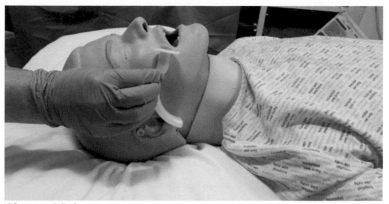

Figure 20.2. Estimating the correct size of an oropharyngeal airway.

is rotated through 180°. It is then inserted until it lies in the oropharynx. The rotation technique reduces the chance of pushing the tongue backwards and downwards. Correct positioning of the airway is indicated by an improvement in airway patency and by the seating of the flattened reinforced section of the airway between the patient's incisors:

- If the oropharyngeal airway is too small, it can push the tongue backwards and worsen the airway obstruction. An oropharyngeal airway that is too large can bypass the glottic inlet and fail to correct the airway obstruction.
- Vomiting or laryngospasm can occur if the glossopharyngeal and laryngeal reflexes are intact.
- Damage to teeth, dislodgement of caps and crowns, mucosal trauma and bleeding can occur.

Nasopharyngeal airway

The nasopharyngeal airway is passed through the nose, as the name implies, and ends behind the tongue, above the epiglottis and again relieves the obstruction from the tissues in the oropharynx. It is a soft rubber or plastic tube (Figure 20.3). It is beveled at one end and with a flange at the other, and is better tolerated than an oropharyngeal airway in a patient who is semi-conscious. It may be the best choice in patients with restricted mouth opening due to trismus or maxillofacial injuries. The airway is sized in millimeters according to the internal diameter and the length increases with increasing diameter. Commonly used adult sizes are 6-7mm.

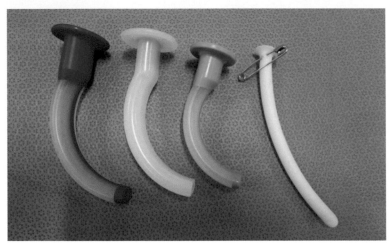

Figure 20.3. Oropharyngeal airways of various sizes and a nasopharyngeal airway.

Technique of inserting a nasopharyngeal airway

After checking the patency of the nostril, a well-lubricated airway is inserted vertically along the floor of the nose with a slight twisting action. If any obstruction is felt, it should be removed and the other nostril can be tried.

Nasopharyngeal airway insertion can be associated with trauma to the nasal mucosa, turbinates and adenoids. There is also a risk of bleeding. It is contraindicated in patients with a bleeding diathesis and a suspected base of skull fracture.

Ventilation

Artificial ventilation should be initiated in patients with inadequate or absent ventilation. The most simple form of providing artificial ventilation includes squeezing the self-inflating bag connected either to a face mask (bag mask), laryngeal mask or tracheal tube. The self-inflating bag should be connected to an oxygen source. As the bag is squeezed, the contents are delivered to the patient's lungs. On release, the expired gas is diverted to the atmosphere via a one-way valve and the bag then refills automatically via an inlet at the opposite end. Using this bag-mask device, the lungs can be ventilated with air alone (FiO_2 0.21), but the addition of oxygen of 5-6L/min, directly to the self-inflating bag adjacent to the air intake, would increase the FiO_2 to 0.45. The FiO_2 can be increased to 0.85 by attaching a reservoir bag connected to an oxygen flow of 15L/min.

Airway management techniques

The different techniques available to manage the airway include:

- Face mask ventilation.
- Insertion of a supraglottic airway device (SAD).
- Laryngoscopy and tracheal intubation.
- Tracheostomy.
- Cricothyroidotomy.

The choice of technique depends on the individual clinical scenario and the experience of the attending medical or paramedical personnel.

Face mask ventilation

This involves delivering ventilation through a tightly fitting face mask (Figures 20.4 and 20.5). In order to deliver effective ventilation of the lungs, a patent airway should be established.

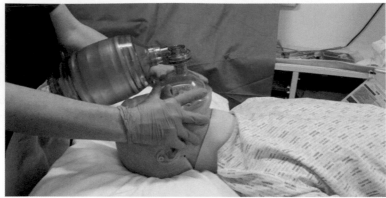

Figure 20.4. Technique of face mask ventilation.

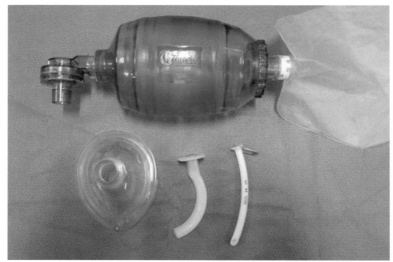

Figure 20.5. Equipment required for face mask ventilation: self-inflating bag, face mask, an oropharyngeal airway and a nasopharyngeal airway.

One-person face mask ventilation

Following an appropriate head and neck position, a jaw thrust is performed, and the mask is held with one hand and the bag is squeezed with the other hand. Frequently this may fail to provide an airtight seal and any leak will result in hypoventilation.

Two-person face mask ventilation

In order to achieve an airtight seal, a jaw thrust is performed and maintained with both hands. A self-inflating bag is squeezed by a second person. In the operating theatres, the bag-squeezing function can be performed with the assistance of a ventilator. Poorly applied cricoid pressure may also make it more difficult to ventilate, as also incorrectly applied airway opening techniques or airway adjuncts.

Airway adjuncts such as an oropharyngeal or a nasopharyngeal airway may be required to establish a patent airway.

Face mask ventilation following induction of general anaesthesia

It is important to establish adequate mask ventilation soon after administration of the induction agent. All measures should be taken to maintain a patent airway. Choosing a face mask of an appropriate size, an adequate depth of anaesthesia and ensuring an adequate seal are important elements of optimum face mask ventilation. During face mask ventilation, tidal volume, peak airway pressure and end-tidal CO_2 concentration should be monitored.

Supraglottic airway device (SAD)

Airway patency can be secured with the use of a supraglottic airway device (SAD). Several SADs have been introduced into clinical practice, e.g. i-gel®, intubating laryngeal mask airway (ILMA), LMA Classic™, LMA ProSeal™, LMA Supreme®, and the laryngeal tube to name just a few (Figure 20.6). In this section we will focus on the technique and use of a SAD in general.

Generally, they can be classified into two groups:

- First-generation SADs (e.g. LMA and LMA Classic™).
- Second-generation SADs (e.g. i-gel®, LMA ProSeal™).

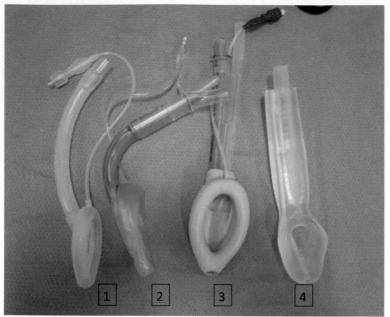

Figure 20.6. Supraglottic airway devices. 1) Laryngeal mask airway; 2) LMA Supreme®; 3) LMA ProSeal™; 4) i-gel®.

Second-generation SADs have additional features such as an integrated bite block, a gastric drainage port and a higher seal pressure. When they are correctly placed, the distal aperture of the gastric drainage tube should open to the oesophagus and this facilitates the drainage of gastric contents in case regurgitation occurs. Therefore, they minimise the risk of aspiration.

The LMA Classic™ was introduced into clinical practice in 1988, devised to provide and maintain a seal around the laryngeal inlet to allow spontaneous ventilation and controlled ventilation at moderate levels of positive pressure. Initially used primarily in the operating room, their use was subsequently expanded to the emergency department and the pre-hospital setting.

It is shaped like an endotracheal tube at the proximal end connecting to an elliptical mask at the distal end. It is designed to sit in the hypopharynx and cover the supraglottic structures, therefore allowing relative isolation of the trachea.

The widespread use of the LMA coincided with the development and use of propofol, as propofol obtunded the laryngeal reflexes enough to allow the passage of the LMA in non-paralysed patients. Therefore, LMA insertion in the peri-operative period requires an adequate depth of anaesthesia before its insertion.

Technique of inserting a SAD (LMA or i-gel®)

A SAD of appropriate size should be chosen (Table 20.1) and if it is an LMA, the cuff should be checked by inflating with an appropriate volume of air. Then the cuff is deflated and the outer surface of the cuff is lubricated using a water-soluble jelly. Ideally, the head and neck should be aligned with the neck slightly flexed and head extended at the atlanto-occipital joint (the classical 'sniffing' position). This position is

Table 20.1. Selection of an appropriate sized LMA and i-gel® according to the patient's weight.

Patient's weight (kg)	<5	5-10	10-20	20-30	30-50	50-70	70-100
LMA size	1	11/2	2	21/2	3	4	5
Max. cuff inflation volume for LMA (ml)	4	7	10	14	20	30	40
Patient's weight (kg)	2-5	5-12	10-25	25-35	30-60	50-90	>90
i-gel® size	1	1.5	2.0	2.5	3	4	5

contraindicated in patients with a suspected cervical spine injury or unstable cervical spine where the SAD can be inserted in a neutral head position with manual in-line stabilisation.

The SAD insertion technique is based on an imitation of the swallowing mechanism, with the aim of avoiding collision with highly innervated anterior pharyngeal structures such as the epiglottis, larynx and arytenoids. It is introduced into the patient's mouth with the aperture facing forward, held between the index finger and thumb at the junction of the mask and tube. The tip of the SAD is held behind the upper incisor (Figure 20.7A), pressed against the hard palate, then gently advanced into the oropharynx. The right index finger is used to guide the mask along the palato-pharyngeal axis and gently pushed forwards until a firm resistance is encountered (no force should be used in advancing the SAD as this may result in incorrect placement and trauma). The index finger is then gently withdrawn from the oropharynx, grasping the tube part of the LMA with the other hand. The cuff is then inflated and if the position is satisfactory the tube will lift 1 or 2cm out of the mouth as the cuff finds its correct position. When correctly inserted the tip of the SAD (LMA) rests against the upper oesophageal sphincter (Figure 20.7B). If the SAD can't be inserted after 30 seconds, the patient needs reoxygenation before another attempt at the insertion of a SAD. The confirmation of a patent airway is done by auscultating the chest during inspiration, noting bilateral chest movement and by capnography. The second-generation SADs have an integrated bite block which prevents airway obstruction; in the vent the patient bites the SAD tube. If an LMA is used, a bite block should be inserted alongside the LMA to avoid the patient biting on the LMA tube and causing complete airway obstruction.

Advantages of SADs

- Muscle relaxants can be avoided.
- The problems associated with laryngoscopy and tracheal intubation can be minimised.
- The sympatho-adrenal response is less than tracheal intubation.
- The recovery phase is smooth with fewer incidences of airway problems in recovery.

- LMAs have been used in the management of a difficult airway both in elective and emergency situations.

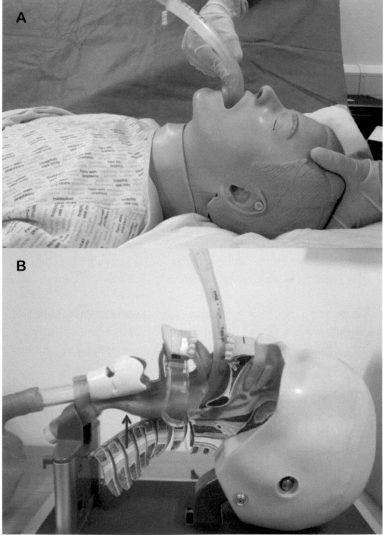

Figure 20.7. A) Technique of inserting a SAD (i-gel®). B) A correctly positioned LMA with the tip (arrow) resting against the upper oesophageal sphincter.

The use of an LMA and other SADs is not without its problems. Because of the fact that it produces an incomplete seal around the laryngeal inlet, its elective use is contraindicated in some situations.

Contraindications

Absolute contraindications (in all settings, including an emergency) are:

- Cannot open mouth.
- Complete upper airway obstruction.

Relative contraindications (in the elective setting) to the use of a SAD are:

- Increased risk of aspiration:
    - prolonged bag-valve-mask ventilation;
    - morbid obesity;
    - second or third trimester pregnancy;
    - patients who have not fasted before ventilation;
    - upper gastrointestinal bleed.
- Suspected or known abnormalities in the supraglottic anatomy.
- The need for a high airway pressure to achieve adequate ventilation.

With increasing use, problems have been reported. Rare complications due to laryngeal mask airway (LMA) insertion occur in the operating room. The rate of complications is 0.15%, but the rate is likely to be higher in the emergency setting. Such complications include the following:

- Aspiration of gastric contents.
- Local irritation.
- Upper airway trauma:
    - pressure-induced lesions;
    - nerve palsies.
- Mild sympathetic response.
- Negative pressure pulmonary oedema.
- Complications associated with improper placement:
    - obstruction;
    - laryngospasm.

Laryngoscopy and tracheal intubation

Tracheal intubation involves the placement of a tube into the trachea. The most widely used route is the orotracheal route; however, nasotracheal intubation is required in some situations (e.g. limited mouth opening or surgery in the oral cavity). After the trachea has been intubated, a balloon cuff is typically inflated, to prevent leakage of respiratory gases, and to prevent aspiration of regurgitated stomach contents. The tube is then secured and connected to the anaesthesia breathing system or a self-inflating bag or to a mechanical ventilator to commence ventilation.

Tracheal intubation is considered to be superior to other advanced airway management techniques for the following reasons:

- The airway is reliably isolated from foreign material in the oropharynx.
- Suction of inhaled particles and secretions from the lower respiratory tract is possible.
- It provides more effective ventilation of the lungs.

The basic indications for intubation in the operating room and intensive care unit are:

- Airway protection.
- Airway patency.
- Maintenance of adequate oxygenation.
- Positive-pressure ventilation.
- Respiratory suctioning/toilet.

Technique of direct laryngoscopy

For successful direct laryngoscopy, a direct line of sight from the maxillary teeth to the glottis must be obtained by optimal positioning of the head and neck. Therefore, it is imperative that the patient is positioned appropriately. The sniffing position has been recommended as optimal for patient intubation and airway management. Historically, the definition of this position is credited to an Irish-born anaesthetist, Sir Ivan Magill, who described it as "sniffing the morning air" or "draining a pint of beer".

The equipment for direct laryngoscopy and intubation is shown in Figure 20.8.

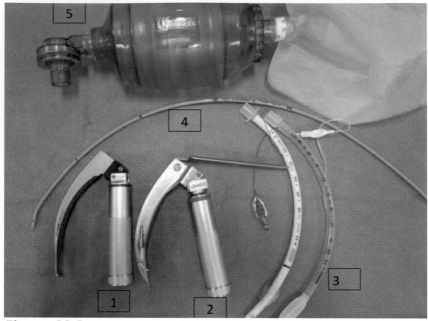

Figure 20.8. Equipment for direct laryngoscopy and intubation. 1) Macintosh laryngoscope; 2) McCoy laryngoscope; 3) Tracheal tube; 4) Bougie; 5) Self-inflating bag.

After Magill described the "sniffing the morning air" position, Bannister and MacBeth in 1944 analysed the angles of the oral, pharyngeal, and laryngeal axes with the head in different positions for the purpose of identifying the best possible alignment of the three axes to expose the glottis and facilitate endotracheal tube insertion. They identified the following key components:

- Flexion of the lower cervical spine.
- Extension of the upper cervical spine.
- Extension of the atlanto-occipital joint.

The main advantage of this position is the optimal exposure of the glottis for the purpose of intubation with a Macintosh blade. Also, the position is advantageous for the anaesthesia provider to facilitate the approach to the airway in the non-obese population (i.e. optimal patency of the airway;

ideal for mask ventilation). This position is contraindicated in patients with known or suspected cervical spine injuries where a neutral position should be used.

Another position frequently used is the so-called 'ramped' position, which has been proposed to facilitate ventilation and visualisation of the glottis for intubation in obese patients. The position may be achieved by placing blankets or other devices, e.g. Oxford pillow, underneath the patient's head and torso so that the external auditory meatus and sternal notch are aligned horizontally. The aim is to achieve the same best alignment of the three axes (oral, pharyngeal, and laryngeal) in obese patients that is achieved with the sniffing position in non-obese patients.

Both ventilation and the laryngoscopic view appear to be improved with the head-elevated position leading to potential advantages, including increased rates of successful intubation and decreased rates of morbidity and mortality related to airway management.

Once the patient is optimally positioned they are anaesthetised and paralysed. The anaesthetist opens the patient's mouth by separating the lips and pulling on the upper jaw with the index finger as well as using their right hand to press on the patient's forehead in a semicircular downward motion. Holding a laryngoscope in the left hand they insert it into the mouth of the patient with the blade directed to the right tonsil. Once the right tonsil is reached, the laryngoscope is swept to the midline, keeping the tongue on the left to bring the epiglottis into view. The laryngoscope blade is then advanced until it reaches the angle between the base of the tongue and the epiglottis, the vallecula (Figure 20.9). Next, the laryngoscope is lifted upwards and forwards to bring the vocal cords into view, with caution not to pivot on the teeth. The anaesthetist then takes the tracheal tube in his right hand and inserts it through the vocal cords. Finally, the tracheal tube cuff is inflated to a volume just enough to stop the audible leak whilst squeezing the bag up to a pressure of 20cm H_2O. The cuff pressure should be measured using a manometer and should be less than 30cm H_2O. In the majority of cases, where a Grade 1 or 2 view of the glottis (Figure 20.10) is obtained, tracheal intubation is likely to be easy.

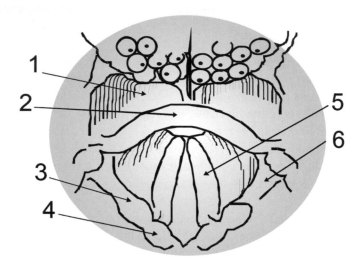

Figure 20.9. Structures visualised during direct laryngoscopy. 1) Vallecula; 2) Epiglottis; 3) Cuniform cartilage; 4) Corniculate cartilage; 5) Vocal cords; 6) Aryepiglottic fold.

The correct placement of the tracheal tube should be confirmed using continuous waveform capnography and by the presence of bilateral breath sounds on auscultation.

The success of tracheal intubation at first attempt depends on the following factors:

- Experience of the operator.
- Optimal head and neck position.
- Adequate depth of anaesthesia.
- Selection of appropriate laryngoscope blade.
- Use of external laryngeal manipulation and a bougie.

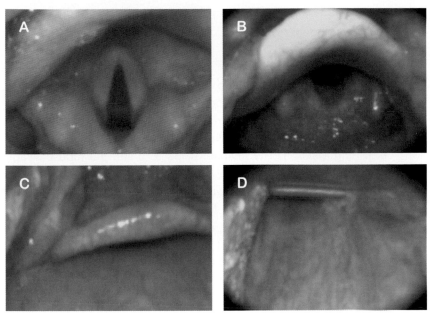

Figure 20.10. A laryngoscopic view of the glottis (Cormack and Lehane grading).
A) Grade 1 view; B) Grade 2 view; C) Grade 3 view; and D) Grade 4 view.

As multiple attempts can increase morbidity, when a difficulty is experienced, help should be summoned and an alternative technique of airway management should be chosen.

Videolaryngoscopy

A number of new indirect laryngoscopes are now available. They are frequently referred to as videolaryngoscopes (VL) because of a video camera positioned near the tip of the blade, which captures the image of the glottis in real time and transmits it to a video screen.

VLs offer several advantages over conventional direct laryngoscopy. Videolaryngoscopy does not require the alignment of oral, pharyngeal and laryngeal axes. Therefore, it requires less force to be applied and comparatively less haemodynamic changes. They provide a superior view of the glottis and improve the success rate of intubation.

There are three different types of videolaryngoscopes that are used in clinical practice (Figure 20.11):

- Macintosh type (e.g. C-Mac® videolaryngoscope). These devices have a Macintosh-type blade and an insertion method similar to conventional direct laryngoscopy. The glottis is visualised either directly or on the video screen.
- Anatomically shaped blade with a tube guide (channelled blade, e.g. King Vision®). The channel helps to guide the tube passage through the glottis.
- Anatomically shaped blade without a tube guide (non-channelled blade, e.g. GlideScope®, C-Mac® with D-Blade™). The curved shape of the blade allows a view of the glottis without flexing or extending the head and neck; however, directing the endotracheal tube toward the glottis may be difficult. Therefore, they require either a bougie or a pre-formed stylet to facilitate the passage of the tube.

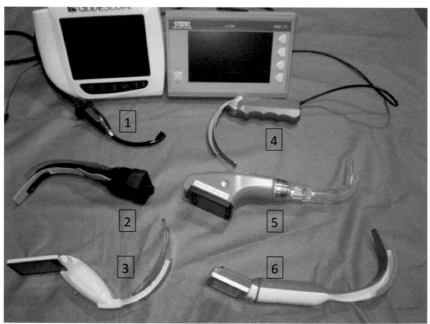

Figure 20.11. Channelled and non-channelled videolaryngoscopes. 1) GlideScope®; 2) Airtraq™; 3) McGrath®; 4) C-Mac®; 5) Pentax AWS®; 6) King Vision®.

Complications

Although intubation is often a rapid and simple technique, it is associated with complications (Table 20.2). The incidence and occurrence of complications may depend on several factors outlined below.

Patient factors:

- Complications are likely in infants, children and adult women, as they have a relatively small larynx and trachea and are more prone to airway oedema.
- Patients who have a difficult airway are more prone to injury as well as hypoxic events.

Table 20.2. Complications of intubation.

At time of intubation	While patient is intubated	After intubation
Trauma to lips, teeth, tongue, nose	Aspiration	Sore throat
Failed intubation	Airway obstruction	Hoarseness
Oesophageal intubation	Endobronchial intubation	Laryngeal oedema
Laryngospasm	Disconnection	Vocal cord granuloma
Bronchospasm	Pneumothorax	Nerve injury
Trauma to laryngeal structures		Tracheal stenosis
Tracheal		Tracheo-oesophageal fistula
Cervical spine injury		
Tachycardia and hypertension		

- Complications are more likely during emergency situations.

Anaesthesia-related factors:

- The knowledge and experience of the anaesthetist play a vital role in the occurrence and outcome of complications during airway management.
- A hurried intubation, without adequate evaluation of the airway or preparation of the patient or the equipment is more likely to cause complications.

Equipment:

- Large size of tracheal tube and prolonged duration of intubation may predispose to a postoperative sore throat.
- The use of stylets and bougies predispose to trauma.

Cricothyroidotomy

This is an emergency access to the airway through the front of the neck. The cricothyroid membrane is located between the cricoid and thyroid cartilage and is the most superficial and less vascular structure. A cannula or tube inserted through the cricothyroid membrane acts as access to the airway below the level of the vocal cords.

The main indication includes the 'can't intubate, can't oxygenate' scenario (severe facial injury and failed intubation followed by failed face mask ventilation and failed oxygenation through a supraglottic airway device).

Three different techniques are available:

- Needle or narrow-bore cannula cricothyroidotomy. There are purpose made cannulae (Ravussin cannula) available, but they require a high-pressure ventilation device such as a jet injector (2-4 bar pressure) to facilitate ventilation. Exhalation is passive and must occur through the pharynx and larynx. In the case of complete airway obstruction, a second cannula through the cricothyroid membrane may be required to facilitate exhalation. Complications include failure due to kinking, malposition or displacement of the cannula. In addition, barotrauma due to high pressure and surgical emphysema are possible complications.

- Large purpose-made cannula with an internal diameter of 4mm or more. The lungs can be ventilated using an anaesthetic breathing system. Two available devices include the QuickTrach® cannula over the needle technique and Melker™ (Seldinger technique; 4mm/6mm cuffed and uncuffed cannulae).

- Surgical cricothyroidotomy. The 2015 Difficult Airway Society (DAS) guidelines recommend a scalpel surgical cricothyroidotomy (www.das.uk.com). This requires three simple pieces of equipment: a scalpel with a broad blade (size 10), a bougie with an angled tip and a size 6mm cuffed tracheal tube.

If the cricothyroid membrane is palpable, a transverse stab incision is performed on the cricothyroid membrane, the scalpel is rotated and a bougie is inserted along the side of the scalpel. Subsequently, a cuffed tube is railroaded over the bougie. In situations where the cricothyroid membrane cannot be identified using anatomical landmarks, a midline vertical incision on the front of the neck is required to dissect the midline structures and identify the cricothyroid membrane. The choice of technique depends on the clinical experience of the anaesthetist and the team. Regular training for anaesthetists and theatre team members is essential to ensure a high success rate in this rescue technique.

Complications include failure, haemorrhage, surgical emphysema, oesophageal perforation, tracheal laceration, misplacement, vocal cord paresis, subglottic stenosis, and laryngeal stenosis.

Tracheostomy

A tracheostomy is a surgical procedure that creates access to the trachea through the front of the neck. A tube is inserted into the opening and connected to an oxygen supply and ventilator to assist with breathing.

This may be performed surgically but anaesthetists and intensive care physicians usually perform the procedure using a percutaneous technique, inserting a tube from the outside of the neck into the trachea, using various devices and commonly under endoscopic guidance.

Tracheostomies are used in two broad situations:

- Acute setting — usually in an emergency to secure the airway.
- Chronic or elective setting — usually when the patient is to be ventilated for the longer term:
  - to secure an airway in patients with injuries or surgery to the head and neck area;
  - to facilitate weaning from positive pressure ventilation in acute respiratory failure or prolonged ventilation;
  - to facilitate the removal of respiratory secretions;
  - to protect/minimise the risk of aspiration in the patient with a poor or absent cough reflex.

In certain circumstances the tracheostomy may facilitate:

- Improved oral hygiene for a patient requiring ventilation.
- Decreased requirement for sedation in the intubated patient.
- Oral movement for communication, nutrition and hydration (with manipulation).
- Reduction in damage to the larynx, mouth or nose from prolonged endotracheal intubation.
- Vocalisation (with manipulation).
- Improved patient comfort.

Complications of tracheostomies

Historically, tracheostomies were associated with a high risk of complications and a significant mortality rate.

- Immediate (post-insertion):
  - haemorrhage (minor or severe);
  - misplacement (pretracheal tissues or to main bronchus);
  - pneumothorax;
  - surgical emphysema;

- occlusion of the tube by cuff herniation;
- oesophageal perforation.
- Delayed (post-insertion):
  - tube blockage with secretions (may be sudden or gradual);
  - infection of the stoma site;
  - infection of the bronchial tree;
  - tracheal ulceration;
  - tracheal necrosis;
  - tube migration to the pretracheal space;
  - risk of occlusion of the tracheostomy tube in obese or fatigued patients who have difficulty extending their neck;
  - tracheo-oesophageal fistula formation;
  - accidental decannulation;
  - haemorrhage (minor or severe).
- Late (post-decannulation):
  - granulomata of the trachea may cause respiratory difficulty when the tracheostomy tube is removed;
  - persistent sinus at the tracheostomy site;
  - tracheal dilation;
  - tracheal stenosis at the cuff site;
  - scar formation requiring revision;
  - tracheomalacia.

Types of tracheostomy tubes (Figure 20.12)

Single-lumen tubes

A single-lumen tube maximises the inner lumen of the tracheostomy tube, therefore, decreasing airway resistance. They are mostly for short-term use. The lumen may become blocked with secretions and it requires replacement every 5-7 days.

Double-cannula tracheostomy tubes

A double-cannula tracheostomy tube has a removable inner cannula which can be removed and cleaned. The presence of an inner tube reduces the internal diameter, thereby increasing the resistance. However, it can be used in the longer term (27 days).

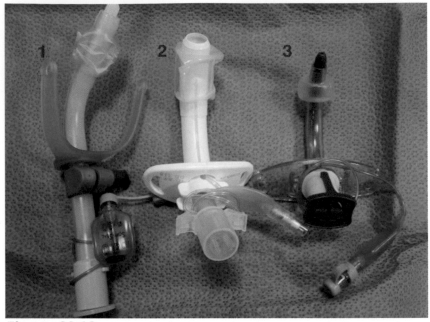

Figure 20.12. Different types of tracheostomy tubes. 1) Adjustable flange tracheotomy tube; 2) Double-cannula tracheostomy tube; 3) Cuffed tracheostomy tube.

Uncuffed tracheostomy tubes

Uncuffed tracheostomy tubes are suitable for patients in the recovery phase of critical illness who have returned from intensive care and may still require chest physiotherapy and suction via the trachea. In the event of the tracheostomy becoming blocked, the patient may be able to breathe around the tube.

Fenestrated tracheostomy tubes

Fenestrated tracheostomy tubes assist in directing airflow to pass through the patient's oropharynx/nasopharynx.

Adjustable flange tracheostomy tubes

Adjustable flange tracheostomy tubes with adjustable flanges are specifically designed for patients who have a deep-set trachea. They can be adjusted to the desired length.

Peri-operative airway management

The main goal in airway management is to safely enable the delivery of oxygen to the patient. The 4th National Audit Project in the United Kingdom (NAP4) in 2011 showed that inadequate skill and poor judgment in airway management continued to lead to potentially avoidable morbidity.

The main causes for airway-related morbidity included deficiencies in airway assessment leading to inadequate preparation, under-utilisation of awake intubation techniques and the inappropriate use of supraglottic airway devices (SAD). In a review of litigation related to anaesthesia in National Health Service (NHS) hospitals in the UK from 1995 to 2007, airway and respiratory-related events accounted for 12% of all anaesthesia claims, 53% of deaths and 27% of cost, and were involved in 10 out of the 50 most expensive claims.

Pre-operative airway assessment

During the pre-operative airway assessment, anaesthetists need to answer the following questions:

- Is there a difficulty with face mask ventilation?
- Is there a difficulty with insertion of a SAD?
- Is there a difficulty with laryngoscopy and tracheal intubation?
- Is the front of the neck access/tracheotomy possible?

Airway assessment includes a history, clinical examination and special investigations.

Any previous history of difficulty in face mask ventilation, laryngoscopy or intubation should immediately arouse concern regarding a patient's airway and should not be dismissed. Airway management can be difficult in certain congenital diseases such as Pierre-Robin, Treacher-Collins and Klippel-Feil syndromes, in rheumatoid arthritis, ankylosing spondylitits, fixation of the cervical spine, facial trauma, head and neck irradiation, and head and neck pathology.

Clinical examination

The first consideration is whether a seal can be obtained with the face mask. A history of snoring, or obstructive sleep apnoea (OSA), a beard, obesity, age over 55 years, poor Malampatti grade, a thyromental distance less than 6.5cm, and poor mandibular protrusion are all associated with difficult face mask ventilation.

Poor dentition, loose teeth, and protuberant teeth can make laryngoscopy difficult. Patients should be warned of possible dental damage to loose, diseased or restored teeth.

Mouth opening is largely a function of the temporomandibular joint, is important to allow the passage of a laryngoscope to allow a glottic view and also in the case of a failed intubation to allow the passage of a SAD to allow oxygenation. The normal lower limit of mouth opening for young adults is 3.7cm (about three fingerbreadths). Mandibular protrusion should be assessed by asking the patient to put their lower teeth in front of their upper teeth. This gives an indication of whether the tongue and the oral soft tissues will be able to be pushed out of the way during laryngoscopy to enable viewing of the glottis opening.

With the Mallampati test, the patient is asked to open their mouth maximally and protrude their tongue without phonation while the examiner sits opposite them at the same level. The oropharynx is inspected and depending on what is seen, there are four classes:

- Class 1: posterior pharyngeal wall visible, including the posterior pillars and the whole of the uvula including the tip.
- Class 2: posterior pharyngeal wall visible, including the posterior pillars and part of the uvula.
- Class 3: posterior pharyngeal wall not visible and soft palate visible.
- Class 4: soft palate not visible and hard palate visible.

The combination of Malampatti Class 3 or 4, interincisor distance of less than 3.7cm and a thyromental distance of less than 6.5cm has been shown to have 85% sensitivity and 95% specificity for a difficult tracheal intubation.

A thyromental distance of less than 6.5cm indicates a possible difficult intubation.

Craniocervical extension is a vital part of airway management for basic airway control and direct laryngoscopy. It is difficult to assess atlanto-occipital and atlanto-axial joint movement clinically. Poor craniocervical extension has also been associated with poor mouth opening.

No tests are perfect by themselves but by combining all the information above from the history and examination will identify groups of patients who will present a challenge in their airway management.

Special investigations

In selected patients it can be useful to examine cervical spine X-rays (to assess craniocervical mobility), or CT and MRI scans (to assess airway patency and the extent of pathology) or even flexible fibreoptic endoscopy (to assess pathology).

Intra-operative airway management

Any airway management plan should include a plan A — primary plan, plan B — back-up plan, and even plan C — back-up of the back-up plan. The primary plan is the plan with the highest probability of success and is safe for the nature of the airway identified at the pre-operative visit.

Any anticipated difficulty in airway management should be communicated with the team members (surgeons, the anaesthetic practitioner and the rest of the team) during the team brief.

During the sign-in part of the WHO surgical safety check list, an anaesthetic machine check and availability of other necessary equipment should be confirmed.

Pre-oxygenation

Following positioning on the operating table, patients are preoxygenated to denitrogenate the functional residual capacity (FRC) while observing the expired oxygen concentration, and anaesthesia is induced depending on the anaesthetic plan. Following induction of anaesthesia, a selected muscle relaxant is administered and laryngoscopy is performed. If a poor laryngoscopic view (Grade 2, 3 or 4) is initially obtained, external manipulation of the larynx is the first response. A 'backwards, up, rightward pressure' is often used to improve the laryngoscopic view.

Management of the difficult airway

As mentioned earlier in the chapter, during the airway assessment, anaesthetists may be able to predict the airway management. In certain situations, they may not be able to predict a difficulty or all pre-operative tests may appear normal, but following induction of anaesthesia, airway management may become unexpectedly difficult.

Once we know what problems we may encounter, we can tailor our technique accordingly. Moreover, anaesthetists manage the difficult airway differently depending on whether or not there is upper airway obstruction.

Anticipated difficult airway with no upper airway obstruction

This situation refers to patients with anticipated difficulties in airway management with conventional techniques. This includes patients with anatomical or pathological problems who are generally symptom-free in their day-to-day lives.

Once the potential problem is recognised, every anaesthetist in that situation will try to answer the following questions:

- Can the surgery proceed with local or regional anaesthesia?
    - need to make sure that a plan is in place in case the local or regional technique is unsuccessful or it wears off in the middle of the operation;
    - the airway should be easily accessible.
- If a GA is needed then can I secure the airway with an awake technique?
    - awake intubation is the gold standard in this scenario because:

     i. spontaneous breathing and ventilation are maintained until the airway is secured;

     ii. the airway is protected from aspiration;

     iii. if things go wrong then there is a way out.

- Is paralysis and intubation necessary or can I use a supraglottic airway and a spontaneous breathing technique?
  - a back-up plan is paramount;
  - the anaesthetist should be experienced in establishing the airway with the proposed back-up plan.

Anticipated difficult face mask ventilation

Mask ventilation is the most basic, yet the most essential, skill in airway management. It is the primary technique of ventilation before tracheal intubation or insertion of any airway device. Its most unique role, however, is as a rescue technique for ventilation should tracheal intubation fail or proves difficult. The ability to establish adequate mask ventilation has, therefore, become a major branch point in any difficult airway algorithm. Anaesthetists should acquire the skill of mask ventilation, the knowledge of the causes of difficult mask ventilation or impossible mask ventilation, and develop alternative management options when the mask ventilation is difficult or impossible.

An inability to establish adequate mask ventilation may result from different underlying mechanisms that can be broadly divided into technique and/or airway-related:

- Technique-related:
  - operator — lack of experience;
  - equipment — wrong mask size, difficult fit due to anatomy;
  - position — suboptimal head and neck position;
  - cricoid pressure — incorrectly applied;
  - drug-related — inadequate depth of anaesthesia, lack of relaxation.
- Airway-related:
  - upper airway obstruction:
    - i. epiglottis and tongue;
    - ii. excess soft tissue due to obesity, sleep apnoea;

     iii. tonsillar hyperplasia;

     iv. laryngospasm;

     v. tumours — oral, maxillary, pharyngeal, laryngeal;

     vi. external compression — neck haematoma, neck mass;

  - lower airway obstruction:

     i. bronchospasm;

     ii. mediastinal mass;

     iii. tracheal/bronchial tumour.

- Chest wall deformity restricting chest expansion.

Difficult mask ventilation can also be associated with difficult intubation. In such situations, an awake intubation technique should be preferred.

Anticipated difficult tracheal intubation

Appropriate planning is crucial to avoid morbidity and mortality when a difficulty is anticipated with airway management.

The options available when a difficult tracheal intubation is anticipated include:

- Avoiding general anaesthesia.
- Avoiding tracheal intubation and maintaining the airway using a face mask or supraglottic airway device.
- Tracheal intubation using an awake technique (awake fibreoptic intubation or awake videolaryngoscopy).

When avoiding general anaesthesia, a local or regional anaesthetic technique can be used; however, the following provisions should be made:

- The anaesthetist should be able to establish the airway in case the local anaesthetic or nerve block fails or wears off.
- All airway equipment should be available and ready to use in case complications of the block result in a loss of consciousness or respiratory compromise.

- During the team brief and during the sign-in part of the WHO check list, the anaesthetist's planned strategy for conversion to general anaesthesia should be discussed.

The technique of general anaesthesia using a supraglottic airway or face mask ventilation may be considered provided the patient is at low risk of aspiration and a plan has been made for managing intra-operative failure of ventilation or oxygenation.

Deciding on awake or post-induction tracheal intubation

With an anticipated difficult tracheal intubation that cannot be avoided, the clinician must decide if intubation can proceed safely after induction of general anesthesia or if it would be achieved more safely in the awake patient. An awake approach can potentially confer a safety benefit by having the patient maintain airway patency, gas exchange, and protection of the airway against aspiration of gastric contents or blood during the intubation process.

Two primary questions should be addressed:

- If general anesthesia is induced, is tracheal intubation predicted to succeed with the chosen technique?
- If tracheal intubation fails, will oxygenation by face mask or supraglottic airway succeed?

The cooperative elective surgical patient must be optimised pre-operatively and managed in the safest way possible. When a difficult tracheal intubation is anticipated in this population, proceeding with post-induction tracheal intubation should occur only with an estimated margin of safety equivalent to that of an awake intubation. Special situations where intubation following induction of general anaesthesia may have to be considered include an uncooperative or agitated patient or a child with a difficult airway. In such situations, the judicious use of sedation or general anaesthesia with spontaneous ventilation should be used.

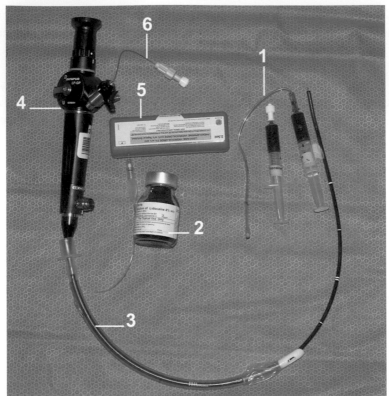

Figure 20.13. Drugs and equipment used for awake fibreoptic intubation. 1) Mucosal atomisation device; 2) 4% lidocaine; 3) Tracheal tube loaded on the fibreoptic scope; 4) Fibreoptic scope; 5) 5% lidocaine with 0.5% phenylephrine; 6) Epidural catheter.

An awake intubation under topical anaesthesia with/without sedation can be performed using a fibreoptic scope or videolaryngoscope. Awake intubation using a fibreoptic scope is considered as the gold standard because of its wider application and it can be used in both the oral and nasal routes and also in the presence of upper airway pathology. The minimum equipment required for an awake intubation is as described in Figure 20.13. The technique of awake intubation involves premedication using an antisialogogue, preparation of equipment, monitoring, oxygen administration, airway preparation, endoscopy, tracheal intubation and the confirmation of correct tube placement.

Anticipated difficult airway with upper airway obstruction

This can be a life-threatening emergency and the presence of a senior anaesthetist and anaesthetic assistant, the theatre team, and an ENT surgeon is absolutely necessary for the safe management of the airway. Untreated, this will lead to hypoxia and all the consequences thereof. The management of this airway depends on the clinical situation, site, severity and progression of the obstruction, as well as the expertise of the anaesthetist. Examples of this would be upper airway trauma, rapidly progressing infections of any aspects to the upper airway (acute epiglottitis, croup, tonsillar abscesses), and the all too common foreign bodies stuck in the upper airways.

Although anaesthetists will encounter very rapidly progressing emergencies, most often there is time to plan the safest way of airway management. When the patient is being examined the questions to be considered should be as follows:

- What is the site, extent and pathology of the lesion causing upper airway obstruction?
- How much time do we have?

The fine detail of the management plans are beyond the scope of this chapter but the basic principles are mentioned above.

Unanticipated difficult tracheal intubation

Airway management, ensuring uninterrupted oxygenation and ventilation, is a fundamental part of the practice of anaesthesia and of emergency and critical care medicine. A difficult intubation is defined by the American Society of Anesthesiologists as tracheal intubation requiring more than three attempts, in the presence or absence of tracheal pathology. An unanticipated difficulty with endotracheal intubation may result in catastrophic outcomes, including cerebral hypoxia and death.

The Difficult Airway Society (DAS) guidelines for the management of an unanticipated difficult tracheal intubation (Figure 20.14) are based on a series of escalating management plans: if Plan A does not work, back-up plans B, C, or D must be executed. The plans are as follows:

- Plan A is tracheal intubation. When it fails, plan B should be implemented. The probability of first-attempt success can be maximised by the familiarity with and attention to equipment and

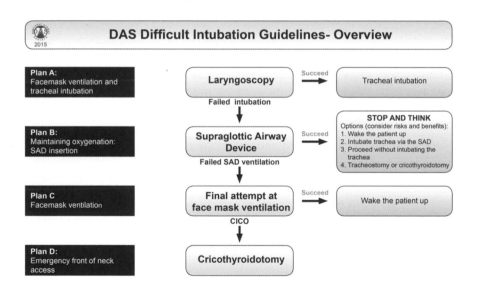

Figure 20.14. Difficult Airway Society difficult intubation guidelines: overview. *Reproduced with permission from the Difficult Airway Society 2015 guidelines for the management of an unanticipated difficult intubation in adults. Frerk C, Mitchell VS, McNarry AF, Mendonca C, Bhagrath R, Patel A, O'Sullivan EP, Woodall NM, Ahmad I. Difficult Airway Society intubation guidelines working group. Br J Anaesth 2015; 115 (6): 827-8.*

adjunct (e.g. gum elastic bougie) preparation, patient positioning, and optimal drug dosage.

- Plan B involves maintaining oxygenation using a supraglottic airway. Once the supraglottic airway device is inserted successfully, the decision should be made as to whether to wake the patient up or to intubate the trachea through the supraglottic airway. An experienced anaesthetist can perform tracheal intubation through the supraglottic airway. In some situations, the decision to continue a life-saving surgery using a supraglottic airway may be essential. In other rare scenarios, a tracheostomy may be required at this stage.
- Plan C involves an optimum attempt at oxygenation using a face mask and adjuncts.
- Plan D involves rescue techniques for a 'can't intubate, can't oxygenate' situation.

When the above methods are unsuccessful, when the patient cannot be successfully oxygenated using a face mask or supraglottic airway, the patient requires rapid surgical access to the trachea for adequate ventilation and oxygenation. Three corrective measures are vital: immediate recognition, a call for help, and preparation for a surgical/transtracheal airway, most commonly a cricothyroidotomy.

In the event that intubation unexpectedly becomes difficult or impossible, a predetermined plan will allow anaesthesia providers to manage the airway and ensure uninterrupted oxygenation and ventilation of the patient. An unanticipated difficult intubation, if associated with a difficult mask ventilation, allows only a short period of time to solve the problem before hypoxaemia, hypercarbia, and haemodynamic instability occur. Early skilled assistance is critical, followed by advancement through a series of predetermined and rehearsed strategies. Evidence continues to emerge that patient morbidity increases with the number of failed attempts at tracheal intubation.

Extubation

Tracheal extubation is a high-risk phase of anaesthesia. The majority of problems that occur during extubation and emergence are of a minor nature, but a small number may result in injury or death.

In contrast to tracheal intubation, extubation is almost always elective, and therefore careful planning is possible. This should include identification of patients at risk of failed tracheal extubation, and those with anatomic features that place them at a higher risk of difficult reintubation should this prove necessary. The goal is to ensure uninterrupted oxygen delivery to the patient's lungs, avoid airway stimulation, and have a back-up plan, that would permit ventilation and reintubation with minimum difficulty and delay should extubation fail.

Premature extubation during emergence is more likely to be associated with complications such as breath holding, aspiration, laryngospasm, and hypoxaemia.

No single extubation technique covers all clinical scenarios and no technique is without risk. The ultimate decision to remove the tracheal tube or supraglottic airway device or to postpone the procedure is primarily based on experience. Adequate staffing and communication are essential, and an anaesthetist must always be immediately available.

Planning for extubation begins with ensuring optimal conditions, including adequate oxygenation and minute ventilation and intact protective reflexes, and excluding probable causes of airway obstruction. The patient should be haemodynamically stable and normothermic. Recovery from any administered neuromuscular blocking agents should be confirmed using neuromuscular monitoring. Tracheal extubation of at-risk patients requires expert judgment to ensure that appropriate circumstances and resources are in place to provide continuous post-extubation oxygenation.

If tracheal intubation had been difficult or circumstances at the end of surgery suggest that reintubation would be difficult, a short-term maintenance of tracheal access using an airway exchange catheter is recommended.

Case scenario 1

A 50-year-old female patient suffering from hypertension presents for an elective knee arthroscopy. Her weight is 89kg and she has a body mass index (BMI) of 37. She has no history of reflux. Ten years ago she had a general anaesthetic for infertility investigation. On examination she has good mouth opening, a Mallampati score of 3, good jaw protrusion and a thyromental distance of 6.5cm, and normal movements of the cervical spine.

What would be the airway management plan in this patient?

This patient has presented for a short surgical procedure. During the team brief, the duration and nature of the surgery should be confirmed.

Considering the short duration of the procedure, a SAD can be considered. i-gel® or LMA Supreme™ are second-generation SADs, more suitable in this case as compared to an LMA. In this case, an i-gel® is chosen as it allows positive pressure ventilation and if required fibreoptic assisted tracheal intubation can be performed through an i-gel®.

In this case, following pre-oxygenation and monitoring, anaesthesia is induced using 100μg of fentanyl and 200mg of propofol. Following loss of verbal contact, a size 4 i-gel® supraglottic airway is inserted with ease on the first attempt. Anaesthesia is maintained with sevoflurane in a room air/oxygen mixture. There is no leak noted from the i-gel® airway at any stage of the operation, which lasts 45 minutes and proceeds uneventfully. At the end of the operation the patient is woken up, and the i-gel® is removed. There are no signs of traumatic insertion, and the inner aspect of the device is dry.

Case scenario 2

A 65-year-old female suffering from COPD, hypertension, hyperlipidaemia and Type II diabetes presented for an emergency laparotomy for small bowel obstruction due to intra-abdominal adhesions. Her weight is 62kg and her body mass index (BMI) is 24. Her past anaesthetic history consists of a laparoscopic appendicectomy 7 years previously. On examination she has good mouth opening, a Mallampati score of 1, good jaw protrusion and a thyromental distance of greater than 6.5cm and normal movements of the cervical spine. A nasogastric (NG) tube is in place with 150ml of bilious aspirate present in the drainage bag.

Induction of anaesthesia and airway management

This patient needs rapid sequence induction as she is at high risk of aspiration during induction because of her pathology and the presence of NG aspirate.

On arrival to the anaesthetic room, a wide-bore intravenous access is established and the necessary monitoring is commenced. Suction is applied to the end of the NG tube and is detached when no more aspirate is obtained. Following pre-oxygenation through a tight fitting mask with 100% oxygen, a FiO_2 of above 0.8 is achieved. A modified RSI is carried out by administering 100µg of fentanyl, 200mg of propofol and 50mg of rocuronium. The operating department practitioner (ODP) applies appropriate cricoid pressure. Direct laryngoscopy is performed and reveals a Grade II Cormack and Lehane laryngeal view and the trachea is intubated quickly on the first attempt. When intubation is confirmed, the ODP releases the cricoid pressure. The operation proceeds uneventfully and the patient is extubated fully awake, discharged to the ward an hour later and home 3 days later feeling well.

Rapid sequence induction

Rapid sequence induction (RSI) is an established method of inducing anaesthesia in patients who are at risk of aspiration of gastric contents into the lungs because they either are inadequately starved, have impaired gastric emptying or are known to have a history of gastric reflux. The classical technique of RSI involves pre-oxygenation, intravenous induction of anaesthesia with an agent with rapid onset and neuromuscular blockade (paralysis), and the application of cricoid pressure followed by tracheal intubation without face mask ventilation. Over the years the classical technique has been modified with the introduction of new drugs. Fentanyl is most commonly used, along with induction agents such as propofol and thiopentone. Both suxamethonium and rocuronium have been used as the muscle relaxants of choice due to their rapid onset of action. However, suxamethonium has a higher incidence of side effects and therefore rocuronium has been increasingly used. In addition, sugammadex at a dose of 16mg/kg rapidly reverses the neuromuscular blockade of rocuronium. Inappropriately applied cricoid pressure can lead to a poor glottis view during laryngoscopy and may also interfere with inserting a supraglottic airway. In view of maintaining oxygenation during the apnoeic period, gentle face mask ventilation can be used.

RSI is not indicated in a patient who is unconscious and apnoeic. This situation is considered a 'crash' airway, and immediate mask ventilation and endotracheal intubation without pretreatment, induction, or paralysis is indicated.

Factors associated with a high risk of aspiration include:

- Abdominal pathology, especially obstruction or ileus.
- Delayed gastric emptying (e.g. pain, trauma, opioids, alcohol).
- Incompetent lower oesophageal sphincter, hiatus hernia, gastro-oesophageal reflux disease.
- Altered conscious level resulting in impaired laryngeal reflexes.
- Neurological or neuromuscular disease.
- Pregnancy.
- Difficult airway.
- Metabolic disturbances.

The risk of aspiration in these patients is present throughout the peri-operative period, especially during induction and emergence from anaesthesia.

RSI should be approached with caution in a patient with a suspected difficult airway. If difficulty is anticipated, then an awake technique or the use of airway adjuncts (e.g. fibreoptic intubation) is recommended.

Case scenario 3

A 41-year-old lady, with a BMI of 30, presents for urgent incision and drainage of a lower right molar tooth abscess. She is a life-long smoker with a 20-pack/year history. She suffers from hypertension and diet-controlled diabetes.

She had completed a week-long course of antibiotics given to her by her dentist; however, the infection hadn't cleared and for the past 2 days she was feeling hot and flushed, with increasing pain on the right side of her mouth and when she swallows.

On examination, she appears flushed, tachycardic at 100bpm, with a normal blood pressure. Respiratory examination is unremarkable. On airway examination, she is unable to open her mouth more than one fingerbreadth, and to protrude her jaw. Thyromental distance is more than 6.5cm. There is erythema and swelling on the anterior aspect of her neck and it crosses the midline.

In view of the findings, the anaesthetist decides that the best way to proceed with airway management is an awake fibreoptic intubation. The reasons for the choice of this technique are:

- If problems arose during induction of general anaesthesia, it would not be possible to insert a SAD into her mouth, due to the limited mouth opening, to ensure adequate oxygenation.
- Normal anatomy may be distorted as indicated by erythema and swelling.

- Mask ventilation is expected to be difficult due to the underlying pathology, making holding of the mask and ensuring airway patency difficult.

Before the procedure

- The anaesthetist needs to be familiar with using the fibreoptic scope.
- All resuscitation equipment should be to hand.
- The patient should be fully monitored throughout the procedure.
- Calculation of the local anaesthetic dose beforehand is essential. A maximum dose of 9mg/kg of lidocaine, based on lean body weight, for topical anaesthesia in adults is recommended.
- Nasal topical vasoconstrictors are applied.
- Obtain intravenous access and connect to fluids. Antisialogogues can be used but keep in mind they take 20-30 minutes to have an effect.
- Administer oxygen to the opposite nostril using a nasal cannula (sponge plug with a central orifice for oxygen tubing).
- Communication with the patient throughout the procedure is of vital importance.

During the procedure, the anaesthetists need to know the anatomy, and be able to recognise what they are looking at and what they are hoping to see next. Manipulation of the endoscope needs to be in a gentle manner, to avoid mucosal trauma.

Awake fibreoptic intubation (FOI)

Awake fibreoptic intubation (FOI) is a technique which allows a flexible oral or nasal route to provide a clear visualisation of the vocal cords, and subsequent passage of an endotracheal tube into the trachea under direct vision.

Awake FOI is an essential skill in the management of a patient with a known difficult airway (who has previously required awake FOI or other procedures and adjuncts aside from normal airway adjuncts for ventilation and intubation), or who has an anticipated difficult airway as found during the airway assessment pre-operatively.

Indications

- Previous difficult airway, intubation or awake FOI.
- Previous difficulty in mask ventilation.
- Anticipated difficult airway as found on pre-assessment.
- To avoid iatrogenic injury — such as patients with an unstable C-spine as a result of trauma, rheumatoid arthritis.

Contraindications

- Lack of airway skills.
- Difficult airway with impending airway obstruction.
- Allergy to local anaesthetic agents.
- Infection/contamination of the upper airway — blood, friable tumour, open abscess.
- Grossly distorted anatomy.
- Fractured base of the skull (contraindication to the nasal route).
- Penetrating eye injuries — increased intraocular pressure.
- Patient refusal or uncooperative patient.

Further reading

1. Jeon YS, Choi JW, Jung HS, *et al*. Effect of continuous cuff pressure regulator in general anaesthesia with laryngeal mask airway. *J Int Med Res* 2011; 39: 1900-7.
2. Brindley PG, Simmonds MR, Needham CJ, Simmonds KA. Teaching airway management to novices: a simulator manikin study comparing the "sniffing position" and "win with the chin" analogies. *Br J Anaesth* 2010; 104: 496-500.
3. Law JA, Broemling N, Cooper RM, *et al*. The difficult airway with recommendations for management - part 1. Difficult tracheal intubation encountered in an unconscious/induced patient. *Can J Anaesth* 2013; 60: 1089-118.

4. Law JA, Broemling N, Cooper RM, *et al*. The difficult airway with recommendatioins for management - part 2 - the anticipated difficult airway. *Can J Anaesth* 2013; 60: 1119-38.

5. 4th National Audit Project of The Royal College of Anaesthetists and The Difficult Airway Society. Major complications of airway management in the United Kingdom, Report and Findings, March 2011.

6. Popat M, Mitchell V, Dravid R, *et al*. Difficult Airway Society Guidelines for the management of tracheal extubation. *Anaesthesia* 2012; 67: 318-40.

7. Frerk CM, Mitchell VS, McNarry AF, *et al*. Difficult Airway Society 2015 guidelines for the management of unanticipated difficult intubation in adults. *Br J Anaesth* 2015; 115: 827-48.

21 Head and neck procedures

Aleksandra Nowicka and Cyprian Mendonca

Introduction

Oral and maxillofacial surgery is a challenging area of anaesthesia. It involves a wide spectrum of operative procedures, the complexity of which ranges from simple dental extractions to prolonged reconstructions with a transfer of a free tissue flap. Anaesthetists are often faced with complex airway issues, and particularly the urgent cases are regarded with apprehension by many.

The risk of airway problems in the population undergoing head and neck procedures is high. Patients present for surgery with a multitude of pathologies (e.g. neoplasms or facial fractures), many of which alter the anatomy of the airway. The problem which is a reason for surgery may cause airway obstruction, difficult bag and mask ventilation or impede the view of the larynx during intubation. The fact that 40% of cases reported to the Fourth National Audit Project of the Royal College of Anaesthetists (NAP4) had head and neck pathology highlights the importance of careful airway planning in this population to avoid the most feared scenario of loss of airway on induction of anaesthesia, leading to a 'can't intubate, can't oxygenate' scenario.

The importance of meticulous airway assessment in this group of patients cannot be overestimated. It should be followed by formulating an airway strategy which takes into consideration the failure of the primary plan. Having a plan for extubation is just as important as a plan for intubation, as the surgical procedure may have an impact on the patient's airway, e.g. by causing airway oedema or bleeding. Therefore, with many procedures, there is a distinct possibility of airway obstruction after extubation.

435

A shared airway is another aspect of maxillofacial surgery not relevant to most other anaesthetic specialties. There are several implications of a surgeon working close to, or within the airway:

- Adequate surgical access is required; therefore, the nature of the surgical procedure will influence the choice of the airway device.
- The airway device may become obstructed, dislodged or damaged during surgery. This is particularly relevant to laryngeal mask airways (LMAs) but may also be the case with endotracheal tubes.
- The patient's head is usually positioned away from the anaesthetic machine limiting the access to the airway. Long breathing circuits and intravenous extensions are needed.
- The surgeon is working near the eyes, so meticulous care needs to be taken to ensure eye protection.

In all head and neck cases, good communication between the surgeon and the anaesthetist is vital. It is important to discuss the operating plan, the choice of the airway device, the strategy for securing the airway in cases of predicted difficulties, and the plan for postoperative care. Any problems during the procedure should be promptly communicated between the anaesthetic and surgical teams.

Dental extractions

Surgical considerations

Dental extractions are usually brief procedures with high-turnover operating lists. Similarly to other head and neck procedures, judicious decisions will need to be made regarding airway management. A standard set up of the operating theatre for head and neck procedures is shown in Figure 21.1.

Unrestricted access to the oral cavity

An oral route with the use of a reinforced or north facing Ring-Adair-Elwyn (RAE) tube may provide adequate access; however, in many cases the surgeon will require unrestricted access to the oral cavity provided by a nasal endotracheal tube.

The choice of airway

The choice of airway will depend on patient factors, the experience of the anaesthetist and surgeon, and the duration and complexity of the surgery. It is best discussed with the surgeon at the team brief, before starting the theatre list. Simple dental extractions can be carried out with a reinforced LMA *in situ*. For more complex procedures, such as wisdom teeth extractions, tracheal intubation is required.

Throat packs

Throat packs are often used to absorb blood and secretions accumulating in the oropharynx. They are particularly useful during conservative procedures, where a large volume of water is spilled by the drill along with particulate matter. Problems associated with throat packs include the possibility of trauma to the pharyngeal mucosa and, more importantly, the risk of retention. Therefore, whenever a throat pack is used, steps need to be taken to ensure that it is removed at the end of the surgery.

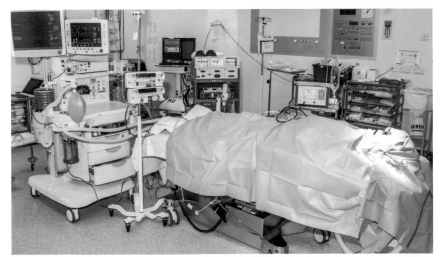

Figure 21.1. Standard set up of the operating theatre for head and neck procedures. Note that the head end of the patient is away from the anaesthetic machine limiting the access to the airway.

Patient position

The position is usually supine with or without a head-up tilt. Attention should be paid to the care of the eyes, as they are close to the surgical field.

Local anaesthetics and vasoconstrictors

A mixture of a local anaesthetic and a vasoconstrictor is usually injected at the start of the procedure to aid haemostasis and postoperative pain relief. It can cause temporary tachycardia and hypertension. Even though halothane is no longer in widespread use, arrhythmias still occur more commonly during anaesthesia for dentistry. The use of vasoconstrictors added to the local anaesthetic mixture is one of the contributing factors. Other factors include the patient's anxiety and high levels of endogenous catecholamines and trigeminal nerve stimulation during extractions.

Anaesthetic considerations

Shared airway

Cases of a shared airway always raise the possibility of a displacement of airway devices and airway obstruction. Vigilance and close cooperation with the surgeon is needed through the duration of the case, particularly if an LMA is used, as airway devices may need to be moved to facilitate access to all four quadrants of the mouth.

Choice of muscle relaxant

The brief nature of most dental extractions has implications on the use of a muscle relaxant if tracheal intubation is planned. Historically, suxamethonium was used for very short procedures. However, it is associated with many undesired effects such as myalgia and suxamethonium apnoea. Mivacurium is a short-acting non-depolarising muscle relaxant popular with some anaesthetists. A technique of administering a reduced dose of muscle relaxant that permits early reversal of neuromuscular blockade is also widely used. Rocuronium, if used, can be reversed by sugammadex at any stage.

Maintenance of anaesthesia

Maintenance of anaesthesia with an inhalational agent is preferred by most anaesthetists. Taking into consideration the balance between the cost of the agent and the recovery profile, sevoflurane is currently regarded as the agent of choice for day-case patients.

Analgesia

Paracetamol and non-steroidal anti-inflammatory drugs are usually sufficient for postoperative analgesia. They can be administered orally, as a premedication, or intravenously during the procedure. Appropriate steps should be taken to prevent postoperative nausea and vomiting. Dexamethasone is useful in this respect as it also reduces swelling associated with the extractions.

Dental extraction in children

A large proportion of patients requiring general anaesthesia for dental extractions are children, and in these cases, one has to consider all implications of paediatric anaesthesia.

In dental hospitals, brief dental procedures in children are often carried out with the use of a nasal mask. In these cases, inhalational induction is performed with a standard face mask, which is then exchanged for a nasal mask, allowing the surgeon unrestricted access to the oral cavity. The airway is maintained by the anaesthetist by the application of a jaw trust. This type of anaesthesia is historically performed in a sitting position (chair dental anaesthesia), which facilitates maintenance of the airway and limits accumulation of blood and debris in the pharynx. It is, however, associated with pooling of blood in the lower body, reduced venous return, and the possibility of hypotension and cerebral hypoperfusion. A semi-supine position can be a good compromise in this situation.

Special care dentistry

As the vast majority of dental procedures in adults can be carried out under local or regional anaesthesia, adult patients usually present for general anaesthesia for a reason. This may be because of a fear of dental procedures or needles, an allergy to local anaesthesia, or the presence of infection impeding the use of local anaesthesia. Anxiety levels are usually high in these patients and sedative premedication, topical anaesthesia for intravenous access or inhalational induction may be requested.

Patients with learning difficulties and behavioural problems also present commonly due to poor oral hygiene and an inability to comply with dental treatment. This group of patients can be particularly challenging to the anaesthetist. Poly-pharmacy and coexisting medical problems are common. Sedative premedication is often required. However, its effects may be difficult to predict. As these patients are likely to return for repeat

Table 21.1. Summary of problems encountered during anaesthesia for special care dentistry.

- Consent — the patient may not have the capacity to consent for treatment. The Mental Capacity Act 2005 may need to be employed.
- Mental health problems.
- Challenging behaviour.
- Presence of coexisting disease:
  - epilepsy;
  - congenital heart disease;
  - musculoskeletal deformities;
  - syndromes associated with a difficult airway;
  - obesity;
  - deafness and visual loss;
  - gastrointestinal problems — reflux, dysphagia, feeding through a gastrostomy.
- Poly-pharmacy, often includes sedatives.
- Sedative premedication is often used; the response is variable.
- Transport will be required.
- Additional time the during operating list is needed.

dental treatments, it is important to avoid negative experiences during admission. This can be done by early planning and an individual approach to each patient. Challenging behaviour will require the anaesthetist to adapt a pragmatic approach, e.g. when certain interventions such as ECG monitoring are declined.

It is usual for dental extractions to be carried out as day-case procedures. However, patients with severe coexisting diseases may require overnight hospitalisation.

A summary of the problems encountered during anaesthesia for special care dentistry are outlined in Table 21.1.

Dental abscesses

Surgical considerations

Dental abscesses result from the extension of dental caries from the root and apex of the tooth to the surrounding alveolar bone. In the majority of cases, dental abscesses can be treated with antibiotics and drained under local anaesthesia and do not require hospital admission or anaesthetic input. However, untreated odontogenic infections can spread to the soft tissues of the head and neck, along the facial planes. Upward spread of an infection arising from maxillary teeth may result in sinusitis and orbital cellulitis. Infection arising from molar teeth extending posteriorly may affect the masseter muscle, causing trismus, or reach the retropharyngeal space or the epiglottis, at which point they may present a major challenge to the anaesthetist.

The key aspects of the management of a patient with a dental abscess include identifying any airway compromise or potential airway difficulties, decisions on the method of inducing anaesthesia and securing the airway, the treatment of infection with a surgical procedure and appropriate antibiotics, and the supportive management of systemic sepsis and septic shock if present.

Problems that may cause difficulties in the management of the airway are summarised in Table 21.2. Experienced help may be required. An

Table 21.2. Possible causes of airway difficulties in patients with dental infections.

Problem	Comments
Trismus	Caused by spread of infection to the masseter muscle
	Present in approximately 20% of patients requiring hospital admission
Retropharyngeal abscess, inflammation of supraglottic structures	Due to posterior spread of infection from molar teeth
Osteomyelitis of mandible	May cause bone deformation and limited mouth opening
Ludwig's angina	Cellulitis of the soft tissues of the floor of the mouth
	Causes elevation of the tongue and impaired swallowing

airway plan should be formulated after a careful assessment and consultation with the surgeon. The method of securing the airway will depend on the airway evaluation, patient's cooperation, and experience of the anaesthetist. The techniques that may be employed include awake fibreoptic intubation, intravenous induction and muscle relaxation or a tracheostomy under local anaesthesia depending on the anticipated severity of airway difficulty.

Trismus cannot reliably be expected to improve after induction of general anaesthesia. Mouth opening is more likely to improve in cases of superficial space abscesses, and if the duration of symptoms is short. One study of 100 patients with trismus secondary to a dental abscess found that after induction of anaesthesia and muscle relaxation, improvement in mouth opening of more than 9mm was found in all patients with symptom duration of less than 3 days. If mouth opening is severely restricted or if direct laryngoscopy is expected to be difficult, there should be a low threshold for an awake fibreoptic intubation and it is the most safe option for securing the airway. The airway may need to be secured urgently if there are signs of early airway compromise, such as a change of voice, odynophagia, a rapid progression of swelling or lack of tongue protrusion. If the airway compromise is severe, a tracheostomy under local anaesthesia may be necessary.

The surgical procedure itself involves dental extractions and either oral or extra-oral drainage of abscesses. Drains may need to be inserted. Dental infections are caused by the microorganisms constituting the normal oral flora, and are therefore always polymicrobial. The choice of antibiotics should be dictated by local protocols, but both aerobic and anaerobic cover are required.

If the original presentation was with airway obstruction or severe sepsis or if significant swelling is present, a period of ventilation on the intensive care unit may be needed before extubation. The decision on the timing of extubation should be made jointly with the surgeon.

Anaesthetic considerations

Odontogenic infections have the potential for causing systemic sepsis. It is important to look for signs of a systemic inflammatory response and, if present, careful assessment of the patient's fluid status and organ function should be made. Fluid resuscitation may be necessary. Intensive or high dependency care admission may be required to provide organ support in cases of septic shock and multi-organ failure.

Severe complications of dental infections include osteomyelitis, intracranial spread with cavernous sinus thrombosis and descending mediastinitis. They are well recognised and associated with increased mortality and morbidity. Other rare complications such as haemorrhage from the erosion of major vessels of the neck or formation of a cerebral abscess have also been described.

Severe odontogenic infections only rarely complicate unsuccessful dental treatment. The vast majority results from poor oral hygiene, lack of routine dental treatment, and failure to seek emergency treatment early. Patients are likely to have low socioeconomic status. Substance abuse and mental health problems such as schizophrenia or severe depression, which are associated with inadequate dental care, may be an issue. Diabetes mellitus and an immunocompromised state are factors predisposing to the rapid spread of odontogenic infections.

Maxillofacial trauma

Anaesthetists may encounter patients with maxillofacial injuries in two different settings: in the emergency department, in the context of trauma resuscitation, or in theatre, providing anaesthesia for definitive procedures.

Approximately 30% of trauma patients with severe injuries admitted to the emergency department also have maxillofacial trauma. Airway management in this group of patients can be difficult for a number of reasons:

- The cervical spine needs to be protected whenever the mechanism of trauma suggests a possible injury or is not known. Manual in-line stabilisation of the cervical spine can lead to a poor view of the glottis during direct laryngoscopy.
- Anatomy may be disrupted. Blood clots and debris, dislodged teeth, secretions and gastric contents may be present in the airway obstructing the view during laryngoscopy.
- Facial injuries may produce an airway obstruction. This may be caused by posterior displacement of the maxilla in cases of Le Fort III fractures, posterior displacement of the tongue in bilateral mandibular fractures, foreign bodies, soft tissue swelling, major haemorrhage, or a disruption of the airway, such as a ruptured larynx or transected trachea.
- A full stomach risks aspiration of gastric contents.
- The patient may be uncooperative and agitated limiting the use of techniques such as awake intubation or even making pre-oxygenation difficult.

- The incidence of other injuries in patients with maxillofacial trauma is reported as 55-70%. If cardiovascular compromise is present, it may be exacerbated by the induction of anaesthesia.
- There is usually limited time for preparation, and the anaesthetist will be working in a less familiar environment, outside the comfort zone of the operating theatres.

Rapid sequence induction of anaesthesia and oral intubation using direct laryngoscopy is the most commonly used technique for securing the airway. If a difficulty in airway management is anticipated, a videolaryngoscope and a clinician experienced in its use should be immediately available. Other techniques such as intubation through the LMA, fibreoptic intubation, or an awake tracheostomy may sometimes be necessary. In difficult cases, the anaesthetist should use the technique they are familiar with and, if needed, experienced help should be called early. Whenever intubation is undertaken in the emergency department, the standards of monitoring and the assistance available should be the same as in theatre. A clear plan for failure of the initial technique should be in place and communicated to the team. Intubation adjuncts and rescue airway devices should be available.

Facial fractures

Surgical considerations

The timing of repair of facial wounds will depend on the presence and severity of other injuries. In severely injured trauma patients, only damage control surgery is performed, followed by definitive surgery after the patient's condition has stabilised. Ocular injuries and open wounds take priority over facial fractures. Fixation of mandibular fractures should ideally be performed within 24-48 hours. Repair of other facial fractures is usually undertaken semi-electively, after other serious injuries have been addressed and the swelling has settled.

In all cases of facial fractures, it is essential to discuss the operating plan with the surgeon. Generally, tracheal intubation through the nasal route will be required for fixation of mandibular fractures, and an oral south-facing RAE tube for fractures of the zygomatic complex. In some cases, the surgeon may need to stabilise the bone with the use of intermaxillary fixation, wiring together the mandible and maxilla. If this technique is required, it precludes oral intubation. The fixation may remain in place for the postoperative period, in which case it also prevents postoperative access to the oral cavity with implications for emergency airway management. Very rarely, in cases of complex fractures, unobstructed surgical access to the nasal and oral cavity may be required and either an intra-operative tube exchange or a tracheostomy may be needed. Submental intubation where the endotracheal tube is exteriorised through the incision in the floor of the mouth has also been described.

The level of monitoring will be dictated by the condition of the patient and the presence of other injuries. The patient should be positioned supine and their head stabilised in a head ring. Anaesthesia can be maintained with either a remifentanil infusion used in combination with an inhalational agent or total intravenous technique. The use of remifentanil is popular, as it allows good control of blood pressure, suppression of respiration and

Table 21.3. Types of facial fractures.

- Frontal sinus.
- Nasal bones.
- Zygomatic/zygomaticomaxillary fractures.
- Maxillary fractures:
  - Le Fort I — transverse fracture of the maxilla above the level of the root apices and through or below the level of the nose;
  - Le Fort II — fractures traverse the nose, infra-orbital rim, and orbital floor and then proceed laterally through the lateral buttress and posteriorly through the pterygomaxillary buttress;
  - Le Fort III — high level, suprazygomatic fractures, also known as craniofacial disjunction, are the result of the mid-face being separated from the cranial base.
- Mandibular fractures:
  - fractures of symphysis, body, angle, ramus, condyle, and subcondyle regions.

airway reflexes, and smooth emergence. If the surgeon plans to leave the intermaxillary fixation in place after the surgery, all possible measures should be taken to prevent nausea and vomiting.

During the surgical elevation of a fractured zygoma, severe bradycardia may occur. If it is the case, the surgeon should be asked to stop the manipulation, which usually resolves the problem. Nevertheless, atropine and glycopyrrolate should be immediately available during these procedures.

The types of facial fractures are outlined in Table 21.3.

Anaesthetic considerations

During the pre-operative assessment, the presence and severity of other injuries should be assessed. The most common injuries coexisting with facial trauma are intracranial haematomas and cervical spine injuries. If such injuries are present, steps need to be taken to optimise the intracranial pressure and cerebral perfusion during anaesthesia. The presence of spinal fractures may affect the patient's handling and the management of the airway.

A detailed airway assessment is of great importance. Details of facial fractures should be noted along with the degree of soft tissue swelling. If major oedema is present, awake intubation needs to be considered. Limitation of mouth opening is common. In cases of isolated mandibular fractures and in the absence of the temporomandibular joint involvement, trismus is usually due to pain and disappears on induction of anaesthesia. In zygomatic fractures, however, the compressed zygoma may impinge on the temporalis muscle or the coronoid process of the mandible and mouth opening may not improve on induction. If there is any doubt, it is useful to ask the surgeon if there is any mechanical reason for trismus.

Extubation needs to be carefully planned, particularly if the patient was difficult to intubate, or significant oedema is present. Hyoid bone fractures and Le Fort II and III fractures are at particular risk of postoperative swelling and airway obstruction. If intermaxillary fixation is in place, equipment to release the fixation should be available at all times and the patient should be nursed in the high dependency unit.

The postoperative pain, however, is usually mild, and opioids are not necessary, with the exception of fractures of the mandible and orbital fractures extending behind the eye, where the pain is more severe.

Radical neck dissection

Surgical considerations

Radical neck dissection is an integral part of the treatment of metastatic head and neck cancers. Malignancies, which most commonly spread into the cervical lymph nodes, arise from the mucosal areas of the upper airway, in particular the larynx, oropharynx, hypopharynx, and oral cavity. The operation in its classic form involves removal of cervical lymph nodes along with the sternocleidomastoid muscle, internal jugular vein, and spinal accessory nerve. Multiple modifications of the classic procedure, aimed at preserving some of the above structures, are commonly performed. Radical neck dissection is often performed alongside other procedures aimed at the resection of the primary tumour or its recurrence and reconstruction of the tissue defect. Anaesthetic management will largely depend on these additional procedures.

For neck dissection alone, the reinforced tracheal tube is the usual choice of airway. The tube should be directed north — away from the surgical field.

The patient is positioned supine, with a sandbag under the shoulders and a head-up tilt to aid drainage of venous blood from the neck and improve the operating field. The head is placed in a head ring and tilted away from the operative side.

A manipulation of the carotid sinus by the surgeon can cause bradycardia and severe hypotension. This response can be minimised by injecting local anaesthetic around the sinus prior to the manipulation.

The blood loss varies between surgeons and the techniques used, and is usually between 200-300ml, but there is a potential for substantial blood loss. Haemorrhage from major neck vessels is a possibility. Even in the absence of brisk bleeding, the blood loss from slow venous oozing may be considerable. Cross-matched blood should be available.

Bilateral radical neck dissection carries a significant risk of cerebral oedema. If bilateral dissection is required, either the internal jugular vein is preserved on one side, or two separate procedures are carried out several weeks apart, to allow a collateral circulation to form. It has been shown that staged second neck dissections carry the risk of increased intracranial pressure even if the subsequent operation is undertaken many years after the initial surgery. Even in cases of bilateral neck dissections where one internal jugular vein is preserved, postoperative imaging demonstrates thrombosis in up to 30% of cases.

Although rare, venous air embolism is a possibility during this operation. A high index of suspicion for this complication should be maintained. Pneumothorax is another rare complication.

It is desirable to avoid excessive coughing and straining during emergence from anaesthesia, as it increases the head and neck venous pressure and may precipitate bleeding. Achieving smooth emergence is challenging, and no single technique guarantees success. Simple steps that can be taken include adequate analgesia, the avoidance of transfer from the operating table to the bed in light planes of anaesthesia, and leaving the patient undisturbed, with the cuff of the endotracheal tube deflated until consciousness is regained. Advanced techniques include extubation with remifentanil infusion and laryngeal mask exchange.

The usual time taken for an isolated unilateral dissection is between 2-4 hours but it may be significantly longer if neck dissection is performed alongside other procedures such as a laryngectomy, pharyngectomy, glossectomy, and oral and maxillofacial resections. During these operations the usual precautions for long surgery should be observed. Additional procedures will also influence other aspects of anaesthetic management. Nasal intubation will be needed if the surgeon requires access to the oral cavity. A nasogastric tube should be inserted and appropriately secured if swallowing difficulties are expected. Reconstruction of a tissue defect may be performed with a rotational or free flap with all the anaesthetic implications of a tissue transfer. If reconstruction with a radial free flap is planned, intravenous or arterial cannulae must not be inserted in the same arm. Tracheostomy should be considered if the surgery is likely to cause postoperative airway compromise. Alternatively, delayed extubation may be performed on the intensive care unit after the operative site oedema has settled.

Anaesthetic considerations

Patients with head and neck cancer are known to have a high incidence of a difficult airway. This may be due to the distortion of the anatomy caused by the tumour or surrounding oedema, scar tissue from previous surgery or post-radiotherapy changes. The overall incidence of difficult intubation in this population is approximately 12%, but may be as high as 30% in patients who have undergone previous major head and neck surgery and 40% following head and neck radiotherapy. Bag and mask ventilation and ventilation with an LMA are also more likely to be difficult.

Careful airway assessment is crucial. Symptoms and signs of airway obstruction should be actively sought. CT scans and nasoendoscopy under local anaesthesia add value to the clinical assessment in cases of an obstructed airway. Previous anaesthetic charts may be of limited value in predicting the grade of laryngoscopy, as the airway may deteriorate significantly between procedures due to the presence of scar tissue or post-radiotherapy fibrosis. These can cause oedema, induration of tissues, and limitation of neck and jaw movement. If trismus is present, it is unlikely to resolve with the induction of anaesthesia.

An airway strategy which includes the failure of the initial plan for intubation needs to be developed for each case. There should be a low threshold for a fibreoptic intubation. Awake fibreoptic intubation is a gold standard for the management of an anticipated difficult airway; however, it is also not without problems, e.g. it may precipitate an airway obstruction in cases of tracheal stenosis or bleeding from friable tumour tissue.

Smoking and alcohol consumption are risk factors for squamous cell carcinoma, which is the most common type of head and neck cancer. Both are associated with intra-operative and postoperative problems. A history of alcohol consumption should be actively sought. Alcohol withdrawal syndrome may occur in patients who cease alcohol consumption in hospital. The consequences of delirium in this context, such as pulling out surgical drains and intravenous cannulae, or refusing oxygen can be life-threatening. Alcohol-dependent patients should undergo detoxification before the surgery.

Patients with head and neck malignancies may be treated with neoadjuvant chemotherapy. The adverse effects of chemotherapeutic agents are common and in many cases include organ dysfunction. The history of chemotherapeutic agents used and clinical features of toxicity should be sought. Routine investigations such as a full blood count and urea and electrolytes are helpful in evaluating organ dysfunction. Additional investigations may also be required depending on the agent used.

It is usual to insert an arterial line, as these procedures have the potential for significant blood loss as well as intra-operative hypotension and arrhythmias. Although central venous access is usually not required, it may be useful for patients with significant comorbidities. It is important to remember that following the resection of an internal jugular vein, the drainage of blood from head and neck depends on the contralateral internal jugular vein. It is, therefore, prudent to avoid this site for central venous access, as it may cause compression by an incidental haematoma or stenosis of the vessel. If required, the femoral vein should be utilised. The urinary catheter should be inserted for prolonged procedures. Temperature monitoring is essential.

The patient should receive balanced anaesthesia, aimed at reducing sympathetic activity and avoiding intra-operative hypertension. Inhalational or intravenous maintenance can be used. A remifentanil infusion is useful, particularly if intra-operative use of a nerve stimulator is planned, as it suppresses respiration and airway reflexes, and supplemental doses of muscle relaxant are normally not required. It is safe to use a muscle relaxant for intubation, as it would normally wear off by the time the nerve identification is required. This should, however, be confirmed with a train-of-four count.

The postoperative analgesic requirements are moderate. Analgesia with paracetamol and oral or intramuscular morphine is usually sufficient. Patient-controlled analgesia is rarely required.

Thyroidectomy

Surgical considerations

Indications for surgery include the treatment of thyroid cancer, the presence of goitre and hyperthyroidism resistant to medical treatment. The complexity of surgical procedures varies from simple excision of a thyroid nodule to complex operations involving removal of a malignant or retrosternal goitre.

Thyroidectomy can be performed under regional anaesthesia. A deep and superficial cervical plexus block can be utilised; however, this technique is not popular in the UK as a sole anaesthetic technique, and patients normally undergo general anaesthesia. A reinforced tracheal tube is the usual choice of airway.

The eyes should be lubricated and padded. This is of particular importance in patients with Graves' disease who may suffer from exophthalmos. The patient's position is supine, with a sandbag under the shoulders, head on a head ring, and arms by their sides. The table is tilted head up to optimise venous drainage from the head and neck. For the same reason, an endotracheal tube should be secured with a tape, rather than tied around the neck.

Thyroid surgery involves a degree of tracheal manipulation which may precipitate coughing. This can be avoided by spraying the vocal cords with local anaesthetic on intubation and full muscle relaxation throughout the surgery. Alternatively, a remifentanil infusion can be used to suppress airway reflexes, particularly when neuromuscular monitoring is required.

Injury to the recurrent laryngeal nerve is a recognised complication and may occur by several mechanisms including ischaemia, contusion, traction, entrapment and transection. The risk of nerve damage is greater during surgery for malignancy and reintervention. The surgeon may wish to monitor the function of the recurrent laryngeal nerve intra-operatively by monitoring evoked electromyography (EMG) potentials from the vocalis muscle. This involves the use of a tracheal tube with integrated EMG electrodes positioned at the level of the vocal cords. In these cases, it is important to ensure that the effects of neuromuscular blocking drugs are no longer present when monitoring is undertaken.

Retrosternal goitres can usually be excised through the cervical route. A tracheal compression may temporarily worsen when the surgeon manipulates the retrosternal part of the gland but is normally relieved after the goitre is removed. In a small number of cases, a medial sternotomy may be required, which is usually performed jointly with thoracic surgeons.

Intra-operative hypertension should be avoided, as it exacerbates bleeding from the surgical field. However, at the end of the procedure, normal or even supranormal blood pressure should be achieved to ensure adequate homeostasis and prevent postoperative bleeding. A Trendelenburg position and Valsalva manoeuvre are often employed for the same reason.

Anaesthetic considerations

Patients should be euthyroid prior to surgery. Operating on a patient with uncontrolled hyperthyroidism risks a hypermetabolic state known as a 'thyroid storm'. A hypothyroid state predisposes to peri-operative respiratory and cardiovascular depression, hypoglycaemia, electrolyte imbalance, hypothermia and, in most severe cases, myxoedematous coma.

Patients presenting with goitre may prompt worries about the ease of airway management. This is particularly the case if the goitre is retrosternal, symptomatic or particularly large causing tracheal deviation and compression. The duration of the goitre and the presence of symptoms should be determined in addition to the routine airway assessment. The patient may give a history of positional dyspnoea, dysphagia, dysphonia or stridor and show signs of superior vena caval obstruction.

The main areas of concern are a difficult bag and mask ventilation, difficult intubation, and tracheomalacia causing postoperative airway obstruction.

The overall incidence of a difficult endotracheal intubation in thyroid surgery is approximately 5-6%. It has been reported that the presence of a large goitre alone is not associated with a higher incidence of difficult intubation. However, the presence of a malignant goitre and Mallampati Grade III or IV have been identified as two independent risk factors for a difficult intubation. Nasoendoscopy is routinely performed by surgeons before a thyroidectomy to assess the function of the vocal cords. An inability to visualise the larynx with this method also predicts a difficult intubation.

Although controversy exists regarding the appropriate method of induction of anaesthesia in cases of a large goitre causing tracheal compression, in experienced hands intravenous induction followed by muscle relaxation and laryngoscopy (direct or videolaryngoscopy) is an appropriate technique. However, if there is a suspicion that the airway may be lost during induction of anaesthesia, the awake intubation technique is the method of choice. While planning the strategy for the management of the airway, it is important to remember that rescue techniques, such as emergency cricothyroidotomy or tracheostomy, are likely to be difficult in the presence of a large goitre. If problems are encountered during induction, ventilation via a rigid bronchoscope may be a useful technique of achieving oxygenation.

Tracheomalacia precipitating airway collapse is another feared complication of a longstanding goitre. Recent evidence, however, suggests that this complication is very rare in the Western world, even in cases of retrosternal goitre. Most cases are believed to occur in developing countries, in the areas of endemic goitre. In a case series which included 62 patients with significant tracheal compression by goitre, there were no cases of tracheomalacia reported. In cases of a large or retrosternal goitre, the surgeon may feel the tracheal rings before extubation. A lack of leak around the endotracheal tube after deflating the cuff may alert the anaesthetist about the possibility of this complication.

The incidence of airway complications during emergence and in the postoperative period is generally higher than on induction of anaesthesia.

Airway obstruction may be caused by laryngeal oedema, bilateral recurrent laryngeal nerve palsies, or haemorrhage or tracheomalacia. Emergency reintubation and tracheostomy may be necessary.

Postoperative analgesia with regular paracetamol and NSAIDs, and intermittent morphine is usually sufficient. The superficial cervical plexus block is effective at reducing postoperative pain.

Case scenario 1

A 30-year-old male with a severe learning disability and behavioural problems is scheduled for dental extractions. He requires 24-hour care and lives in a residential institution. His verbal communication is very limited and he often becomes extremely agitated and aggressive, especially in unfamiliar situations. His medications include chlorpromazine and diazepam. There is no other past medical history of note and the airway assessment and physical examination are unremarkable.

How would you manage this patient?

Pre-operative management

During the pre-operative assessment, it is established that he is very unlikely to cooperate with venous cannulation and that he gets scared by new faces, too many people in the room, and people wearing head covers.

After consultation with the carers regarding the needs of the patient, a detailed plan for hospital admission and induction of anaesthesia should be formulated. Inhalational induction should be explained to the patient. A face mask and photographs of the anaesthetist and the ODP should be given to him to take home so that he becomes familiar with the anaesthetic room environment.

This patient should be placed first on the operating list and additional time during the list should be allowed due to the complexity of the case. Theatre staff are advised not to wear hats while with the patient as this may trigger anxiety and challenging behaviour.

On the morning of the surgery, the patient should be admitted to the side room directly from the ambulance, accompanied by his carers. Oral midazolam 15mg can be administered as sedative premedication.

Intra-operative management

The patient should be accompanied into the anaesthetic room by his carers. Initially, only a pulse oximeter is applied as a means of monitoring. The application of ECG electrodes or a blood pressure cuff can be done after induction of anaesthesia. An inhalational induction can be performed with the use of nitrous oxide and sevoflurane. Although most patients comply well with the application of the face mask some may require a brief period of physical restriction. Following loss of consciousness, standard monitoring and intravenous access, atracurium 0.5mg/kg is administered. A nasal intubation is preferred for surgical access. Topical application of phenylephrine 0.5% and lignocaine to nasal mucosa provides vasoconstriction and minimises bleeding. Anaesthesia can be maintained with sevoflurane. Paracetamol and ketorolac can be administered for postoperative pain relief, and dexamethasone to prevent postoperative nausea and to reduce oedema.

Postoperative management

The patient should be extubated awake and transferred into the recovery room. The carers are allowed into the recovery room. He can be safely discharged home a few hours later.

Case scenario 2

A 57-year-old female presents for a total thyroidectomy for a multinodular goitre. She has a 2-year history of thyroid enlargement. She also reports a 4-week period of breathing difficulties when supine.

Her past medical history includes hypertension and Type 2 diabetes mellitus controlled with diet. The only regular medication is amlodipine.

On examination she is obese with a BMI of $31kg/m^2$. She is comfortable and not in apparent respiratory distress but becomes short of breath with inspiratory and expiratory stridor when positioned supine. There is a firm, midline neck mass measuring 5cm obscuring the thyroid cartilage. The inter-incisor distance is 5cm, the Mallampati Grade is 2, and the jaw protrusion and neck movements are normal.

The flexible fibreoptic laryngoscopy in the ENT clinic a week ago was normal. The laboratory tests showed normal thyroid function, electrolytes, and full blood count. The results of a previous fine-needle aspiration were benign. A CT of the neck and chest showed a markedly enlarged heterogeneous thyroid gland without substernal extension but with compression of the trachea by 50% of the baseline diameter. No suspicious lymphadenopathy was noted and the findings were consistent with a multinodular goitre.

How would you manage this patient?

Airway management plan

As based on the airway assessment, the view of the larynx on direct laryngoscopy is expected to be good. An intravenous induction of anaesthesia with propofol and rocuronium can be planned. A videolaryngoscope is kept ready in the anaesthetic room. Ventilation through the rigid bronchoscope by the ENT surgeon is planned as a rescue technique in case of a loss of airway at any stage. In addition, ensuring immediate availability of sugammadex allows reversal of neuromuscular blockade in the event of a difficult intubation. As the thyroid cartilage is obscured by the mass, one should exercise caution as an emergency cricothyroidotomy may not be possible in the event of a can't intubate, can't oxygenate scenario.

Intra-operative management

An arterial line is useful, in addition to the standard monitoring. Following pre-oxygenation, anaesthesia can be induced and maintained using a TIVA technique (propofol and remifentanil target-controlled infusion). Rocuronium 0.1mg/kg is the muscle relaxant of choice. Postoperative pain relief can be provided with a combination of local infiltration, paracetamol and morphine. Dexamethasone and ondansetron should be given to prevent postoperative nausea and vomiting.

At the end of the procedure, the leak test should be performed to rule out tracheomalacia. The patient is then transferred onto the bed, the muscle relaxation reversed with neostigmine and glycopyrrolate and anaesthesia discontinued. After the return of spontaneous respiration, the tracheal cuff is deflated and the patient is left undisturbed until consciousness is regained, and then extubated. To ensure smooth extubation, a remifentanil infusion is continued until extubation.

Postoperative management

Regular paracetamol and an intermittent oral morphine solution are prescribed for postoperative analgesia.

Case scenario 3

A 28-year-old female is admitted for emergency drainage of a dental abscess under general anaesthesia. She presented to hospital with pyrexia and a left-sided facial swelling lasting for 24 hours. She is 18 weeks' pregnant. The pregnancy has been uneventful and there is no other past medical history of note.

On examination, she is comfortable. Her temperature is 37°C (admission temperature was 38°C), heart rate is 90 beats per minute, and blood pressure is 110/65mmHg. There is significant swelling and erythema of the left cheek extending over the masseter muscle, and the submandibular space. The patient also has severe trismus, with an inter-incisor distance of 8mm. Tongue protrusion is impossible. The breathing pattern is comfortable and no dysphonia is present.

The full blood count shows leucocytosis and mild microcytic anaemia. Urea and electrolytes are normal. A CT scan was not performed.

How would you manage this patient?

Pre-operative management

Intravenous antibiotics are started on admission to the hospital. As the patient demonstrates severe trismus and the infection involves multiple facial spaces, the mouth opening is unlikely to be improved significantly following induction of anaesthesia. Therefore, an awake fibreoptic intubation through the nasal route is the preferred option.

Potential airway difficulties during anaesthesia along with the conduct of an awake intubation, possible implications of a severe infection and of general anaesthesia on pregnancy should be explained to the patient. The management plan should be discussed with the surgeons and the theatre team. The obstetric team should also be informed about the admission.

Intra-operative management

Following awake nasal intubation, anaesthesia can be induced and maintained with sevoflurane and remifentanil. Adequate muscle relaxation for surgical access can be provided with atracurium. The surgical procedure involves intra-oral drainage of the abscess and tooth extraction. The tooth extraction can be challenging due to the trismus.

Paracetamol and morphine should provide adequate postoperative pain relief. Dexamethasone and ondansetron can be administered for prophylaxis of postoperative nausea and vomiting.

At the end of the surgery, careful suction of the pharynx is performed, and the patient is placed in a semi-sitting position. After the reversal of the neuromuscular blockade, sevoflurane should be discontinued, but the remifentanil infusion should be continued with the target of 2ng/ml until extubation. The patient should be extubated when awake and cooperative.

Postoperative management

Regular paracetamol and an oral morphine solution should provide adequate analgesia. The patient should be monitored on the ENT ward.

Further reading

1. Association of Paediatric Anaesthetists of Great Britain and Ireland/Association of Dental Anaesthetists. Guidelines for the management of children referred for dental extractions under general anaesthesia, August 2011.

2. Cantlay K, Williamson S, Hawkings J. Anaesthesia for dentistry. *Br J Anaesth CEACCP* 2005; 5: 71-5.

3. Uluibau I, Jaunay T, Goss A. Severe odontogenic infections. *Aust Dent J Med Suppl* 2005; 50: 4.

4. Schumann M, Biesler I, Börgers A, *et al*. Tracheal intubation in patients with odentogenous abscesses and reduced mouth opening. *Br J Anaesth* 2014; 112: 348-54.

5. Curran J. Anaesthesia for facial trauma. *Anaesth Intensive Care Med* 2008; 9(8): 338-43.

6. Juneja R, Lacey O. Anaesthesia for head and neck cancer surgery. *Curr Anaesth Crit Care* 2009; 20: 28-32.

7. Dempsey GA, Snell JA, Coathup R, Jones TM. Anaesthesia for massive retrosternal thyroidectomy in a tertiary referral centre. *Br J Anaesth* 2013; 111: 594-9.

22 Anaesthesia and ENT surgery

Alexander Philip and Cyprian Mendonca

Introduction

Ear, nose and throat (ENT) surgeries are among the most commonly performed surgical procedures in the UK. They include day-case procedures such as adenoidectomy and myringotomy to complex prolonged procedures that are performed in specialist centres such as laryngectomy and tracheal resection. About a third of all ENT procedures are performed on children.

The major concerns in ENT surgery are those related to the airway; this may stem either from the disease process or from the shared airway, or both. A joint plan between the surgeon and the anaesthetist is essential on deciding the best airway control option. An intra-operative airway problem may necessitate interruption of the surgery to rectify the problem.

The most commonly performed ENT procedures include:

- Adenotonsillectomy.
- Nasal and sinus surgery.
- Ear surgery.
- Microlaryngoscopy.
- Laser ENT surgery.
- Tracheostomy.
- Laryngectomy.

Adenotonsillectomy

Surgical considerations

Anatomically, the palatine tonsils and the adenoids form part of the Waldeyer's ring of lymphoid tissue which encircles the pharynx; this also includes the lingual tonsils. They are most prominent between the age of 4 and 7 years and subsequently regress. In the UK, tonsillectomy is one of the most frequently performed surgical procedures.

The surgical indications for tonsillectomy for recurrent acute sore throat in children and adults (Scottish Intercollegiate Guidelines Network [SIGN] guidelines 2010) include:

- The episodes of sore throat are disabling and prevent normal functioning.
- Seven or more well-documented and clinically significant, but adequately treated, sore throat episodes in the preceding year; or
- Five or more such episodes in each of the preceding 2 years; or
- Three or more such episodes in each of the preceding 3 years.

Anaesthetic considerations

Obstructive sleep apnoea (OSA)

Pre-operatively, inquiries must be made as to the suggestive features of OSA. These include day-time somnolence, apnoeic episodes during sleep, interrupted and restless sleep, snoring and, in more severe cases, behavioural changes, neurocognitive impairment and cor pulmonale.

In adults, the STOP-BANG questionnaire (Table 22.1) is validated as a screening tool in the pre-operative period in order to detect the presence of OSA. Answering yes to three or more questions suggests a high probability of OSA.

Children and adults suffering from OSA have a higher incidence of peri-operative and postoperative complications including desaturation, airway irritability leading onto laryngospasm and obstructed airway during anaesthetic induction. They will be more sensitive to respiratory depression

Table 22.1. STOP BANG questionnaire as a screening tool for obstructive sleep apnoea. *From: Chung F, Subramanyam R, Liao P, et al. High STOP-BANG score indicates a high probability of obstructive sleep apnoea. Br J Anaesth 2012; 108: 768-75. This is an open access article under the terms of the Creative Commons Attribution Non-Commercial License (http://creativecommons.org/licenses/by-nc/2.5/uk/).*

Snoring — Do you snore loudly? (louder than talking or loud enough to be heard through doors)	Yes/No
Tired — do you often feel tired, fatigued or sleepy during daytime?	Yes/No
Observed — Has anyone observed you stop breathing during your sleep?	Yes/No
Blood **P**ressure — Do you have or are you being treated for high blood pressure?	Yes/No
BMI — more than 35kg/m^2?	Yes/No
Age— Age more than 50 years old?	Yes/No
Neck circumference — greater than 40cm?	Yes/No
Gender — Male?	Yes/No

caused by general anaesthetics, sedatives and opiates. Hence, they may require HDU/ICU care postoperatively and may be unsuitable as day-case procedures. This must be highlighted in the anaesthetic plan.

Routine pre-operative investigations are not indicated for this procedure, hence underlying the importance of a detailed history of the parents. Nocturnal polysomnography is expensive and the performance of the test and its interpretation vary between centres. In longstanding cases, right heart strain on ECG and polycythemia on a full blood count may be seen.

Shared airway management

A secure airway is vital, as access is limited once surgery commences. The choice is between a laryngeal mask airway (LMA) and an endotracheal (ET) tube, either a reinforced or an oral RAE (Ring-Adair-Elwyn) tube (Table 22.2; Figure 22.1).

Table 22.2. Comparison between an endotracheal tube and a laryngeal mask airway as an airway for adenotonsillectomy.

Endotracheal tube (ET tube)	LMA
Definitive airway	Avoids use of muscle relaxation
Surgical access better	Smoother emergence
Need for muscle relaxation/deep anaesthesia	Less traumatic
	May interfere with surgical access
	Less secure, may dislodge intra-operatively

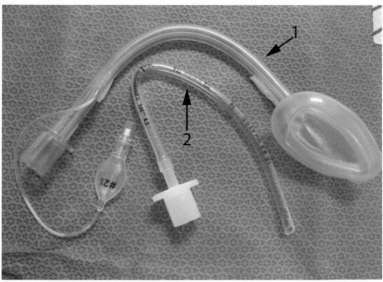

Figure 22.1. Flexible single-use LMA (1) and RAE (2) tube.

Induction and maintenance of anaesthesia

- Standard intravenous induction, e.g. propofol with short-acting opioid/inhalational induction with O_2/N_2O/sevoflurane, depending on patient acceptability.
- Spontaneous or controlled ventilation.

The Boyle-Davis mouth gag (Figure 22.2) is commonly used by surgeons to keep the mouth open, depress the tongue and facilitate surgical access. The blade has a central groove to accommodate the ET tube, a gag to keep the mouth open and a suspension assembly to maintain its position. Application of the gag may be particularly stimulating. The anaesthetist should be vigilant during application of the mouth gag to prevent compression, displacement or accidental displacement of the airway device.

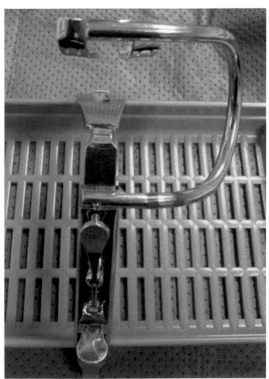

Figure 22.2. Boyle-Davies mouth gag.

Extubation and recovery

Prior to extubation, 100% oxygen should be delivered, the oral cavity should be suctioned under direct vision and the post-nasal space should be suctioned using a soft catheter. Most prefer to extubate children in the lateral head-down position. Adult patients can be extubated in the supine, head-up position once they are fully awake.

Patients with OSA may need high-dependency monitoring and an overnight stay. The following considerations should be given for these children while they have their surgery: preferably on the morning list, inhalational induction, anticipate the possibility of airway obstruction and laryngospasm during induction and the avoidance of long-acting opioids.

Analgesia

A judicious combination of paracetamol, NSAIDs (both are known to have an opioid-sparing effect) and opioids should be used. The simple oral analgesics may be given pre-operatively, ensuring peak plasma levels at the conclusion of surgery. They may also be given rectally after inducton. Regular doses of paracetamol and NSAIDs along with rescue opioids provide good postoperative analgesia.

Postoperative nausea and vomiting (PONV)

The incidence of PONV is high after adenotonsillectomy. A multimodal approach works well, consisting of minimising the fasting period, avoiding nitrous oxide and the use of antiemetics, for example, ondansetron 0.1mg/kg and dexamethasone 0.1mg/kg. Dexamethasone has also been shown to reduce analgesic requirements.

The 'bleeding' tonsil

A post-tonsillectomy bleed is the most serious postoperative complication, and may be classified as primary (within the first 24 hours postoperatively) or secondary (bleeding occuring within 28 days of surgery). The commonest cause in the first instance is surgical and in the second is infection. The incidence tends to be higher in adults, for infectious indications of surgery, e.g. recurrent tonsillitis and the use of diathermy.

Anaesthetic issues

Anaesthetic considerations include:

- Hypovolaemia is easy to underestimate due to swallowing and spitting of blood, and haemodynamic compensation in an otherwise healthy patient.
- A 'full stomach' due to swallowed blood and the consequent risk of aspiration.
- The possibility of a difficult intubation due to bleeding in the oral cavity and airway oedema.
- Frightened child and stressed parents.

Anaesthetic management

Pre-operative fluid resuscitation should be done prior to induction of general anaesthesia. This includes securing IV access with a wide-bore cannula, checking the haemoglobin concentration and transfusion of blood and blood products as indicated. Anaesthesia should not be induced until hypovolaemia is deemed to have been corrected.

Pre-induction preparation should include keeping ready a selection of ET tubes, including a few sizes smaller than predicted and a choice of suction catheters. Pre-oxgenation followed by a rapid sequence induction should be performed with a slight head-down tilt. Once haemostasis is achieved, the stomach should be emptied with a large-bore gastric tube. The trachea should be extubated with the child fully awake in the left lateral position. The child should be closely observed in recovery for further signs of bleeding.

Adult tonsillectomy

The same general principles apply, but a controlled ventilation technique with muscle relaxation and ET intubation is more common. The procedure tends to be more painful in adults, hence, intra-operative morphine will be required.

Nasal and sinus surgery

Surgical considerations

The range of procedures includes septoplasty, rhinoplasty, functional endoscopic sinus surgery (FESS), polypectomy and sinus washout, with many common anaesthetic issues.

The aim of septoplasty is to straighten the cartilage and bone in the nasal septum with the aim of reducing airflow obstruction and improving airflow through the nasal passages. Rhinoplasty may be done concurrently as a cosmetic procedure to improve the shape of the nose. The indications for this procedure include:

- Nasal obstruction arising from a deviation of the nasal septum in patients who have failed medical therapy. Other causes of nasal obstruction like polyps, chronic lung disease and allergies should be excluded before surgery is offered.
- Epistaxis — to gain access to a posterior bleeding vessel.
- Traumatic tearing/dislocation of the nasal septum.
- As part of a cosmetic procedure.

FESS is usually performed for the surgical treatment of sinusitis, polyps and chronic sinus infections. It involves removing the diseased mucosal lining and facilitating a pathway for drainage. FESS may be combined with septoplasty to allow the surgeon to gain better access.

Anaesthetic considerations

Patients for these surgeries will usually present with sinusitis, allergic rhinitis, obstructive sleep apnoea, previous nasal surgery or recent nasal trauma. It is important to ascertain from the history the degree of nasal obstruction and the possibility of obstructive sleep apnoea (OSA). Also, enquire about daytime somnolence and question the patient's partner about snoring and nocturnal apnoeic spells. In patients with a strong history of nocturnal hypoxia, the possibility of pulmonary and systemic hypertension, ventricular hypertrophy and heart failure must be considered, especially if combined with obesity. If the pre-operative history suggests OSA, the patient should be referred for polysomnography studies. An ECG is useful to identify any chamber hypertrophy.

Other routine anaesthetic history should be taken including information about any other systemic problems, anaesthetic history and allergies. Airway examination should concentrate on determining the extent of nasal obstruction as this can interfere with mask ventilation.

The patient should be counselled about the possibility of needing an overnight stay in the high-dependency unit for monitoring and nocturnal continuous positive airway pressure (CPAP). If already using a CPAP machine, the patient should be asked to bring in the machine on admission.

Intra-operative management

Anaesthetic options include a local anaesthetic +/- sedation or a general anaesthetic. A general anaesthetic affords the anaesthetist more control, with the ability to provide an optimal surgical field using moderate hypotension (discussed later). A local anaesthetic may be preferable in patients with multiple medical issues.

Face mask ventilation is likely to be difficult in patients with nasal obstruction and may require a Guedel airway. In common with other ENT surgeries, they involve sharing the airway in some form. The aim should be to direct the airway away from the surgical field, to enable maximal surgical exposure. The choices include either a south-facing RAE tube or, more increasingly, flexible LMAs. The risk with the latter is inadvertent surgical displacement. Communication between the surgeon and anaesthetist is particularly important, with surgery needing to be necessarily interrupted to correct any airway issues. Intra-operative access to the head is restricted; hence, secure fixation of the airway device and protection of pressure points (especially the eyes) are important. The surgeon may ask for the eye on the operative side to be left untaped. The head can be stabilised on a head ring.

Controlled ventilation is usually unnecessary for these procedures. Total intravenous anaesthesia (TIVA) techniques are very suitable, with combinations of propofol, alfentanil and remifentanil. Moderate hypotension produced by these short-acting opioids will assist in decreasing blood loss, as will a 15-20° head-up tilt.

The use of throat packs is popular to absorb collected upper airway blood during nasal surgeries. Continued posterior trickling of blood from the surgical site is well absorbed by throat packs. Appropriate precautions should be taken to ensure removal of the throat pack at the end of surgery. Suggested safety systems include clear communication between theatre staff, sticking a label on the patient's forehead, tying the throat pack to the airway device and including the throat pack in the swab count.

Nasal vasoconstriction is frequently requested by surgeons to obtain a clear surgical field. Care must be taken not to exceed toxic doses. The options include:

- Cocaine 4-10%.
- Phenylephrine 0.5%.
- Co-phenylcaine (lignocaine 5% and phenylephrine 0.5%).
- Moffat's solution prepared using a combination of 2ml cocaine 10%, 2ml sodium bicarbonate 1% and 1ml of 1:1000 adrenaline.
- Oxymetazoline or xylometazoline (topical vasoconstrictors).

The local anaesthetic injected by the surgeon at the operative site, paracetamol and NSAIDs provide intra-operative analgesia. These may be continued in the postoperative period. Strong opioids are usually not required and should be avoided in a patient with OSA.

As the area of surgical exposure is minimal, intra-operative fluid requirements need only to address overnight fasting requirements. Care should be taken not to 'over' warm the patient, and temperature should be monitored intra-operatively.

At the end of surgery, throat pack removal and thorough suction are essential. The patient should be placed in a left lateral or head-down position with a Guedel airway in place until the airway reflexes return following a deep extubation. The use of newer anaesthetic agents allow smooth and awake extubation. A head-up or sitting position is more often used with awake extubation.

The nasal cavities are usually packed following these procedures; this may be uncomfortable for the patient. Consider a higher level of monitoring in a patient with a strong pre-operative history of OSA.

Ear surgery

Surgical considerations

A wide range of surgical procedures are performed on the ear (Table 22.3).

Table 22.3. Commonly performed surgical procedures on the ear.

External ear	Removal of lesions, foreign bodies, cosmetic procedures (e.g. bat ear correction)
Middle ear and mastoid	Myringotomy and grommet insertion, myringoplasty, tympanoplasty, mastoidectomy
Inner ear	Surgeries on labyrinth, endolymphatic sac and cochlear apparatus

Otitis media is the commonest reason for surgical procedures on the ear. Children have a short Eustachian tube; this may cause reflux of nasopharyngeal secretions (due to recurrent upper respiratory infections) into the middle ear and cause repeated infections of the middle ear. This is exacerbated by mucosal oedema of the Eustachian tube and enlarged adenoids frequently blocking the orifice of the Eustachian tube. Chronic middle ear disease leads to sequelae like deafness, tympanic perforation, damage to middle ear ossicles and cholesteatoma (an abnormal, non-cancerous skin growth in the middle ear).

Myringotomy and insertion of a grommet (also called a tympanostomy tube, or T-tube) are performed to keep the middle ear aerated for a prolonged period and to prevent fluid accumulating in the middle ear. Myringoplasty aims to close a persistent tympanic membrane perforation using temporalis muscle, fat, fascia or tragal perichondrium. Tympanoplasty is a longer, more extensive process involving reconstructive repair of the damaged tympanic membrane and the ossicular chain. A postaural approach is preferred due to better surgical access.

A mastoidectomy is commonly performed in patients with chronic suppurative otitis media (CSOM) to enable removal of a cholesteatoma or diseased air cells. In addition, it may be performed as part of a more complex non-ENT procedure. These include neurosurgical removal of lateral and temporal lobe malignancies like schwannomas and meningiomas. Mastoidectomy is also performed to allow surgical access to place a cochlear implant in patients with sensorineural hearing loss.

Anaesthetic considerations

Myringotomy/grommet insertion

The child may have a history of frequent upper respiratory tract infection and so may show evidence of OSA due to adenoid hypertrophy. Usually performed as a day case, anaesthetic options include spontaneous ventilation via a face mask or LMA. Postoperative pain is usually mild, and simple analgesics (paracetamol, NSAIDs) are usually sufficient.

Myringoplasty, tympanoplasty and mastoid surgery

The main issues of anaesthetic interest are:

- Prolonged anaesthetic.
- Surgical requirement for a bloodless field.

- Effect of nitrous oxide diffusion on middle ear pressures.
- Facial nerve monitoring.
- High incidence of PONV.

Prolonged anaesthetic

These procedures can run into several hours. Due care must be given to secure the airway which will be inaccessible once surgery commences. Options include controlled ventilation with an endotracheal tube or a reinforced LMA. Anaesthesia can be maintained with propofol and remifentanil or remifentanil with a volatile anaesthetic agent.

Remifentanil has a number of advantages in middle ear surgery:

- It helps to provide a smooth, balanced anaesthetic, and a smooth emergence is beneficial to prevent graft displacement.
- It provides potent intra-operative analgesia.
- It can be used as part of a multimodal approach to provide relative hypotension to decrease bleeding in the surgical field.
- It can be used as part of total intravenous anaesthesia along with propofol which reduces the incidence of PONV.

Care must be taken to maintain normothermia. As the area of surgical exposure is small, it is very easy to overwarm the patient. Also, third space fluid loss is minimal, so fluid to cover for overnight fasting requirements is sufficient. Arms and pressure points should be well padded.

Surgical requirement for a bloodless field

Simple measures help greatly in reducing bleeding in the surgical field. A 15° head-up tilt helps to reduce venous ooze. A smooth, balanced anaesthetic technique using remifentanil prevents excessive haemodynamic disturbance and careful ventilation prevents hypercapnia. Adrenaline infiltration of the surgical field and providing relative hypotension (mean arterial pressure 10-20% less than normal) will ensure optimal surgical conditions.

The provision of induced hypotension (lowering of blood pressure during anaesthesia by 30% of resting value) is usually unnecessary and should only be undertaken after carefully balancing the risk versus benefit. It should be avoided in patients with preexisting cardiovascular compromise and cerebrovascular insufficiency. Drugs that may be used include metoprolol, labetalol, clonidine, vasodilators (sodium nitroprusside, glyceryl trinitrate [GTN]) and remifentanil.

Effect of nitrous oxide (N₂O) diffusion on middle ear pressure

As N_2O is considerably more soluble than nitrogen in blood, it will diffuse into the middle ear cavity more rapidly than nitrogen can leave and can cause an increase in middle ear pressure. The consequences of this include displacement of surgically placed grafts, tympanic membrane rupture and an increased incidence of PONV. Options include discontinuing N_2O 15-20 minutes prior to placing the graft or avoiding N_2O completely.

Facial nerve monitoring

The facial nerve runs within the middle ear in close proximity to the ossicular chain and through the mastoid during its course through the temporal bone. The surgeon may wish to monitor the facial nerve intra-operatively, especially if the disease process has made anatomical identification difficult. Depending upon the available technology, an audible or visual signal from the monitor will serve to identify the nerve by detecting nerve activity using electrodes attached to the face. This nerve activity is attenuated or completely abolished by neuromuscular blockade; hence, this must be completely reversed (as demonstrated by a peripheral nerve stimulator) before surgery in the vicinity of the facial nerve or avoided altogether by using a TIVA technique with propofol and remifentanil.

Postoperative nausea and vomiting (PONV)

Procedures on the middle ear are frequently implicated in the causation of PONV and a multimodal approach works well to prevent this. Non-pharmacological approaches, such as avoiding prolonged starvation and adequate hydration, supplemented by prophylactic antiemetics (ondansetron and dexamethasone), avoiding N_2O and the use of propofol as part of TIVA, significantly reduces the incidence of PONV.

Balanced analgesia with regular paracetamol, NSAIDs, infiltration of local anaesthetic at the surgical site and avoiding strong opioids will also help to decrease PONV.

Microlaryngoscopy

Surgical considerations

Microlaryngoscopy involves examination of the larynx using an operating microscope. It may be purely diagnostic or may involve excision of abnormal tissue or biopsy, e.g. for laryngeal cancers. The procedure may be combined with laser surgery to remove abnormal tissue. Microlaryngoscopy can be employed to inject Teflon® into paralysed vocal cords to improve phonation. The surgical requirements are:

- Good access to the larynx, i.e. without visual interference from the airway device.
- Immobility of airway structures.
- A need to interrupt ventilation at various points intra-operatively.

Anaesthetic considerations

Patients are usually elderly with multiple comorbidities. They are likely to be long-term smokers and may have recently received radiotherapy. Radiation to the anterior aspect of the neck has particular implications in posing a potentially difficult intubation due to radiation-induced fibrosis of anterior neck structures. Many of these patients present for repeat anaesthetics as a means of assessing progress of their disease process.

The airway should be carefully assessed for signs of obstruction from the history, clinic notes (nasal endoscopy may have been performed) and radiological investigations.

The main concerns during the peri-operative phase are the options for ventilation. These are outlined below.

Conventional ventilation using a microlaryngeal (MLT) tube

An MLT tube is a long (31cm) 5mm to 6mm ID cuffed oral ET tube with a high-volume low-pressure cuff. Volatile-based anaesthesia is possible and the inflated cuff protects against the aspiration of blood and resected airway debris. An MLT may restrict the surgical view. Due to the narrow lumen, there is high internal resistance, so long slow inspiration should be used during controlled ventilation.

Jet ventilation techniques (Figure 22.3)

This is achieved with a Sanders injector or Manujet using oxygen and entrained air. There are many portals to provide the jet ventilation:

- An operating laryngoscope is inserted and correctly aligned with the larynx. The jet injector needle is then attached to its proximal end. Airway debris and smoke may be blown into the larynx during ventilation.
- A cricothyrotomy cannula is inserted through the cricothyroid membrane under local anaesthetic or with the patient under GA via an LMA. Various commercially available cricothyrotomy kits exist; a 16G cannula may also be used. There is the risk of subcutaneous injection of gas if the needle is incorrectly placed or displaced.

The source of oxygen is the high-pressure centrally supplied oxygen at 4 bar pressure. This pressure is reduced when it passes through pressure-reducing valves and can be further adjusted by operating a regulator attached to the handset to attain a pressure that will produce adequate chest expansion and hence maintain gas exchange and oxygenation. A Luer lock connection is required to connect the handset to the cannula. A ventilatory rate of 8-10/min, allowing adequate time for elastic recoil of the lungs and chest wall, will enable stable ventilatory dynamics.

Although jet ventilatory techniques provide an excellent surgical view due to the absence of airway devices, it has certain disadvantages:

- Assessment of tidal volume and minute ventilation is difficult.
- Barotrauma is possible if there is obstruction to expiration.

- The trachea remains unprotected.
- A volatile-based anaesthetic is not possible.
- Ventilation may need to be interrupted mid-surgery to enable surgical work to proceed.

Good communication between surgeon and anaesthetist is essential. A total intravenous technique (propofol and remifentanil) is required to maintain anaesthesia. Muscle relaxation is usually essential for these procedures and a local anaesthetic spray to the vocal cords reduces the risk of laryngospasm, but this will have an effect on airway reflexes, so recovery must be performed in the left lateral, head-down position.

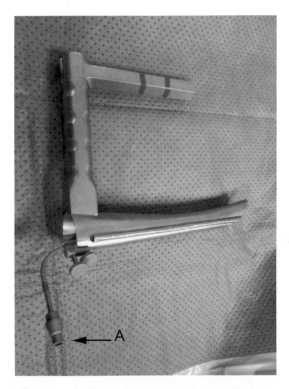

Figure 22.3. Operating laryngoscope with a jet ventilation needle (A).

When surgery concludes, jet ventilation may be continued until spontaneous ventilation resumes or it may be discontinued and ventilation may be continued by a face mask or LMA.

Postoperative analgesia may be provided with paracetamol and NSAIDSs if not contraindicated by medical issues. Dexamethasone is useful as an antiemetic and also to prevent any postoperative airway oedema.

Laser ENT surgery

Surgical considerations

Laser consists of a beam of high-energy, monochromatic light capable of producing vapourisation of tissue. In ENT surgery, the use of lasers is now widespread and finds its application in the treatment of airway tumours, e.g. bronchial carcinomas, vocal cord tumours and head and neck tumours.

The lasers commonly used in ENT surgery are carbon dioxide (CO_2) lasers and neodymium-yttrium aluminium garnet (Nd-YAG) lasers:

- The carbon dioxide laser (wavelength 10,600nm) is a gas laser suitable for precise cutting and coagulation. As it has a long wavelength, the penetration is relatively shallow and so tissue damage can be directly visualised by the surgeon. They are popular for vocal cord and airway lesions.
- The Nd-YAG laser is a solid-state laser that has a shorter wavelength (1064nm). It has a greater penetration (about 1cm) than the CO_2 laser and, hence, can be used for photocoagulation and debulking of airway tumours.

General considerations

All hospitals using lasers should have their own local safety protocols. In general these should reflect the Department of Health's "Guidance on the Safe Use of Lasers in Medical and Dental Practice 1995". The important points to note are:

- Every clinical area that uses laser should have a designated laser protection officer whose responsibilities include ensuring the safe use of the laser and staff education.
- Appropriate eye protection to be worn by staff. The goggle colour should be suitable for the type of laser used (clear glass for CO_2, green for Nd-YAG). The goggles should have lateral shields to protect the lateral aspect of the eyes.
- Appropriate notification outside theatres using lasers must be provided.

Anaesthetic considerations

The key issues specific to laser airway surgery include:

- Risk of airway fire.
- Preventing damage to the eyes and skin.
- Concerns about laser plume.

Risk of airway fire

A major anaesthetic issue in laser airway surgery is the risk of a fire in an oxygen-enriched environment when a high-energy source is used. All the three elements of the 'fire triangle' are present in airway laser surgery (Figure 22.4):

- The ET tube and breathing system act as a source of fuel.
- Oxygen present in the fresh gas delivered through the ET tube is the oxidising agent.
- The laser acts as a source of heat energy.

As all these elements are necessary for laser surgery, the emphasis is on decreasing the risk of an airway fire. Steps that can be taken to minimise the risk of airway fires include:

- Using a gas mixture of air and oxygen. N_2O should be avoided as it is flammable.

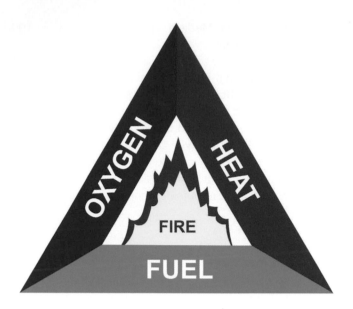

Figure 22.4. Three elements of the fire triangle.

- Use of as low an inspired oxygen concentration (FiO_2) as possible.
- Keeping a 50ml syringe of saline on hand (to flood the operative field in the event of an airway fire).
- Use of instruments that have a matt surface, which will not reflect the laser beam onto normal tissue, unlike shiny surfaces.
- Choosing the right ventilation strategy. Options include:
  - jet ventilation. This involves the use of a Sanders injector placed within a rigid laryngoscope. During inspiration, oxygen enriched with entrained air is delivered and egress of carbon dioxide happens in expiration. A TIVA technique and muscle relaxation will be required;
  - the use of an endotracheal tube. Standard, unmodified endotracheal tubes are unsuitable as they support combustion. A non-flammable laser tube with a flexible stainless steel body and with a double cuff (Laser-Flex® tube — Figure 22.5) is commonly used. The proximal cuff may be inflated with saline mixed with methylene blue to provide a visual indicator of cuff rupture. The cuff should be protected by saline-soaked pledgets.

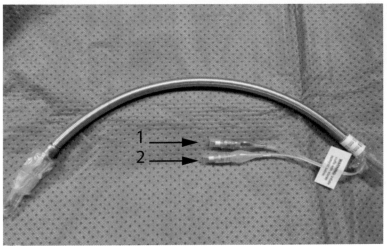

Figure 22.5. Laser-Flex® tracheal tube. 1) Pilot balloon leading to proximal cuff; 2) Pilot balloon leading to distal cuff.

Preventing damage to the eyes and skin

Retinal and corneal damage can occur. Goggles should be used (see above). These should have side shields to protect the lateral side of the eyes. The patient's eyes should be potected by non-flammable tape, moist swabs or goggles.

Moistened swabs should be placed on skin adjacent to the operative site. All areas of exposed skin should be covered with non-plastic non-combustible drapes. The use of flammable skin preparation solutions should be avoided.

Concerns about laser plume

A plume consists of the smoke and particulate debris resulting from the vapourisation of biological tissue by the laser.

Plume smoke has been shown to contain viruses, bacteria, and blood and tissue fragments. They also contain various chemicals like carbon monoxide, hydrogen cyanide, formaldehyde and benzene. They may also contain certain carcinogens and mutagens.

There is currently no reliable evidence of any short- or long-term adverse effects of exposure to laser plume.

A plume scavenging system (PSS) must be maintained close to the operative site to ensure efficient removal of the plume from the theatre environment.

Management of an airway fire

- Switch the laser off immediately.
- Flood the surgical site with saline.
- Disconnect from the anaesthetic circuit, extubate and ventilate by face mask using a self-inflating bag with as low an FiO_2 as practicable to avoid reigniting any smouldering debris in the airway.
- The surgeon should inspect the airway with a rigid bronchoscope.

As airway fire can lead to airway oedema and lung injury with hypoxaemia in the first 48 hours after the incident, it would be advisable to keep the patient intubated and ventilated in the critical care unit (CCU) to enable serial assessment of respiratory function. Dexamethasone can be used to reduce airway oededma. The airway should be examined bronchoscopically after 48 hours.

Surgical tracheostomy

Surgical considerations

Most CCU patients, who are deemed to require prolonged ventilation, will have a percutaneous tracheostomy performed on the CCU itself, using a percutaneous technique. Sometimes it is considered prudent to perform the procedure surgically. This may be due to technical issues such as a short neck and obesity that make it difficult to identify anatomical landmarks.

Anaesthetic considerations

Most CCU patients presenting for surgical tracheostomy will invariably be intubated and ventilated. Full preparation should be made in the CCU for transfer of the patient to the operating theatre and a TIVA technique used. During the intra-operative phase, anaesthesia can be maintained using the TIVA technique or a volatile agent.

Prior to the patient's arrival in theatre, ensure that the appropriate sized tracheostomy kit is available in theatre and the integrity of the cuff has been checked. An emergency cricothyroidotomy kit should also be kept handy. A sterile catheter mount should also be available to enable connection of the breathing system to the tracheostomy tube once inserted.

The patient should be positioned on the operating table supine with a pad placed between the scapulae to enable neck extension and hence improving surgical access. The head should be supported in a head ring to maintain stability.

A laryngoscopy should be performed, the oropharynx should be suctioned, and the laryngoscopic view should be assessed prior to starting the procedure. All airway equipment necessary for laryngoscopy and reintubation should be readily available in the operating theatre. The *in situ* endotracheal tube should be taped away from the surgical field with the pilot balloon readily visible to enable cuff deflation when required. Ensure good muscle relaxation during the procedure. Long breathing circuits and sampling lines will be required.

100% oxygen should be delivered for 3-5 minutes prior to inserting the tracheostomy tube. This is particularly beneficial if there were any technical problems during insertion of the tracheostomy tube. The cuff on the ET tube should be deflated prior to surgical incision on the trachea to prevent cuff rupture and to enable reinflation and continued ventilation if problems ensue.

The ET tube should be withdrawn to a point just above the tracheotomy site, taking care not to accidentally extubate the trachea. The surgeon can provide a visual guide to the extent to which the tube needs to be withdrawn. The new tracheostomy tube is then inserted and connected to the anaesthetic circuit using the sterile catheter mount. Its position should be confirmed by end-tidal CO_2 monitoring. In the event of any problems, the ET tube should be advanced back into position.

After completing the procedure, the patient should be transferred back to the CCU. A chest X-ray should be performed in the CCU to confirm the position and rule out any subcutaneous emphysema or pneumothorax.

Tracheostomy to relieve airway obstruction

Tracheostomy may be performed as an urgent procedure to relieve airway obstruction. In this scenario, there are many options to secure the airway depending on the site of the obstruction, clinical urgency and experience of the anaesthetist. The options are:

- Local anaesthesia to the airway followed by fibreoptic bronchoscopy or videolaryngoscopy ('awake intubation').
- Induction of general anaesthesia and tracheal intubation.
- Tracheostomy under local anaesthetic infiltration.

Each of these techniques has their own disadvantages, which must be carefully considered.

Awake intubation may not be easy in a very anxious and hypoxic patient with critical airway obstruction. At the level of the glottis, complete airway obstruction may occur whilst passing the fibreoptic scope. Friable tumours may bleed on contact with the scope.

Inhalational induction may also be difficult in the presence of airway obstruction. As the anaesthetic plane deepens, the airway can obstruct resulting in further hypoxia. Attempts at insertion of the oropharyngeal airway and airway manipulation can result in laryngospasm.

Although tracheostomy under local anaesthetic can be uncomfortable and may not be well tolerated by an anxious patient, it may be the only safe option in certain scenarios.

The decision is taken based on the experience of the anaesthetist and available help. If it is planned to induce general anaesthesia, an ENT surgeon should be present and ready to perform emergency tracheostomy.

The patient may find it difficult to tolerate the tracheostomy tube. Local anaesthetic infiltration at the surgical site and topical lidocaine into the trachea may help the patient to tolerate the tube. Humidified oxygen should be delivered through the tracheostomy tube to prevent drying of respiratory secretions.

Laryngectomy

Surgical considerations

Laryngeal cancers are four times commoner in men and three-quarters of all cases diagnosed are in patients over the age of 60. A vast majority of newly diagnosed cases (80%) tend to be smokers, with long-term alcohol intake implicated in 25%.

The surgical approach chosen is usually determined by the site of the lesion and extent of local spread (Table 22.4).

Table 22.4. Anatomical classification of the larynx.

Supraglottic region	Arytenoids, false cords, epiglottis, aryepiglottic folds
Glottis	True vocal cords, anterior and posterior commissures
Infraglottic region	Extending up to the lower border of the cricoid cartilage

Partial laryngectomy

This involves resection of the cancerous tissue, but an attempt is made to preserve some part of the vocal cords. The surgery is combined with a temporary tracheostomy. Various options are available:

- Cordectomy — removal of one vocal cord.
- Anterior frontal laryngectomy — removal of the anterior aspect of both vocal cords.
- Hemilaryngectomy — removal of half of the larynx.

Supraglottic laryngectomy

This approach is used when the tumour is confined to the supraglottic region. The false vocal cords and the epiglottis are resected by the endoscopic approach or the open approach. A temporary tracheostomy is created at the end of the procedure.

Total laryngectomy

The entire laryngeal apparatus is removed. Some part of the pharynx is also removed. The surgery may also involve a neck dissection to remove involved lymph nodes. A permanent tracheostomy is created.

Anaesthetic considerations

Pre-operative

Most patients presenting for laryngeal surgery will be elderly, male and long-term smokers. Underlying cardiovascular disease, alcohol consumption and chronic obstructive airway disease are likely. Stabilisation of any major reversible factors, e.g. unstable coronary syndromes and arrhythmias, should be carried out in association with a pre-optimisation program consisting of chest physiotherapy, pre-operative steroids, cessation of smoking, bronchodilators, patient motivation and education. Pulmonary function tests and arterial blood gas analysis will help in guiding the progress of optimisation.

If long-term alcohol consumption is an issue, then the problems of malnutrition, enzyme induction resulting in altered drug handling, deranged coagulation, electrolyte abnormalities and postoperative alcohol withdrawal should be considered.

Airway assessment is crucial to successful anaesthetic management. The causes for a potentially difficult airway are:

- Mechanical obstruction due to the tumour. This produces symptoms such as hoarseness of the voice (usually in glottic tumours), dysphagia and cough. In some patients, shortness of breath will be exacerbated on lying flat, due to mobile pedunculated tumours obstructing the glottis when supine.
- Suboptimal view during laryngoscopy.
- Potential for airway bleeding due to tumour friability.
- Fixed anterior neck structures due to radiation.

In addition to standard airway examination, the anterior aspect of the neck must be examined for radiation-induced fibrosis and fixation of anterior neck structures, previous surgical scars and any prominent masses.

A pre-operative nasoendoscopy (easily performed in the outpatient clinic under local anaesthetic) is invaluable in planning airway management. The size and location of the tumour, airway calibre and vocal cord movement can be assessed. Further information can be derived from a CT scan or MRI to assess airway compression and the extent of spread of the disease.

Intra-operative

The options for securing the airway are:

- Conventional laryngoscopy and intubation.
- Awake fibreoptic-guided intubation.
- A transtracheal catheter inserted via the cricothyroid membrane to provide jet ventilation of the lungs with oxygen while the airway is secured.
- Surgical tracheostomy.

A nasogastric tube is required for postoperative feeding. It can be either inserted after induction of anaesthesia or can be inserted by the surgeon near the end of the procedure.

The patient is positioned supine on the operating table, with a pad under the shoulders, a 15° head-up tilt (to reduce venous ooze) and their head supported in a head ring. Anaesthesia is maintained by a volatile agent or TIVA technique using propofol and remifentanil.

Considering this is a prolonged surgical procedure and the lack of access to the airway during the intra-operative period, the following measures should be taken:

- Padding of eyes and peripheral nerves.
- Extra long anaesthetic circuits and sampling line.
- Large-bore peripheral venous access. Bleeding can be significant from dissection around the neck and it is easy to underestimate blood lost under the drapes.
- Warm fluids and body warmer and temperature monitoring.
- Invasive blood pressure monitoring using an arterial line and urinary catheter.

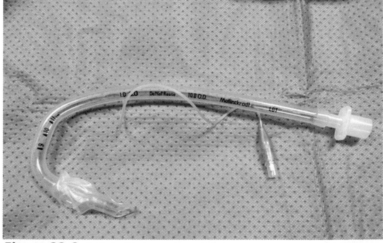

Figure 22.6. J-shaped laryngectomy tube.

Once the end stoma has been created, a J-shaped laryngectomy tube (Figure 22.6) is placed in the trachea and the breathing circuit is connected to the laryngectomy tube.

Postoperative

An extubation strategy should be planned for patients in whom an end stoma has not been created. Extubation over an airway exchange catheter is a prudent option. A temporary tracheostomy is inserted in some cases to facilitate immediate postoperative management.

Postoperative care should be managed in a high dependency unit with staff experienced in tracheostomy care. The tracheostomy should be regularly suctioned to clear blood and secretions. Humidifed oxygen should be provided to prevent drying of airway secretions.

Analgesic requirements are met by a multimodal approach using intravenous morphine patient-controlled analgesia (PCA), supplemented by paracetamol and NSAIDs. Antiemetics are prescribed as required.

Case scenario 1

A 2-year-old child weighing 13kg with obstructive sleep apnoea and a history of recurrent bouts of tonsillitis is scheduled for a tonsillectomy.

How would you manage this patient?

Pre-operative

Establish rapport with the child and parents. Information should be elicited about any medical problems, previous anaesthetics, allergies, details regarding a history of obstructive sleep apnoea and any recent upper respiratory infections. An explanation of the anaesthetic plan, including a rectal suppository for postoperative analgesia, is given. Eutectic mixture of lidocaine and prilocaine (EMLA®)/Ametop™ should be prescribed. Hands should be examined for venous access which can be difficult.

Intra-operative

Routine monitoring can then be attached including the ECG, pulse oximeter and non-invasive blood pressure (NIBP) monitor. The child at this age may not be cooperative for ECG and NIBP monitoring prior to the induction of anaesthesia. However, the pulse oximeter should be attached prior to the induction of anaesthesia.

If IV access can be secured easily, intravenous induction of anaesthesia can be performed following IV access. In cases where IV induction is difficult, inhalational induction with oxygen and sevoflurane would be the choice in children. In this scenario, airway obstruction can worsen as the child is induced. Following induction of anaesthesia, fentanyl 1µg/kg and a muscle relaxant (atracurium 0.5mg/kg) can facilitate tracheal intubation. The airway is secured with a size 4.5mm ID south-facing RAE tube. Controlled ventilation is best achieved with pressure-controlled ventilation.

The patient is positioned with their neck extended and padding placed under the shoulder, taking care to ensure that the tube is not kinked by the Boyle-Davis mouth gag.

During the procedure, further analagesia is provided with 12.5mg of per rectal diclofenac and intravenous paracetamol 15mg/kg. Ondansetron 0.1mg/kg and dexamethasone 0.1mg/kg should be given intravenously as an antiemetic. Intravenous fluid (lactated Ringer's solution or Hartmann's solution) 10ml/kg body weight is administered to maintain hydration and further IV fluid can be administered to supplement blood loss.

Postoperative

Prior to extubation the oral cavity should be suctioned under direct vision and the nasopharynx should be suctioned using a soft catheter.

Neuromuscular blockade should be reversed and the child can be extubated once fully awake. If deep extubation is planned, the patient should be extubated in a deep plane of anaesthesia after reversal and achievement of adequate spontaneous ventilation, in a left lateral head-down position and maintained in this position until the airway reflexes return.

Postoperative pain is managed using paracetamol, NSAIDs and small doses of oral morphine (0.1 to 0.2mg/kg) as needed. Care should be taken to avoid postoperative respiratory depression. The child may need to be monitored in a paediatric high dependency unit.

Case scenario 2

A mastoidectomy is planned in a 35-year-old female patient with a past history of postoperative nausea and vomiting (PONV) following a previous anaesthetic.

How would you manage this patient?

Pre-operative

Enquiring about any medical problems, particularly hypertension, is important. Medications, including previous anaesthetic problems, need to be addressed. Also, ask for a history of any allergies and then the anaesthetic plan can be explained.

Intra-operative

Routine monitoring should be applied including the ECG, pulse oximeter and NIBP monitor.

IV induction should be with propofol and remifentanil, followed by a non-depolarising muscle relaxant to facilitate laryngoscopy and tracheal intubation. The use of remifentanil will help in reducing the dose of muscle relaxant required for facilitating intubation. As this patient has a previous history of PONV, maintenance of anaesthesia using a TIVA technique (target-controlled infusion of [TCI] propofol and remifentanil) would be helpful in minimising the risk of PONV. The surgeon is likely to use facial nerve monitoring; hence, further doses of muscle relaxant should be avoided. The patient should be positioned on the table with a slight head-up tilt. Controlled hypotension is achieved with remifentanil.

Analgesia is provided by local anaesthetic infiltration by the surgeon and intravenous paracetamol. Morphine IV is usually not required and can be administered in the immediate recovery period following the assessment of pain. Regular paracetamol and NSAIDs should be prescribed for postoperative analgesia.

A multimodal approach at antiemesis is provided by avoiding nitrous oxide, adequate hydration and a combination of antiemetics (ondansetron and dexamethasone).

Postoperative

The patient should be extubated awake at the end of surgery.

Analgesia is provided by regular paracetamol and NSAIDs, and rescue oral morphine. Antiemesis is covered by ondansetron and cyclizine.

Further reading

1.	Flory S, Appadurai IR. Special considerations in anesthesia for laryngeal cancer surgery. *Otorhinolaryngol Clin Int J* 2010; 2: 185-90.

2.	Ravi R, Howell T. Anaesthesia for paediatric ear, nose and throat surgery. *Br J Anaesth CEACCP* 2007; 7: 33-7.

3.	Kitching AJ, Edge CJ. Lasers and surgery. *Br J Anaesth CEACCP* 2003; 3: 143-6.

4.	Roberts F. Ear, nose and throat surgery. In: Allman KG, Wilson IH, Eds. *Oxford Handbook of Anaesthesia*, 2nd ed. Oxford University Press, 2006: 603-32.

5.	English J, Norris A, Bedforth N. Anaesthesia for airway surgery. *Br J Anaesth CEACCP* 2006; 6: 28-31.

6.	Chung F, Subramanyam R, Liao P, *et al.* High STOP-BANG score indicates a high probability of obstructive sleep apnoea. *Br J Anaesth* 2012; 108: 768-75.

23 Neurosurgical procedures

Ilyas Qazi and Cyprian Mendonca

Introduction

Anaesthesia for neurosurgical procedures in a rapidly evolving subspecialty can be highly challenging and complex. The timely provision of an efficient neuroanaesthetic and neurocritical care service can have a significant impact on peri-operative patient outcomes. The risk of patient morbidity/mortality could relate both to the patient's underlying neurological condition and the neurosurgical procedure performed.

The majority of neurosurgical procedures are performed under general anaesthesia. The key objectives are thorough pre-operative assessment and optimisation, meticulous peri-operative planning, execution of the neuroanaesthetic technique and postoperative recovery of the patient in a high dependency area. Maintenance of a stable cardiorespiratory status within clinically acceptable limits is crucial during neuroanaesthesia, as even transient compromises in cerebral or spinal perfusion can hugely impact upon operating conditions and outcomes.

The types of neurosurgical procedures can be broadly classified into classic neurosurgical procedures and interventional neuroradiological procedures (Table 23.1).

Table 23.1. Commonly performed neurosurgical procedures.

Classical neurosurgery procedures	Interventional neuroradiology procedures
Craniotomy for a space-occupying lesion	Digital subtraction angiography
Ventriculoperitoneal shunt	Endovascular coiling of intracranial aneurysms
Evacuation of traumatic intracranial haematoma	Embolisation of cerebral or spinal arteriovenous malformations
Pituitary surgery	Catheter-directed thrombolysis
Insertion of an ICP monitoring device	
External ventricular drain insertion	
Clipping of intracranial aneurysms	
Spinal surgical procedures	

Cerebral circulation

The brain derives its arterial blood supply from the circle of Willis (Figure 23.1), an arterial network formed by the anastomosis of the internal carotid and vertebral arteries at its base. Cerebral venous drainage occurs via cerebral veins into the dural venous sinuses, which further drain into the jugular venous bulb.

The cerebral blood flow (CBF) is normally 50ml/100g/min of brain parenchymal tissue which correlates to about 15% of the cardiac output received by the brain. The normal intracranial pressure (ICP) is 5-15mmHg. The cerebral perfusion pressure (CPP) which effectively is the

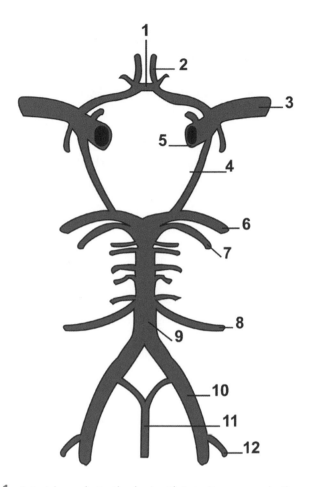

Figure 23.1. Arterial supply to the brain. 1) Anterior communicating artery; 2) Anterior cerebral artery; 3) Middle cerebral artery; 4) Posterior communicating artery; 5) Internal carotid artery; 6) Posterior cerebral artery; 7) Superior cerebellar artery; 8) Anterior inferior cerebellar artery; 9) Basilar artery; 10) Vertebral artery; 11) Anterior spinal artery; 12) Posterior spinal artery.

pressure at which blood flows to the brain is given by the following equation:

$$CPP = MAP - (ICP + VP).$$

As the venous pressure (VP) at the jugular bulb is usually zero, the CPP is normally calculated as the difference between the mean arterial pressure (MAP) and the ICP.

The CBF is normally autoregulated and kept constant between mean arterial pressures of 50-150mmHg (Figure 23.2). Outside these limits, the normal autoregulatory mechanisms are impaired (e.g. in traumatic brain injury) and the CBF varies passively with the perfusion pressures. In patients with chronic hypertension, the cerebral autoregulatory threshold is shifted to the right (Figure 23.2).

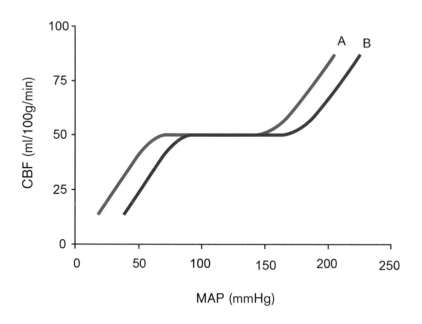

Figure 23.2. Cerebral blood flow autoregulation. A) Normal autoregulatory level; B) Autoregulatory level in patients with chronic hypertension.

CBF is governed by the following factors:

- Cerebral metabolism — CBF is directly related to the rate of cerebral metabolism. CBF is increased in seizure states and vice versa reduced in brainstem death.
- $PaCO_2$ — CBF is linearly related to $PaCO_2$ within a range of 3.5 to 10kPa. CBF approximately doubles with a $PaCO_2$ rise from 4 to 8kPa.
- PaO_2 — there is little to no change in CBF above a PaO_2 of >8kPa. There is cerebral vasodilatation if PaO_2 drops to less than 8kPa, thereby increasing CBF.
- Temperature — cerebral metabolism is reduced by approximately 5% per °C drop in temperature.

Control of intracranial pressure (ICP)

The intracranial constituents, namely, brain substance (85%), cerebrospinal fluid (CSF)(10%) and blood (5%), are held within the confines of the bony skull. As stated in the Monro-Kellie doctrine, with the skull being a rigid box, any alteration in the volume of its intracranial contents results in the compensatory changes of these constituents. The compensatory changes include displacement of the CSF into the spinal subarachnoid space, increased absorption of CSF and reduction in the intracranial blood volume. It a critical volume is reached, these compensatory mechanisms become overwhelmed leading to a sharp rise in the ICP. If a space-occupying lesion (SOL) has developed quickly, it allows little time for compensation with consequent detrimental effects, when compared to a SOL which has evolved more slowly.

Factors causing a raised ICP are:

- Increased intracerebral blood volume. Various factors such as hypercarbia, hypoxia, increased cerebral metabolic rate and volatile anaesthetic agents in concentrations of >1 minimum alveolar concentration (MAC) can increase cerebral blood volume. The factors that reduce venous drainage (compression of neck veins, a head-down position, coughing and increased intrathoracic volume) lead to an increased cerebral venous volume.

- Increased extracellular fluid volume leading to cerebral oedema.
- Increased CSF volume as a result of hydrocephalus, benign intracranial hypertension and blocked ventriculoperitoneal shunt.
- Increased brain volume from intracranial haemorrhage, abscess and tumour.

Clinical features of a raised ICP are:

- Early: headache, vomiting, papilloedema, seizures, focal neurological signs.
- Late: agitation, drowsiness, Cheyne-Stokes respiration, rising blood pressure and bradycardia (Cushing's reflex), ipsilateral or bilateral pupillary dilatation, decorticate or decerebrate posturing.

Management of a raised ICP

A raised ICP can lead to impairment of cerebral perfusion resulting in areas of focal or global cerebral ischaemia. With exhaustion of compensatory mechanisms, the raised ICP can cause compression and herniation of brain tissue. The principles of management include:

- Avoid hypoxia, hypercarbia, hypertension and hyperthermia. Control of $PaCO_2$ and adequate oxygenation can be achieved by controlled ventilation.
- Avoid increases in venous pressure, prevent coughing and straining, avoid the head-down position and pressure on neck veins from tracheal tube ties.
- Ensure CPP is >70mmHg.
- Minimise cerebral oedema by avoiding hypotonic fluids.

Specific strategies to reduce ICP

- A 30° head-up position to encourage venous drainage and reduction in central venous pressure.
- Aim for a $PaCO_2$ between 4.5-5kPa. Hyperventilation to <4kPa may cause cerebral ischaemia secondary to excessive cerebral vasoconstriction.

- Insertion of an external ventricular drain (EVD) or a lumbar drain for CSF drainage.
- Consider corticosteroids to reduce cerebral oedema in patients with brain tumours.
- Cautious use of osmotic diuretics (mannitol) or loop diuretics (furosemide) to reduce cerebral oedema.
- Maintain normothermia and normoglycaemia to avoid worsening of neurological outcomes.
- Treatment of seizures with antiepileptics such as phenytoin or levetiracetam.

Effect of anaesthetic agents on ICP

The most currently used volatile anaesthetic agents (isoflurane, sevoflurane, desflurane), when used in concentrations of <1 MAC, have beneficial effects on reducing the cerebral metabolic rate of oxygen consumption ($CMRO_2$). At a concentration >1 MAC, they are known to increase cerebral blood flow and inhibit cerebral autoregulation. Nitrous oxide is associated with cerebral vasodilatation and increases in CBF and is generally avoided.

Most intravenous induction agents (thiopentone, propofol), with the exception of ketamine, have beneficial effects on the $CMRO_2$, CBF and ICP.

Suxamethonium can cause a clinically insignificant transient rise in ICP, although it can be used in a rapid sequence induction. Non-depolarising muscle relaxants such as atracurium, rocuronium and vecuronium do not have any effect on CBF and ICP.

Opioids have little to no effect on CBF and ICP.

Neurosurgical intervention to control ICP

- A surgical intervention should be considered based on an initial patient assessment if there is compelling evidence of benefit in reducing the mass effect from a SOL such as a haematoma, intracranial tumour or an abscess.

501

- A decompressive craniectomy may be considered in refractory cases, where conservative strategies have failed to reduce ICP.
- An external ventricular drain and lumbar drains can be considered for controlled CSF drainage.
- ICP can be monitored using an intraventricular catheter or intraparenchymal device.

General considerations in neuroanaesthesia

Pre-operative assessment

A focused and systematic pre-operative assessment of the presenting neurological condition and any underlying comorbidities should be undertaken.

A detailed airway assessment must be carried out to identify potential airway difficulties including any cervical spine instability. An airway management strategy may then be planned appropriately including the need for an awake fibreoptic intubation. Patients who have depressed consciousness may have compromised gag reflexes and are prone to aspiration, chest infection and atelectasis.

Careful consideration should be given to agree and achieve set targets for MAP, CPP and ICP, in discussion with the neurosurgical team.

Patients are prone to developing diabetes insipidus (DI), the syndrome of inappropriate ADH (SIADH) secretion and cerebral salt wasting syndrome secondary to disturbances of the hypothalamic-pituitary-adrenal axis (HPA axis). Therefore, renal function and urine output should be closely monitored. Any electrolyte imbalance should be corrected and hyperglycaemia should be treated.

The Glasgow Coma Scale (GCS) score and any existing neurological deficits need to be documented pre-operatively. The complexity and duration of the surgery is dependent on the site, size and vascularity of the SOL being removed. Reviewing the radiological imaging such as CT and MRI scans may provide useful information.

Sedative premedication is generally avoided to prevent any further compromises in neurological function.

Deep vein thrombosis (DVT) prophylaxis is reliant upon the use of graduated compression stockings and pneumatic compression devices peri-operatively. Low-molecular-weight heparins (LMWHs) are relatively contraindicated due to an increased risk of intracranial haemorrhage. Anticipated blood loss and the availability of cross-matched blood should be checked during the sign-in process. Planned admission to a neurocritical care area would need to be organised pre-operatively.

Intra-operative management

The key intra-operative goals during neurosurgery are smooth induction, maintenance of stable haemodynamic parameters, the provision of optimal surgical conditions, minimising cerebral oedema, maintenance of CPP and the use of anaesthetic agents that allow rapid recovery and neurological assessment.

Intracranial surgeries are predominantly carried out under general anaesthesia. Minor procedures, e.g. burr hole evacuation of a chronic subdural haematoma, may be performed with a local anaesthetic scalp infiltration technique in a compliant patient. Awake craniotomies are now being increasingly performed in specialist centres and rely on theatre team coordination and patient cooperation.

The routine intra-operative monitoring includes ECG, pulse oximetry, end-tidal carbon dioxide ($EtCO_2$) and temperature. Intra-arterial blood pressure monitoring provides dynamic beat-to-beat information on blood pressure. A central venous cannulation is indicated in cases such as posterior fossa surgery, clipping of cerebral aneurysms and in situations where inotropic support is required. Urinary bladder catheterisation allows hourly urine output monitoring and the use of osmotic or loop diuretic use for ICP management. When a neuromuscular blocking agent is administered, objective monitoring of neuromuscular function should be carried out.

Venous access should be secured using a wide-bore cannula. The following precautions should be taken during the induction phase:

- A smooth induction avoiding coughing, straining and maintaining haemodynamic stability is key to minimising an ICP rise at induction.
- Both propofol and thiopentone have beneficial effects on $CMRO_2$, CBF and ICP.
- Opioids such as fentanyl, alfentanil and remifentanil can obtund the stress response associated with laryngoscopy and tracheal intubation.
- Cervical spine control during intubation is mandatory if there is underlying cervical spine instability.
- A reinforced endotracheal tube is used for intubation to avoid kinking, and is secured with tape. Avoid tracheal tube ties to prevent compression of neck veins.
- Protection of eyes with tapes and eye pads.
- Positioning a patient on an operating table is a paramount consideration in operative planning and is the key to easy surgical access. Besides supine positioning, other patient positions employed are prone, sitting, park bench and lateral positions. Because of the lengthy duration of these procedures, careful attention must be paid to prevent compression injuries to eyes, skin, soft tissues, joints and nerves.

During the maintenance phase, the following principles are useful in maintaining a good CPP and avoiding any rise in intracranial pressure:

- A total intravenous anaesthesia (TIVA) technique incorporating propofol and a remifentanil target-controlled infusion (TCI) provides an ideal pharmacokinetic profile which enables a smoother maintenance, optimum operating conditions, haemodynamic stability and an ability to rapidly titrate the anaesthetic and analgesic depth during stimulating periods, such as the application of the Mayfield® clamp. It also facilitates rapid recovery and neurological assessment. Infiltration of the scalp with local anaesthetic minimises the cardiovascular response to the scalp incision.

- Nitrous oxide is preferably avoided as it increases CBF due to its cerebral vasodilatory properties and can also lead to an increase in the size of pneumocephalus by expanding air-filled spaces.
- Controlled intermittent positive pressure ventilation (IPPV) helps to maintain the $EtCO_2$ levels between the recommended limits of 4-4.5kPa. Application of positive end-expiratory pressure (PEEP) is generally avoided as it can increase the intrathoracic pressure and impede cerebral venous drainage.
- The blood pressure is generally maintained to achieve a target CPP >70mmHg with the help of vasopressors if needed. Vasopressors such as metaraminol are best used as a continuous intravenous infusion rather than intermittent boluses.
- Hypotonic and dextrose-containing IV fluids should be avoided as they are associated with poor neurological outcomes secondary to cerebral oedema.
- Temperature control is important during neurosurgery. Warming devices such as air warming blankets and warming IV fluids help to maintain normothermia.

Reversal and extubation

Adequate reversal of the neuromuscular blockade should be confirmed with a neuromuscular monitor (train-of-four ratio >0.9) prior to awakening the patient. A remifentanil TCI aids in an overall smoother extubation by minimising coughing and bucking. Uncontrolled transient hypertension during awakening can be treated with titrated doses of labetalol. A rapid recovery is crucial in allowing an early neurological assessment in the immediate postoperative period. If a decision has been made to continue sedation and ventilation following surgery, then ICP monitoring is recommended in the postoperative period.

Postoperative pain control

Most neurosurgical procedures result in mild to moderate postoperative pain. In addition to local anaesthetic infiltration to the surgical wound site, pain control in the majority of cases can be achieved with simple analgesics such as paracetamol and codeine phosphate. Oral or parenteral morphine administration might be resorted to in a minority of cases. NSAIDs are generally avoided due to the risk of increased bleeding.

Postoperative care

Most neurosurgical patients are recovered in a neurocritical care area or a specialist neurosurgical ward, where they are closely monitored for the development of any neurological deficits. A thorough documentation and detailed handover is extremely important to ensure continuity of patient care.

Anaesthesia for specific neurosurgical procedures

Traumatic brain injury and emergency surgery

Traumatic brain injury (TBI) accounts for 34% of all trauma in the UK. The severity of TBI is assessed using the Glasgow Coma Scale (Table 23.2).

Table 23.2. Glasgow Coma Scale.

Eye opening response	Score	Verbal response	Score	Motor response	Score
Spontaneous	4	Oriented	5	Obeys commands	6
To verbal stimuli	3	Confused	4	Localises pain	5
To pain	2	Inappropriate words	3	Withdraws from pain	4
None	1	Incoherent	2	Flexion to pain	3
		None	1	Extension to pain	2
				None	1

TBI includes a plethora of injuries such as cerebral contusion, diffuse axonal injury, subarachnoid haemorrhage, subdural or extradural haematoma. The key objective in the management of TBI is to prevent secondary brain injury. The Brain Trauma Foundation outlines the following measures in TBI management:

- Maintain systolic BP ≥100mmHg for 50 to 69 years of age and ≥110mmHg for 15 to 49 years or over 70 years of age.
- Maintain CPP between 60-70mmHg.
- Maintain ICP ≤20mmHg.
- Maintain normocapnia, normoxia, normoglycaemia and normothermia to minimise adverse outcomes following TBI.

Other considerations

- Associated cervical spine injuries will need a careful assessment and an airway management plan.
- Extracranial injuries must not go unnoticed and should be managed in a timely manner.
- Seizures lead to a significant increase in cerebral metabolism and must be treated with the utmost priority.
- Mannitol, as an osmotic diuretic, may be administered to temporarily stabilise a profound rise in ICP, when there is associated pupillary dilatation secondary to loss of pupillary reflexes and a rapid deterioration in the GCS score.
- Patients must be haemodynamically stabilised before transferring to a specialist neurosurgical centre.

Evacuation of intracranial haematomas

Surgical considerations

Intracranial haematomas may be classified into extradural, subdural, or intracerebral. The key features of intracranial haematomas are described in Table 23.3. Acute extradural and subdural haematomas require immediate surgical intervention (Figures 23.3. and 23.4).

Table 23.3. Key features of different types of intracerebral bleeding.

Extradural haematoma	Subdural haematoma	Intracerebral haematoma
Usually secondary to a skull fracture	Results from tearing of the bridging vessels within the subdural space	Results from trauma or haemorrhagic stroke
Located between the dura and the skull periosteum	Located between the pia and arachnoid mater	In many cases bleeding is present in both the brain parenchyma and the ventricles
Results from a middle meningeal artery or a dural sinus tear	Chronic subdural haematoma, commonly seen in the elderly, can occur even with a minor head injury and has a better prognosis if managed appropriately	Could be a complication of anticoagulation therapy
Lucid interval is followed by deterioration in the patient's condition		
Biconvex (lentiform) appearance on the CT scan	Acute subdural haematoma is usually life-threatening and needs early evacuation	
	Crescent-shaped appearance on the CT scan	

Intracerebral haematomas may result in a stroke and initial management involves haemostatic therapy and measures to control ICP, blood pressure and prevention of aspiration. Surgical intervention may include insertion of an external ventricular drain, craniotomy and evacuation of the haematoma or a decompressive craniectomy. Patient positioning on the

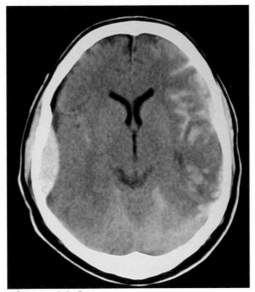

Figure 23.3. CT scan of the head showing an extradural haematoma on the right side.

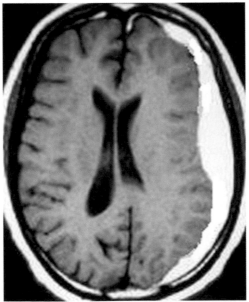

Figure 23.4. CT scan of the head showing a subdural haematoma on the left side.

operating table depends on the site of the haematoma. In the case of a haematoma involving the frontoparietal region, the patient is positioned in a supine position with the head turned opposite to the side of the operation and the neck slightly extended. The position is fixed using a three-point Mayfield® clamp. In the case of a haematoma involving the posterior temporal or occipital regions, a more posterior approach is planned, with the patient positioned supine, the ipsilateral shoulder elevated on a roll, and the head turned into the lateral position and fixed in a three-point Mayfield® clamp. In the case of an infratentorial haematoma, the patient is turned to the prone position with the neck slightly flexed. The position is fixed using a three-point Mayfield® clamp.

Anaesthetic considerations

These procedures are performed as an emergency; hence, there is very limited time available for pre-operative assessment and optimisation. Most often, patients with a head injury are already intubated in a peripheral hospital or at the scene of injury and transferred to the neurosurgical theatre. It is important to have a mini team brief to discuss the proposed surgical procedure, anticipated problems and postoperative care. If already intubated, tracheal tube position and ventilatory parameters should be assessed on arrival into the anaesthetic room. In addition, the patient requires catheterisation of the bladder to monitor urine output. The patient should be positioned according to the site of the craniotomy in the anaesthetic room. Some patients may require the use of a Mayfield® head clamp and others a horseshoe-type head rest. Prior to starting the surgery, the availability of blood and blood products should be confirmed. Venous access should be secured with a wide-bore cannula and a facility for rapid blood transfusion and fluid administration should be available. The key principles of anaesthetic management include preservation of CPP, control of ICP and optimum oxygenation and ventilation. Invasive arterial pressure measurement enables continuous monitoring of mean arterial pressure.

Ventriculoperitoneal shunt

Surgical considerations

Shunt surgeries are performed as a treatment modality for hydrocephalus. The majority of these procedures are carried out in children. A commonly performed shunt is the ventriculoperitoneal (VP) shunt which allows drainage of the CSF from the lateral ventricle into the peritoneal cavity. It is usually performed on the right side. Following induction of general anaesthesia, the patient is positioned supine with the head turned to the left. An abdominal incision is made to access the peritoneal cavity. A cranial incision is made over the right parieto-occipital region. The lateral ventricle is accessed via a small burr hole. A further surgical procedure involves creating a subcutaneous pocket for a reservoir and valve, followed by creating a subcutaneous tunnel between the skull and abdominal incision.

Anaesthetic considerations

During the pre-operative assessment, particular attention should be paid to associated respiratory and cardiac comorbidities, symptoms of raised ICP and the level of consciousness. During induction, routine precautions should be taken to avoid a rise in ICP. Invasive monitoring is not usually indicated. The process of tunnelling the shunt tube is intensely stimulating, hence maintaining an adequate anaesthetic depth is essential. There is a danger of intracranial haemorrhage with very rapid CSF fluid shifts, hence a controlled CSF drainage is vital.

Craniotomy for space-occupying lesions

Surgical considerations

Common indications for a craniotomy include excision or debulking of intracranial tumours, evacuation of haematomas and drainage of intracranial abscesses. Patient position is dictated by the location and size of the tumour. SOLs in the posterior fossa may require a park bench, prone or sitting position. The sitting position is less commonly used due to the risk of venous air embolism. In addition, posterior fossa surgery can be complicated with associated haemodynamic instability due to proximity to the vasomotor centre.

Anaesthetic considerations

The routine precautions should be taken to minimise any effect on intracranial pressure. In addition to routine monitoring, invasive blood pressure monitoring is essential to control blood pressure during the periods of intense stimulation such as the application of head pins to fix the Mayfield® clamp. Central venous catheterisation is usually used for aspiration of air from the right atrium in cases of venous air embolism. A TCI of propofol and remifentanil allows easy titration of the anaesthetic depth during stages of intense surgical stimulation and a better pharmacokinetic recovery profile to allow early postoperative neurological assessment. Depth of anaesthesia monitoring (Bispectral Index and entropy) is recommended during TIVA-based techniques. The depth of neuromuscular blockade can be monitored using a neuromuscular monitor. Good venous access and the availability of blood and blood products are crucial for managing sudden unexpected intra-operative bleeding. During the intra-operative phase, once the dura is opened following a craniotomy, there is minimal surgical stimulation. An intravenous infusion of vasopressors such as metaraminol should be used to maintain blood pressure within normal limits. Hypertensive episodes during emergence are usually managed with titrated doses of labetalol.

Clipping of intracranial aneurysms

Surgical considerations

Intracranial aneurysms are localised abnormal dilatation of cerebral blood vessels. They are classified as saccular, fusiform and dissecting aneurysms. The most common sites include the internal carotid, anterior communicating and posterior communicating arteries, and middle cerebral arteries.

Arteriovenous malformations are characterised by a nidus forming the transition between the feeding cerebral artery and draining vein without an interconnecting capillary network. They may be associated with surrounding cerebral ischaemia (vascular steal phenomenon) and high-output cardiac failure.

With advances in interventional radiological techniques, a major proportion of intracranial vascular lesions are now amenable to neuroradiological interventions.

The surgical procedure involves positioning the patient appropriately for a craniotomy using a Mayfield® head clamp. Following a craniotomy, access is gained to the neck of the aneurysm and clips are applied to the neck of the aneurysm. The procedure is performed under an operating microscope, hence an immobile surgical field is very essential. Intra-operative rupture of the aneurysm is associated with a high mortality. Immediate measures to control the hypertensive crisis and cerebral protection with barbiturates (thiopentone) and hypothermia may be needed during surgical control of aneurysmal bleeding.

Anaesthetic considerations

The main goals include:

- Prevention of aneurysm rupture during induction and intra-operatively.
- Maintenance of adequate CPP and cerebral oxygenation.
- Smooth and rapid emergence from anaesthesia to allow full neurological assessment.
- Use of balanced anaesthesia with muscle relaxation.

This procedure often presents as an emergency following a failed radiological intervention (coiling) or following acute subarachnoid haemorrhage. Those aneurysms that are not suitable for radiological intervention are scheduled for elective clipping. In either situation, a focused neurological examination should be performed and recorded. Blood group and availability of cross-matched blood should be checked. Aspirin and any anticoagulant drugs should be stopped appropriately.

Peripheral venous access should be secured using two large-bore cannulae. Monitoring during anaesthesia includes peripheral oxygen saturation using pulse oximetry, continuous ECG, invasive arterial blood pressure, central venous pressure, body temperature (nasopharyngeal), urine output, neuromuscular blockade, blood loss estimation and intermittent blood gases, glucose and a haematocrit.

Induction and maintenance

Pre-oxygenation followed by smooth induction with obtundation of the hypertensive response to laryngoscopy is essential to avoid rupture of the aneurysms. Intravenous induction using propofol and a target-controlled infusion of remifentanil allows smooth induction. Anaesthesia is maintained with total intravenous anaesthesia (propofol and remifentanil) or with a suitable volatile agent (desflurane, sevoflurane or isoflurane). Nitrous oxide should be avoided due to the risk of venous air embolism.

Controlled hypotension is less commonly used, as it decreases regional cerebral blood flow. In patients with subarachnoid haemorrhage, normal autoregulation is impaired due to cerebral vasospasm.

Mannitol at a dose of 0.5-1mg/kg reduces the intracranial pressure. The peak effect is usually seen approximately 30-45 minutes after the start of the intravenous infusion. Dexamethasone (8-10mg) also can be administered intravenously to reduce cerebral oedema. Prophylactic anticonvulsant phenytoin or levetiracetam is usually administered during the intra-operative period.

Emergence and recovery

In an elective case, provided there are no intra-operative complications and the aneurysm is successfully clipped, the patient should be woken up at the end of surgery. This allows neurological assessment and reduces respiratory complications associated with postoperative ventilation. During extubation and recovery, hypertension, coughing, straining and hypercarbia should be avoided. Before discontinuing remifentanil (in view of its shorter duration of action), ensure adequate postoperative analgesia using long-acting opioids (titrated doses of morphine 0.1 to 0.15mg/kg) and intravenous paracetamol.

Postoperative care

The patient should be monitored in a neurosurgical intensive care unit. Blood pressure should be maintained very close to the normal range (at least within 20% of the patient's normal blood pressure). Relative hypervolaemia and relative haemodilution should be maintained in the postoperative period. Neurological observations (level of consciousness, size and reactivity of the pupils, limb movements) along with blood pressure, heart rate, temperature, urine output, sedation score and pain score should be monitored regularly.

Postoperative analgesia includes regular administration of paracetamol 1g (oral or IV) four times a day and codeine phosphate 30 to 60mg (oral or IM) four times a day. Patient-controlled analgesia with morphine or titrated doses of intravenous morphine can also be used whilst monitoring the patient in neurosurgical intensive care or a high dependency care unit.

Cervical spinal surgery

Surgical considerations

Most surgeries are undertaken to relieve compression of the spinal cord or spinal nerve roots. This may involve trauma, malignancy, congenital anomalies and infection (e.g. vertebral abscess). Surgery on the cervical spine involves excision and replacement of intervertebral discs and decompression of nerve roots or the spinal cord. In some cases, this may involve fusion of the cervical vertebrae to stabilise the cervical segments. An anterior approach is usually used for lower cervical vertebrae. A posterior approach is used for procedures involving the upper cervical vertebrae; occipito-cervical fixation for atlanto-axial subluxation and decompression for spinal canal stenosis/cervical myelopathy. Posterior decompression is usually accompanied with lateral mass fixation with the aid of screws and rods.

Anaesthetic considerations

During the pre-operative assessment, the site and extent of the surgery should be confirmed.

Most often, posterior decompression is performed to limit the progression of cervical myelopathy, hence patients presenting for this procedure are usually in the elderly age group, so they may have associated comorbidities.

A thorough airway assessment is essential. In situations where a difficult airway is anticipated, awake intubation is the technique of choice. In cases of an unstable cervical spine, all precautions should be taken to minimise movement of the cervical spine during airway management. Manual in-line stabilisation and videolaryngoscopes may help to minimise cervical spine movement during tracheal intubation. For posterior decompression, the patient should be positioned in the prone position with their head fixed onto the Mayfield® clamp with the help of head pins. Careful attention should be given when securing the airway to avoid accidental intra-operative extubation.

In addition to standard monitoring, arterial blood pressure monitoring is useful when a prolonged duration of surgery is anticipated (e.g. decompression and fixation at multiple levels and posterior decompression).

Intra-operative management involves measures to maintain spinal cord perfusion by maintaining blood pressure at normal levels, ensuring an immobile surgical field during the critical stages of the surgery. Blood loss is usually minimal; however, group and save for the electronic issue of blood should be confirmed prior to starting the case. Surgery involving the upper cervical spine, especially at the atlanto-axial region, may lead to cardiovascular instability due to vagal stimulation.

During emergence from anaesthesia, care should be taken to minimise coughing and bucking, as this may increase blood pressure and venous pressure in the neck leading to bleeding at the surgical site. Retropharyngeal haematomas may also compromise the airway, leading to acute airway obstruction. Postoperative pain is usually managed using regular administration of paracetamol, codeine phosphate and oral morphine.

Transnasal transsphenoidal excision of pituitary adenomas

Surgical considerations

The surgical approach to the suprasellar space is used for excision of pituitary tumours. The MRI scan and intra-operative imaging are used to guide the instrumentation. In addition, an operative microscope is used to magnify the surgical field. The surgery can also be performed with the aid of an endoscope and is facilitated by the use of an intra-operative navigation system using MRI or CT scans. Important anatomical structures around the surgical field include the optic chiasma, cavernous sinus and internal carotid artery. For this procedure the patient is positioned supine, with their head slightly elevated.

Anaesthetic considerations

During the pre-operative assessment, particular attention should be given to associated endocrine disease such as acromegaly or Cushing's syndrome. Some patients may also have associated hypothyroidism and hypoadrenalism. Any replacement hormones should be continued and advice from an endocrinologist is helpful in the management of peri-operative hormone replacement.

During induction, patients may require supplementary hydrocortisone. Urine output and temperature should be monitored during the intra-operative period. The airway is secured using a reinforced tracheal tube. A throat pack is used to absorb the trickling of blood from the surgical site. Appropriate precautions should be taken to ensure removal of the throat pack at the end of the surgery. Suggested safety systems include clear communication between theatre staff, sticking a label on the patient's forehead, tying the throat pack to the tracheal tube and including the throat pack in the swab count. During surgical preparation, in order to minimise bleeding, the nose is packed with pledgets soaked with lidocaine and epinephrine, or 2% lidocaine and epinephrine 1: 80,000 may be infiltrated to the mucosa. Hence, blood pressure and heart rate should be closely monitored.

During the procedure, there is a possibility of vascular injury leading to sudden blood loss, hence vascular access should be secured using a wide-bore cannula and intra-operative invasive blood pressure monitoring is useful.

In the postoperative period, the patient should be monitored in the high dependency unit. Steroid supplementation should be continued for 48-72 hours. Urine output and fluid balance should be closely monitored. As a result of surgical oedema there is reduced antidiuretic hormone (ADH) secretion in the postoperative period leading to diabetes insipidus. Occasionally, the patient may develop the syndrome of inappropriate ADH secretion. Therefore, urine specific gravity, sodium and serum electrolytes should be monitored.

Interventional neuroradiological procedures

Surgical considerations

With rapid advances in interventional neuroradiology, a wide spectrum of procedures is being carried out using this technique. Some examples include diagnostic angiography, coil embolisation of cerebral aneurysms (elective and emergency), glue embolisation of cerebral arteriovenous malformations, thrombolysis and thrombectomy following stroke.

Stereotactic-guided neurosurgical procedures include deep brain stimulation for movement disorders, implantation of intracranial electrodes for telemetry and temporal lobe resections for epilepsy. A surgical requirement is for a motionless field, as any movement would lead to catastrophic complications.

Anaesthetic considerations

A pre-operative assessment should include the details of the presenting neurological condition and associated comorbidities. A thorough neurological examination should be performed to identify and document existing neurological deficits. As the procedure involves exposure to radiation, pregnancy testing in women of child-bearing age is essential. Pre-operative blood tests should include renal function as patients are prone to contrast-induced nephropathy.

A blood group and cross-match should be available. Any allergy to radiocontrast dyes should be elicited.

Monitoring should include invasive arterial BP, temperature and hourly urine output.

A large-bore IV access is required as there is potential for intra-operative bleeding. For procedures involving coiling of an aneurysm, the systolic BP target should be 100-160mmHg (avoid hypertension and hypotension to minimise the risk of rebleeding and ischaemia, respectively). Vasopressors may be needed to achieve the target BP. Usually the patient is positioned supine so that the patient's head is away from the anaesthetic machine, hence the need for long infusion lines and breathing tubes. Interventional procedures are relatively painless (following local anaesthetic infiltration at the catheter insertion site).

Other considerations include:

- Radiation safety for the patient and staff.
- Contrast-induced nephropathy — minimise the risks by adequate hydration, limiting the total dose of radiocontrast dyes used. Renal function should be monitored for 72 hours post-procedure.
- Heparin is administered to minimise thromboembolic complications. The activated clotting time (ACT) should be monitored with heparin treatment.

Smooth emergence and extubation with the avoidance of coughing and straining are key to preventing a precipitous ICP rise and risk of rebleeding and rupture of unprotected or partially protected aneurysms. Postoperatively, the patient should be monitored in a high dependency area to facilitate neurological observations and monitoring of potential complications.

Case scenario 1

A 22-year-old male patient was brought to the emergency department by the paramedics following a road traffic collision. He presented in a combative state with a GCS score of 11, is tachycardic, hypotensive and hypothermic, and with multiple bruises to his head, chest, abdomen and limbs. A trauma series whole body CT revealed an undisplaced skull fracture with an extradural haematoma measuring 12mm in the right temporoparietal region with an associated midline shift of >5mm. His GCS subsequently drops to 7 with an abnormal flexor response to pain and right pupillary dilatation with a sluggish reaction to light. The neurosurgeons are keen to take him to theatre for an emergency evacuation of the extradural haematoma.

How would you manage this patient?

Pre-operative management

- A rapid ABCDE (ATLS® principles) assessment of the patient with simultaneous stabilisation is key to preventing secondary brain injury.
- Events surrounding the mechanism of injury and any pre-existing comorbidities are confirmed.
- This patient would need airway protection in the form of a secure flexo-metallic tracheal tube as he is at risk of aspiration secondary to his low GCS.
- Cervical spine control in the form of manual in-line stabilisation (MILS) should be adhered to whilst performing a rapid sequence induction to avoid a pressor response to laryngoscopy.

- Ensure large-bore IV access and send bloods for an FBC, U&Es, clotting profile and blood group/cross-match.
- Maintain normoxia (PaO$_2$ >12kPa, SpO$_2$ >97%) and normocapnia (PaCO$_2$ 4.5-5kPa).
- Monitor invasive BP, avoid hypotension (MAP >80mmHg); he may need intravascular volume replacement and vasopressors to achieve the target BP.
- Maintain normothermia and normoglycaemia.
- Promptly treat any associated seizure activity with antiepileptics, e.g. phenytoin.
- Because of a rapid drop in GCS with pupillary signs, administer mannitol in consultation with the neurosurgeon to control ICP and to prevent brain herniation.

Intra-operative management

- Maintain oxygenation and ventilation as discussed in the pre-operative management.
- Ensure that the ET tube is firmly secured with sleek tapes to avoid dislodgement/accidental extubation.
- Encourage venous drainage with a slight head-up position and by avoiding compression of neck veins.
- As the patient's head end is away from the anaesthetic machine, long breathing system tubings and IV extension lines are required.
- Maintain BP as per the set targets in discussion with the neurosurgeons.
- Monitor blood loss and replace blood/blood products as necessary.
- Maintain normoxia, normocapnia, normothermia and normoglycaemia.
- Careful logrolling with spinal precautions during positioning.
- Adequate padding of pressure areas and eye protection.
- Use of a pneumatic compression device (Flowtron®) to prevent DVT.
- Maintenance of anaesthesia with a TCI of propfol and remifentanil may allow easy titration of anaesthetic depth, haemodynamic stability, cerebral protection and a better pharmacokinetic recovery profile facilitating early neurological assessment.

Postoperative management and recovery

- Postoperatively, this patient may need to be ventilated in the neurocritical care unit.
- Blood pressure should be maintained to ensure an adequate cerebral perfusion pressure.
- Hypothermia and hyperglycaemia should be avoided.
- Avoid the administration of NSAIDs as their use is associated with an increased risk of bleeding.
- Steroids have no role in the management of traumatic brain injury (TBI).
- Continue mechanical measures of DVT prevention.

Case scenario 2

A 78-year-old male patient is brought to the emergency department with a history of headache, increasing confusion and sleepiness. His wife reports that he had a fall a few weeks ago but did not seek medical attention at the time. His other comorbidities include hypertension and atrial fibrillation (AF). He is on antihypertensives and takes warfarin for his AF. A CT scan of the head reveals a chronic subdural haematoma (CSDH) in the left frontoparietal area with an associated sulcal effacement and midline shift.

How would you manage this patient?

Pre-operative management

- A thorough pre-operative history focusing on the patient's presenting neurological condition and any underlying comorbidities is undertaken.
- Any associated risk factors such as advancing age, a history of falls, head injury, indirect trauma, treatment with anticoagulants and

- antiplatelets, a bleeding diathesis, alcohol excess, epilepsy or haemodialysis are identified.
- It is important to seek a collateral history from the patient's relatives/carers to confirm the patient's symptoms and establish a timeline of events, as the patient is likely to miss out on vital information because of potentially associated memory loss.
- Besides a routine examination, a thorough neurological examination is conducted to identify any neurological deficits.
- The most important step in the diagnosis of CSDH is a high index of suspicion.
- Routine bloods including an FBC, U&Es and clotting profile, and an ECG need to be reviewed.
- This patient is on warfarin for his AF and is likely to have a raised INR. Depending on the urgency of the procedure, he may need a reversal of his warfarin therapy with either vitamin K or prothrombin complex concentrates after discussion with the haematology and neurosurgical team to minimise the risk of further peri-operative bleeding.
- Ensure an adequate availability of blood and blood products before the start of surgery.

Intra-operative management

- Commonly performed surgical procedures include drainage by a mini-craniotomy or burr hole evacuation.
- A burr hole evacuation of the CSDH may be performed under local anaesthesia in a cooperative patient.
- Intra-operative monitoring includes ECG, $EtCO_2$, SpO_2, NBP +/- arterial BP monitoring, temperature, urine output monitoring and neuromuscular monitoring.
- Venous access using a wide-bore cannula.
- Ensure a smooth induction, avoid the hypertensive response to laryngoscopy with opioids, short-acting beta-blockers (esmolol) or IV lignocaine. Vasopressors may be needed to maintain haemodynamic stability at induction.
- Cerebral protection strategies include maintenance of CPP and ICP.

- Monitor for signs of venous air embolism.
- DVT prevention by using pneumatic compression devices.
- Monitor and replace intra-operative blood loss.

Postoperative management

- Ensure smooth extubation, postoperative analgesia and an early neurological assessment.
- Patients need to be recovered in a specialist neuro ward or high dependency area depending on the complexity of the procedure performed.
- Monitor for complications such as rebleeding, seizures and tension pneumocephalus.

Further reading

1. James E, Cottrell JE, Newfield P. *Handbook of Neuroanaesthesia*, 5th ed. Lippincott Williams and Wilkins, 2012.
2. Basil FM, David KM, Smith M. *Core topics in Neuroanaesthesia and Neurointensive Care.* Cambridge University Press, 2011.
3. Tameem A, Krovvidi H. Cerebral physiology. *Br J Anaesth CEACCP* 2013; 13: 113-8.
4. Dinsmore J. Anaesthesia for elective neurosurgery. *Br J Anaesth* 2007; 99: 68-74.
5. Patel S, Reddy U. Anaesthesia for interventional neuroradiology. *BJA Education* 2016; 16: 147-52
6. Nowicki RWA. Anaesthesia for major spinal surgery. *Br J Anaesth CEACCP* 2014; 14: 147-52.
7. Dinsmore J. Traumatic brain injury: an evidence-based review of management. *Br J Anaesth CEACCP* 2013; 13: 189-95.
8. Al-Rifai Z, Mulvey D. Principles of total intravenous anaesthesia: basic pharmacokinetics and model descriptions. *Br J Anaesth CEACCP* 2016; 16: 92-7.

24 Thoracic procedures

Nagendra Prasad and Narotham R. Burri

Introduction

General anaesthesia for thoracic surgery, as for other sub-specialty procedures, involves the management and maintenance of airway, breathing and circulation whilst providing the triad of general anaesthesia, i.e. unconsciousness, pain relief and reflex suppression. Thoracic surgical or diagnostic procedures that are performed on the tracheobronchial tree, pleura, mediastinum, lungs and chest wall require the anaesthetist to possess the relevant knowledge of anatomy and physiology, and apply this knowledge appropriately, to conduct an uneventful anaesthetic for the indicated thoracic surgery. Thoracic procedures range from a minor diagnostic rigid/flexible bronchoscopy to a major operation such as a thoracotomy. Most thoracic procedures require a general anaesthetic with or without regional anaesthesia. However, procedures such as a flexible diagnostic bronchoscopy or insertion of a chest drain can be done under a local anaesthetic.

The sharing of airway and lungs between the anaesthetist and the surgeon, the lateral decubitus position, an open chest and the requirement to collapse the non-dependent pathological lung that requires surgery and positive pressure ventilation of the normal dependent lung all pose a unique challenge to the anaesthetist.

The following is an account of the relevant anatomical and physiological aspects pertinent to conducting anaesthesia for thoracic procedures, in the context of the above-mentioned factors.

Shared airway and lung

Rigid and flexible bronchoscopy are performed as a sole procedure or, most often, as part of the surgical procedure. After induction of anaesthesia, a rigid bronchoscope is passed through the vocal cords by the surgeon to inspect the tracheobronchial tree before proceeding with the intended surgery. At this point, the airway remains unprotected, whilst the surgeon is performing the bronchoscopy. This is a highly stimulating procedure that can lead to sympathetic stimulation causing hypertension. A low-pressure ventilation circuit, as in paediatric practice (ventilating bronchoscope), cannot be used in adults to provide ventilation or to deliver a volatile anaesthetic. Oxygenation is maintained using a Venturi injector connected to the rigid bronchoscope and anaesthesia is maintained using an intravenous anaesthetic (intermittent boluses or continuous infusion of propofol).

Collapse of the lung that is being operated on, using either a double-lumen tube (DLT) or a bronchial blocker, provides room for the surgeon to operate and facilitates surgery, but this contributes to shunt causing hypoxaemia. The application of continuous positive airway pressure (CPAP) to this collapsed lung or resumption of ventilation may be required to maintain oxygenation in situations of unacceptable saturation or oxygenation.

The lateral decubitus position

Ventilation and perfusion are not homogeneous in the lungs. Ventilation and perfusion increase independently from the apex to the base of an upright lung in an erect position. Considering the changes in ventilation and perfusion independently, the magnitude of increase in perfusion from the top to the bottom of the lung is much greater than the increase in ventilation, leading to a high ventilation/perfusion (V/Q) ratio in the apex and a low V/Q ratio in the base. High V/Q zones contribute to dead space or wasted ventilation (high ventilation and low perfusion) and low V/Q zones contribute to shunt (low ventilation and high perfusion).

The anterior and posterior parts of the lung in the supine position, the top and the bottom lungs in the lateral decubitus position, behave like the apex and base of an upright lung, respectively. The top collapsed lung of the patient undergoing thoracic surgery thus contributes to a significant increase in the shunt.

In an awake patient, in the lateral decubitus position, the dependent lung is better ventilated due to the more efficient contraction of the dependent hemidiaphragm and receives a greater proportion of perfusion due to gravity.

Hypoxic pulmonary vasoconstriction (HPV) is a protective mechanism which reduces the magnitude of the shunt by decreasing blood flow to the non-ventilated lung through vasoconstriction and diverting this blood flow to the ventilated part of the lung. This protective HPV reflex is preserved with intravenous anaesthetic agents and this is impaired when volatile agents are used in excess of 1 minimum alveolar concentration (MAC).

Apart from an inequality in ventilation and perfusion between the dependent bottom and non-dependent top lung, the potential damage to structures secondary to pressure should be addressed. Corneal abrasions, and injury to the brachial plexus and common peroneal nerves should be prevented through adequate eye protection, sufficient support to the head, neck and chest, and padding between the legs.

Open chest wall and positive pressure ventilation

A breach in the chest wall causes the lung to collapse on that side due to the elastic recoil of the lung and the loss of negative pleural pressure. The negative pleural pressure is responsible to keep the lungs expanded and preventing collapse.

The relationship between ventilation and perfusion is significantly altered when the non-dependent chest is open in the lateral position. The onset of spontaneous respiration in an open chest results in two major changes: a mediastinal shift and paradoxical breathing (pendelluft effect), producing hypercarbia and hypoxia.

During spontaneous breathing, the inspiratory negative pleural pressure in the intact dependent lung causes the downward shift of the mediastinum and the opposite in expiration, resulting in a decrease in tidal volume. It also results in a to-and-fro gas flow between the two lungs, with inspiration increasing the pneumothorax and collapse of the non-dependent lung due to gas flowing into the dependent lung. The opposite occurs in expiration.

Controlled positive pressure ventilation favours the non-dependent (top) lung in the lateral position, as it is more compliant than the dependent lung. Neuromuscular blockade further accentuates this effect as the dependent lung compliance is reduced by the raised abdominal contents against the dependent hemidiaphragm, impeding the dependent lung ventilation. The open pneumothorax on the non-dependent side enhances the differential ventilation, as the upper lung is less restricted in movement as the pressure of the abdominal contents pressing against the upper lung is minimal (Figure 24.1); thus, a ventilation/perfusion mismatch is worsened causing hypoxia.

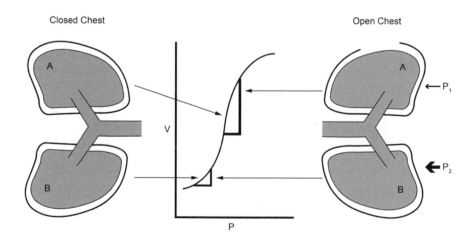

Figure 24.1. Compliance curve demonstrating the position of the dependent lung on the curve following induction of general anaesthesia and positive pressure ventilation. A) Top, non-dependent lung; B) Bottom, dependent lung; P) Pressure; V) Volume; P1) Indicating minimal pressure on the non-dependent lung; P2) Indicating larger pressure on the dependent lung from abdominal contents.

Collapse of the operated or non-dependent lung

A single-lumen cuffed endotracheal tube is commonly used for securing the airway to provide positive pressure ventilation and to maintain anaesthesia in patients undergoing non-thoracic general surgery.

In thoracic surgery, one or both the lungs having pathology and requiring surgery, makes it obligatory to consider the right and the left lungs as independent units for the purposes of isolation and ventilation. Hence, special equipment such as a DLT or a bronchial blocker is used either to ventilate/collapse each lung independently or to collapse the desired lung, respectively.

The indications for insertion of a DLT can be categorised into those that aim to prevent contamination of the lung, those that aim to control ventilation of the lung and finally to those that aim to provide surgical access. Whilst the former two categories are considered as absolute indications, the latter category (surgical access) is considered as a relative indication (Table 24.1).

Table 24.1. Indications for one-lung anaesthesia or lung isolation.

To prevent contamination

Infection (lung abscess)
Haemorrhage

To control ventilation

Bronchopleural fistula
Giant lung cyst/bulla on one side
Surgery involving the main bronchus

To provide surgical access

Lobectomy
Pneumonectomy
Oesophagectomy
Video-assisted thoracoscopic surgery (VATS)

Double-lumen tubes

A simple way to understand the construction of a double-lumen tube (DLT) is to consider the DLT as two single-lumen tubes (SLTs) fused together side by side with their lengths unequal. When inserted into the airway, the shorter tube serves as the tracheal tube and the longer tube serves as the bronchial tube. The DLT not only has a pair (tracheal and bronchial) of lumens but also has several other paired characteristics (Figure 24.2).

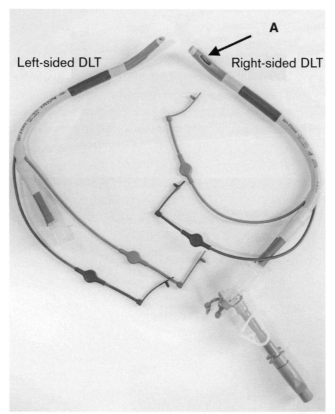

Figure 24.2. Left- and right-sided double-lumen tubes. Bronchial cuffs are in blue and tracheal cuffs are in red with the same colour-coding for the pilot balloons and the tracheal and bronchial limbs. The right DLT has a slot in the cuff (A) for right upper lobe ventilation.

The DLT has a pair of curves, cuffs, pilot tubes and balloons, and limbs for both the tracheal and bronchial lumens (Figure 24.3). The DLT, when held with its proximal concave tracheal curve facing up, points its bronchial end to the side of its intended use, i.e. the left DLT points to the left and the right DLT points to the right.

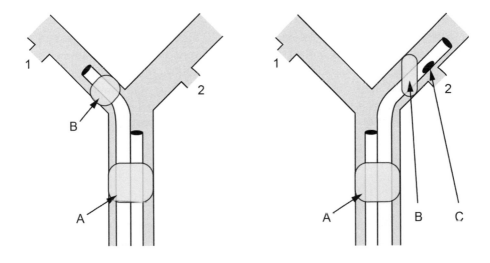

Figure 24.3. Correct placement of a double-lumen tube. The tracheal lumen is correctly placed in the trachea and the bronchial lumen is correctly placed in the respective main bronchi. A) Tracheal cuff; B) Bronchial cuff; C) Lumen for the right upper lobe bronchus; 1) Left upper lobe bronchus; 2) Right upper lobe bronchus.

The cuffs are a high-volume low-pressure type with colour-coding. The bronchial cuff, pilot balloon and the limb are blue in colour, whereas the tracheal cuff, pilot balloon and the limb are transparent in the Bronch-Cath™ and red in the Robertshaw-type DLTs. Unlike the left DLTs, the bronchial cuff of the right DLTs has a hole to facilitate the ventilation of the right upper lobe (RUL). This hole needs to be aligned with the RUL bronchus meaning that a fibreoptic scope and skill are required to achieve this.

The disposable DLTs made of PVC (Bronch-Cath™, Mallinckrodt™) or red rubber (Robertshaw) are commonly used in practice. Bronch-Caths are available in sizes of 28, 32, 35, 37, 39 and 41 French gauges (FG) with an internal diameter ranging from 3.1 to 5.4mm and the corresponding outer diameters are 9.3 to 13.7mm. Robertshaw tubes are available in extra-small, small, medium and large sizes. Bronch-Caths with a 37/39 FG, and medium/large Robertshaw DLTs usually fit an average-sized adult male and 35/37 FG Bronch-Caths and small/medium Robertshaw DLTs usually fit an average-sized adult female. Broncho-Caths sized at 41 FG and large-sized Robertshaw DLTs are used for larger patients.

Bronchial blockers

A bronchial blocker (Figure 24.4) is a narrow long tube with a lumen and balloon at the tip. The blocker is inserted into the main bronchus of the lung to be isolated and the balloon is inflated via the pilot balloon. The blocker, coupled to a fibreoptic bronchoscope with the help of a monofilament loop, is passed through a multiport adaptor attached to a single-lumen endotracheal (ET) tube placed in the trachea and guided into the chosen bronchus using the fibreoptic scope. The cuff is inflated once the blocker is seated in the bronchus and the loop removed. In situations where it is difficult to insert a DLT either due to distorted anatomy or a difficult airway, bronchial blockers can be passed through a single-lumen ET tube in order to achieve lung isolation.

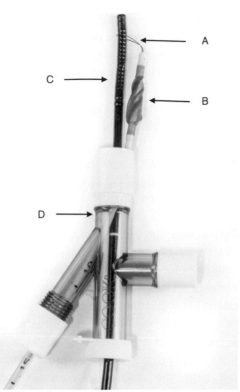

Figure 24.4. Bronchial blocker. A fibreoptic bronchoscope (black) and Arndt bronchial blocker (yellow) are shown coupled together using the loop of the blocker after passing them through the multiport adapter individually. The side arm of the multiport adapter connects to the breathing circuit. A) Loop on the blocker; B) Balloon; C) Fibreoptic bronchoscope; D) Multiport adapter.

Management of one-lung anaesthesia

Following induction of the anaesthetic and achieving muscle relaxation, laryngoscopy, as for routine endotracheal intubation, is performed and the DLT is inserted with the tracheal curvature facing the opposite side. The tip of the tube (bronchial end) is passed through the vocal cords with the stylet in place (Robertshaw DLTs are more rigid and do not have a stylet).

After passing through the vocal cords, the stylet is removed, the DLT (left-sided DLT) is turned 90° anti-clockwise or clockwise (right-sided DLT) and advanced until resistance is met with at the level of the carina, to enter the left or right bronchus, respectively (Figure 24.3).

A bronchial blocker is inserted through a single-lumen ET tube, using a multiport adapter and the technique depends on the type of blocker used, as described earlier.

Isolation and control of ventilation

After the DLT is inserted, the tracheal cuff is inflated and ventilation of both lungs confirmed by bilateral auscultation and capnography. The tracheal limb of the catheter mount is then clamped, the tracheal lumen opened to the atmosphere whilst manually ventilating via the bronchial limb and the bronchial cuff is inflated with a few millilitres of air until the leak through the open tracheal lumen disappears. Clamping of the tracheal limb of the catheter mount and open tracheal lumen should allow ventilation of the lung that is intubated and collapse of the lung on the non-intubated side; the reverse occurs with clamping of the bronchial limb and opening of the bronchial lumen to the atmosphere. The fibreoptic scope is used to check the correct placement of the DLT and confirm the above clinical findings.

Inadvertent advancement of the DLT too far to one side, failure of the bronchial limb to enter the bronchus and entry of the bronchial limb to the unintended opposite side are identified and rectified through auscultation and fibreoptic bronchoscopy, prior to positioning the patient in the lateral decubitus position. It is imperative that correct placement of the DLT is confirmed prior to commencing the surgery.

When a bronchial blocker is used, the balloon is inflated and the correct position of the blocker in the intended bronchus is confirmed using the fibreoptic scope. The lumen of the blocker is opened to the atmosphere to facilitate the collapse of that side. To reinflate/ventilate the collapsed lung, the balloon is deflated and ventilation via the single-lumen tube is continued.

Management of hypoxia during one-lung ventilation

During one-lung ventilation, adequate muscle paralysis is ensured and the lung is ventilated with tidal volumes of 10-12ml/kg. The peak airway pressures must be limited to less than $35cmH_2O$, with either mode. Prevention and treatment are the two strategies to address hypoxia during one-lung anaesthesia. Oxygen at 100% and two-lung ventilation for as long as possible are a few preventative measures.

Treatment involves a few therapeutic measures to address intra-operative hypoxia: ruling out malposition of the DLT, suction of the DLT lumens to clear any blockage, relief of bronchospasm, reducing high airway pressures through adequate relaxation, maintenance of cardiac output, positive end-expiratory pressure (PEEP) to the ventilated lung, CPAP to the collapsed lung, intermittent two-lung ventilation, clamping of the pulmonary artery on the operative side and abandoning one-lung anaesthesia.

Removal of the DLT/blocker

Prior to closure of the chest and after completion of the surgery, the bronchial lumen should be sucked to clear off any secretions, re-expansion of the collapsed lung must be confirmed and the bronchial cuff should be deflated after the cessation of one-lung ventilation. A DLT or SLT with the blocker are removed following reversal of neuromuscular blockade and when fully awake and the extubation criteria are met.

Pre-operative assessment of thoracic surgical patients

This includes a detailed history, clinical examination and investigations.

Through case notes and patient interview, any history of smoking, cardiac disease, respiratory disease, renal disease, medications for concurrent illnesses, weight loss and nutritional state should be explored. Peri-operative cardiac morbidity is increased in this group of patients when accompanied by certain cardiac risk factors (Table 24.2).

Table 24.2. Factors contributing to increased peri-operative cardiac morbidity.

- Unstable coronary syndromes.
- Decompensated heart failure.
- Significant arrhythmias.
- Severe valvular heart disease.

Paraneoplastic syndromes in patients with lung neoplasms may present as endocrine, haematological, metabolic or neuromuscular disturbances. In patients with a thymoma, 30% are known to have myasthenia gravis.

Clinical examination of the respiratory system is undertaken through inspection, palpation, percussion and auscultation, to assess the severity of the presenting respiratory/lung problem. Signs of any superior vena cava (SVC) obstruction, airway obstruction secondary to mediastinal pathology such as engorgement of neck veins, the use of accessory muscles and stridor should be identified. Any findings of endocrine disturbances secondary to paraneoplastic syndromes during the systemic examination should warrant appropriate investigation. Signs of anaemia, poor nutrition, respiratory failure and heart failure must be looked for.

Airway assessment, and assessment of the upper back for any planned regional technique must be done as a routine.

Pre-operative investigations

As per the National Institute for Health and Care Excellence (NICE) guidelines, thoracic surgery falls into the major grade of surgery.

A full blood count is done in all patients whilst renal function and an ECG are performed in patients who score greater than ASA Grade 2. Coagulation testing is recommended in patients on anticoagulants or those with coexisting liver or clotting disorders. In addition, a blood group and save and cross-matching may be required.

More specific tests are performed to assess respiratory function and imaging to assess the extent of disease and pulmonary pathology. Respiratory function is assessed using spirometry, arterial blood gases and the diffusing capacity of the lungs for carbon monoxide (DLCO).

Assessment of cardiopulmonary interaction

Cardiopulmonary interaction is assessed using cardiopulmonary exercise testing. This test is done in the laboratory by subjecting the patient to incremental exercise using a treadmill or bicycle, until the maximal predicted heart rate is reached, if symptoms do not limit the exercise. Patients scheduled for thoracic surgery have less complications when the VO_{2max} is >20ml/kg/min, whereas the risk of morbidity and mortality is high if VO_{2max} is <15ml/kg/min.

Alternatives to exercise testing have been demonstrated to have potential as replacement tests for a pre-thoracotomy assessment. The six-minute walk test (6MWT) shows an excellent correlation with VO_{2max} and requires little or no laboratory equipment. A 6MWT distance of <200m correlates to a VO_{2max} <15ml/kg/min and also correlates with a fall in oximetry (SpO_2) during exercise.

An algorithm based on lung function tests has been developed by the British Thoracic Society and American College of Chest Physicians (ACCP) to help decision-making with regards to proceeding with a lung resection (Table 24.3).

Table 24.3. Algorithm for the assessment of lung resection.

1) FEV_1 >1.5L (for lobectomy) and >2L (for pneumonectomy), proceed with the surgery

2) If FEV_1 <1.5L (for lobectomy) and <2L (for pneumonectomy), measure the ppo-FEV_1 and the ppo-DLCO

    If ppo-FEV_1 and ppo-DLCO are >40%, proceed with the surgery

3) If ppo-FEV_1 and ppo-DLCO are <40%, perform CPET

    If VO_{2max} from the CPET is >15ml/kg/min, proceed with the surgery

    If $VO_{2\ max}$ from the CPET is <15ml/kg/min, consider non-surgical options

CPET = cardiopulmonary exercise testing; DLCO = diffusing capacity of the lungs for carbon monoxide; FEV_1 = forced expired volume in first second; ppo = predicted postoperative.

Radiological investigations

- Chest X-rays (CXR) are useful to identify any lung collapse, consolidation, pleural effusion, pneumothorax, tracheobronchial tree abnormality and mediastinal masses, metastatic lesions, ribs and lungs.
- Computed tomography (CT) scans help in differentiating between benign and malignant diseases.
- Positron emission tomography (PET) scans are performed using 2-Deoxy-2-fluoro-D-glucose as a tracer to indicate the uptake of glucose by the tumour. A PET scan is valuable in assigning the 'T' stage for TNM classification.

Endoscopic procedures for diagnosis and staging

- Rigid and flexible bronchoscopy allow for visualisation of the tracheobronchial tree and also to obtain samples of tissue.

- Mediastinoscopy is performed for lymph node staging apart from other indications. N1 stage disease is suitable for surgery, N2 stage disease is controversial for surgery and N3 stage disease precludes surgery.
- Video-assisted thoracoscopic surgery (VATS).

The in-hospital mortality rate in the UK for lobectomy and pneumonectomy ranges between 2-4% and 6-8%, respectively. The British Thoracic Society and Society of Cardiothoracic Surgeons of Great Britain and Ireland recommend the assessment of respiratory function, cardiovascular fitness, performance status, nutritional status and age prior to undertaking lung resection to treat lung cancer.

Risk stratification

In 2007, using the data from the database, EPITHOR, from the French Society of Thoracic and Cardiovascular Surgery, THORACOSCORE was developed to predict in-hospital mortality after thoracic surgery. The various factors included in the THORACOSCORE are gender, age, ASA Class, priority of surgery, type of procedure, associated comorbidities, performance status and dyspnoea score. The performance status and dyspnoea score are described in Tables 24.4 and 24.5.

Table 24.4. Performance status: (World Health Organisation [WHO]).

Performance status	Description of the activity
0	Normally active
1	Cannot carry out heavy physical tasks
2	Is active more than 50% of the time
3	Is at rest more than 50% of the time
4	Is at rest 100% of the time

Table 24.5. Dyspnoea score: (Medical Research Council [MRC]).

Grade	Dyspnoea
0	No dyspnoea
1	Dyspnoea during strenuous exercise (2 flights of stairs)
2	Dyspnoea when hurrying or walking up a slight hill (1 flight of stairs)
3	Dyspnoea when walking at own pace (walking on level)
4	Dyspnoea after walking on level ground for a few minutes or 100m
5	Too dyspnoeic to leave the house, dyspnoea when dressing/undressing

Pre-operative interventions and premedication

Medications taken for coexisting medical conditions must be continued. Cessation of smoking, continuation of the use of bronchodilators and steroids in patients with chronic obstructive pulmonary disease (COPD) and asthma, institution of antibiotics to treat any chest infection, provision of physiotherapy, weight loss in obese patients and adequate nutrition for malnourished patients constitute the key pre-operative interventions.

Oral antacids in the form of H_2-blockers or proton pump inhibitors are prescribed if the patient has oesophageal reflux. Sedatives or analgesics as a routine premedication are avoided. However, short-acting intravenous sedatives and an antisialagogue (glycopyrrolate/atropine) can be administered in the operating theatre to facilitate insertion of lines and to dry the respiratory tract to both facilitate bronchoscopy and prevent atelectasis, respectively.

Anaesthesia for specific thoracic procedures

Thoracic surgical procedures involve procedures on the chest wall, tracheobronchial tree, pleura, lungs, diaphragm, oesophagus, great vessels and the mediastinal structures (Table 24.6).

Table 24.6. List of thoracic surgical procedures.

Tracheobronchial tree	Pleura	Lung
Rigid bronchoscopy	Pleural biopsy	Wedge resection
Removal of foreign body	Pleurodesis	Segmentectomy
Dilatation/insertion of tracheal stent	Decortication	Lobectomy
Tracheal repair and reconstruction	Pleurectomy	Sleeve resection
	Extended pleurectomy and decortication	Pneumonectomy
Endobronchial stents and coils		Bullectomy
Bronchoplasty (sleeve resection)		Lung volume reduction surgery (LVRS)
Repair of bronchopleural fistula		

Chest wall	Others
Insertion of chest drain	Oesophagectomy
Resection of chest wall tumours	Repair of tracheoesophageal fistula
Repair of chest wall/sternal deformity	Thoracic sympathectomy
	Surgery on thoracic aorta (aneurysm)
Diaphragmatic repair	Repair of ruptured oesophagus, diaphragm or tracheobronchial tree

Endoscopy or opening the chest wall (thoracotomy) enables the conduct of thoracic surgical procedures.

The tracheobronchial tree, mediastinum, oesophagus, and the thoracic cavity can be approached endoscopically for performing diagnostic and therapeutic procedures through bronchoscopy, mediastinoscopy, oesophagoscopy and thoracoscopy (video-assisted thoracoscopic procedures).

A brief account of surgical and anaesthetic considerations for these procedures is provided below.

Bronchoscopy

Bronchoscopy means inspection of the tracheobronchial tree. It can be performed using either a rigid or flexible scope.

Surgical considerations

A rigid bronchoscope is a stainless steel tube that is passed through the vocal cords. A flexible scope is passed through the rigid bronchoscope to inspect the lower tracheobronchial tree. Brushing, bronchoalveolar lavage, endobronchial biopsy and transbronchial biopsy procedures are facilitated by the flexible bronchoscope that is passed through the rigid bronchoscope

Following induction of anaesthesia, the surgeon passes the rigid bronchoscope through the mouth whilst guarding the upper teeth of the patient with their thumb, visualises the epiglottis and vocal cords through the scope and advances the scope into the trachea.

Anaesthetic considerations

An unprotected airway is at risk of aspiration. Premedication with omeprazole or ranitidine the night before and on the morning of the surgery helps in reducing gastric volume and acidity.

Problems related to a shared airway include maintenance of ventilation and anaesthetic. Intermittent insufflation through the side port of the bronchoscope and the use of jet ventilation are options to provide oxygenation. Total intravenous anaesthesia is used to maintain the anaesthetic. Boluses of propofol/midazolam and alfentanil with a short-acting muscle relaxant or target-controlled infusions of propofol and remifentanil can be used to maintain the anaesthetic and obtund the cardiovascular responses like hypertension. Lidocaine spray to the vocal cords can be useful but may impair the cough reflex postoperatively for a few hours. Suxamethonium with repeat doses or short-acting non-depolarising relaxants like mivacurium or rocuronium with reversal by sugammadex are a few options to achieve and maintain the required muscle paralysis for this highly stimulating procedure.

Airway injury, hypoxia, hypercapnia, bleeding and pneumothorax are potential complications of rigid bronchoscopy. However, these procedures can be done as day cases.

Cervical mediastinoscopy

Cervical mediastinoscopy means inspection of the mediastinal contents through the neck.

Surgical considerations

The thoracic inlet and diaphragm form the upper and lower limits of the mediastinum. An imaginary line passing through the lower border of T4 divides the mediastinum into the superior and inferior levels. The inferior mediastinum is further divided into the anterior, middle and posterior compartments. The great vessels, trachea, oesophagus, thoracic duct and the phrenic and vagus nerves lie in the superior mediastinum.

The anterior mediastinum accommodates the thymus gland and lymph nodes along with the sternopericardial ligaments. The pericardium, heart, great vessels and phrenic nerve are in the middle mediastinum, whilst the oesophagus, descending aorta, thoracic duct, azygos veins and lymph nodes are found in the posterior mediastinum.

Cervical mediastinoscopy allows sampling of paratracheal and pretracheal lymph nodes and obtaining a biopsy of tissue from tumours such as a sarcoid or lymphoma and examination of the middle mediastinum.

A right anterior mediastinoscopy via the second right intercostal space, parasternally, allows assessment of the right mediastinum, SVC and right hilum. A mediastinotomy is performed for accessing large anterior mediastinal masses. About a 1.5cm-length transcervical incision is made one fingerbreadth above the suprasternal notch for cervical mediastinoscopy. A parasternal incision is made in the second right intercostal space, for a right anterior mediastinoscopy. A mediastinoscope is passed along the anterior aspect of the trachea after dissection of the pretracheal fascia and retraction of the strap muscles. Visualisation of mediastinal structures through the scope and sampling of the tissue with the help of instruments passed through the scope constitute the procedure.

Anaesthetic considerations

Any SVC obstruction, tracheal deviation or compression must be ruled out pre-operatively. General anaesthesia with tracheal intubation using a single-lumen cuffed endotracheal tube and positive pressure ventilation is common practice.

Standard monitoring including pulse oximetry, ECG and non-invasive blood pressure (NIBP) monitoring are used.

A pulse oximeter is placed on the right hand and an NIBP cuff is applied to the left arm. Compression of the brachiocephalic artery can compromise perfusion to the right arm and brain. Pulse oximetry on the right hand allows for monitoring of the perfusion of the fingers on the right arm. NIBP measurements from the left arm remain unaffected.

A second cannula is secured in the leg after induction of general anaesthesia. A potential for massive haemorrhage from the neck vessels may need a median sternotomy. Cannulation of a vein in the lower limb (in the territory of the inferior vena cava) helps in resuscitation. Boluses of fentanyl are usually sufficient for intra-operative analgesia. Local infiltration of the incision, paracetamol and NSAIDs are used to offer postoperative analgesia. Most of these patients are suitable for same-day discharge.

Oesophagoscopy

This involves inspection of the oesophagus.

Surgical considerations

Oesophagoscopy is performed for diagnostic and therapeutic indications. Removal of foreign bodies, diagnosis of a stricture and haematemesis are a few indications. Rigid oesophagoscopy requires a general anaesthetic whereas flexible oesophagoscopy can be performed under sedation.

Following induction and intubation of the trachea, the rigid oesophagoscope is passed under direct vision into the oropharynx and upper oesophagus. The rigid scope allows larger instruments and insertion of stents through it, in contrast to the flexible scope.

Anaesthetic considerations

General anaesthetic with endotracheal intubation with an SLT and positive pressure ventilation remains common practice. Performing a rapid sequence induction can avert the risk of aspiration in cases of gastro-oesophageal reflux disease. Care should be taken to avoid any airway obstruction and disconnection of the breathing system during the procedure.

Thoracoscopy and VATS

Thoracoscopy means inspection of the thoracic cavity. VATS is video-assisted thoracoscopy and surgery.

Surgical considerations

The lateral decubitus position, with the back of the patient parallel and close to the edge of the table supported by rolls or tape, is used for VATS procedures. The upper arm is positioned in an arm-rest and the lower arm is flexed and positioned in front of the head. In order to open up the intercostal spaces, a table break position is achieved using a slight head-down tilt and feet-down tilt.

The following incisions are required for port sites:

- For the camera: a 0.5-1cm incision at the midaxillary line in the 7th or 8th intercostal space.
- For the working port: a 3-5cm incision along the inframammary crease in the 5th or 6th intercostal space. Additional incisions for extra ports may be placed posteriorly or in the axilla. Single-port VATS surgery is gaining popularity.

A 30° or 45° angled or flexible scope is passed through the camera port to gain a panoramic view of the interior of the hemithorax. A working port is used to pass forceps, scissors, suction, dissection instruments, stapling devices and other instruments to carry out the video-assisted thoracoscopic surgery. A specimen pouch is used to extract the resected

---

Table 24.7. Procedures performed through VATS.

- Drainage of pleural effusions.
- Biopsy of pleura and lung.
- Pleurectomy.
- Pleurodesis.
- Pericardial window/biopsy.
- Resection of lung: wedge resection, segmentectomy and lobectomy.
- Thymectomy.
- Thoracic sympathectomy.

tissue at the end of the procedure. The pulmonary vein and artery, and the bronchus of the corresponding lung lobe or segment, are mobilised, stapled and divided. A specimen is removed using a pouch, intercostal drains (apical/basal) are placed and the incision sites are closed. VATS is performed for many procedures, which were done via a thoracotomy in the past (Table 24.7).

Anaesthetic considerations

Assessment of these patients should be as for a thoracotomy. The management options for postoperative analgesia should be made clear to the patient and consent must be obtained for any planned regional (intercostal/paravertebral/epidural) technique.

A balanced general anaesthetic and positive pressure ventilation with a DLT or an endobronchial blocker to collapse the lung on the operated side is common practice.

The surgeon performs a rigid/flexible bronchoscopy, following the induction of general anaesthesia. This informs the anaesthetist about any intraluminal pathology and calibre of the proximal tracheobronchial tree. Anaesthesia at this point is maintained with intravenous agents (propofol and opiates using either boluses or a continuous infusion). Following completion of bronchoscopy, a DLT is inserted to intubate the main bronchus of the lung that will be ventilated (dependent lung, non-operated lung) or a bronchial blocker is inserted into the main bronchus of the lung that will be collapsed (non-dependent, operated lung). Anaesthesia is maintained using oxygen, air and a volatile anaesthetic agent or using total intravenous anaesthesia.

If the patient has a chest drain, chest drain removal is done only after the lung on that side is collapsed so as to prevent an inadvertent iatrogenic pneumothorax. Complete collapse of the lung that is being operated on provides good surgical access for the surgeon. The principles of one-lung anaesthesia and management of hypoxia as discussed earlier in the previous section must be applied.

A regional anaesthetic would reduce the need for postoperative opiates and enhance postoperative recovery. Postoperatively, a CXR should be performed to confirm re-expansion of the lung. Supplemental oxygen and good analgesia should be ensured.

The surgeon, at the end of the VATS procedure, under direct vision, can insert a paravertebral catheter into the paravertebral space.

A local anaesthetic bolus and infusion through the paravertebral catheter provides good postoperative pain relief. The technique has less complications and side effects in comparison to a thoracic epidural and is gaining popularity.

Thoracotomy

This involves an incision between the ribs and access to the thoracic cavity, and is commonly performed for lung resection, repair of a bronchopleural fistula and decortication of the lung.

Surgical considerations

Following induction of anaesthesia, the patient is positioned in the lateral decubitus position with the operating side being uppermost. A curvilinear incision is made extending from the anterior axillary line to a point midway between the medial border of the scapula and the spinous processes, passing 3-4cm below the tip of the scapula. The latissimus dorsi and serratus muscles are divided to enter the chest cavity. A lateral muscle-sparing (preserves latissimus dorsi), French and axillary incisions are other alternate incisions.

Lung resections range from obtaining a sample tissue for biopsy to removal of part of the lung or the whole lung. Types of lung resection are as follows:

- Lobectomy — removal of a single lobe.
- Sublobar resection — non-anatomical (wedge resection) and anatomical (segmentectomy).

- Sleeve resection — removal of a lobe with the bronchus (bronchoplasty).
- Pneumonectomy — removal of the whole lung.

Anaesthetic considerations

A thorough pre-operative assessment, optimisation and risk stratification should take place pre-operatively. Lung cancer is the most common indication. Non-small cell cancers are amenable for surgery, whereas small cell cancers are not. Be aware of any paraneoplastic syndromes and resulting endocrine/metabolic disturbance.

Any airway difficulty or difficulty in DLT insertion should be anticipated and a strategy must be in place to troubleshoot considering the use of a videolaryngoscope, fibreoptic bronchoscope, rigid bronchoscope and bronchial blocker as part of this strategy. Ensure that a group and save is done and two units of cross-matched compatible red cells are available.

Options for postoperative analgesia include a thoracic epidural, paravertebral block or intrathecal opiates. These techniques should be discussed with the patient and consent obtained. Although thoracic epidural analgesia is considered as the gold standard for pain relief following a thoracotomy, paravertebral analgesia is gaining popularity because of a better side effect profile and comparable pain relief. A sample regimen for an epidural involves a test dose of 3ml 0.5% levobupivacaine followed by 0.1ml/kg of 0.25% levobupivacaine to establish the block. A continuous infusion (0.1% levobupivacaine and 2-5μg/ml fentanyl) can be started at 0.1ml/kg/h. In the elderly, the dose needs to be reduced as they exhibit an increased epidural spread.

A large-bore peripheral venous cannula should be placed in the hand or forearm on the operated non-dependent side. An arterial line is placed in the dependent arm. A central venous catheter (CVC) is not routinely used but if required it should be inserted on the same side as the thoracotomy.

A balanced general anaesthesia with muscle relaxation, positive pressure ventilation and one-lung ventilation in combination with a regional anaesthetic (thoracic epidural or paravertebral) is a common technique. A left-sided DLT offers a higher margin of safety and can be used for surgeries not involving the left main bronchus.

Both the lumens of the DLT should be sucked and re-expansion of the collapsed lung ensured prior to closing of the chest. A 'leak' test is done on the bronchial suture line through manual inflation of the lung to 40cm H_2O.

The ability to follow commands, the return of airway protective reflexes, adequate reversal of neuromuscular blockade, adequate pain control, normothermia, haemodynamic stability and normal electrolyte values allow successful extubation at the end of the surgery.

Extubation of patients whenever possible at the end of the surgery aids in good recovery. The need for postoperative ventilation in these patients increases pulmonary morbidity through stressing the suture lines and causing a risk of air leaks and chest infections.

Although extubation at the end of the surgery is encouraged, some patients may require postoperative ventilatory support. Factors that may predispose to prolonged postoperative oxygen supplementation include age above 70 years, the presence of fibrotic lung disease, poor pre-operative lung function, surgery lasting more than 4 hours and a PaO_2 of <8kPa. Meticulous fluid balance and the avoidance of excessive IV fluid therapy reduces peri-operative pulmonary morbidity.

Bronchopleural fistula

A bronchopleural fistula is a communication between the bronchus and the pleural space resulting in a persistent air leak.

Surgical considerations

Large-bore chest drain insertion, opting for reduced tidal volumes, a lower inspiratory pressure and PEEP, permissive hypercapnia and permissive hypoxaemia constitute the principles of conservative management of a bronchopleural fistula.

Thoracoplasty, lung resection and stapling, pleural abrasion and decortication are surgical procedures for refractory cases of bronchopleural fistula.

Anaesthetic considerations

Lung collapse, loss of delivered tidal volume and the inability to apply PEEP are the main problems with a large fistula in a ventilated patient. A bronchopleural fistula is an absolute indication for lung isolation. Lung isolation becomes essential to generate the tidal volumes necessary to maintain oxygenation and ventilation through the application of positive pressure ventilation to the normal lung.

Empyema and decortication

Empyema is defined as pus in the pleural space.

Surgical considerations

Rib resection and drainage and decortication are the two common surgeries that are performed to treat empyema. Rib resection and drainage is a simpler option and can be performed under general anaesthesia with an SLT or under regional anaesthesia if general anaesthesia carries a high risk. Decortication involves peeling off parietal pleura and this procedure can cause significant bleeding and air leaks.

Anaesthetic considerations

The key considerations are whether there is any air leak, whether the lung isolation facilitates the operation and how to provide pain relief.

A DLT is preferred over a bronchial blocker in order to clear the pus from the airways through suction. Gas induction, an awake fibreoptic intubation and a rapid sequence induction (RSI) are used to achieve lung isolation (to prevent soiling of the healthy lung). RSI is the most commonly used approach.

Surgical access is improved with a collapsed lung. The lung may not collapse in empyema due to adhesions. A collapsed lung contributes to shunt and worsens any pre-existing hypoxaemia. The option of two-lung ventilation can be discussed with the surgeon and instituted with the surgeon's acceptance.

An intercostal block and patient-controlled analgesia, a paravertebral catheter and patient-controlled analgesia and thoracic epidural anaesthesia can be considered for the provision of pain relief. Patients with empyema are likely to have systemic sepsis. Although a thoracic epidural is seen as the gold standard for pain relief in thoracotomy, a risk benefit analysis should inform decision-making.

Postoperative care for thoracic surgery patients

Oxygen supplementation should be provided using humidified oxygen to maintain the peripheral oxygen saturation above 96%.

A multimodal postoperative analgesic regimen can be chosen using a combination of the following techniques:

- Oral analgesics — paracetamol, NSAIDs and opiates.
- Systemic opiates — patient-controlled analgesia.
- Intercostal block.
- Paravertebral block
- Interpleural block.
- Thoracic epidural analgesia.
- Intrathecal opiates.

In addition to routine postoperative care, additional attention should be given to the following aspects of postoperative management.

Fluid balance

Administration of IV fluids is limited postoperatively in this group of patients with a view to prevent complications such as acute lung injury secondary to excessive fluid administration. Hartmann's solution at 1ml/kg/hr, with an upper limit of 70ml/hr, is a commonly used postoperative fluid regime.

Physiotherapy and mobilisation

Chest physiotherapy provided by the physiotherapy team helps in early mobilisation and in turn reduces the risk of atelectasis and postoperative hypoxaemia. Apart from incentive spirometry, therapy with bronchodilators and mucolytics help in the clearance of lower airway secretions. A mini-tracheostomy and institution of CPAP/BPAP are used as preventative measures for postoperative atelectasis and hypoxaemia.

Chest drainage

Chest drainage with an underwater seal and suction allows re-expansion of the lung postoperatively.

Antibiotics

Antibiotics are administered for surgical prophylaxis and for treating any chest infection as per the local institutional policy.

The following are possible complications in the postoperative period:

- Respiratory complications include atelectasis, pneumothorax, pulmonary haemorrhage and bleeding into the airways and the formation of a bronchopleural fistula.
- Cardiac complications include arrhythmias (atrial fibrillation after pneumonectomy), low cardiac output syndrome, right heart failure and cardiac herniation, particularly after a pneumonectomy.
- Neurologic injuries can also occur in the form of peripheral nerve injury from surgery, and or retraction, positioning from stretching and/or by pressure.

Case scenario 1

A 58-year-old man is scheduled to have a left upper lobectomy for a bronchial tumour. His pre-operative FEV_1 is 1.2L. He has a background history of smoking 30 cigarettes a day for 35 years and also is being treated for hypertension.

Would you proceed with the surgery?

An FEV_1 of >1.5L would be considered acceptable to undergo a lobectomy. In this case it would be better to have a quantitative lung scan to find out about the percentage predicted postoperative (% ppo) FEV_1 and % ppo transfer factor for carbon monoxide (TLCO). Values >40% for % ppo-FEV_1 and % ppo-TLCO indicate the patient's suitability for surgery.

His % ppo-FEV_1 and % ppo-TLCO results come back as less then 30%.

What would you do?

This patient will have to undergo exercise testing to find out his VO_{2max}. It is acceptable to proceed with the surgical option if the VO_{2max} is >15ml/kg/min.

This patient has an increased risk of respiratory morbidity. He has a ppo-FEV_1 of less than 40%. In the postoperative period, he needs respiratory support in the intensive care unit and a staged extubation should be performed. Postoperative pain should be managed using a multimodal analgesic approach that includes a combination of a thoracic epidural or paravertebral analgesia along with regular paracetamol and NSAIDs.

Case scenario 2

A 45-year-old woman is scheduled for a right-sided lobectomy. She has been stable intra-operatively from a haemodynamic and ventilatory point of view with an SpO_2 of 96%, an acceptable blood gas on FiO_2 of 0.6, with the right lung collapsed and left lung ventilated. Despite increasing FiO_2 to 100%, the saturation is now 87%.

What would you do next?

Check the monitoring equipment for disconnection and immediately check the tube position with a fibreoptic bronchoscope for displacement and malposition. Any secretions and blood should be suctioned and cleared and the ventilator parameters reassessed.

After increasing the FiO_2 to 100% and clearing the secretions, the oxygen saturation has increased to 91%.

What would be your next plan of action?

Continue with one-lung ventilation, but in order to improve oxygenation, measures should be taken to optimise ventilation and perfusion.

In order to optimise ventilation, the plan would be to do a manual re-expansion recruitment manoeuvre or PEEP on the ventilated lung, followed by CPAP on the non-ventilated lung if oxygenation is not improving.

If there is still no improvement, inhaled nitric oxide or prostaglandin I_2 (PGI_2) can be used to improve perfusion. As a final measure, following discussion with the surgeon, intermittent two-lung ventilation can be considered.

Further reading

1. Slinger PD, Johnston MR. Preoperative assessment: an anesthesiologist's perspective. *Thorac Surg Clin* 2005; 15: 11-25.

2. Campos JH. An update on bronchial blockers during lung separation techniques in adults. *Anesth Analg* 2003; 97: 1266-74.

3. Anesthesia for thoracic surgery. In: Barash PG, Cullen BF, Steolting RK, Cahalan MK, Eds. *Clinical Anesthesia*, 6th ed. Lippincott Williams & Wilkins, 2009.

4. Slinger P, Ed. *Principles and Practice of Anesthesia for Thoracic Surgical Procedures*. Springer, 2011.

5. Falcoz PE, Conti M, Brouchet L, *et al*. The Thoracic Surgery Scoring System (Thoracoscore): risk model for in-hospital death in 15,183 patients requiring thoracic surgery. *J Thorac Cardiovasc Surg* 2007; 133: 325-32.

6. Lim E, Baldwin D, Beckles M, *et al*. Guidelines on the radical management of patients with lung cancer. British Thoracic Society and the Society for Cardiothoracic Surgery in Great Britain and Ireland. *Thorax* 2010; 65(iii): 1-27.

7. Gould G, Pearce A. Assessment of suitability for lung resection. *Br J Anaesth CEACCP* 2006; 6: 97-100.

8. Paramasivam E, Bodenham A. Air leaks, pneumothorax, and chest drains. *Br J Anaesth CEACCP* 2008; 8: 204-9.

9. Ng A, Swanevelder J. Hypoxaemia during one-lung anaesthesia. *Br J Anaesth CEACCP* 2010; 10: 117-22.

25 Cardiac procedures

Narotham R. Burri

Introduction

Cardiac surgery involves procedures that are performed on the surface of the heart, on great vessels (closed heart procedures) and within the cavities of the heart (open heart procedures). A coronary artery bypass graft (CABG) and repair of an aortic dissection are examples of closed heart procedures. Replacement or repair of a valve is an example of an open heart surgery procedure. Planning and provision of a safe and appropriate anaesthetic for these surgeries requires knowledge of the background pathophysiology, surgery planned and the functional status of the patient. Cardiac procedures differ from other surgeries peri-operatively because of the requirement of a third dimension in the form of cardiopulmonary bypass (CPB) in addition to anaesthetic and surgery. The principles of provision of cardiac anaesthesia are covered under the following headings:

- Physiological considerations.
- Pre-operative work-up for cardiac surgery.
- Conduct of anaesthetic for routine cardiac surgery and CPB.
- Routine postoperative care.
- Anaesthesia for specific cardiac procedures:
    - coronary artery bypass grafting (CABG);
    - aortic valve surgery;
    - mitral valve surgery;
    - aortic surgery;
    - pericardectomy;
    - redo heart surgery.

Physiological considerations

Physiological goals are set during a cardiac anaesthetic for a given cardiac condition targeting preload, afterload, contractility, rate and rhythm in order to achieve an adequate cardiac output (CO) in the context of an existing cardiac pathophysiology. A brief description of these physiological variables is provided below.

Preload

Preload is the stretching of cardiac ventricular muscle at end-diastole, i.e. just before the initiation of ventricular contraction. Left ventricular end-diastolic volume is representative of left ventricular preload. The Frank Starling Law states that an increase in preload increases cardiac output, up to a certain point.

Preload is assessed by measuring central venous pressure (CVP), pulmonary capillary wedge pressure (PCWP), transthoracic echocardiography (TTE), transoesophageal echocardiography (TOE) and direct examination of the heart during surgery. Factors that influence preload are left ventricular compliance, circulating blood volume, the presence of atrial systole and length of the diastole.

Afterload

Afterload is the tension generated by the left ventricle during contraction. Left ventricular end-systolic pressure is representative of left ventricular afterload. Measurement of systemic vascular resistance (SVR) through a pulmonary artery catheter (PAc) is indicative of afterload. Factors influencing afterload are SVR, area of aortic valve and left ventricular outflow tract, and left ventricular wall stress.

Contractility

Contractility is the ability of the cardiac muscle to contract at a given preload and afterload. Assessment of contractility is done by TTE, TOE and direct examination of the heart during surgery. Factors that increase or decrease contractility are as follows:

- Autonomic nervous system: ↑ by sympathetic stimulation, ↓ by parasympathetic stimulation.
- Drugs: ↑ by inotropes, ↓ by beta-blockers.
- Local metabolites: ↓ by hydrogen ions, hypercapnia and hypoxia.
- Bowditch effect: ↑ contractility with ↑ heart rate (HR) (force-frequency effect).

Cardiac output, blood pressure and systemic vascular resistance relationship

BP = CO x SVR and CO = SV x HR
BP = blood pressure, CO = cardiac output (normal: 4-6L/min)
SVR = systemic vascular resistance (normal: 1500-2500 $dyne.s.cm^{-5}$)
SV = stroke volume (normal: 60-100ml), HR = heart rate

Stroke volume is determined by preload, afterload and contractility of the heart.

Pre-operative work-up for cardiac surgery

History, examination and investigations

History

Exploration into the onset and progress of the presenting condition that requires surgery, along with probing and review of the case notes for any additional risk factors, forms the core of history taking (Table 25.1). Chest pain (angina), shortness of breath (dyspnoea) and episodes of fainting attacks (syncope) constitute the main symptoms of cardiac disease. The severity of angina is graded using the Canadian Cardiovascular Society (CCS) classification (Table 25.2) and dyspnoea is graded using the New York Heart Association (NYHA) classification (see Table 25.5 later on in the chapter).

Table 25.1. Factors contributing to a higher risk for cardiac surgery.

- Hypertension.
- Diabetes mellitus.
- Renal insufficiency.
- COPD.
- Cardiac failure.
- Previous cardiac surgery.
- Neurological disease.
- Body mass index <20 or >35kg/m^{-2}.
- Peripheral vascular disease.
- Acute coronary syndrome.

Table 25.2. Canadian Cardiovascular Society classification of angina.

CCS class	Association with ordinary physical activity	Description
CCS I	Unaffected	Walking or climbing stairs does not cause angina Exertion causes angina
CCS II	Slight limitation	Walking >2 blocks, climbing >1 flight of stairs causes angina
CCS III	Marked limitation	Walking 1-2 blocks, climbing 1 flight of stairs causes angina
CCS IV	Angina at rest	Inability to carry out any physical activity without discomfort

CCS = Canadian Cardiovascular Society.

Examination

A minimum set of examinations is listed below which is not exhaustive:

- Cardiovascular system: palpate the central and peripheral pulses, assess the jugular venous pressure (JVP), heart rate and rhythm, auscultate the heart sounds and any murmurs, and measure the blood pressure.
- Peripheries: check the lower limbs for varicosities and pedal oedema.
- Respiratory system: obtain the respiratory rate and auscultate the lung fields.
- Abdomen: look for any distension, hepatomegaly and ascites.
- Nervous system: check for any disease or deficit (transient ischaemic attack/stroke) and document.
- Airway: assess mouth opening, dentition, and neck and jaw movements.
- Note the height, weight and BMI. The body surface area is obtained from a nomogram and this is required to calculate the appropriate flow by the pump during bypass.

Investigations

Routine tests
- Full blood count.
- Coagulation.
- Blood group and cross-match.
- Blood urea, creatinine and electrolytes.
- Liver function tests.

Specific tests and the information obtained
- CXR: detects cardiomegaly, gross pathology and proximity of the heart to the sternum in redo surgeries.
- ECG: diagnosis of ischaemia, pericarditis, rhythm and conduction disturbances.
- TTE: provides qualitative and quantitative assessment of cardiac structure and function. Calculation of the ejection fraction (EF) allows quantification of left ventricular systolic function (Table 25.3).

Table 25.3. Left ventricular systolic function and ejection fraction.

Left ventricular function	Ejection fraction
Normal	>55%
Mild impairment	45-54%
Moderate impairment	36-44%
Severe impairment	≤35%

- TOE: provides qualitative and quantitative assessment of cardiac structure and function. TOE provides more detailed evaluation of mitral valve and thoracic aortic disease (aneurysm/dissection) and has become an expected standard of monitoring peri-operatively for most cardiac surgeries.
- Coronary angiography: determines the presence, location, severity of the coronary artery disease and suitability for CABG. Left heart catheterisation, ventriculography and aortography can be done at the same time (Table 25.4).
- Stress testing (echo/nuclear): differentiates between myocardial stunning and hibernation. The former is amenable for revascularisation and the latter is not. Stress testing identifies viable myocardium.
- Cardiac/thoracic CT scan: indicated in thoracic aortic disease, coronary artery disease and cardiac masses.
- Cardiac/thoracic MRI: evaluates cardiac function. MRI is the most sensitive examination for the assessment of myocardial viability and thoracic aortic disease.
- Pulmonary function tests: spirometry and diffusion capacity assess lung function and help in quantifying the lung disease. COPD adds to the risk.
- Ultrasonography of the carotid arteries: examination of the carotid arteries for any stenosis. Extra cardiac arteriopathy adds to the risk for cardiac surgery.

Table 25.4. Haemodynamic values obtained from left and right heart catheterisation.

Parameter	Measurement	Normal value
Systemic arterial pressure	Systolic/diastolic (mean)	100/60-140/90mmHg (70-105mmHg)
LV pressure	Systolic/end diastolic	100-140/12mmHg
Ra pressure		2-6mmHg
RV pressure	Systolic/end diastolic	25/2mmHg
Pulmonary arterial pressure	Systolic/diastolic (mean)	25/12(16)mmHg
PA wedge pressure	Mean	6-12mmHg
Cardiac Index	Range	2.5-4.2L/min/m^2
Systemic vascular resistance (SVR)	Range	800-1200 dyne/s/cm^5
Pulmonary vascular resistance (PVR)	Range	100-200 dyne/s/cm^5

Assessment of functional status

Functional capacity of patients presenting for cardiac surgery is expressed in terms of the New York Heart Association classification (Table 25.5) or in METs (metabolic equivalents of tasks) as in the Duke Activity Status Index (Table 25.6). NYHA class along with the disease severity guides the indications for surgery provided by the American Heart Association (AHA).

Table 25.5. Functional capacity — NYHA classification.

NYHA class	Cardiac disease and affect on OPA	Description
NYHA I	Unaffected	No fatigue, palpitations, dyspnoea or angina with OPA
NYHA II	Slight limitation of OPA	OPA results in fatigue, palpitations, dyspnoea or angina
NYHA III	Marked limitation of OPA	Less than OPA results in fatigue, palpitations, dyspnoea or angina
NYHA IV	Symptoms at rest	Fatigue, palpitations, dyspnoea or angina at rest

NYHA = New York Heart Association; OPA = ordinary physical activity.

Table 25.6. Duke Activity Status Index.

Activity status	Example activity	METs
Poor	Able to walk indoors, take care of self, light work around the house	<4
Intermediate	Able to walk 1 or 2 blocks, do moderate work, play golf or doubles tennis	4-7
Good	Able to run short distance, heavy work, singles tennis	>7

One MET (metabolic equivalent of task) = 3.5ml/kg/min of oxygen consumption by the body.

Risk stratification

Risk stratification is provided by the EuroSCORE tool, an additive model of risk, where the sum of the points for risk factors equals the predicted mortality in percentage. Points are allotted to patient-related, cardiac-related and operation-related factors (Table 25.7).

Table 25.7. European system for cardiac operative risk evaluation (EuroSCORE).
From: Nashef SA, Roques F, Michel P, et al. Eur J Cardiothorac Surg 1999; 16: 9-13.

Factors	Comments	Points
Patient-related factors		
1 Age	Per 5 years or part thereof over 60.	1
2 Sex	Female.	1
3 Chronic obstructive pulmonary disease	Long-term use of bronchodilators/steroids for lung disease.	1
4 Extra cardiac arteriopathy	Any one or more of claudication, carotid occlusion >50% stenosis. Previous or planned intervention involving the abdominal aorta, limb arteries or carotids.	2
5 Neurologic dysfunction	Severely affecting ambulation or day-to-day functioning.	2
6 Serum creatinine	> 200µmol/L pre-operatively.	2
7 Previous cardiac surgery	Requiring opening of the pericardium.	3
8 Active endocarditis	Patient still under antibiotic treatment for endocarditis at the time of surgery.	3
9 Critical pre-operative state	Any one or more of the following: VT/VF/aborted sudden death, pre-operative cardiac massage, pre-operative ventilation before arrival in anaesthetic room, pre-operative inotropic support, IABP or pre-operative acute renal failure (anuria or oliguria <10ml/h).	3

Continued

Table 25.7 *continued*. European system for cardiac operative risk evaluation (EuroSCORE). *From: Nashef SA, Roques F, Michel P, et al. Eur J Cardiothorac Surg 1999; 16: 9-13.*

Factors	Comments	Points
Cardiac-related factors		
1 Unstable angina	Rest angina requiring IV nitrates until arrival in anaesthetic room.	2
2 LV dysfunction	Moderate or LVEF 30-50%.	1
	Poor or LVEF <30%.	3
3 Recent infarct	(<90 days).	2
4 Pulmonary hypertension	Systolic PA pressure >60mmHg.	2
Operation-related factors		
1 Emergency	Carried out on referral before the beginning of the next working day.	2
2 Other than isolated CABG	Major cardiac procedure other than or in addition to CABG.	2
3 Surgery on thoracic aorta	For a disorder of the ascending or descending aorta or the aortic arch.	3
4 Post-infarct septal repair		4

LV = left ventricle; PA = pulmonary artery; LVEF = left ventricular ejection fraction; CABG = coronary artery bypass grafting; VT = ventricular tachycardia; VF = ventricular fibrillation.

Advice regarding the patient's regular medications

Cardiac patients are not uncommonly on multiple medications and require review before the surgery (Table 25.8).

Table 25.8. Pre-operative medications and management.

Medication	Management
Antihypertensives	Continue till the morning of surgery Hold ACE inhibitors and ARBs on the morning of surgery Hold diuretics on the morning of surgery
Anti-anginal	Continue to the morning of surgery
Antiplatelets	Aspirin: variable, stop for 5 days pre-operatively Clopidogrel: stop for 5-7 days pre-operatively GPIIb/IIIa inhibitors: stop for one half life of the drug
Anticoagulants	Warfarin: stop for 4 days pre-operatively Dabigatran: stop for 24 hours pre-operatively LMWH (enoxaparin): stop 12-24 hours pre-operatively Heparin infusion: stop 4 hours pre-operatively
Hypoglycaemics	Omit oral hypoglycaemics (biguanide: metformin) on the morning of surgery

ACE = angiotensin converting enzyme; ARB = angiotensin receptor blocker; GPIIb/IIIa = glycoprotein IIb/IIIa; LMWH = low-molecular-weight heparin.

Conduct of anaesthesia for routine cardiac surgery and cardiopulmonary bypass

Premedication

Premedication remains a common practice in cardiac anaesthesia. The rationale is to reduce anxiety, and prevent tachycardia and hypertension, so as to minimise the risk of cardiac ischaemia. Commonly used premedicants are benzodiazepines, antacids, alpha-2-agonists, antisialogogues and opiates. Oral temazepam 10-20mg or lorazepam 2-4mg and omeprazole 20mg, 1-2 hours prior to induction, or intramuscular morphine 0.2-0.3mg/kg with 200-400μg hyoscine, 1 hour prior to induction, along with administration of oxygen, are example regimes.

Preparation prior to commencing anaesthetic

Ensure there is availability of the necessary equipment and drugs. Draw up the anaesthetic drugs, inotropes, vasopressors, and heparin. Make sure that the surgeon, perfusionist and nursing staff are present. Conditions such as a tight left main stem stenosis, critical/severe aortic or mitral stenosis and severely impaired LV function or cardiogenic shock pose a higher risk of decompensation and warrant the presence of the surgeon during induction.

Induction

- Transfer premedicated patients with oxygen supplementation to the operating theatre.
- Perform a team brief and WHO surgical safety checks prior to induction.
- Establish pulse oximetry and a 12-lead ECG (lead II and V5 display).
- Gain large-bore (14G/16G) peripheral venous access under LA.
- Cannulate the radial artery under LA. Avoid the radial artery if it is to be harvested for grafting. Bilateral radial arterial cannulations may be done in surgery for dissection of the aorta to determine pre-ductal and post-ductal arterial pressures.
- Establish a depth of anaesthesia monitor, if available.
- Unconsciousness, analgesia and muscle relaxation constitute the triad of a balanced general anaesthetic and the triad is achieved through the use of a combination of an induction agent, opiate and non-depolarising muscle relaxant, respectively. A combination of propofol, fentanyl and rocuronium to achieve a balanced anaesthetic is a commonly used regime and there are several alternative medications. Institution of CPB necessitates endotracheal intubation and ventilation of these patients.

Post-induction and maintenance

Post-induction events

- Intubate the trachea and fix the endotracheal tube to the corner of the mouth.
- Commence IPPV with a tidal volume of 6-8ml/kg, FiO_2 of 0.6 in air and avoid N_2O.
- Maintain anaesthesia using a volatile agent or intravenous agent (TIVA). Isoflurane and propofol are common choices for maintenance.
- Secure additional venous access/invasive monitoring. Insert a central venous catheter (CVC) under ultrasound guidance. The practice of using a pulmonary artery flotation catheter is declining but a sheath can be inserted alongside the CVC to have an additional line for volume infusion or to float a PAc, if necessary.
- Administer antibiotic prophylaxis and perform urinary catheterisation.
- Establish temperature monitoring via a nasopharyngeal probe.
- Protect pressure points through adequate padding.
- Insert a transoesophageal echocardiography (TOE) probe.
- Transfer the patient from the anaesthetic room into the operating theatre carefully, paying attention to the lines to avoid any accidental avulsions.
- Reconnect to the ventilator on arrival to the operating room.
- Re-establish pulse oximetry, capnography, ECG and invasive monitoring.
- Perform a baseline ABG and activated clotting time (ACT).
- Check the patency of venous access and maintain the anaesthetic.

Maintenance

- Volatile agents at a concentration of 0.5-1 minimum alveolar concentration (MAC) or a propofol infusion either by an infusion at a rate of 3-4mg/kg/hr or by a target-controlled infusion to deliver a target site concentration of 1.5-3µg/ml are the available options to maintain anaesthesia following induction and whilst on CPB. However, the measurement of end-tidal concentration of volatile agents or MAC is not possible currently whilst on CPB.
- Anaesthetic preconditioning may confer some cardioprotection with the use of volatiles for maintenance.

- Anaesthetic and surgical stimuli at certain stages (laryngoscopy, tracheal intubation, skin incision, sternotomy) can trigger the sympathetic system or parasympathetic system (sternal retraction, sternal elevation, pericardial stretch), leading to undesirable haemodynamic consequences such as an increase in heart rate and systemic vascular resistance or a decrease in heart rate or asystole, respectively. Titrated doses of opiate, an adequate depth of anaesthetic and the judicious use of vasopressors address these problems.

A median sternotomy via a skin incision extending from three fingerbreadths below the suprasternal notch to the tip of the xiphisternum is performed using a sternal saw. The surgeon may request to stop ventilation briefly during this sternal split to prevent damage to the pericardium and pleura. Following systemic heparinisation, the surgeon cannulates the aorta first and the right atrium or bicaval cannulation, next. Arterial hypertension should be avoided by maintaining the systolic pressure at <100mmHg at the time of aortic cannulation to prevent aortic dissection. The aortic and venous cannulae are then connected to the arterial and venous pipes of the CPB circuit.

Cardiopulmonary bypass: equipment, conduct and management

Cardiopulmonary bypass provides cardiac surgeons with a still and bloodless surgical field to perform complex surgeries on the surface of the heart or within the heart chambers. The perfusionist remains in charge of CPB and conducts the bypass maintaining close communication with the cardiac surgeon and the anaesthetist throughout the procedure.

Brief details of the CPB equipment are provided below, followed by the conduct of the CPB.

Equipment

CPB consists of an extracorporeal circuit with a venous reservoir, an oxygenator and pump (Figure 25.1). A polyvinylchloride (PVC) tubing of varying diameter interconnects all these components. The venous pipe drains venous blood from the right heart or a systemic vein into the venous reservoir and the mechanical pump pumps this venous blood into an oxygenator and heat exchanger, returning the oxygenated blood via the arterial pipe into the systemic artery (ascending aorta commonly).

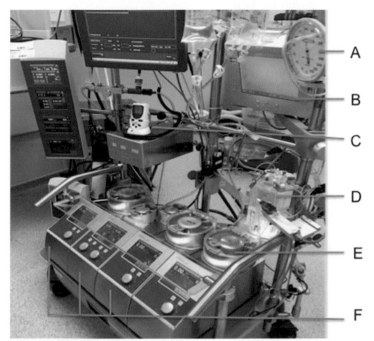

Figure 25.1. Cardiopulmonary bypass circuit. A) Arterial line pressure gauge; B) Monitor of in-line analyzer; C) Oxygen analyzer; D) Venous reservoir; E) Arterial pump; F) Pumps for suction, cardioplegia and venting.

Components of the CPB circuit

Arterial (aortic), venous and cardioplegia cannulae
The size of the arterial cannula depends on the vessel cannulated and ranges from a 15.6- to 24-French gauge. The distal ascending aorta is the most common site to be cannulated.

Venous access to the heart is gained through either a single two-stage venous cannula or bicaval venous cannulae. A two-stage venous cannula is inserted into the right atrium to drain blood from the SVC, right atrium and IVC, where the right atrium is not opened for surgery. The SVC and IVC are cannulated separately, if the right atrium is opened for surgery with a Y connector joining the both.

Cardioplegia cannulae are available for insertion into the aortic root, coronary ostia or coronary sinus for antegrade or retrograde delivery of cardioplegia (Figure 25.2). A double-limb cannula inserted into the aortic root above the aortic valve not only allows delivery of cardioplegia but also serves as a vent to keep the left ventricle empty offering additional

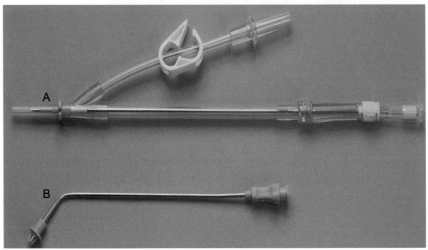

Figure 25.2. Cardioplegic cannulae. A) Double-limb aortic root cardioplegia cannula; B) Coronary ostial cannula for cardioplegia.

myocardial protection. Coronary sinus cannulation is done to provide retrograde cardioplegia in cases of aortic regurgitation (AR) or severe coronary artery disease.

Perfusion tubing

PVC tubing connects the components of the extracorporeal circuit.

Venous reservoir

The venous reservoir comprises a hard shell or collapsible bag that collects the venous return. The level of blood within the reservoir is maintained during CPB to facilitate not only an adequate return but also to prevent inadvertent pumping of air.

Mechanical pump heads

The mechanical pump performs the pumping function of the heart.

The roller pump (flow generator) has two rollers and squeezes blood through the tubing using a peristaltic motion that provides either a pulsatile or non-pulsatile flow with an output dependent on the number of rotations and diameter of the tubing.

Membrane oxygenator

The membrane oxygenator functions as an artificial lung and consists of a hollow fibre with micropores made of polypropylene. The oxygen and air mixture flows through the fibres and the venous blood flows outside of the fibres. Gas exchange is facilitated by the concentration gradient obeying Fick's law of diffusion (diffusion α partial pressure difference/distance).

Heat exchanger

A heat exchanger is integral to most oxygenators. An external unit pumps temperature-controlled water into the heat exchanger to aid the control of temperature of the blood. A highly thermal conductive material separates the heat exchanger from the blood.

Gas supply system

Gas supply to the CPB unit consists of oxygen, air and carbon dioxide. A blender, a flow meter and an oxygen analyser allow the mixing of air, control of flow and oxygen concentration, respectively. An anaesthetic vapouriser added to this assembly of gas supply allows delivery of volatile agents whilst on CPB.

Filters

Filters ranging from 0.2µ for a gas line to 40µ for an arterial line are incorporated into the extracorporeal circuit at several segments.

Suckers and vents

Blood in the surgical field is drained into the venous reservoir via suckers aided by roller pumps (Figure 25.1). The vent suckers drain venous blood that is not drained by the venous cannula. Venting of the heart prevents distension of the heart, reduces myocardial rewarming, evacuates air from the cardiac chambers during de-airing and improves surgical exposure through creation of a dry surgical field.

The extracorporeal system is assembled, primed and prepared by the perfusionist. The PVC tubing of the extracorporeal system is primed with around 1500ml of priming solution, which could be crystalloid, colloid, blood or a combination of these depending on the patient's requirement and institutional policy. Heparin and mannitol added to the prime serve the purposes of anticoagulation and osmotic diuresis and free radical scavenging, respectively. The perfusionist takes a note of the patient's body weight and height to calculate the required blood flow rate for a given patient based on the patient's body surface area.

Conduct of CPB

CPB equipment is commonly referred to as an artificial heart lung machine. The gas exchanger within the CPB circuit facilitates oxygen uptake and carbon dioxide removal, performing the function of the lung, whilst the mechanical pump within the circuit pumps the blood into the systemic circulation, performing the function of the heart (Figure 25.3). The following steps are commonly followed during the initiation of CPB:

- The surgeon connects the aortic cannula to the arterial pipe and the venous cannula to the venous pipe of the extracorporeal circuit. Clamps are placed on both the arterial and venous pipes by the perfusionist at this stage.
- The gas supply on the circuit is switched on to deliver oxygen, air and the volatile agent.
- The surgeon then communicates to the perfusionist to commence CPB. The perfusionist explicitly confirms the commencement of

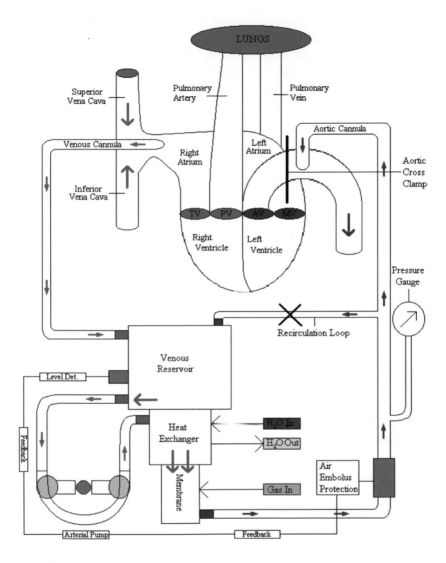

Figure 25.3. A simplified schematic of the cardiopulmonary bypass circuit. Extracorporeal circulation is shown commencing at the venous cannula (follow blue arrows from the SVC, IVC, Ra) to enter the venous reservoir, from which the blood is pumped into an oxygenator and heat exchanger and returned via the arterial side (follow red arrows after the membrane) through an aortic cannula distal to the cross-clamp in the distal ascending aorta.

bypass and initiates the process. Closed loop communication is the norm in cardiac theatres.

- The clamp on the arterial pipe is removed and the pump speed is gradually increased to achieve the desired flow rate, whilst monitoring the level of the prime fluid/blood in the venous reservoir.
- The venous clamp is then gradually removed on the extracorporeal circuit to achieve full flow calculated for the patient.
- When the desired flow is achieved, the perfusionist confirms it stating that the patient is on "full flows".
- The anaesthetist discontinues the IV fluid infusion and stops ventilation at this stage and chooses the CPB mode on the anaesthetic machine.
- The surgeon applies a cross-clamp proximal to the aortic cannula. Cardioplegia is delivered via the aortic root cannula placed proximal to the cross-clamp in antegrade delivery of the cardioplegia or via the cannula in the coronary sinus in retrograde delivery of the cardioplegia to achieve diastolic cardiac arrest.

Maintenance and management of CPB

During CPB, blood bypasses the heart and lung, and mechanical ventilation is discontinued. Hence, volatile agent cannot be administered via ventilation of the lungs. An intravenous infusion of propofol or administration of volatile agent via the oxygenator of the extracorporeal circuit remains as standard practice currently.

Anticoagulation
A heparin dose of 300U/kg (3mg/kg) is administered to achieve systemic anticoagulation prior to cannulation of the aorta or an alternative artery. An activated clotting time (ACT) of >450 seconds is required to go onto CPB. The ACT is monitored every 30 minutes during CPB and is maintained at 400-480 seconds. After CPB is terminated, heparin is reversed with protamine and the ACT is restored to +/-10% from the baseline value.

Heparin
Unfractionated heparin is a highly negative polyanionic mucopolysaccharide with molecules that weigh between 5-30kDa. Heparin

increases the affinity of antithrombin to thrombin by more than a thousand-fold to exert the anticoagulant activity. Failure to achieve an ACT of more than 480 seconds with a dose of 500 units/kg of heparin indicates heparin resistance. The resistance could be due to either an antithrombin deficiency or increased protein binding of heparin. Administration of fresh frozen plasma (FFP) to raise the antithrombin III levels is a strategy to address this issue.

Protamine

Protamine is a polycation prepared from fish sperm. Polycationic protamine combines with anionic heparin to form a stable salt that is devoid of anticoagulant property; 1mg of protamine neutralises 1mg of heparin. Adverse effects secondary to protamine administration include a decrease in both systemic and pulmonary arterial pressures, anaphylactoid reactions, pulmonary vasoconstriction and antihaemostatic effects. Slow administration (not in less than 3 minutes, titrating it over 10 minutes), irrespective of a peripheral or central route of administration, prevents adverse haemodynamic consequences.

Coagulation monitoring and conservation of blood

Apart from the ACT monitor, near-patient coagulation monitors such as thromboelastography (TEG®) or rotational thromboelastometry (RoTEM®) are commonly used to study clot kinetics, i.e. speed of initiation, strength and stability of the clot. Management of peri-operative coagulopathy with blood products is rationalised through the use of these monitors.

Tranexamic acid, aprotinin and epsilon-aminocaproic acid are the antifibrinolytics that are currently in use to address fibrinolysis and coagulopathy that occurs during CPB.

The blood that is not returned during CPB is washed, filtered and centrifuged providing a concentrate of red cells for transfusing back into the patient.

In-line monitoring

An in-line monitor integral to the CPB circuit continuously monitors pH, $PaCO_2$, PaO_2, potassium, arterial and venous oxygen saturation, haematocrit, haemoglobin, and temperature during CPB.

Cardiovascular management

Ideal targets for cardiovascular management are yet to be defined. The following physiological targets are used as a standard practice during CPB:

- Mean arterial pressure (MAP): 50-70mmHg.
- Central venous pressure: 5mmHg.
- Pump flow: 2.2-2.5L/min/m^2.
- Mixed venous oxygen saturation (SvO$_2$): >65%.
- Haematocrit: 0.20-0.25.
- Acid base balance: alpha-stat approach during hypothermia.
- Plasma glucose: 5-9mmol/L.

Maintenance of temperature and acid base control

Temperatures ranging from 15-37°C are used during CPB. Normothermia or systemic hypothermia (25-32°C) is maintained during CPB excluding the condition of deep hypothermic circulatory arrest (DHCA). Hypothermia reduces cerebral and myocardial metabolism and oxygen consumption and for every 1°C fall in temperature, cerebral metabolism drops by 6-7%.

Solubility of a gas increases as the temperature decreases. The gases are more in dissolved form rather than in gaseous form. The partial pressure of carbon dioxide (PaCO$_2$) in the blood falls as temperature decreases and the pH increases giving rise to alkalosis. The pH-stat (addition of CO$_2$ to blood) and alpha-stat (allowing pH and PaCO$_2$ to drift) approaches are the two available options to manage acid base homeostasis during hypothermia. The alpha-stat approach is the commonly used approach.

Myocardial protection

Myocardial protection is achieved through either administration of cardioplegia or through non-cardioplegia techniques.

Cardioplegia literally means 'heart paralysis'. Potassium-rich cardioplegia solutions infused via the coronary arteries antegradely or via coronary veins retrogradely, lead to a rapid diastolic arrest of the ischaemic heart following cross-clamping of the aorta above the level of the coronary arteries. This state of cardioplegia limits energy consumption and metabolite accumulation within the cardiac myocyte during the ischaemic period and protects the heart. The cardioplegia technique continues to be the preferred method for prolonged intracardiac procedures.

Potassium is the main component of cardioplegia solutions. A rapid infusion of cardioplegia solution inactivates the sodium channels preventing depolarisation (upstroke of myocyte action potential) and leads to diastolic arrest of the heart. A cold cardioplegia solution at 4-10°C is infused initially and the heart is simultaneously cooled topically with ice or cold saline. Infusion of warm blood cardioplegia before and after cardioplegic arrest preserves myocardial ATP levels.

Non-cardioplegia myocardial protection strategies include the cross-clamp and fibrillation, hypothermic systemic perfusion with prolonged ventricular fibrillation and deep hypothermic circulatory arrest (DHCA) techniques.

Filtration

Haemofiltration and ultrafiltration incorporating hollow fibre semipermeable membranes are used in CPB circuitry not only to remove excess fluids, electrolytes, and inflammatory mediators, but also to raise the haematocrit.

Systemic adverse effects of CPB

CPB contributes to several systemic adverse effects, which include systemic inflammatory response syndrome (SIRS), organ dysfunction, coagulopathy, haemolysis, renal and splanchnic hypoperfusion, and cerebrovascular accident (stroke). SIRS may be reduced by the use of membrane oxygenators, heparin-coated circuits, centrifugal pumps, intra-operative steroids and leukodepletion filters.

Weaning

The patient is weaned off the CPB after the surgical procedure is finished.

The patient is rewarmed to normothermia, the cardiac chambers are de-aired if opened, and the lungs are ventilated to expel any air from the pulmonary circulation. TOE examination helps in confirming adequacy of de-airing. Removal of the cross-clamp from the ascending aorta may be followed by ventricular tachycardia or ventricular fibrillation. This leads to myocardial damage and is averted by prompt defibrillation via internal paddles using 5-10J of direct current. Insulated pacing wires are sutured to the epicardium and tunnelled through the chest wall to get connected to the pacemaker box. Commonly, atrial and ventricular epicardial wires are placed. Atrial wires are redundant in the situation of atrial fibrillation.

The perfusionist gradually occludes the venous limb on the surgeon's request to come off bypass. This increases the right ventricular preload and reduces venous drainage. To match against dropping venous return, the pump flow is gradually reduced letting the heart eject. The perfusionist confirms that the patient is "off bypass". At this point, if a volatile has been administered via the CPB circuit, the anaesthetist must reintroduce it via the vapouriser on the anaesthetic machine. After adequate filling of the heart (preload), if adequate blood pressure is not achieved, a vasopressor may be needed to maintain SVR and haemodynamics if the contractility of the heart is good (direct inspection of RV and visualisation of LV on TOE).

Fixed rate dual-chamber pacing (DOO) at 80-100/min is initiated whilst in theatre to be insensitive to diathermy and this is changed to the physiological atrioventricular sequential pacing (DDD) mode before transfer to the ICU.

Decannulation

The venous cannula and vents are removed after terminating the CPB. Residual blood in the pericardium and pleura is drained into a cardiotomy reservoir and suction is discontinued. Protamine is administered slowly to reverse heparin; 1mg of protamine neutralises 100 units/1mg of heparin. The aortic cannula is removed after administration of protamine. Hypertension is avoided during decannulation of the aorta.

Failure to wean from CPB

Impaired myocardial contractility, myocardial infarction, dysrhythmia, hypothermia, inadequate or excessive preload, extremes of systemic vascular resistance, haemorrhage, inadequate surgical correction and malfunction of the prosthetic valve are some of the causes of failure to come off bypass.

Corrective measures are undertaken and reinstitution of CPB for a brief period to stabilise the situation may be required. Pharmacological or mechanical support are instituted in order to facilitate weaning from CPB and also to support the heart during the operative phase until it resumes independent function.

Pharmacological support in the form of inotropes, vasopressors, inodilators or mechanical support in the form of an intra-aortic balloon pump (IABP) is not an uncommon requirement in the initial postoperative phase. A brief account of this support is provided below.

Pharmacological support

Adrenaline
- Catecholamine — inotrope.
- Action: stimulates α and β adrenoceptors.
- Haemodynamic effect: increase in HR, cardiac output (CO) and MAP.
- Dose: IV infusion 0.005-0.1µg/kg/min.
- Indications: cardiac arrest, anaphylaxis, cardiogenic shock, post-cardiac surgery, low CO syndrome
- Adverse effects: arrhythmias, pulmonary, renal and splanchnic vasoconstriction, increase in glucose and lactate, decrease in potassium.

Dopamine
- Catecholamine — inotrope.
- Action: stimulates DA_1, β_1 and α receptors in a dose-dependent fashion.
- Haemodynamic effect: renal and splanchnic vasodilation, increase in HR, CO.
- Dose: 1->10µg/kg/min.
- Indications: weaning from CPB and post-cardiac surgery augmentation of CO.
- Adverse effects: dose-dependent arrhythmias.

Dobutamine
- Catecholamine — inotrope.
- Action: stimulation of β_1 and β_2 receptors.
- Haemodynamic effect: increase in HR and CO, decrease in SVR and PVR.
- Dose: 1-20µg/kg/min.
- Indications: cardiogenic shock (low CO with high SVR).
- Adverse effects: dose-dependent arrhythmias.

Noradrenaline
- Catecholamine — vasopressor.
- Action: stimulates α and β_1 adrenoceptors.
- Haemodynamic effect: increase in SVR, PVR and MAP.
- Dose: IV infusion 0.01-0.2µg/kg/min.
- Indication: low CO unresponsive to fluids and inotropes, decreased MAP and SVR in post-cardiac surgery, vasoplegic syndrome and septic shock.
- Adverse effects: renal, hepatic and mesenteric ischaemia.

Metaraminol
- Catecholamine — vasopressor.
- Action: predominantly α_1 stimulation and some β stimulation.
- Haemodynamic effect: increase in SVR and MAP, increase or decrease in CO.
- Dose: IV bolus 3-15µg/kg.
- Indications: decrease in MAP secondary to a decrease in SVR.
- Adverse effects: decrease in CO and increase in SVR and PVR.

Phenylephrine
- Catecholamine and vasopressor.
- Action: stimulation of α_1 adrenoceptors.
- Haemodynamic effect: increase in SVR, PVR and MAP, decrease in HR.
- Dose: IV bolus 1-10µg/kg, IV infusion 0.05-3µg/kg/min.
- Indications: decrease in MAP secondary to a decrease in SVR.
- Adverse effects: decrease in CO and increase in SVR and PVR.

Phosphodiesterase (PDE) III inhibitors (inodilators)
- Action: inhibition of PDE III and preventing breakdown of cAMP.

- Haemodynamic effect: increase in HR and CO, decrease in SVR and PVR (inodilator).
- Dose:
  - milrinone: loading dose 25-75μg/kg, IV infusion 0.37-0.75μg/kg/min;
  - enoximone: loading dose 0.5-1.0mg/kg, IV infusion 3-10μg/kg/min.
- Indications: weaning from CPB, low CO syndrome, RV dysfunction and pulmonary hypertension.
- Adverse effects: hypotension, tachycardia, ventricular arrhythmia, thrombocytopenia, fever, nausea and vomiting.

Levosimendan
- Calcium sensitizer — inotrope.
- Action: stabilises Troponin C in its active state.
- Haemodynamic effect: increase in CO and HR, decrease in SVR and PVR.
- Dose: loading dose 12-24μg/kg, IV infusion 0.05 to 0.6μg/kg/min for 24 hours.
- Indications: acute heart failure, severe LV dysfunction, acute coronary syndromes.
- Adverse effects: increased myocardial contraction without increasing oxygen demand.

Vasopressin
- Endogenous ADH — vasopressor.
- Action: stimulates V_1 and V_2 receptors.
- Haemodynamic effect: increase in SVR.
- Dose: IV infusion 0.01-0.1 units/min.
- Indications: decreased SVR, catecholamine-resistant vasoplegia post-cardiac surgery and septic shock.
- Adverse effects: skin necrosis after extravasation, increase in the risk of thrombosis, hyponatraemia, anaphylaxis and ischaemia of the gastrointestinal tract.

Calcium
- Action: increase in intracellular calcium, increase in muscle contraction.
- Haemodynamic effect: increase in SVR, MAP and CO.
- Dose: IV bolus 0.5-1g (6.8-13.6mmol).

- Indications: decreased Ca^{2+}, Mg^{2+} and MAP, increased K^+.
- Adverse effects: potentiation of ischaemia reperfusion injury.

Mechanical support

Intra-aortic balloon pump (IABP)

An intra-aortic balloon pump (IABP) is used to augment myocardial function in combination with pharmacological therapy or when pharmacological support has failed. The device consists of a balloon with a 30-40ml capacity, which is deployed in the descending thoracic aorta distal to the origin of the left subclavian artery, through femoral arterial access. An IABP improves LV performance by increasing cerebral perfusion pressure (CPP) and decreasing left ventricular end-diastolic pressure (LVEDP). The balloon is inflated with helium at the onset of diastole and deflated at the end of diastole. This is achieved by timing inflation and deflation to the invasive BP trace or R wave on the ECG. An IABP augments LVEDP, increases CPP, decreases SVR during systole and improves LV performance. Systemic anticoagulation and timing of inflation/deflation cycles are vital.

Extracorporeal membrane oxygenation (ECMO)

Veno-arterial extracorporeal membrane oxygenation (VA-ECMO) provides cardiopulmonary support and veno-venous extracorporeal membrane oxygenation provides pulmonary support. These supports can be provided on intensive care units that have the necessary resources and staff.

Assist devices

Univentricular, i.e. left ventricular or right ventricular (LVAD/RVAD), or biventricular (BiVAD) assist devices are advanced mechanical devices to assist and support the LV, RV or both. These are used as a bridge to recovery, transplant or destination therapy.

Transfer to the ICU

Following successful weaning from CPB, the patient is kept sedated, ventilated and supported haemodynamically as appropriate and transferred to the intensive care unit for further postoperative care.

On arrival to the ICU, adequate ventilation is confirmed, along with a stable heart rate and rhythm, transducers are re-zeroed and adequate arterial and venous pressures are ensured. Epicardial pacing is changed from a fixed rate to demand mode. Hand over of the patient to the ICU staff should cover all the patient details including allergies, surgical details including the procedure, complications, ease of weaning from CPB, haemodynamic support, and anaesthetic details including vascular access, grade of laryngoscopy, fluids, blood and products administered, post-CPB blood gases and ACT, pending investigations, acceptable haemodynamic targets for postop care and expected duration of sedation and ventilation.

Routine postoperative care

Day 0: immediate postoperative course

Sedation and ventilation are continued for 2-4 hours to allow rewarming and exclude postoperative bleeding. Intravenous morphine and nurse-controlled analgesia is common practice. Haemodynamic goals are set aiming for a heart rate of 60-80/min, preservation of sinus rhythm, MAP of 60-80mmHg, CVP of 6-10mmHg, good peripheral perfusion and urine output of >0.5ml/kg/hr.

Common early postoperative problems are listed in Table 25.9.

Blood loss up to 3ml/kg/hour in the first hour, 2ml/kg/hour in the second to fourth hour and 1ml/kg/hr during the fifth to twelve hours postoperatively is considered acceptable postoperatively. Output from the chest drain, haemodynamic and metabolic status, bedside ECHO and a near-patient coagulation monitor (TEG®) facilitate efficient management of postoperative bleeding. The patient may need blood and products if the bleed is secondary to coagulopathy or if the patient has to return to theatre for securing haemostasis if the bleed is surgical. Hypokalaemia and hyperkalaemia contribute to dysrhythmias and need correction. Oliguria is addressed through adequate volume loading, increasing MAP and a diuretic. Metabolic acidosis is indicative of a low cardiac output in the absence of renal impairment. Abdominal distension and postoperative nausea and vomiting (PONV) are addressed by insertion of a nasogastric tube and antiemetics. Failed extubation requires reintubation and a gradual wean from ventilation is done as tolerated.

Table 25.9. Common early postoperative problems following cardiac surgery.

Haemodynamic/ ventilatory	Fluid and electrolytes	Renal and metabolic	Gastrointestinal tract
Haemorrhage	Positive fluid balance	Oliguria	Abdominal distension
Hypertension	Hypokalaemia	Acidosis	Postoperative nausea and vomiting
Hypotension	Hyperkalaemia	High lactate	
Dysrhythmias			
Inadequate gas exchange			
Failed extubation			

Day 1 and later

Chest drains are removed if the drainage is <25ml/hour for 2 hours. Invasive arterial blood pressure monitoring can be continued in a high dependency unit. A urinary catheter may be retained for a day or two. A central venous catheter is left *in situ* for 3-4 days. Epicardial pacing wires are taken out after 5-6 days, if not required.

Anaesthesia for specific cardiac procedures

Coronary artery bypass grafting (CABG)

Surgical considerations

The right and left coronary arteries arise from the sinuses of Valsalva located above the right and left aortic cusps of the aortic valve. The left main stem (LMS) divides into the left anterior descending (LAD) artery and circumflex (Cx) artery which run along the anterior interventricular and atrioventricular grooves, respectively. The right coronary artery (RCA) runs along the posterior atrioventricular groove. Branches of the coronary arteries and the territory of distribution are listed in Table 25.10.

Table 25.10. Branches of the coronary arteries supplying the heart.

Left anterior descending (LAD)	Circumflex (Cx)	Right coronary artery (RCA)
Branches:	Branches:	Branches:
• Diagonal arteries (2-6) • Septal arteries (3-5) • Right ventricular branches	• Obtuse marginal artery • Left atrial branch • SA nodal artery (45%) • AV nodal artery (10-15%) • Posterior descending artery (10-15%)	• Sinoatrial nodal artery (55%) • Conus (infundibular) branch • Acute marginal branch • Anterior right ventricular branches • AV nodal artery (85-90%) • Posterior descending artery • Posterior left ventricular artery
Supply:	Supply:	Supply:
Anterior wall of the left ventricle	Lateral wall of the left ventricle	Sinoatrial node
Anterior two-thirds of the ventricular septum	Anterolateral papillary muscle of the mitral valve	Atrioventricular node
Anterior surface of the right ventricle	Left atrium	Right ventricle
	To the nodes as above	Posterior third of the ventricular septum

AV = atrioventricular; SA = sinoatrial.

Coronary blood flow is around 4-5% of the cardiac output, i.e. 200-250ml/min. But, the oxygen consumption of the myocardium is disproportionately higher at 10% indicating the requirement for a constant and adequate blood supply. A loss of 50% in diameter for a coronary artery results in a 75% loss in cross-sectional area and 70% loss in diameter results in a 90% loss in cross-sectional area. Stable exertional angina and unstable angina tend to occur with 75% and 90% degrees of stenosis, respectively.

Pre-operative ECG will indicate the ischaemic territory and diseased vessel (Table 25.11). Coronary angiography reveals the exact location and severity of the stenosis.

Table 25.11. ECG: localisation of myocardial territory and diseased coronary artery.

Lead	Infarct	Artery
II, III and aVF	Inferior	RCA
V1 and V2	Anteroseptal	Proximal LAD
V3 and V4	Anteroapical	Distal LAD
V5 and V6	Anterolateral	Circumflex

A knowledge of the factors influencing myocardial oxygen supply and demand helps in providing favourable conditions peri-operatively, so as to increase the oxygen supply and reduce the demand for preventing further insult to the ischaemic myocardium (Table 25.12).

Coronary artery bypass graft surgery is performed to revascularise the myocardium by bypassing all the severe stenotic lesions in the coronary arteries. The surgery is performed to provide symptom relief and improve survival.

Table 25.12. Determinants of myocardial oxygen supply and demand.

Factors increasing oxygen supply	Factors increasing oxygen demand
Increase in aortic pressure	Increase in heart rate
Low LVEDP	Increase in myocardial contractility
Low coronary vascular resistance	Increase in wall tension
Adequate haemoglobin	

Indications for CABG include:

- Left main stem stenosis >50%.
- Triple-vessel disease with ejection fraction (EF) <50%.
- Triple-vessel disease with EF >50% and inducible ischaemia.
- Two-vessel disease with involvement of the proximal LAD artery and EF <50%.
- Non-stentable lesions.

Saphenous venous grafts are commonly used. Long-term patency of the coronary artery bypass conduits depends on the vessel chosen for grafting. Ninety-five percent of left internal mammary artery (LIMA) grafts are patent at 10 years after surgery and this drops to 80% for free RIMA, radial artery and long saphenous vein grafts. The LIMA should be used to bypass the LAD artery when possible, and the RIMA is used when the LIMA is unavailable or unsuitable for harvesting.

CABG is usually performed utilising CPB, but can be performed on a beating heart without using CPB termed as 'off-pump' CABG (OPCABG).

On-pump CABG entails the following key steps: a median sternotomy, harvesting of the conduits (LIMA, saphenous vein), systemic anticoagulation, cannulation of the aorta and right atrium, CPB, cross-clamp of the aorta, cardioplegic diastolic cardiac arrest, distal anastomosis of the LIMA to the LAD and vein grafts to the target vessels during arrest and CPB, release of the cross-clamp, recovery of cardiac arrest, proximal anastomosis of the conduits to the ascending aorta, weaning off bypass, reversal of anticoagulation, and surgical haemostasis.

Anaesthetic considerations

The anaesthetic goals for a patient undergoing CABG are as follows:

- Heart rate: avoid tachycardia.
- Heart rhythm: sinus rhythm.
- Preload, afterload and contractility should be maintained at normal levels.
- Prevention of ischaemia: balance the oxygen supply and demand.

Off-pump CABG

Off-pump CABG avoids the complications of CPB such as SIRS, coagulopathy, neurological injury and renal impairment. Aortic cannulation and cross-clamping are not required.

Surgical considerations

The challenges are two-fold: firstly, to gain adequate exposure of the heart with minimal cardiac motion and, secondly, to protect the myocardium from ischaemia. The surgeon places a tissue stabiliser device on the heart. Graft conduits (artery/vein) are harvested as in on-pump CABG. The cardiac wall is stabilised by placing the stabiliser device (Octopus® stabilisation system) over the epicardium at the intended site of arteriotomy and anastomotic suturing. Deep pericardial retraction sutures or the use of a stockinette sutured into the oblique sinus (present between the left and right pulmonary veins behind the left atrium) facilitate lifting of the heart. An intracoronary shunt is used to prevent bleeding from the arteriotomy site during anastomosis of the grafts.

Anaesthetic considerations

Anaesthetic goals for off-pump CABG include maximal cardiac protection, maintenance of haemodynamics with monitoring and pharmacologic support, early emergence and excellent postoperative analgesia.

Good premedication, avoidance of tachycardia and good communication between the surgeon and the anaesthetist are essential. The use of volatile agents such as isoflurane and sevoflurane for maintenance of anaesthetic offer the benefit of preconditioning and protection against ischaemia. Monitoring should include a 12-lead ECG with simultaneous lead II monitoring and continuous ST segment analysis to aid in the detection of peri-operative ischaemia. Anaesthetic maintenance is achieved with either a volatile or intravenous agent. Cardiac displacement increases the risk of intra-operative arrhythmias. Serum potassium is maintained at >4.5mmol/L and 5g of magnesium is administered prophylactically. Anticoagulation is achieved with 1-2mg/kg of heparin to maintain an ACT at 250-300 seconds. Hypothermia is avoided through the administration of warm IV fluids, warming blankets and a heat and moisture exchanger (HME) filter on the anaesthetic circuit.

Haemodynamic disturbances are due to displacement of the heart during the anastomosis; the pressure exerted by the stabilisation device on the wall of the ventricle and vertical positioning of the heart leads to mitral and tricuspid regurgitation.

Maintenance of a high perfusion pressure (MAP >70mmHg) and low myocardial oxygen consumption are required to counter the impact of displacement of the heart. The Trendelenburg position and administration of IV fluids and vasopressors facilitate the maintenance of haemodynamics. Tachycardia is treated using a beta-blocker, and bradycardia is addressed by pacing the right atrium. TOE helps in the rapid detection of regional wall motion abnormalities, but displacement of the heart and the presence of swabs makes it difficult to obtain good images and to interpret them. OPCABG is shown to reduce the need for transfusion along with a reduction in ventilatory support and ICU stay.

Aortic valve surgery

Surgical considerations

The aortic valve has an area of 2.5-3.5cm^2 and is a tricuspid valve separating the aorta from the left ventricle. It has three cusps, namely the right coronary, left coronary and the non-coronary. The right and left coronary arteries arise from the sinuses of Valsalva located at the right and left coronary cusps, respectively.

Aortic stenosis and regurgitation are caused by rheumatic fever, calcific degeneration and a bicuspid valve. Infective endocarditis, aortic root dilation (Marfan syndrome), dissection and trauma may cause aortic regurgitation.

Angina, dyspnoea and syncope are the symptoms of aortic stenosis. Chronic aortic regurgitation presents as non-exertional angina or congestive heart failure.

Aortic stenosis causes obstruction to LV outflow and increases LV afterload. The left ventricle undergoes concentric hypertrophy secondary to pressure overload. Left ventricular thickness is inversely related to LV compliance and exposes it to a higher risk of myocardial ischaemia. Decreased LV compliance leads to diastolic dysfunction. Decompensation leads to subendocardial ischaemia, pulmonary congestion and reduced EF with LV dilation causing angina, dyspnoea and syncope, respectively.

The onset of symptoms indicate a reduced mean survival in the order of 2 years for dyspnoea, 3 years for syncope and 5 years for angina. Echocardiography is the key pre-operative investigation. ECG assesses left ventricular hypertrophy (LVH), ischaemia, and the rhythm. An MRI or a CT scan is indicated if the aortic root is seen to be dilated on echocardiography.

Aortic regurgitation of blood into the LV causes LV volume overload and enlargement. An enlarged LV increases wall stress and results in an increase in LV mass leading to eccentric hypertrophy. An echocardiogram quantifies the severity of aortic regurgitation.

Aortic valve stenosis is the commonest indication for valve replacement in the Western world. Valve replacement is the gold standard and when the risks for surgery are prohibitive, a transcatheter aortic valve implantation (TAVI) is considered.

Indications for surgery for aortic valve disease

The American Heart Association's guidelines for valve replacement are outlined below.

Aortic stenosis (AS):

- Class I:
  - severe AS with symptoms;
  - severe AS undergoing other cardiac surgery (CABG, mitral valve);
  - severe AS with LV systolic dysfunction (EF <50%).
- Class IIa: moderate AS undergoing other cardiac surgery (CABG, mitral valve).
- Class IIb: severe AS with rapid progression of aortic stenosis.

Aortic regurgitation (AR):

- Class I: severe AR with severe symptoms or LV systolic dysfunction.
- Class IIa: severe AR with LV dilation (end-systolic dimension [ESD] >50mm/end-diastolic dimension [EDD] >65mm).
- Class IIb: severe AR with rapid progression.

The key steps involved in aortic valve surgery are as follows: a median sternotomy, systemic anticoagulation, cannulation of the aorta and right atrium, CPB, cross-clamp of the aorta, cardioplegic diastolic cardiac arrest, aortotomy proximal to the cross-clamp, excision of the native valve, insertion of a prosthetic valve, closure of the aorta, recovery from cardioplegic arrest, and weaning off CPB.

Anaesthetic considerations

Pre-operative assessment should include quantification of risk to assess suitability of the patient for surgery. Non-surgical options for high-risk patients are TAVI and balloon valvuloplasty of the aortic valve (BAV). Careful administration of premedication reduces anxiety-induced tachycardia. The anaesthetic goals are summarised in Table 25.13.

Table 25.13. Anaesthetic goals for aortic stenosis and aortic regurgitation.

Heart rate	Aortic stenosis	Aortic regurgitation
Heart	60-80/min	70-90/min
Rhythm	Sinus	Sinus
Preload	Maintain	Maintain high enough PCWP
Afterload	Maintain and avoid reduction	Reduce
Contractility	Maintain	Maintain

PCWP = pulmonary capillary wedge pressure.

Aortic stenosis

An arterial line is inserted before induction. The use of a pulmonary artery catheter has become less common. Patients with aortic stenosis have a fixed cardiac output. From the relation, BP = CO x SVR and CO = SV x HR, we know that the blood pressure depends solely on the systemic vascular resistance because the stroke volume is fixed. Avoidance of hypotension at the time of induction and until CPB is initiated is crucial to avoid adverse haemodynamic compromise. Titrated opiate-based induction is recommended. Vasodilation should be avoided and a vasopressor used to control hypotension. Maintenance of coronary perfusion pressure is needed to prevent subendocardial ischaemia. External defibrillation pads are applied if a mini- or redo-sternotomy is planned. A hypertrophied left ventricle may suffer suboptimal protection during CPB and this can cause post-CPB LV dysfunction. An hypertrophied interventricular septum can cause dynamic LV outflow tract obstruction postoperatively.

Aortic regurgitation

In contrast to the goals for stenosis, mild tachycardia and a drop in SVR maintain forward flow in AR and are beneficial. Bradycardia may result in myocardial ischaemia.

TOE examination should assess the valve lesion, confirm the diagnosis and exclude other pathologies. Post-bypass TOE examination checks for adequacy of de-airing, assesses the valve and left ventricular function.

Mitral valve surgery

Surgical considerations

The mitral valve has an area of 4-6cm^2 and is an atrioventricular valve located between the left atrium and left ventricle. It is bicuspid and has two leaflets, an anterior leaflet and a posterior leaflet. The posterior leaflet has scallops on it, which are three in number. These scallops are assigned numbers P1, P2 and P3 (Carpentier classification) on the posterior leaflet; a similar numbering is assigned to the corresponding areas on the anterior leaflet though it does not have any scallops (A1, A2 and A3). This classification helps in localisation of pathology of the valve and is useful in planning and performing the surgical repair. The mitral valve is composed of five components, namely the mitral annulus, leaflets, chordae tendinae, papillary muscles and left ventricular wall. All these five components function as one unit.

A valve area of <2cm^2 is considered as stenosis and an area of <1cm^2 is classed as severe stenosis. Mitral stenosis is most often caused by rheumatic heart disease and it takes 10-20 years from the onset of rheumatic fever to the onset of signs, a further 10-20 years for the onset of mild symptoms, and decompensation sets in after another 10-20 years. The 10-year survival rate is 80% in patients who are in the NYHA I/II functional class and drops to 10-15% for those in the NYHA III/IV functional class.

Primary mitral regurgitation (MR) is due to myxomatous degeneration, rheumatic disease, endocarditis and mitral valve prolapse. Secondary MR is due to ischaemia of papillary muscles or LV and dilated cardiomyopathy. Based on the mitral leaflet motion and the direction of the regurgitant jet, MR is classified into Type I, Type II and Type III categories. Echocardiography quantifies the MR. MR progresses slowly and patients may remain asymptomatic for many years. Detection of a pansystolic murmur incidentally may be the first sign. Asymptomatic patients with MR are at risk of sudden death and irreversible left ventricular dysfunction. Left atrial dilation, atrial fibrillation and pulmonary hypertension are other consequence of MR. Surgery is performed to prevent death and progression of LV dysfunction.

In mitral stenosis (MS), reduced left ventricular inflow results in increased left atrial pressure, and back pressure on pulmonary circulation leads to dyspnoea, pulmonary hypertension, right ventricular failure and subsequent left ventricular failure. Fatigue, dyspnoea, orthopnoea, paroxysmal nocturnal dyspnoea, hoarseness of voice, dysphagia, left lung collapse and atrial fibrillation may be present secondary to a distended left atrium. Pulmonary hypertension and right heart failure manifest as pulmonary oedema, ascites and haemoptysis.

In MR, there is retrograde blood flow from the LV into the LA during systole. Excess volume in the LA then flows forward into the LV. Increased flow into the LV leads to increased LV end-diastolic volume, volume overload, eccentric hypertrophy, mitral valve annular dilatation, LA dilation, increased left atrial pressure, pulmonary artery pressure, RV systolic pressure and RV failure. An EF less than 60% in patients with MR is indicative of left ventricular systolic dysfunction unlike in patients without MR.

Indications for mitral valve surgery

The American Heart Association's guidelines for mitral valve surgery are outlined below.

Mitral stenosis (MS):

- Class Ia: moderate to severe MS with symptoms (NYHA III/IV).
- Class IIa: severe MS with severe pulmonary hypertension or NYHA I/II Class.

- Class IIb: moderate to severe MS with recurrent embolic events on anticoagulation.

Mitral regurgitation (MR):

- Class I: severe MR with NYHA Class II-IV or LVESD >40mm/ LVEF <60%.
- Class IIa: severe MR in asymptomatic patient with a likelihood of repair >90%.
- Class IIIa: severe MR with AF or pulmonary hypertension.
- Class IIIb: severe MR, poor LV function despite maximal anti-failure treatment.

The surgical treatment option for mitral valve stenosis is mitral valve replacement and the surgical treatment options for mitral valve regurgitation are either a valve repair or valve replacement. Replacement is done when repair is not possible as in papillary muscle rupture. The advantages of repairing mitral valve over replacement are a decreased mortality and reduction in valve deterioration, reoperation, infective endocarditis and haemorrhage. Left ventricular dysfunction is less with mitral valve repair due to a preserved subvalvular apparatus and LV geometry.

The key steps involved in mitral valve surgery are as follows: a median sternotomy, systemic anticoagulation, cannulation of the aorta, bicaval cannulation, CPB, cross-clamp of the aorta, cardioplegic diastolic cardiac arrest, access to the mitral valve via a left atriotomy or biatrial transseptal incisions, repair or replacement of the mitral valve, closure of the atria, recovery from cardioplegic arrest, weaning off CPB.

Anaesthetic considerations

The anaesthetic goals for mitral stenosis and regurgitation are summarised in Table 25.14. Avoidance of tachycardia is an important goal for mitral stenosis. Pre-operative beta-blockade, opiate-based induction and titrated analgesia with adequate depth facilitate stable haemodynamics. Fluid overload should be avoided but preload should be maintained exercising caution not to overload the RV.

Table 25.14. Anaesthetic goals for mitral stenosis and mitral regurgitation.

Parameter	Mitral stenosis	Mitral regurgitation
Heart rate	60-80/min	80-100/min
Heart rhythm	Sinus	Sinus
Preload	Maintain high enough PCWP	Maintain high enough PCWP
Afterload	Maintain	Reduce
Contractility	Maintain	Maintain
PCWP = pulmonary capillary wedge pressure.		

Reduction of regurgitant fraction through reduction of SVR and maintenance of a moderate tachycardia are the goals for MR. Premedication should be avoided if the pulmonary artery pressure (PAP) is high. Hypoxia, acidosis and hypercapnia should be avoided to prevent a rise in PAP. Six independent predictors of the need for inotropic support when weaning off bypass have been identified. They are as follows:

- Wall motion abnormalities on TOE.
- Combined mitral valve and CABG surgery.
- Left ventricular ejection fraction (LVEF) <35%.
- Reoperation.
- Moderate to severe MR.
- Aortic cross-clamp time.

PAc placement allows rationalisation of inotropes if required while coming off bypass or during the postoperative period. The choice of inotrope is either catecholamine (adrenaline) or a PDE III inhibitor (milrinone). Milrinone is an inodilator that causes a reduction in SVR and PVR whilst improving contractility. Intra-operative TOE plays an important role in mitral valve surgery. The left atrium provides a good acoustic window for the TOE to visualise the mitral valve. Pre-bypass TOE provides new information in 9-13% cases and post-bypass TOE identifies valve dysfunction in 6-11% cases. Pre-bypass TOE is done systematically to assess the location, mechanism severity and reparability of the regurgitation. The information is passed on to the surgeon. Measurement of PAP and LV function helps in planning inotropic support. TOE examination is done post-bypass and before the administration of protamine to assess the surgical repair.

Aortic dissection

Surgical considerations

Dissection of the aorta involves separation of the intima from the medial wall as a result of a small tear. Progression of dissection along the length of the aorta may occlude the arterial branches arising from the aorta and compromise blood supply to the organs.

Aortic dissection is caused by arterial hypertension, connective tissue disorders, pregnancy, iatrogenic injury, hereditary vascular disease and aortic aneurysms. The aorta is divided into four segments: the ascending aorta, aortic arch, descending thoracic aorta and abdominal aorta.

Dissection is classified based on the anatomical location and duration of symptoms. Diagnosis of aortic dissection made within 2 weeks from the onset of symptoms is termed as acute and if the diagnosis is made later than 2 weeks, then it becomes chronic.

Anatomical location is outlined in Table 25.15

Dissection of the aorta carries a high mortality; Type A dissection is managed surgically (mortality of 27%) and Type B dissection is managed conservatively. Type A dissections are surgical emergencies and carry a poor prognosis with a 1% mortality per hour for the first 48 hours.

Table 25.15. Classification of aortic dissection.

Anatomical location	DeBakey classification	Stanford classification
Ascending aorta, arch, descending thoracic aorta	Type I	Type A
Ascending aorta	Type II	Type A
Descending thoracic aorta	Type III	Type B

The key surgical steps constitute a median sternotomy, exposure and preparation of the groin for possible femoral cannulation, full anticoagulation, conventional atrio-aortic CPB establishment (note: femoral artery cannulation prior to a median sternotomy to allow sucker CPB if aorta cannot be cannulated), selective antegrade or retrograde cerebral perfusion where deep hypothermic circulatory arrest (DHCA) is planned, and repair of the ascending aorta with an interposition graft/aortic valve or aortic root replacement (Bentall procedure).

DHCA is the technique of combining core cooling of the body and cessation of blood flow. Most cardiac operations are performed using cardioplegic arrest and CPB but some procedures require DHCA (Table 25.16).

Circulation can only be safely arrested for a minute at 36°C but this can be increased to 30-40 minutes and 45-60 minutes at deep hypothermic temperatures such as 20°C and 16°C, respectively.

The sequence of events for DHCA is as follows:

- CPB is established after arterial and venous access are gained for the circuit.
- The patient's core temperature is dropped to the desired level (15-18°C).

Table 25.16. Indications for DHCA.

- Surgery on the aortic arch: aortic dissection/aneurysm.
- Need for bloodless field: thoracoabdominal aneurysm.
- Impossible to clamp ascending aorta: distal ascending aorta aneurysm.
- To control and repair massive haemorrhage: blood loss during sternotomy.

- Maintain 15-18°C for 10-15 minutes to achieve a steady state.
- The arterial limb is clamped.
- Circulating volume is drained into the venous reservoir.
- The pump is switched off.
- After completion of the procedure the patient is placed in the Trendelenburg position.
- Extracorporeal circulation is then resumed at a slow rate initially.
- After CPB is reestablished, gradual rewarming is achieved at a rate of 0.2°C to 0.5°C per minute. It is important not to rewarm at a faster rate to prevent neurological injury.

Complications of DHCA include coagulopathy and platelet dysfunction, SIRS (CPB+DHCA) and neurological injury.

Anaesthetic considerations

Aortic dissection is presented with a diverse range of symptoms and signs, and a high index of suspicion is necessary for diagnosis. Pain, syncope, dyspnoea, stroke, pulse deficit and a murmur of aortic regurgitation are some relevant findings.

Amongst the diagnostic tools, MRI has the highest sensitivity (95-100%) and specificity (95-100%), closely followed by TOE and a CT scan. Surgery is expedited once the diagnosis is made.

The initial management aims at control of blood pressure under invasive monitoring with vasodilators, beta-blockers and analgesics. Six units of blood should be cross-matched and the need for blood products should be anticipated. Anaesthetic technique aims to maintain haemodynamic stability. Left upper limb arterial cannulation is done because of possible involvement of the brachiocephalic artery. A femoral arterial line is secured if the arch vessels are to be isolated. A large-bore CVC for rapid transfusion, TOE monitoring, nasopharyngeal and bladder temperature monitoring constitutes standard practice.

Pericardectomy

Surgical considerations

The pericardium is the sac that covers the heart, consisting of fibrous and serous layers.

The serous pericardium is further divided into visceral and parietal pericardium with 5-10ml of pericardial fluid present between these two layers. Infections, radiotherapy, cardiac surgery, tumours, drugs and connective tissue diseases can affect the pericardium causing constrictive pericarditis.

Diastolic dysfunction secondary to a fibrosed and calcified pericardial sac around the heart is the key feature of constrictive pericarditis. Signs of impaired RV filling predominate. Cardiac volume is fixed with equal end-diastolic pressure in all four chambers and dissociation between intrathoracic and intracardiac pressures. Hepatomegaly and ascites are presenting features. The condition must be differentiated from restrictive cardiomyopathy.

A surgical pericardectomy, involving complete removal of the thickened pericardium from the left and right ventricle and the diaphragm, is the definitive treatment and carries a reported mortality of 6%. Most surgeons, in view of better exposure and easy access for cannulation, prefer a median sternotomy. CPB is required for the clearance of the posterior pericardium. However, an anterolateral thoracotomy is an alternative approach and requires lung isolation.

Anaesthetic considerations

Patients are often in poor physiological condition, prone to major haemorrhage and haemodynamic instability during the procedure. CPB may be required on standby. Airway pressures are kept to a minimum and positive end-expiratory pressure (PEEP) avoided to counter the effects of positive pressure ventilation on left ventricular filling. Pressure-controlled ventilation is preferred over volume- controlled ventilation. Impaired diastolic filling, increased atrial pressures, tachycardia and reduced stroke volume are the features of the condition.

Haemodynamic goals for constrictive pericarditis are:

- Preload: increase.
- Afterload: maintain.
- Contractility: maintain. Inotropic support may be needed.
- Heart rate: high in view of the fixed stroke volume.
- Rhythm: sinus rhythm preferred though there is little dependence on late diastolic filling of the ventricles.

Redo heart surgery

Surgical considerations

Redo cardiac operations are more complex and prolonged. There are increased chances of damage to the right ventricle, previously placed grafts, bleeding and coagulopathy. The possibility of haemorrhage and haemodynamic instability before going on to conventional CPB necessitates establishing CPB rapidly by implementing an alternate/back-up strategy involving non-conventional CPB. The sternum tends to be adherent to the aorta, brachiocephalic vein, Ra, RV and previous grafts, posing a significant risk of damage to these structures which can lead to catastrophic haemorrhage and haemodynamic instability.

The groin is prepared and exposed for gaining femoral access to establish CPB, if needed. A sternotomy with a special oscillating saw may reduce substernal tissue damage. Coronary, aortic and Ra cannulation may be difficult for the surgeon.

Redo surgery without having to do a sternotomy is an option. Mitral surgery via a right thoracotomy, limited CABG via a left thoracotomy and AV replacement via a mini-sternotomy or transcatheter approach (TAVI) via a transfemoral or transapical approach are a few examples.

Anaesthetic considerations

Pre-operative

A lateral chest X-ray, CT chest and CT angiography may help in the assessment of structures behind the sternum and the risk of damage. It is important to discuss this with the surgeon and perfusionist to agree on strategies for reducing bleeding.

Induction

Good venous access before a sternotomy is essential. External defibrillator/pacing electrodes should be attached. TOE monitoring and PAc placement are recommended. A CPB circuit should be primed and ready with the perfusionist and surgeon available in the operating room. A head-up position (reverse Trendelenburg) should be considered to reduce RV volume during a sternotomy. It is important to check with the surgeon regarding discontinuation of ventilation. The need for haemodynamic support and difficulties with haemostasis following CPB should be anticipated.

Case scenario 1

A 65-year-old gentleman weighing 80kg with a history of hypertension, hypercholesterolaemia, 30-pack years of smoking and stable angina was diagnosed with triple-vessel disease. His pre-op Hb was 14gm/dL and routine test results were unremarkable. He stopped aspirin and clopidogrel for 5 days pre-operatively and had no known allergies. He underwent an uneventful elective on-pump CABG. He was transferred to the ICU with minimal noradrenaline support. After 4 hours on the ICU, he became hypotensive with a systolic pressure of 90mmHg whilst being paced on AAI mode at 90/min, requiring increased doses of noradrenaline and adrenaline, and volume replacement. Chest drainage was 400ml, 260ml, 200ml and 0ml in the last 4 hours. ABG reveals adequate gas exchange on an FiO_2 of 0.6 and positive pressure ventilation, with a pH of 7.25, lactate of 6, base deficit of 8.0mEq/L; Hb on the ABG is 8g/dL. Urine output in the previous hour was 15mL. TEG® is performed which shows an elevated R-time in the non-heparinase sample at 12 seconds. Protamine 50mg is administered IV but the patient remains hypotensive with a CVP of 20mmHg.

How would you manage this patient further?

This patient is in the immediate postoperative phase. The problems identified with this patient are hypotension, increased doses of noradrenaline and adrenaline, raised lactate, metabolic acidosis, oliguria, low Hb, raised CVP, decreasing chest drainage and a raised CVP at 20mmHg.

Causes for postoperative hypotension include hypovolaemia, arrhythmia, rewarming, ischaemia, low cardiac output syndrome, SIRS secondary to CPB, cardiac tamponade and LV or RV failure.

He is treated with IV fluids, vasopressors, inotropes and protamine but this has not improved the situation.

Management should follow an ABC approach. Senior help should be sought. Adequate gas exchange with ongoing positive pressure ventilation rules out problems with the airway and breathing. Hypotension and metabolic acidosis with oliguria suggest problems with circulation. Hence, the focus should be on addressing this issue. The ABG shows a low Hb. The FBC, coagulation screen and TEG® should be repeated. The R-time on TEG® indicates the reaction time and this is prolonged with anticoagulants and coagulation factor deficiency. Note that the extra dose of protamine has not addressed the issue.

Increased chest drainage with a sudden drop and a raised CVP is indicative of cardiac tamponade. A bedside echocardiogram is a useful confirmatory examination, which will show a pericardial collection and diastolic collapse of the right atrium and right ventricle.

A return to theatre for exploration and control of the bleed and to evacuate the clot to release tamponade with volume resuscitation, using blood and blood products as appropriate based on TEG®, is an appropriate management strategy.

Further reading

1. Moorjani N, Viola N, Ohri SK. *Key Questions in Cardiac Surgery*, 1st ed. tfm publishing Ltd., 2011: 255-350.

2. Mackay JH, Arrowsmith JE. *Core Topics in Cardiac Anesthesia*, 2nd ed. Cambridge University Press, 2012.

3. Hensley FA, Martin DE, Gravlee GP. *A Practical Approach to Cardiac Anesthesia*, 5th ed. Lippincott Williams & Wilkins, 2013.

4. Chikwe J, Cooke DT. *Oxford Specialist Handbook of Cardiothoracic Surgery*, 2nd ed. Oxford University Press, 2013.

5. Jason TP, Vegas A. *Cardiac Anesthesiology Fellow's Manual*, 7th ed. UHN Toronto General Hospital, 2011: 6-9.

6. Machin D, Allsager C. Principles of cardiopulmonary bypass. *Br J Anaesth CEACCP* 2006: 6: 176-81.

7. Jameel S, Colah S, Klein Andrew A. Recent advances in cardiopulmonary bypass techniques. *Br J Anaesth CEACCP* 2010; 10: 20-3.

8.   Looney Y, Quinton P. Mitral valve surgery. *Br J Anaesth CEACCP* 2005; 5: 199-202.

9.   Chacko M, Weinberg L. Aortic valve stenosis: perioperative anaesthetic implications of surgical replacement and minimally invasive interventions. *Br J Anaesth CEACCP* 2012; 12: 295-301.

10. European Society of Cardiology recommendations for the management of patients after heart valve surgery. *Eur Heart J* 2005; 26: 2463-71.

26 Abdominal procedures

Mahul Gorecha and Peeyush Kumar

Introduction

Commonly performed elective procedures include gastrectomy, cholecystectomy, laparotomy for bowel resection, anterior resection, Hartmann's procedure, stoma formations and closure, fistula surgery and haemorrhoidectomy. The pathologies involved can be malignancy, inflammation, diverticular disease or obstruction. Also, more frequently, the laparoscopic approach is being used for appendectomy and bowel resections. The advantages of this approach include reduced surgical stress, improved analgesia and a reduced hospital length of stay. Less common and more specialist procedures include liver resection and anti-reflux surgery.

Gastrectomy

The majority of gastric cancers arise in patients over 65 years of age. The main associated risk factors are: genetic (CDH1), smoking, *Helicobacter pylori*, pernicious anaemia, atrophic gastritis and poor socioeconomic class. Staging of gastric cancer is usually based on the tumour, node, metastasis (TNM) classification. Once a patient has been diagnosed with a gastric adenocarcinoma, they should then have peri-operative chemotherapy followed by a gastrectomy with lymph node clearance.

Surgical considerations

Surgical options include a subtotal or total gastrectomy and the deciding factor is the location of the tumour. After a gastrectomy, a Roux-en-Y reconstruction establishes continuity of the GI tract.

Anaesthetic considerations

Many patients are smokers and likely to have multiple comorbidities. They should be advised to stop smoking and a nutritional assessment made. Patients may also suffer from reflux, dysphagia, nausea and vomiting. They should have routine investigations and further assessment of cardiorespiratory disease using pulmonary function and cardiopulmonary exercise testing. Coexisting disease should be optimised and surgery on post-chemotherapy neutropenia is usually postponed for 3 weeks before reassessment. A thoracic epidural is the gold standard for analgesia for upper gastrointestinal surgery. In addition, patients will require large-bore intravenous access. If surgery is to be prolonged or the patient has many comorbidities, then invasive monitoring with central venous pressure (CVP) and arterial lines is recommended. Postoperative nutrition is very important and patients often have a feeding jejunostomy sited so feeding can be commenced after the operation.

Cholecystectomy

Surgical considerations

The incidence of gallstones in women is higher than in men (24%), with the standard treatment involving laparoscopic cholecystectomy. The procedure is carried out mainly laparoscopically, but some are open. The indications for an open procedure are:

- Patient unable to tolerate a pneumoperitoneum.
- Conversion intra-operatively (occurs in about 5% of cases).
- Cholecystectomy carried out at the same time as another procedure.

Anaesthetic considerations

There can be significant haemodynamic changes and there is potential for blood loss so large-bore IV access is recommended. The procedure is carried out electively or acutely and these patients can be acutely unwell, jaundiced or dehydrated. In acute situations, renal function and coagulation status should be checked. Hypovolaemia should be corrected along with antibiotics according to protocol. Due to positioning, patient size and pneumoperitoneum, ventilation may be difficult. Pain can sometimes be severe so multimodal analgesia including NSAIDs and local infiltration of the ports should be considered. In an open procedure, a thoracic epidural is the analgesia of choice.

Laparotomy

Surgical considerations

The procedure can be either elective or an emergency. An emergency laparotomy is usually due to either obstruction or perforation of the bowel and the patient can often be very unwell with haemodynamic instability. In an elective procedure, the patient is generally well and surgery usually involves resection, anastomosis or stoma reversal. The procedure is carried out though a large midline incision with the patient lying supine. These patients will require risk prediction using the P-POSSUM scoring system to identify high-risk patients and those who will benefit from a high dependency unit bed. The P-POSSUM score is a surgical risk prediction tool which makes calculations based on physiological and operative parameters.

Anaesthetic considerations

In an emergency procedure the patient has an increased risk of aspiration. Therefore, a rapid sequence induction should be used to secure the airway. They will require a full pre-operative assessment including a full blood count, electrolytes, coagulation, electrocardiogram and chest X-ray. In an unwell patient, an arterial blood gas analysis will allow measurement of lactate and blood pH. A central venous access direct arterial blood pressure measurement is useful as these patients can have major cardiovascular instability and often have electrolyte derangements. Cardiac output measurement using oesophageal Doppler or pulse wave analysis can also be helpful in guiding fluid management. In addition, hourly urine output, glucose and temperature should be monitored. There are also a variety of analgesic options. A regional technique involving a thoracic epidural or intrathecal opiates is useful for postoperative analgesia; however, care should be taken in patients with deranged coagulation and sepsis. Other options include a transversus abdominis plane (TAP) block and patient-controlled analgesia (PCA).

Laparoscopic abdominal surgery

Surgical considerations

A greater number of operations can now be carried out laparoscopically and the major benefits of this approach include reduced postoperative pain, fewer wound-related complications and a faster recovery time. However, laparoscopic surgery does have its own risks related to the laparoscopic technique and the physiological effects associated with a created pneumoperitoneum. The most significant surgical risk of laparoscopic surgery includes the direct damage to the abdominal organs and blood vessels from the large trocar.

Anaesthetic considerations

Patient positioning to allow surgical access often requires a steep position with associated physiological effects and significant complications can include cerebral and facial oedema, renal failure and compartment syndrome. In order to perform intra-abdominal laparoscopic surgery, a pneumoperitoneum needs to be achieved by insufflating sufficient carbon dioxide. This increases abdominal volume; therefore, the abdominal wall compliance decreases and intra-abdominal pressure rises. This rising pressure can disrupt individual organ systems causing injury and failure. All patients undergoing laparoscopic surgery need a full assessment and particularly those at increased risk of complications from a pneumoperitoneum and also the possibility of converting to an open procedure. The airway is usually secured with a cuffed endotracheal tube and positive pressure ventilation recommended to minimise the risk of gastric aspiration and to facilitate the elimination of CO_2. A nasogastric tube may be required to deflate the stomach and improve the surgical view. The creation of a pneumoperitoneum and steep Trendelenburg position will impair ventilation. The use of pressure-controlled ventilation will limit barotrauma while titrating PEEP will minimise alveolar collapse. The use of opioid-sparing multimodal analgesia combined with regional and local techniques will reduce opiate requirements and enable early mobilisation and discharge. Laparoscopic surgery also has a high incidence of postoperative nausea and vomiting (PONV), so multimodal prophylaxis is important. As these procedures are often performed as day cases, and have an increased incidence of PONV, total intravenous anaesthesia using propofol and remifentanil is an ideal technique allowing smooth, fast oriented wake up and reduced PONV.

Laparoscopic colorectal surgery

Surgical considerations

These procedures are becoming more popular and the benefits include a reduced stress response, better pain control and faster recovery. However, the procedure can often be very lengthy and may be converted to an open procedure.

Anaesthetic considerations

These patients will require general anaesthesia with intubation and muscle relaxation. The problems encountered will be the same as for laparoscopic surgery including hypercapnia, a steep head-down position and a long operating time. Postoperative analgesia should include a multimodal approach with paracetamol and NSAIDs. In addition, PCA and TAP blocks can be used for postoperative analgesia.

Peri-anal surgery

Surgical considerations

Peri-anal surgical procedures are usually very short, often intensely stimulating and can be very painful. Patients are usually discharged home on the same day. Lithotomy or lateral positions are commonly used for surgical access, but a prone position may be needed for some procedures. Painful stimulation and stretch of peri-anal structures may cause laryngospasm and bradycardia via vagal stimulation.

Anaesthetic considerations

Anaesthetic techniques need a sufficient depth of anaesthesia and analgesia to avoid intense surgical stimulation but also allow rapid emergence so that the patient is able to go home on the same day. A laryngeal mask is generally used as long as there are no contraindications. Short-acting opiates such as fentanyl, alfentanil or remifentanil, combined with paracetamol and NSAIDs, are a favourable analgesic regime.

Anti-reflux surgery

Surgical considerations

Anti-reflux surgery is the treatment for acid reflux. It is a condition in which the stomach contents can enter the oesophagus from the stomach and a hiatus hernia can make the condition worse. The symptoms of reflux are a burning sensation in the stomach and throat, gas bubbles and swallowing difficulty. The most common type of procedure is called a fundoplication which involves repairing the hiatal hernia if there is one, tightening the diaphragmatic opening and wrapping the upper part of the stomach around the end of the oesophagus. The procedure can be carried out as either an open or laparoscopic procedure.

Anaesthetic considerations

In the pre-operative assessment it is important to enquire about the symptoms of reflux. As most will have symptoms of reflux, a rapid sequence induction is recommended. An open procedure will require an upper midline laparotomy, so multimodal analgesia, in addition to a rectus sheath block, will provide good analgesia. Laparoscopic surgery will involve all of the problems of a pneumoperitoneum.

Whipple's procedure (pancreaticoduodenectomy)

Surgical considerations

The procedure involves removal of the head of the pancreas, the gallbladder, and part of the duodenum, followed by anastomosis of the remaining pancreas, bile duct and stomach to the jejunum. It is often indicated for resection of a pancreatic adenocarcinoma, or refractory pancreatitis.

Anaesthetic considerations

This is lengthy extensive surgery; therefore, the potential for large fluid shifts and blood loss is likely, so arterial and CVP lines are recommended. The Whipple's resection is performed through a midline abdominal incision so a thoracic epidural is the best option. Other options include abdominal wall blocks (TAP and posterior rectus sheath) or morphine PCA.

Liver resection

Surgical considerations

The most common indication for hepatic resection is for liver metastases from colorectal cancer. The aim of surgery is to excise the diseased part of the liver whilst minimising blood loss and leaving enough healthy liver to avoid liver failure. The surgical procedure is divided into three main phases: the initial phase, resection phase, with confirmation of haemostasis, and closure. In the initial phase, the liver is mobilised and the vascular anatomy exposed. During the second phase, imaging using CT and MRI will help to localise the tumour and vascular anatomy. Intra-operative ultrasound will confirm pre-operative assessments. Blood loss is very likely and can be reduced by temporary occlusion of the blood supply to the liver during parenchymal resection. These techniques to occlude the venous system can cause significant haemodynamic compromise and can reduce cardiac output by up to 60%. During the third phase, haemostasis can be secured using argon beam coagulation and fibrin glue.

The liver is made up of eight segments and in young patients with a normal hepatic parenchyma, it is safe to remove up to four segments, but patients can develop liver failure after apparently safe resections. Most patients presenting for liver resection in the UK have a normal liver parenchyma, but patients with chronic liver disease presenting for liver resection are at high risk of developing postoperative liver failure. The Child-Pugh scoring system is a reliable tool in patients with chronic liver disease.

Anaesthetic considerations

In hepatic resection, sudden catastrophic bleeding is possible, so large-bore IV access including arterial and CVP lines with cardiac output monitoring will allow better haemodynamic control. Hypoglycaemia is possible, so blood glucose should be regularly monitored including coagulation and temperature. General anaesthesia with tracheal intubation and epidural analgesia is a commonly used combination. Blood loss can be a massive problem and patients with cirrhosis and recent chemotherapy are at increased risk of haemorrhage. Postoperatively, patients developing liver failure show signs and symptoms such as jaundice, encephalopathy and coagulopathy, about 72 hours after surgery. About 30% of patients will develop significant postoperative complications including major bleeding, liver failure, renal failure, respiratory failure and sepsis.

Case scenario 1

A 40-year-old female patient with a BMI of 35 is scheduled for an elective laparoscopic cholecystectomy as a day-case procedure. She has no other comorbidities and she is not on any medication.

How would you manage this patient?

Pre-operative management

- Standard pre-operative anaesthetic assessment with routine blood tests including liver function tests and coagulation.
- Enquire about symptoms and signs of jaundice and reflux.

Intra-operative management

- Large-bore IV access.
- Avoid gastric insufflation during mask ventilation. The surgeon may request to deflate the stomach to facilitate surgical access.
- Total intravenous anaesthesia (TIVA) technique using a target-controlled infusion of propofol and remifentanil.
- Tracheal intubation with a cuffed tracheal tube

A multimodal analgesic regimen includes paracetamol, a NSAID and local infiltration of the port sites and a minimal dose of opioid (morphine). The risk of postoperative nausea and vomiting should be minimal with the use of TIVA. Prophylactic dexamethasone and ondansetron further reduce the risk of postoperative nausea and vomiting and facilitate early discharge.

Postoperative management

The patient can be discharged at 6-8 hours following the procedure, with regular paracetamol and ibuprofen. In addition, codeine phosphate can be used as required.

Case scenario 2

A 75-year-old male patient is scheduled for an elective Hartmann's procedure for cancer of the sigmoid colon. His medical history includes hypertension, a previous myocardial infarction 5 years ago treated with coronary angioplasty and Type 2 diabetes mellitus. His current medication includes aspirin 75mg OD, bisoprolol 5mg OD, metformin 1g BD and lisinopril 20mg OD.

How would you manage this patient?

Pre-operative management

- Anaesthethetic assessment with routine blood tests, coagulation, urea, electrolytes, blood glucose, ECG and HbA1c.
- The ECG shows an old inferior MI, left axis deviation and left ventricular hypertrophy; hence, an echocardiogram is requested which shows good biventricular function with no valvular abnormalities.
- Bisoprolol should be continued on the day of surgery but metformin and lisinopril should be omitted on the day of surgery.

Intra-operative management

- Large-bore IV access.
- Invasive monitoring of arterial blood pressure.
- Non-invasive monitoring of cardiac output and intravenous fluid administration titrated to balance the blood loss and to maintain stroke volume within normal limits.
- Thoracic epidural at the T10-T11 level. Low-concentration levobupivacaine (0.1%) with fentanyl 2-4µg/ml as a continuous epidural infusion.

Postoperative management

- Level 2 care in a high dependency unit where he can be closely monitored.

- Epidural analgesia generally continued up to 3 days, in addition to regular paracetamol and codeine phosphate.
- Restrictive fluid therapy and early enteral feeding.

Further reading

1.   Rucklidge M, Sanders D, Martin A. Anaesthesia for minimally invasive oesophagectomy. *Br J Anaesth CEACCP* 2010; 10: 43-7.

2.   Patel S, Lutz JM, Panchagnula U, Bansal S. Anesthesia and perioperative management of colorectal patients - a clinical review. *J Anaesthesiol Clin Pharmacol* 2012; 28: 162-71.

3.   Baldini G, Fawcett WJ. Anaesthesia for colorectal surgery. *Anesthesiology Clinics* 2015; 33: 93-123.

27 Emergency surgical procedures

George Madden

Introduction

Emergency procedures provide some unique circumstances: unlike in elective surgery, there is only limited time to prepare the patient for theatre, they are likely to have a degree of physiological derangement, and there may be uncertainty as to what the procedure itself will be. Patients who present for emergency surgery tend to be older and are at higher risk of death and major morbidity. In a few cases, these may be patients who have been declined elective surgery based on excessive risk, but now present as emergencies.

Compounding these difficulties, there are sometimes complex organisational problems, such as the competing interests of multiple surgical specialties all wanting their patients to take priority, staff who may have limited experience with certain procedures, and uncertainty over what the surgeon will find, what the operative outcome will be, and hence what the required destination for the patient should be.

What is an emergency procedure?

On first inspection, the concept of an emergency procedure may be obvious; however, as with many medical emergencies, there is a spectrum. This is exacerbated by different specialties having somewhat different concepts of what an "emergency" entails — to some it may simply mean "not elective", i.e. something that has presented via an emergency route of admission, regardless of the actual urgency of the case. At the other end of the spectrum is the "true" emergency, such as an actively haemorrhaging patient in a life-threatening situation.

The emergency theatre team needs to be able to rapidly assess and transfer to theatre the true emergency. Significant logistical arrangements may often be required. Many cases will be transferred from other sites, such as a neurosurgical emergency, and examples such as a polytrauma or ruptured abdominal aneurysm will be shocked and in need of massive transfusion. These are cases where rapid access to definitive surgery can be life-saving. To meet this need, there must be spare capacity in the emergency theatre system to allow for an immediate response.

This contrasts with the non-urgent emergency, which may be deferred for several days without suffering any harm. This does, however, pose a number of different problems. Firstly, the apparently stable patient may deteriorate if their condition is left untreated, with the adverse effects of morbidity and mortality that would ensue. Secondly, the stable patient is still likely to be occupying an acute surgical bed, and cannot be discharged until their surgery is done. They therefore constitute a waste of resources if they are deferred. Thirdly, and most importantly, these are patients who are awaiting their procedure with no small measure of anxiety, and will become increasingly distressed the longer they are left. Facilitating the timely management of these patients while ensuring that there is capacity to deal with the true emergency is a common problem.

In 1987, the National Confidential Enquiry into Patient Outcomes and Deaths (NCEPOD) introduced a classification system to rank the urgency of such emergency cases. This was subsequently revised in 2003 (Table 27.1) and it was suggested that only immediate and some urgent cases should take place overnight. In 1995, they identified that only 51% of hospitals ran emergency theatres on weekdays. This led to the creation of the NCEPOD theatre: a dedicated emergency theatre, which ran 24 hours a day, 7 days a week. Though most units now have a dedicated emergency theatre, the policy of restricting overnight operating to only the most urgent cases is more contentious.

Table 27.1. The NCEPOD classification of surgical procedures based on the urgency of surgical intervention. *Adapted from the National Confidential Enquiry into Perioperative Deaths. Classification of intervention, 2004. Available at http://www.ncepod.org.uk/pdf/NCEPODClassification.pdf.*

Code	Category	Description	Target time	Examples
1	Immediate	Immediate life (A) or limb (B) saving procedure	Within minutes	Ruptured aortic aneurysm Major trauma
2	Urgent	Condition that threatens life, limb or organ	Within hours	Perforated bowel with peritonitis Critical organ or limb ischaemia
3	Expedited	Stable patient needing early intervention for a condition that is not an immediate threat to life	Within days	Excision of bowel tumour with potential to obstruct
4	Elective	Planned in advance of admission	Planned	Joint replacement

Common emergency procedures

Despite the inherent unpredictability of an emergency theatre, there are certain procedures that may be commonplace to, and occasionally unique to, the emergency theatre (Table 27.2).

Table 27.2. Common emergency surgical procedures.

Specialty	Common procedures
General surgery	Incision and drainage of abscesses Appendicectomy 'Hot' laparoscopic cholecystectomy Bleeding or perforated peptic ulcers Laparotomy
Vascular surgery	Ruptured abdominal aortic aneurysm repair Limb amputations Vascular bypass procedures
Urology	Repair of phimosis Orchidopexy for testicular torsion Ureteric stent Nephrostomy
Gynaecology	Evacuation or retained products of conception Management of ruptured or bleeding ectopic pregnancy
Trauma	Washout of contaminated wounds Repair of hip fractures Open fixation of fractures

Pre-operative assessment

Pre-operative assessment of the emergency surgical patient follows a similar process to the elective case, with a few special differences.

Urgency

The NCEPOD classification influences the time available for pre-operative assessment and optimisation. A Category 1 case should be in theatre within minutes, and so the anaesthetist should go to assess the patient as soon as able. In these cases, assessment and anaesthesia will often be contemporaneous with resuscitation. By contrast, a Category 3 case may be stable enough for any relevant investigations to be performed prior to surgery, sometimes justifying deferment. In reality, the urgency is not fixed, and a case may become more or less urgent as the patient's condition changes. The essential point is to ensure regular review takes place if a case is delayed.

Medical history

Regardless of the situation, the assessment should include the reasons for the proposed surgery, past medical history, current medications, previous anaesthetics, starvation status and allergies, followed by an airway assessment. A full anaesthetic assessment may be compromised by the dual limitations of an acutely unwell patient whose ability to communicate their history may be hampered, and the lack of availability of medical notes. In some cases, a collateral history may be available from relatives or occasionally their primary care doctor. It must not be forgotten though that the anaesthetist may be at the end of a chain of medical professionals who have had input into the patient, and those other specialists may already have a significant amount of information.

Presenting condition

In most elective cases, the presenting symptoms have relatively little bearing on the anaesthetic technique. In contrast, the emergency patient may have acute physiological derangement as a consequence of the presenting condition, and be at risk of, or be developing complications of that condition. Furthermore, there may be some doubt as to the diagnosis, and a thorough review of the admission notes and the presenting symptoms may lead the anaesthetist to consider other differential diagnoses that may influence further management.

Drug history

In most elective cases, the patient's drug history is what they are taking normally at home. In emergency circumstances it is important to know not just what they were taking prior to admission, but what drugs have been stopped, and what new agents have been started. In patients undergoing neuraxial procedures, it is especially important to know the time of the last dose of prophylactic low-molecular-weight heparin, and in septic patients when the last dose of antibiotics was, and when the next is due.

Anaesthetic history

The main difference with emergency surgery is that deferment and cancellation are generally not possible, whereas an elective case that gives a history suggestive of an adverse reaction to anaesthetic agents can be deferred for further investigation; the emergency cannot. Additionally, the presence of sepsis, recent anticoagulant use, inadequate fasting or other pathologies may severely restrict the mode of anaesthesia.

These problems can often test the skills of an anaesthetist; the morbidly obese patient taking anticoagulants and who describes a reaction to anaesthetic agents may present problems for regional, volatile or even total intravenous anaesthesia. Careful history taking, a thorough knowledge of pharmacokinetics, and skill with ultrasound-guided regional techniques may rescue such a situation.

Physiological assessment

In some emergencies, the need for urgent surgery represents the definitive management, or sometimes part of the resuscitation, of the patient. As such the assessment of the patient's physiological condition can be crucial. In extremis this may involve an Airway-Breathing-Circulation type of assessment with ongoing resuscitation, but more commonly it may involve assessing the need for pre-operative optimisation or anticipating postoperative organ support.

The extent of pre-optimisation is dependent on the time available. In ideal circumstances, any acute hypoxaemia, hypercapnia, hypotension, dysrhythmia or metabolic disturbance should be investigated and treatment established before coming to theatre. Where this is not feasible, treatment may need to be established intra-operatively and continued in a critical care environment

Airway assessment

In the emergency setting, there is a far increased risk of aspiration. This may be due to lack of time available for pre-operative fasting, delayed gastric emptying due to pain or mechanical bowel obstruction causing vomiting. In these cases it is imperative to rapidly secure the airway after induction, and thus an unanticipated difficult airway has the potential to be catastrophic. Therefore, the importance of airway assessment and adequate pre-oxygenation cannot be over-emphasised. It is particularly important to determine fasting status and a recent history of vomiting. In those who have suffered major trauma or have received significant amounts of opioid, there is the possibility of gastroparesis. If this group of patients is adequately fasted but either not hungry or nauseous, one should be alert to that possibility. It is usual, particularly after trauma, to count the hours from the last meal to the time of injury as the fasting time, making the assumption that no further gastric emptying has occurred after the event.

In a few rare instances, there is little time for airway assessment due to extreme urgency. Every effort should be made to make as much assessment as possible, but in these cases the priority should be to have a contingency plan ready should intubation fail. Here, the use of videolaryngoscopes is becoming increasingly common to maximise the chances of success. It should also be noted that in these rare emergency situations, the possibility of waking the patient up may not be feasible.

Risk stratification in emergencies

An area of growing interest is risk stratification in both elective and emergency surgery because of an associated high degree of mortality and morbidity in a small subset of patients. It is generally accepted that a high-risk patient has a predicted mortality of >5%. Prospective identification of these patients, however, is fraught with difficulties. The use of biomarkers remains in the experimental stages, and has yet to enter mainstream practice. Echocardiography has been criticised as being a static measure of cardiac function, thus it gives limited information on dynamic function. Cardiopulmonary exercise testing (CPET) is of greater value, but is not feasible in the emergency setting.

Cardiac surgery has had great success using logistical regression analysis to design a comprehensive risk scoring system. Similar risk assessment models have been described but they suffer from a number of limitations:

- Utility vs. discriminatory value: essentially, the better the model is at predicting the outcome accurately, the more complex it becomes, and the more information it requires. Usually, the most discriminatory models require a logistic equation which requires a computer to calculate. This limits the usefulness, or utility, of it in general practice. The ideal system would be a simple, robust scoring tool which can be easily assigned and calculated at the bedside.
- Dealing with heterogeneity: cardiac surgery has the advantage of a limited number of relatively similar procedures, whereas general surgery has a much broader variation. The choice is to either develop a tool which can be validated across a wide range of procedures, or to create multiple tools which are procedure-specific. The advantage of the former is that it is easier for the user, and more likely to be used routinely at the expense of greater inaccuracy. The latter is more difficult for the user but may yield better results.

A wide number of tools have been proposed, the simplest being the American Society of Anesthesiologists Physical Status (ASA-PS) classification, which is highly subjective and unreliable. Below is a brief summary of some of the more widely used tools (Table 27.3).

Table 27.3. Various risk assessment tools.

Tool	Description
ASA-PS	Developed in 1948, originally used to guide billing for surgical procedures. Highly subjective and not predictive of outcome. However, it is easy to assign and well established.
Surgical Risk Scale	Score based upon ASA-PS, NCEPOD classification, and BUPA severity of surgery scale. Applicable to general surgical procedures and good discrimination. Simple to use.
P-POSSUM	Developed from logistic regression, and originally for risk adjustment for audit purposes. Well validated as a risk prediction tool. Variants exist for oesophageal and vascular surgery. Some of the variables can only be assigned intra-operatively, so the pre-operative score may be inaccurate. It is also complex, requiring computer software.
NSQUIP Surgical Risk Calculator	Complex equation with multiple data points required to be entered into an online calculator. Validated in the US and not widely used in the UK, but based on data collected from more than 1.4 million operations. Gives information on mortality and specific morbidities.
Surgical Outcome Risk Tool	Recently developed with support from NCEPOD. Uses an online calculator, but with fewer data fields than NSQUIP. It has not yet entered mainstream use but may be promising in the future.

The practical value of these risk scores is to anticipate the risk of an adverse outcome so that resources can be directed into prevention or early and aggressive management of complications. This generally translates as postoperative critical care or an equivalent. It can also be used to guide the surgeon in planning which procedure to offer, if more than one choice exists, and probably most importantly, gives the opportunity for a frank discussion to take place with the patient, giving a realistic impression of the risks involved.

Intra-operative management

In many cases, the emergency case may be no different to the elective case; however, there are some common problems that can occur.

Aspiration risk

The patient may present an aspiration risk due to underlying comorbidity, inadequate fasting time, gastroparesis, peritonitis, or mechanical bowel obstruction. The traditional method for management of aspiration risk is the rapid sequence induction (RSI). The traditionally described RSI is now frequently modified, particularly in terms of the drugs used (Table 27.4).

The key to success is anticipation and planning, as with all airway techniques. It is imperative to secure and protect the airway as early as possible, and so careful attention to head position can improve the chance of success. It is equally important to plan for failure, so a trolley that can be easily tipped head-down and ready access to suction equipment is vital. Any nasogastric tubes already in place should be aspirated to empty the stomach. Should intubation fail, proceeding with surgery using a laryngeal mask airway is rarely advisable. The 'Plan B' should usually be to maintain oxygenation with a second-generation supraglottic airway device (SAD) and then depending on the urgency of the situation, to attempt intubation via the SAD or to wake the patient up. Should the latter option be chosen, it should be noted that the use of opioids may delay the process, and so careful thought should be given before their use.

If intubation is successful, it should be remembered that the aspiration risk will continue until the patient fully regains their airway reflexes. It is therefore appropriate to extubate only when the patient is fully awake, muscle relaxation fully reversed as assessed using train-of-four (TOF)

Table 27.4. Various steps involved in classical and modified rapid sequence induction.

	Classical RSI	Modifications
1	Prepare suction, endotracheal tube, laryngoscope, bougie, and optimise the patient's head position	
2	Pre-oxygenate for >3 minutes with 100% oxygen	• Five vital capacity breaths. • Pre-oxygenation until end-tidal oxygen is above 80-90%. • Use of CPAP. • Use 20 to 25° head-up position. • Use high-flow nasal oxygenation.
3	Apply cricoid pressure at 10N	
4	Administer thiopentone 5mg/kg then suxamethonium 1-2mg/kg	• Addition of opioids such as fentanyl, alfentanil or remifentanil. • Use of propofol rather than thiopentone. • Use of rocuronium 1.2mg/kg instead of suxamethonium.
5	Apply cricoid pressure at 30N	• Some choose to not use cricoid pressure as it may distort the laryngoscopy view with little evidence to support it reducing regurgitation.
6	Wait until fasciculations have ceased or 1 minute, without ventilating	• Increasingly, gentle ventilation is accepted. • Nasal oxygen during apnoeic period.
7	Direct laryngoscopy and intubate	• Increasingly, videolaryngoscopes are chosen to improve the chances of success.
8	Confirm position with capnography and auscultation before removing cricoid	

monitoring (TOF ratio >0.9), and the patient is able to respond to commands. The traditional position for this is the left lateral position, though many prefer the patient in the semi-recumbent position instead. In cases where there is significant concern about aspiration, insertion of a nasogastric tube to empty the stomach may be of benefit.

Hypovolaemia

A patient may be hypovolaemic for a number of reasons: they may be actively haemorrhaging, have increased insensible losses due to fever, have lost fluid intra-abdominally due to the underlying disease process, or have simply undergone prolonged fasting.

Wherever possible, adequate fluid resuscitation should occur prior to induction, and particularly in the case of the haemorrhaging patient, rapid blood transfusion to restore the circulating volume can make general anaesthesia much safer.

The hypovolaemic patient will be compensating for their reduced circulating volume by peripheral vasoconstriction, tachycardia, and a low urine output. Elderly patients or those with significant comorbidity may not tolerate these physiological changes well, whereas the younger patient may compensate well enough to mask quite significant hypovolaemia. Biochemical measures that may help include evidence of haemoconcentration such as rising haemoglobin and haematocrit, raised urea, and raised lactate. If a central venous catheter is *in situ*, central venous oxygen saturation will be low (below 70%).

Once general anaesthesia (or neuraxial anaesthesia) is induced, these compensatory mechanisms will cease, as will any underlying sympathetic drive that the patient normally relies on. The consequence is potentially profound hypotension. Vasopressors such as metaraminol or phenylephrine may be used in the short term to maintain an adequate blood pressure, but characteristically, these effects will be short-lived and repeat boluses will be required. Restoration of circulating volume will have a much longer lasting effect. To avoid excessive fluid administration, the use of non-invasive cardiac output monitors may be valuable; however, simple measures such as the straight-leg raise or fluid challenge may be equally valuable indicators of fluid responsiveness.

In circumstances of extreme hypovolaemia, it is advisable to use invasive intra-arterial blood pressure monitoring prior to induction in order to closely monitor and respond to sudden changes that a non-invasive blood pressure cuff will not be able to read. Any significantly shocked patient will also have significant gastroparesis, so rapid sequence induction is routinely advocated. It is also becoming increasingly common to use ketamine 2-3mg/kg as the induction agent of choice. Though this produces a dissociative anaesthesia which takes some experience to confidently use, its vasoconstricting actions can maintain arteriolar tone during induction.

The act of induction may also worsen the problem. In the case of a ruptured abdominal aortic aneurysm, the abdominal wall tone helps to tamponade the bleeding. After induction, this effect is lost, and the patient will continue to bleed. Recognition is crucial, and the availability of a surgeon to immediately intervene is required.

Any sudden change in haemodynamic status associated with significant bleeding should alert the anaesthetist to the potential problem. Close communication with the surgeon is crucial, and the priority should be to rapidly control the bleeding. If this is not immediately possible, the anaesthetist should be prepared to urgently request blood products via a major haemorrhage protocol (refer to Chapter 13, Peri-operative blood transfusion). It is now recommended that where emergency blood is required, that Group O negative is reserved for females, particularly of childbearing age, and that O positive may be used in males. Group-specific blood can be available before a full cross-match is ready, and this should be the next choice. It should be remembered that hypothermia can worsen coagulopathy, so any blood products should be warmed and patient warming measures should be used. Though an arterial line is clearly valuable in this situation, it should not delay securing haemostasis, so in the direst circumstances it is better to proceed with surgery so the surgeon can gain control of the bleeding while a rapid blood transfusion takes place, and then invasive blood pressure monitoring can be instituted as soon as the situation is more controlled.

Specifically in major haemorrhage, there are clear protocols in UK hospitals, underpinned by the Joint United Kingdom Blood Transfusion and Tissue Transplantation Services Professional Advisory Committee (JPAC). In the presence of ongoing severe bleeding and clinical shock, the major haemorrhage protocol is activated. Transfusion of blood and blood products should be guided by haemoglobin concentration and clotting screen results. Where possible, near-patient testing of coagulation parameters should be used to ensure rapid decision-making.

Unstable cardiac disease

Most patients with significant cardiac comorbidity will either be optimised and stable when presenting for elective surgery, or will be deferred for optimisation, or even refused surgery. The emergency setting, therefore, has greater frequency of unstable cardiac disease, due to this, or due to decompensation triggered by acute illness. These patients do represent a high-risk group and should be managed carefully by senior practitioners.

Again, these patients will be dependent on their sympathetic tone to maintain adequate perfusion. They are also dependent on this tone to maintain coronary perfusion, which relies on diastolic pressure and the length of diastole. A fall in diastolic pressure caused by vasodilatation, and excessive tachycardia, can be extremely difficult to rescue. An episode of severe hypotension can worsen myocardial perfusion and lead to ischaemia which then worsens cardiac output, leading to a vicious cycle if not aggressively managed.

These patients are likely to have a 'slow circulation' where an intravenous anaesthetic may take much longer than anticipated to have an effect, leading to inadvertent overdosing. As most induction agents, including ketamine, are direct myocardial depressants, they can worsen myocardial function. Fortunately, these patients tend to be more sensitive to anaesthetic agents, so a careful titrated dose of induction agents can limit these effects.

Invasive arterial monitoring is almost mandatory in such patients. Ideally instituted when awake, the induction agents can be titrated to effect, and immediately or even pre-emptively counteracted with vasopressors. An infusion of vasopressors is often required to maintain a normal blood pressure, and though this may be done peripherally, it is often advisable to site a central venous catheter.

The induction agent of choice is often difficult to choose, and largely relies upon the experience of the anaesthetist. In the trauma setting, it is becoming increasingly common to induce elderly and frail patients using a sevoflurane gas induction. This has the advantage of a gradual and smooth onset, reducing episodes of hypotension. It does, however, require a patient that is not at risk of aspiration. An alternative approach may be learned from the cardiothoracic anaesthetist, where the routine practice is to use large doses of fentanyl, such as 5-10µg/kg, followed by slow titration of an induction agent. Fentanyl has the advantage of having very few cardiovascular effects, but it is not an anaesthetic agent itself; it simply allows for greater haemodynamic stability and much lower doses of anaesthetic agent. Midazolam has the advantage of reducing the incidence of awareness in cases where the amount of anaesthetic given needs to be kept as low as possible. In a few cases it may be the only hypnotic alongside high-dose fentanyl, but this is reserved for the very high-risk case.

During maintenance, most volatile anaesthetic agents cause a degree of myocardial depression and vasodilatation; however, this can be offset using appropriate vasopressors. Avoiding fluid overload is important, but hypovolaemia is more common, and an adequate preload will improve cardiac output. Cautious, ideally goal-directed fluid administration is suggested.

It is worth making special mention of severe aortic stenosis. This is particularly dangerous for the anaesthetist, as this patient essentially has a fixed cardiac output, and is dependent upon their vascular tone. Loss of vascular tone will result in profound hypotension and significantly impaired coronary filling. This scenario can be near impossible to rescue. The principles of management are essentially the same — awake invasive blood pressure monitoring, careful titration of induction agents, and infusion of vasopressors — but the blood pressure must be very carefully maintained.

Sepsis

This is a very common presentation to the emergency theatre. A patient in septic shock is likely to be hypovolaemic, have an element of myocardial depression, but their most significant problem is vasoplegia. Such patients may need quite aggressive vasopressor treatment, and ideally the patient should first go to critical care for this to be established.

Induction of anaesthesia of these patients can cause significant decompensation. Here it is especially important to have a well-resuscitated patient with vasopressors already running and intra-arterial blood pressure monitoring. The induction agent is less important than its careful titration, and in many cases propofol is as good as any other agent, though ketamine, or even a combination of ketamine and propofol can be used.

More commonly, the septic patient may appear relatively stable during induction, but haemodynamic instability develops as the source of sepsis is manipulated by the surgeon. Peritoneal contamination by bowel contents can be particularly potent and the 'septic shower' produced during surgery can cause quite sudden and severe instability. The anaesthetist should be anticipating such events, and be prepared to treat. In these cases, it is sometimes prudent to site a central venous catheter even when the patient appears stable at induction.

It should not be forgotten that sepsis can lead on to multi-organ dysfunction, including impaired gas exchange heralding the acute respiratory distress syndrome. Septic patients can rapidly deteriorate during surgery, and an apparently stable patient may need a period of invasive ventilation.

Arrhythmias

Arrhythmias can pose a problem to the anaesthetist. Most commonly this is a patient with new-onset or worsened atrial fibrillation. Ideally, they should be delayed while control is established; however, there are times when the arrhythmia is being driven by a septic process, and satisfactory control will not be possible until the source of sepsis is dealt with. Here a balance must be struck between the need for surgery and the need to control the arrhythmia.

Analgesia

There are a number of problems associated with the emergency patient and pain control. Firstly, the patient is likely to already be in pain, and thus an element of 'wind-up' may have occurred, making pain control more difficult. Secondly, the operative procedure may be unfamiliar to the anaesthetist so may be difficult to predict, but also the procedure itself may deviate from what was initially intended, and thus the approach to pain management may change accordingly.

This is compounded by the state of the patient. A haemodynamically unstable patient may be worsened by spinal or epidural anaesthesia or analgesia. Any procedure that leaves a foreign body such as a catheter in a sterile compartment, such as an epidural, is contraindicated if there is a bacteraemia. Single injections such as spinal anaesthetics are potentially higher risk and may cause haemodynamic instability in these patients, though regional techniques are generally deemed safe, as long as it is recognised that the use of local anaesthetic in infected, acidotic tissue, is likely to be ineffective.

Coagulopathy should also be considered, both for the patient that may be anticoagulated due to cardiac disease, or simply for prophylaxis in hospital. Reversal of anticoagulants should always be considered, but it may not be easily achievable in some circumstances. Major haemorrhage itself can also cause coagulopathy, and so caution should be exercised in any potentially bleeding patient.

These problems essentially mean that epidural analgesia is often contraindicated. Regional techniques such as transversus abdominus plane (TAP) or rectus sheath blocks may be useful adjuncts, but ultimately the patient will rely on systemic analgesia, usually patient-controlled opioid analgesia. Simple analgesics such as paracetamol should never be forgotten, however.

Postoperative care

The majority of emergency patients are likely to return to ward-level care, and have a reasonable postoperative recovery. However, high-risk patients are more likely to be emergencies, and these patients are at significant risk of suffering complications such as pneumonia, respiratory failure, myocardial ischaemia, paralytic ileus, acute kidney injury, etc. It is likely that the occurrence of these complications is more to do with patient factors than the care that they receive, but that timely and aggressive treatment can improve their outcomes. This is one of the justifications for risk assessment prospectively and arranging critical care postoperatively.

In all cases it is worth considering where the patient will be after surgery. In some cases they may arrive in theatre directly from the emergency department. The location they return to may be limited by their presenting condition, or influence the strategy for analgesia (for instance, it is common for epidurals to only be managed in specific locations). It is important to consider the requirements for the patient postoperatively and ensure that a bed can be made available.

Case scenario 1

A 27-year-old female presents with a 2-day history of worsening right lower quadrant pain, associated with fever and vomiting. She has tenderness and guarding in the right lower quadrant on examination, and raised inflammatory markers. She is booked in for a laparoscopic appendicectomy.

How would you manage this patient?

Pre-operative assessment

She required intravenous morphine in the emergency department and has been taking oral morphine since. She says the pain has been getting worse in the last 24 hours since admission. No diagnostic imaging has been performed.

Drug history: no regular medications, no allergies.

Past medical history: she smokes 20 cigarettes a day on average since the age of sixteen. She had childhood asthma but hasn't used her inhaler for "years" and no longer keeps one. She never had any severe exacerbations.

Anaesthetic history: no previous surgery and denies any anaesthetic problems in first-degree relatives.

Physiological assessment: pyrexia of 37.8° on admission, and since then has been apyrexial. Her heart rate is 96 bpm, blood pressure is 130/76mmHg and respiratory rate is 18 per minute.

Airway assessment: Mallampati Grade 2. Good neck movements and thyromental distance more than 6.5cm. Although she has not eaten for more than 12 hours, she feels nauseous and had vomited twice in the emergency department, but not since.

Investigations: haemoglobin 141g/L, platelets 453 x 10^9/L, white cell count 14.3 x 10^9/L, pregnancy test negative. Blood group and save done.

Risk stratification and urgency

This is an ASA Class 2 patient, undergoing moderate surgery. Assuming all other parameters are normal, P-POSSUM would predict a mortality of 0.8% and a morbidity of 19%. The Surgical Outcome Risk Tool (SORT) predicts a 30-day mortality of 0.67%. Ward level care would be appropriate postoperatively. This would be an NCEPOD Class 3 case, as there is little evidence that she would significantly deteriorate in the coming hours.

Intra-operative management

Standard monitoring as set out by the Association of Anaesthetists of Great Britain and Ireland (AAGBI) is required, and wide-bore intravenous access is recommended, as this will be a laparoscopic procedure.

A rapid sequence induction should be used. Thiopentone and suxamethonium would be acceptable choices, but given her airway examination does not predict difficulty, opioids would be reasonable (as opiods can potentially delay waking should intubation fail). Equally, propofol would be an acceptable choice.

Maintenance could be with any volatile agent, with analgesia provided with either surgical infiltration or bilateral TAP blocks supplemented with intravenous morphine.

Any female patient of childbearing age with iliac fossa pain should raise a suspicion for a gynaecological cause such as ovarian torsion. It is not uncommon at laparoscopy for the surgeon to want a gynaecologist to attend should there be any evidence of this. This has little bearing on the anaesthetic management, except that it may delay the case and result in periods of relatively little sympathetic stimulation.

After surgery, the patient should be extubated only when fully awake.

Postoperative care

The patient is returned to the ward with regular paracetamol and oral morphine, with intramuscular morphine available for 'rescue'. Antiemetics, fluids and oxygen should also be prescribed.

Case scenario 2

A 72-year-old male is admitted into the emergency department with severe abdominal pain and hypotension. A bedside ultrasound demonstrates an abdominal aortic aneurysm. You are called to review the case urgently and the on-call vascular consultant has been called in from home.

How would you manage this patient?

Pre-operative assessment

Past medical history: moderate COPD, hypertension, non-ST elevation MI 3 years ago requiring percutaneous coronary intervention. He is a current smoker with a 60-pack per year history.

Drug history: inhalers for COPD, aspirin, beta-blocker, ACE inhibitor, statin. No allergies.

Anaesthetic history: hernia repair under general anaesthesia many years ago. Uneventful.

Physiological assessment: heart rate 100 bpm, blood pressure 92/63mmHg, SpO$_2$ 97% on 15L/min via a non-rebreathe mask. Looks pale. Peripheries cold, radial pulse is weak.

Airway assessment: upper set dentures, good mouth opening, Mallampati 2.

Investigations: urea and electrolytes, full blood count, clotting screen and cross-match have all been sent urgently, but no results are available.

Risk stratification and urgency

This is a classic NCEPOD Category 1 case. Thirty-day mortality is usually quoted at 50%, and without repair, the mortality approaches 100%. If necessary an elective list would be suspended.

Intra-operative management

Prior to induction, it is vital to ensure there are blood products available. A major haemorrhage protocol should be activated, and the blood bank contacted to ensure they have received the blood samples that were sent. A rapid transfusion system, which heats the blood and transfuses it under pressure should be ready. Two wide-bore intravenous accesses should be secured if not already done so.

In scenarios such as this, it is acceptable to induce with just intravenous access. An arterial line is likely to be difficult in a shocked patient, and this may delay surgery. It is better to proceed with surgery on the understanding that the priority is to control the bleeding first, and to rapidly transfuse blood products until then on the assumption that they will be hypotensive and rapidly exsanguinating. That said, there is often time to insert an arterial line while awaiting a senior surgeon.

Once the patient has been transferred to theatre, they should be placed supine with both arms outstretched in a 'cruciform' position. As induction will cause a loss of tamponade and decompensation, the consultant surgeon should be scrubbed, and the patient should be prepped and draped before induction of anaesthesia.

A modified rapid sequence induction, with a higher dose of fentanyl to spare the amount of induction agent is ideal. Fentanyl or ketamine would be a good choice if used with caution, and midazolam may be considered as such cases have a high risk of awareness. A videolaryngoscope may improve the chance of securing the airway at the first attempt.

As rapid transfusion of blood takes place to maintain the circulating volume, the surgeon will perform a midline laparotomy and aim to cross-clamp above the aneurysm. This will markedly improve the circulation, and allow for a degree of stability where arterial and central venous access can be obtained. The circulation can be restored while the aneurysm is excluded with a graft. The next period of instability is when the 'top end' suture line of the graft is tested, potentially causing a leak and further haemorrhage. This should be rapidly controlled and the leak repaired. The next, and more crucial, stage is when the distal clamps are removed, restoring circulation to the legs that have been ischaemic for some time. This can cause an influx of cytokines into the circulation that can act as vasodilators and myocardial depressants, requiring significant escalation in vasopressor therapy.

Postoperative care

This patient must go to critical care postoperatively, and only the exceptional case will be extubated in theatre. Analgesia will be with a morphine or alfentanil infusion, and they will be sedated with midazolam or propofol. There is significant morbidity associated with a ruptured abdominal aortic aneurysm, including coagulopathy associated with massive transfusion, renal failure related to cross-clamping near the origins of the renal arteries, myocardial ischaemia, respiratory failure, and paralysis related to spinal cord hypoperfusion.

Further reading

1. Cullinane M, Gray AJ, Hargraves CMK, *et al.* The 2003 Report of the National Confidential Enquiry into Perioperative Deaths. NCEPOD, 2003.

2. National Confidential Enquiry into Perioperative Deaths. Who operates when? A Report by the National Confidential Enquiry into Perioperative Deaths 1995. NCEPOD, 1997.

3. Pearse RM, Harrison DA, James P, *et al.* Identification and characterisation of the high-risk surgical population in the United Kingdom. *Crit Care* 2006; 10: R81.

4. Frerk C, Mitchell VS, McNarry AF, *et al.* Difficult Airway Society 2015 guidelines for management of unanticipated difficult intubation in adults. *Br J Anaesth* 2015; 115: 827-48.

28 Obstetric anaesthesia

Llewellyn Fenton-May

Introduction

The obstetric setting provides unique challenges to the anaesthetist relating to both the changes in physiology associated with pregnancy and the dynamic nature of the work.

Physiology of pregnancy

Pregnancy and labour induce significant physiological changes in the parturient. It is essential that the labour ward anaesthetist has a sound understanding of these changes in order to provide safe analgesia and anaesthesia.

Cardiovascular system

At term, increases in both heart rate and stroke volume lead to an increase in cardiac output of up to 50%, with further increases during labour and delivery. The uterus (primarily the placenta) receives approximately 10% of maternal cardiac output (up to 700ml/min) and unlike the other vital organs, the uterine blood flow is not autoregulated, rather it is dependent on maternal blood pressure.

Systemic vascular resistance drops by around 10% due to the development of the low-resistance placental bed and the dilatatory effects of progesterone and oestrogen.

From about 13 weeks' gestation, the uterus will have sufficient mass to begin to cause a degree of aortocaval compression, reducing venous return and thus cardiac output in the supine position. Whilst the aorta is unlikely to be completely obstructed, reduced distal flow can be demonstrated and will reduce uteroplacental blood flow, thus potentially compromising the fetus.

Systolic blood pressure will tend to drop by around 10mmHg during the second trimester.

Left ventricular hypertrophy and dilatation may lead to left axis deviation on the ECG. Mild sinus tachycardia, ST depression and T wave flattening can be found as normal variants in pregnancy.

Respiratory system

Basal oxygen consumption is increased by around 20% at term, with further increases during labour. Functional residual capacity drops by 15-20% due to the upward displacement of the diaphragm by the gravid uterus. Vital capacity remains unchanged due to increases in transverse and anteroposterior lung diameters. In the supine position, closing capacity may encroach on the functional residual capacity.

Minute ventilation is increased by up to 40% (due to an increase in both tidal volume and respiratory rate), with respiratory alkalosis and a corresponding left side shift on the oxygen dissociation curve to improve oxygen delivery to the fetus and carbon dioxide offloading. Arterial pH is maintained by a compensatory decrease in bicarbonate.

Airway

The airway changes through the course of pregnancy and labour, with difficult intubation being more common than in the general population (reports suggest 1:300). Historically, failed oxygenation secondary to failed intubation has been the leading cause of anaesthesia-related maternal mortality in the Confidential Enquiries into Maternal Deaths.

The airway may be more difficult to manage due to anatomical changes including increase in breast size, increased maternal weight and full dentition. Mucosal oedema can cause difficulties due to both narrowing of the airway and an increased tendency to bleeding on instrumentation. The use of a left tilt to reduce aortocaval compression may lead to difficulties if the tilt is not taken into account during the application of cricoid pressure.

Difficulties with intubation are multifactorial; whilst the above anatomical changes occur, general anaesthetics are less commonly used for obstetric procedures. Most often, general anaesthetics are administered for emergency obstetric procedures due to their associated time pressures and when these occur out of hours an experienced obstetric anaesthetist may not always be available.

Gastrointestinal system

Progesterone, amongst other hormones, decreases the pressure of the lower oesophageal sphincter over the course of pregnancy. This combined with the mechanical effects of the gravid uterus both disrupting the sphincter and increasing intra-abdominal pressure can lead to significant reduction in the overall barrier pressure, predisposing to gastro-oesophageal reflux and aspiration. This risk is again increased by the delay in gastric emptying present during labour.

It is unclear exactly when these factors combine to increase the risk of aspiration during general anaesthesia, and probably varies with other patient-specific factors, but it seems sensible to consider a rapid sequence induction to secure the airway from 16-18 weeks' gestation onwards.

Renal

The kidneys increase in size due to an increase in vascularity and a physiological hydronephrosis. There is no increase in the number of nephrons.

Progesterone-mediated relaxation of both the ureters and bladder combined with uterine pressure on the ureters leads to an increase in the residual volume of urine and a susceptibility to urinary tract infections.

Glomerular filtration rate is increased by 50-60% by the increase in blood volume and cardiac output. This leads to a reduction in urea and creatinine of up to 40% from pre-pregnancy levels. The increase in glucose and protein filtration can exceed the maximal tubular reabsorption leading to a physiological glycosuria or proteinuria. Osmolality is lower as a result of an altered threshold for antidiuretic hormone secretion and increased progesterone and renin-angiotensin-aldosterone system (RAAS) activity.

Haematological

Plasma volume rises by up to 50% by term, driven by the above change in RAAS activity. Red cell mass initially dips, but rises again from around 8 weeks' gestation to about 30% above normal levels by term, driven by an increase in erythropoietin. This discrepancy between the rise in plasma volume and red cell mass results in a physiological anaemia.

The white cell count rises slightly during pregnancy, and more significantly during labour (levels of up to 15×10^9/L).

Platelet turnover is increased, and some women develop mild thrombocytopenia beyond that which could be expected from dilutional effects. Platelet activity is probably increased though, resulting in relatively normal function in these women.

Pregnancy is a hypercoagulable state, with increased concentrations of fibrinogen, thrombin and factors VII, VIII, IX, X, XII and von Willebrand factor. Factors XI and XIII are decreased whilst prothrombin and factor V do not significantly change. Protein S concentration drops through pregnancy, but the other anticoagulants do not.

Albumin and total plasma protein concentrations are reduced, resulting in a drop in the binding capacity for various drugs. Plasma cholinesterase concentration is also reduced resulting in a reduction in the metabolism of suxamethonium.

Central nervous system

Increased intra-abdominal pressure and inferior vena cava compression causes an increase in the venous pressure in the lower half of the body. It results in an increase in blood flow through the epidural venous plexus. This reduces the volume of the epidural space increasing the spread of local anaesthetic and also increases the chances of hitting and cannulating an epidural vein. It also causes the pressure in the epidural space (normally slightly negative) to be slightly positive. During contractions the blood flow through these veins and the pressure in the space is even higher. Similarly, the subarachnoid space and thus cerebrospinal fluid (CSF) volume is decreased and pressure increased, resulting in a relatively larger spread of any drugs injected into it.

There is an increase in CNS sensitivity to volatile anaesthetics, resulting in a reduction in minimum alveolar concentration (MAC) requirement during pregnancy to around 60% of normal and also to opioids and local anaesthetics. This is thought to be due to the effects of progesterone and β-endorphins. Progesterone, however, has a stimulatory effect on respiratory drive, providing some protection from opioid-mediated respiratory depression.

The combination of reduced protein binding, increased neuronal sensitivity to local anaesthetics and increased vascularity of the epidural space makes local anaesthetic systemic toxicity a potential concern on the labour ward.

Endocrine system

The anterior pituitary gland increases in size by up to 135% during pregnancy in order to produce more prolactin to drive lactation. This returns to normal soon after delivery even in women who breast feed. Due to this increase in activity and the anterior pituitary gland's portal blood supply, severe hypotension during haemorrhage can occasionally result in necrosis of the gland (Sheehan's syndrome).

Thyroid hyperplasia during pregnancy sometimes results in the development of a goitre. Whilst the production of thyroid hormones is increased, oestrogen stimulates hepatic thyroid binding globulin production, so free hormone levels are normally stable.

Placental corticotropin-releasing hormone stimulates adrenocorticotropic hormone (ACTH) production, which increases cortisol and aldosterone levels, contributing to water retention and a degree of insulin resistance.

Other systems

It is normal for women to gain around 10-15kg during pregnancy as a result of the fetus, placenta, amniotic fluid, water retention and breast engorgement.

Increased production of relaxin results in ligamentous relaxation, which facilitates the passage of the fetus through the birth canal. It can also lead to soft tissue problems during pregnancy such as symphysis pubis dysfunction, which can be quite debilitating. Lower back pain is common both during and after pregnancy. This is probably due to the increased lumbar lordosis required in response to the growing uterus, although positioning during labour and caring for a newborn may also contribute.

Pain relief in labour

Subjective experiences of labour vary widely, with significant psychological and social factors. Given the intermittent nature of the pain and the desire to avoid both maternal and neonatal side effects, the perfect agent has yet to be developed.

Non-pharmacological

Various non-pharmacological techniques are used for labour, including transcutaneous electrical nerve stimulation (TENS), hypnotherapy, relaxation techniques, aromatherapy and water birth. There is limited evidence for these methods, but they appear to be safe. Many of them appear to provide some pain relief during early labour and improve maternal satisfaction.

Pharmacological

Inhaled nitrous oxide as Entonox® (a 50:50 mixture of nitrous oxide with oxygen) is a popular method of labour analgesia. Due to its low solubility, nitrous oxide has a rapid onset and offset of action. Reported analgesic effects vary, with some studies demonstrating superior analgesia to opioids and others showing more limited effects. Some of its reported benefits might be due to distraction and the mother's perception of control of her own analgesia. Peak analgesia is reached after around 50 seconds of constant use, so a degree of maternal training might improve analgesia by ensuring that the peak of the contraction pain coincides with the peak nitrous effects.

Entonox® has many advantages in labour analgesia — it is easily and rapidly available in a variety of settings, does not appear to have significant adverse effects on the mother, fetus or labour and does not require a specialist to provide it. Side effects that can limit its use include a dry mouth, nausea and disorientation. There is a theoretical risk of bone marrow suppression due to nitrous oxide's inactivation of vitamin B12 as a cofactor to methionine synthase.

Non-opioid and weak opioid analgesics have a ceiling effect and tend not to be effective beyond the early stages of labour.

Intramuscular pethidine (a synthetic opioid and phenylpiperidine derivative) can be given by midwives independently in the UK. Thus, it is commonly used for labour analgesia where other methods have failed to provide relief. Despite its popularity across the UK, it is probably inferior to other drugs. Intramuscular diamorphine is becoming popular as an alternative with less sedation and nausea.

Both pethidine and diamorphine probably exert a significant amount of their effects through sedation and amnesia and often have limited effects on pain scores, with significant numbers of women still having moderate to severe pain scores and limited satisfaction. They both cross the placenta and can result in neonatal sedation, with pethidine and its metabolite norpethidine being ion trapped in the fetus. There is limited evidence relating to their effects on labour and breast-feeding, but opioids might be associated with reduced suckling and early abandonment of breast-feeding.

Patient-controlled analgesia (PCA) can be provided with opioid agonists, chiefly remifentanil. Some units report extremely low epidural rates thanks to the use of remifentanil PCA. Remifentanil is a potent opioid agonist, which is broken down by plasma esterases. It has a rapid onset of action and a relatively context insensitive half-life of 3-4 minutes. A certain amount of maternal training is required to ensure that a bolus is delivered as the contractions start so that the peak effect coincides as closely as possible with the peak of the contraction. Even with the short half-life, maternal respiratory depression is a concern and both respiratory and cardiac arrests have been reported, particularly in women with intra-uterine deaths. With this in mind, the technique cannot be recommended without careful midwife training, strict one-to-one care and respiratory monitoring.

Central neuraxial blockade

Pain from the uterus and thus most of the pain in the first stage, is transmitted via fibres returning to T10-L1. During the second stage, the pain is mainly from the cervix and birth canal and is transmitted through S2-4.

A working epidural provides the best analgesia for labour, but is associated with some significant complications and requires trained personnel to insert and monitor it. Beyond the analgesic benefits of epidurals, they may be of benefit in other settings, for example, in situations where it is necessary to rapidly establish anaesthesia for operative delivery such as multiple deliveries and breech presentation, maternal cardiac diseases, maternal respiratory disease and pre-eclampsia.

Contraindications to central neuraxial blockade are common to all areas of anaesthesia and include:

- Patient refusal.
- Abnormalities of coagulation including congenital disorders, use of anticoagulants and antiplatelet agents, acquired disorders associated with hepatic dysfunction and obstetric disorders including pre-eclampsia and HELLP syndrome (haemolysis, elevated liver enzymes and low platelets).
- Uncorrected hypovolaemia.
- Local or systemic infection (bearing in mind the normal elevation in white blood cell count associated with labour).
- Allergy to amide local anaesthetics.

Relative contraindications include:

- Various cardiac diseases resulting in relatively fixed cardiac output states — although the cardiovascular changes involved in taking a pregnancy to term is a good test of cardiovascular reserve and careful epidural analgesia may be safer than the stresses of labour for some women.
- Anatomical abnormalities including previous surgery might make central neuraxial blockade difficult if surface landmarks are obscured, or unpredictable, especially if there is scarring within (previous surgery) or significant abnormalities in the ligaments and meninges (neural tube defects).

The complications of epidurals include hypotension with or without fetal distress, post-dural puncture headache, nerve injury, epidural haematoma or abscess formation, local anaesthetic toxicity, high/total spinal, maternal immobility, urinary retention, prolongation of labour, increased instrumental delivery and possibly maternal pyrexia. Epidural analgesia does not appear to increase Caesarean section rate or the incidence of lower back pain.

Intrauterine fetal death can be associated with significant coagulopathy and sepsis. Hence, coagulation and inflammatory markers should be checked and taken into account. Epidural analgesia can be provided using several techniques. The block can be established using either an epidural bolus or a combined spinal-epidural (CSE). CSEs provide a more reliable and rapid onset of analgesia and if done using a low-dose spinal first may provide a more compliant patient for the epidural insertion. There is some evidence that the epidural component will be more effective, satisfaction is higher and topping up these epidurals for operative delivery is more reliable. This needs to be balanced against a potentially higher complication rate.

Establishing epidural analgesia requires the administration of a bolus of local anaesthetic. There has been a move in recent years from higher to lower concentration local anaesthetics. Traditional test doses are also being used less often, particularly those containing adrenaline (previously used in an attempt to identify intravascular placement through induced tachycardia). Although some units still advocate 2% lidocaine or 0.25% bupivacaine test doses, many now simply use a higher volume of 0.1% bupivacaine as a combined test and loading dose.

The use of lower concentration epidurals (0.1% versus 0.25% bupivacaine) is associated with less motor blockade and lower operative delivery rates. More recently the move has been from infusions of local anaesthetic to patient-controlled boluses (with or without an infusion), which appear to result in lower total anaesthetic doses, less anaesthetic interventions and less motor blockade. They might increase maternal satisfaction. Further work has been done in this area, resulting in more advanced modes like programmed intermittent epidural bolus pumps, which might again improve outcomes.

Operative delivery

Pre-operative assessment

Pre-operative assessment is essential for the safe delivery of any anaesthetic. This is no different in the obstetric setting. Pre-operative assessment aims to identify potential problems that might arise, such that the patient's condition can be optimised and the anaesthetic management altered to minimise the risk to the patient.

Points relevant to obstetric anaesthesia include the indication and urgency of delivery, placental localisation and other risk factors for abnormal implantation and increased blood loss during previous sections. Other elements of the obstetric history that may be important include a history of any hypertensive or cholestatic disorders of pregnancy. A careful assessment of the airway and exploration for any contraindications to central neuraxial blockade must be undertaken. Consent should be obtained from the patient. The Obstetric Anaesthetists' Association provides patient information leaflets in various languages that may help with communication of relevant information.

Recent blood results should be reviewed, particularly the mother's haemoglobin, and a minimum of a group and antibody screen should have been performed prior to operative delivery. Although there are situations where this may not be possible, blood may have to be sent from the operating theatre on obtaining intravenous access.

Urgency

Urgency is normally described using the categories originally described by Lucas *et al* in 2000 and later endorsed by several other groups, including the Royal College of Anaesthetists (RCOA), Royal College of Obstetricians and Gynaecologists (RCOG) and National Institute for Health and Care Excellence (NICE), but is in reality a continuum. NICE suggests that obstetric units should use decision-to-delivery intervals to monitor performance, using 30 minutes for Category 1 and both 30 and 75 minutes for Category 2. Clearly there are occasions where 30 minutes is excessive and others where it is not achievable or will introduce unnecessary risk. More up-to-date guidelines from the RCOG advocate a more individualised approach to determining optimal decision-to-delivery intervals.

The standard definitions of categories of Caesarean section are:

- One: immediate threat to maternal or fetal life.

- Two: maternal or fetal compromise that is not immediately life-threatening.
- Three: no maternal or fetal compromise, but needs early delivery.
- Four: can be delivered at a time to suit the mother and hospital team.

Principles of management

Regardless of the mode of operative delivery, if time and maternal comorbidities allow and the mother is willing, a regional anaesthetic technique is preferred. It minimises the risk of failed intubation/oxygenation and aspiration, provides better postoperative analgesia with less sedation, allows earlier bonding and breastfeeding, and allows the partner (where appropriate) to be present for the delivery.

Studies suggest that an obstetric spinal can be performed and the block ready in around 10-15 minutes. In situations where time is critical, however, one needs to consider how long it would take for the anaesthetist to accept that their spinal has failed to provide adequate anaesthesia, and then perform a general anaesthetic, which might take considerably longer.

Full monitoring and large-bore intravenous access should always be in place prior to commencing an anaesthetic. Where possible women should have received prophylactic antacids prior to their arrival in theatre and where they have not, they should be given parenterally peri-operatively. H_2 antagonists are probably superior to proton pump inhibitors in increasing gastric pH.

There is limited evidence regarding positioning women for Caesarean section. Normally, the women is placed on the operating table with her pelvis tilted by 30° to the left, either using a wedge or by tilting the table in order to reduce the risk of aortocaval compression and supine hypotension. This may be more important in emergency cases where utero-placental perfusion is already reduced.

Prophylactic antibiotics are normally administered, according to local protocols, prior to the first incision. There is some evidence that co-amoxiclav increases the neonatal incidence of necrotising enterocolitis, so it is often avoided for this indication. In cases of general anaesthesia where thiopentone is being used, caution should be exercised to avoid mixing up between the induction agent and the antibiotic. Uterotonic agents should be given following delivery of the baby to reduce the risk of significant post-partum haemorrhage.

In utero resuscitation

Where there is fetal distress, attempts should be made to improve blood flow to the placenta. This involves avoidance of aortocaval compression through positioning (normally left lateral, but where this has not worked, right lateral and head up may be tried) and where appropriate, administration of fluid to improve maternal cardiac output and tocolytic agents (such as terbutaline 250µg subcutaneous injection).

Spinal anaesthesia

A single-shot spinal is the most common mode of anaesthesia for obstetric procedures in the UK. Using narrow-gauge needles with pencil points (Whitacre/Sprotte), the incidence of significant post-dural puncture headaches is around 0.5%. Compared to epidural anaesthesia, both the sensory and motor blocks tend to be denser and postoperative analgesia can be provided by adding a relatively lipid-insoluble opioid to the injectate (diamorphine or morphine). However, hypotension from the sudden, dense sympathetic blockade is a side effect. This has previously been treated with fluids, either crystalloid or colloid, and before or during administration of spinal anaesthesia. Neither is entirely effective. Vasopressor agents are more suitable and traditionally ephedrine was used, but this is less effective at preventing maternal hypotension than phenylephrine or metaraminol, causes maternal tachycardia, and is associated with more fetal acidosis.

For Caesarean delivery (and during instrumental deliveries, the anaesthetist should be prepared for Caesarean), the sensory blockade should be at least at the level of T5 bilaterally in order to cover the peritoneum. There is variation in the method used to assess the block height, including the use of light touch, pinprick, the first sensation of cold and 'icy' cold. The extent of the block as assessed by these different modalities can be several dermatomes apart, in addition to inter-indvidual variation in the identification of specified dermatomes. Whilst surveys demonstrate that a large proportion of anaesthetists use cold to assess block height, studies have demonstrated that this might be insufficient, and blockade of light touch to T5 indicates adequate anaesthesia for Caesarean section. The most important aspect of this is firstly to warn the woman that she will feel sensations of tugging and pressure during the surgery and secondly to offer alternative anaesthesia or additional analgesia where appropriate.

In pregnancy, as mentioned above, the CSF is relatively compressed and thus injectate will tend to spread further than expected, thus a similar block can be achieved with around 60% of the volume used in the non-pregnant population. Given the height of the block aimed for in Caesarean sections, maintenance of the thoracic kyphosis is important in avoiding excessively high blocks.

Epidural anaesthesia

Epidural anaesthesia is rarely used as a sole technique *de novo*, although it may be beneficial in those with significant cardiac or respiratory comorbidities, where the more gradual sympathetic blockade provided by a slowly topped up epidural is better tolerated than the rapid, dense result of spinal anaesthesia. More common are the topping up of labour epidurals for operative procedures and CSE techniques, where an epidural is left *in situ* to allow extension of a spinal block should surgery be prolonged.

Topping up labour epidurals should only be done after assessment of the patient's notes and current block to assess whether it is likely to provide effective anaesthesia for the procedure. If an epidural has only provided intermittent or patchy analgesia or required frequent unexpected interventions, it is sometimes wise to remove it and site a spinal anaesthetic. If an epidural is topped up and the woman is still in pain, the anaesthetist is left with the decision to perform a spinal on top of this, unsure of what is already in various spaces in the back, with the potential for a very high block or perform a general anaesthetic.

Topping up an epidural for operative delivery should be done with the aim of achieving a bilateral block from T5-S5, tested as for a spinal block. This can be achieved using various mixes of local anaesthetics, commonly 10-20ml 0.5% bupivacaine or 2% lidocaine with or without opioids. Other drugs can be added to create a so-called 'quickmix', normally using 2% lidocaine with adrenaline to prolong the block and sodium bicarbonate to speed the onset of action. It is important to note that only preservative-free drugs should be used in epidurals.

When using high-concentration local anaesthetic to extend an epidural block, the risk of catheter migration into the intravascular or subarachnoid spaces should always be considered and it seems prudent to test the epidural with a small volume prior to the full dose.

General anaesthesia (GA)

General anaesthesia is normally reserved for cases where regional anaesthesia is contraindicated or time does not allow for a spinal. Pregnant women should always be considered to have a full stomach and hence a rapid sequence induction (RSI) with cricoid pressure is normally used. There is also an above average chance of a difficult intubation and equipment to deal with this eventuality should be available.

A non-particulate antacid such as 0.3M sodium citrate should be administered immediately prior to induction. Whilst it increases the volume of the stomach, it has been shown to increase the pH, and thus probably reduces the risk of chemical pneumonitis should the patient aspirate during induction.

The traditional RSI of thiopentone and suxamethonium has been challenged, with many advocating the use of alternative drugs. Thiopentone has traditionally been used in obstetrics and has an extensive record of safety; however, as availability in other countries has become scarce, many have moved to propofol without significant problems coming to light.

The drop in pseudocholinesterase levels is enough to prolong the clinical duration of action of suxamethonium in some women, so the anaesthetist must be prepared for situations where the patient does not start breathing in a 'can't intubate, can't ventilate' scenario.

Positive pressure ventilation reduces venous return and therefore cardiac output. This is exacerbated by hypovolaemia and the use of positive end-expiratory pressure. Limiting mean airway pressures will maximise cardiac output and therefore utero-placental perfusion.

Whilst volatile anaesthetic agents cause a degree of tocolysis, the use of up to 1 MAC does not seem to have a significant effect on blood loss, thus there is no real justification to use excessively light anaesthesia. Nitrous oxide equilibrates rapidly across the placenta, and theoretically may cause diffusion hypoxia upon delivery if used in high concentrations.

Long-acting opioids should be withheld until after delivery of the baby, as they can cause respiratory depression. Shorter-acting drugs can be given if they are deemed necessary, but the neonatologists must be informed in case the baby needs naloxone.

Transversus abdominis plane blocks have been shown to have some role in reducing opioid requirements in women who cannot have central neuraxial opioids and so might be usefully administered after completion of surgery if there is no contraindication. Often the surgeon can place the local anaesthetic whilst closing up.

Prior to extubation, consideration should be given to emptying the stomach with a large-bore nasogastric or orogastric tube.

Where a general anaesthetic is deemed necessary in pre-eclamptic women, extra caution must be taken. These women are more likely to have oedematous airways that are prone to bleeding. The hypertensive response to laryngoscopy can also be catastrophic, and efforts shoud be made to obtund it. This can be done using:

- Opioids such as alfentanil or remifentanil, although again, the neonatologists should be informed of the dose.

- Beta-blockers such as labetalol or esmolol, although esmolol again crosses the placenta and can cause neonatal bradycardia and hypoglycaemia.
- Magnesium.

Manual removal of placenta/perineal repair

These are the two most common procedures performed in labour ward theatres. Both retained placentas and perineal tears can be associated with significant blood loss and so a careful assessment of the patient for signs of hypovolaemia is essential prior to anaesthesia. Assuming normovolaemia and no signs of sepsis or coagulopathy, they are amenable to spinal anaesthesia. A spinal block from S5-T8 will suffice for either procedure.

Non-obstetric procedures during pregnancy

Whilst undesirable, other surgical procedures may need to be undertaken during pregnancy. Where possible, they should be undertaken during the second trimester, as risk of teratogenesis is greatest during organogenesis (up to 12 weeks) and risks of injury to the fetus and premature labour are in later pregnancy. If possible, again regional anaesthesia is preferred and if general anaesthesia is needed after 16-18 weeks' gestation, an RSI should be performed. The mother should be warned regarding the potential for miscarriage, although it probably relates to the underlying condition requiring surgery during pregnancy as much as to the anaesthesia. Potentially teratogenic medications should be avoided wherever possible.

Post-partum haemorrhage

The World Health Organisation defines the loss of more than 500ml as a post-partum haemorrhage (PPH), although more that 1000-1500ml is probably more useful. Whilst some PPHs can be predicted, most are unexpected. The Society of Obstetricians and Gynaecologists of Canada suggested that PPHs can be thought of as having one of four causes: tone, tissue, trauma or thrombin; that is uterine atony, retained tissue preventing effective uterine contraction, perineal trauma or coagulopathy. Thus, management of PPH comes down to identifying the cause and medically or surgically remedying it whilst replacing blood loss. Communication between the obstetric, anaesthetic and haematology teams is essential during the management of a massive PPH and every unit should have a protocol to assist the delivery of optimal care during these emergencies.

Replacement of losses should be undertaken in the same manner it would in other groups of patients, bearing in mind that these are usually young, fit patients, who will physiologically compensate until they are significantly hypovolaemic.

During operative delivery, normal practice is to give oxytocin after the delivery of the fetus. This can be given as a slow bolus with or without an infusion. In elective situations, there is evidence that a 0.3-1 international unit is effective at reducing PPH when followed by a 5-10 international unit/hr infusion. Higher doses are needed in labouring women, in the range of 3-5 international units when followed by an infusion. There is limited evidence relating to the optimal dose when no infusion is used, but the Royal College of Obstetrics and Gynaecology recommend a slow bolus of 5 international units. Oxytocin causes maternal vasodilatation and can cause significant cardiovascular compromise when given rapidly, in large doses or to those with a fixed cardiac output.

Other drugs used to manage post-partum haemorrhage include:

- Ergometrine: an ergot alkaloid, which can cause nausea, vomiting and significant vasoconstriction with hypertension, particularly when given intravenously. It can be given as 250-500µg intramuscular injections or a similar dose cautiously titrated 50-100µg/ml given intravenously.
- Carboprost: a prostaglandin F2α analogue given by intramuscular injection which can cause severe bronchospasm, vomiting and diarrhoea. The dose is 250µg by intramuscular injection every 15 minutes as needed to a total dose of 2mg (maximum of 8 doses).

- Misoprostol: a prostaglandin E1 analogue given orally, buccally, sublingually or rectally.
- Carbetocin: a synthetic analogue of oxytocin with a longer half-life. Evidence is still lacking with regards to its superiority to oxytocin and its high cost currently limits use.

Surgical management of PPH may include repair of perineal trauma, removal of retained products, management of atony with bimanual pressure, B-lynch suture, tamponade with balloon insertion, ligation of the uterine arteries and ultimately hysterectomy. Interventional radiology may have a role in certain cases, particularly placenta praevia, but high-quality evidence is still awaited.

Pre-eclampsia

Pre-eclampsia is a systemic disease of pregnancy. It normally develops in the second half of pregnancy and is not fully understood, but is believed to be related to abnormal placentation, with resultant placental ischaemia, release of various placental factors, a maternal inflammatory response and systemic endothelial dysfunction. It is characterised by maternal hypertension and proteinuria.

Diagnosis is made on the basis of a systolic blood pressure >140mmHg or diastolic >90mmHg on two separate occasions 6 hours apart with previously normal blood pressure and proteinuria of 1+ or greater on dipstick or a urinary protein:creatine ratio >0.3. Other signs and symptoms include visual disturbances, headaches, hyper-reflexia, epigastric pain, generalised oedema, intra-uterine growth retardation, oliguria and acute kidney injury.

The treatment of pre-eclampsia is delivery of the placenta. When pre-eclampsia manifests before term, it can often be managed through antihypertensives in order to allow fetal maturation prior to delivery. The drugs ordinarily used are labetalol, nifedipine and methyldopa.

In the presence of severe pre-eclampsia, the mother should be managed on a labour ward high dependency unit. If delivery is planned

663

within 24 hours, magnesium is used to reduce the risk of eclampsia — normally a 4g loading dose followed by a 1g/hour infusion for at least 24 hours. Monitoring of deep tendon reflexes usually suffices; measuring serum magnesium levels is rarely required unless the woman has renal dysfunction.

If the woman has severe hypertension, intra-arterial blood pressure monitoring and intravenous antihypertensives may be required. The normal drugs are:

- Labetalol, given as 50mg boluses and an infusion of 20-160mg/hour.
- Hydralazine, given as 5mg slow boluses up to 20mg — this can unveil significant hypovolaemia, so consideration should be given to a crystalloid bolus with the initial dose.

Severe hypertension should be treated as an emergency, as it can result in intracranial haemorrhage, which is a significant cause of maternal deaths.

Eclamptic seizures are dangerous, and should be treated as an emergency. The fits themselves are normally brief and should be treated with airway support and oxygen whilst magnesium is being given to reduce the incidence of further seizures.

In severe pre-eclampsia, platelet count can drop as a result of consumption and a coagulopathy can occur related to disseminated intravascular coagulation (DIC). This can also be a part of HELLP syndrome. As a result it is sensible to check platelet count and clotting on a regular basis in case of the need for analgesia or operative delivery.

Pre-eclamptic patients are prone to pulmonary oedema because of a degree of both systolic and diastolic dysfunction, vasoconstriction, reduced plasma oncotic pressure and endothelial dysfunction. Care must be taken in assessing their fluid status and in the acute phase they should be fluid restricted.

Case scenario 1

A 25-year-old woman in her first pregnancy with a breech presentation had undergone a failed external cephalic version. She was 76kg with a BMI of 27kg/m² and no allergies. Airway assessment revealed a Mallampati Grade 1 view with good mouth opening and neck movement, a thyromental distance of 7cm and intact dentition. Bloods sent from the antenatal clinic show her Hb was 124g/L, white cell count 8.8 x 10⁹/L, and platelets 158 x 10⁹/L. The obstetricians offered her a Caesarean section, which she accepted. Today her blood pressure is 112/64mmHg and her heart rate is 68/min and regular.

How would you proceed with the anaesthetic plan?

This is an elective scenario and there is adequate time for the patient to be given an explanation on a spinal anaesthetic. After confirming that she arrived on the day appropriately starved, having taken ranitidine 150mg last night and this morning, she should be moved to theatre, where non-invasive blood pressure, ECG and oxygen saturation monitoring should be instituted and a 16G cannula placed in a vein in the dorsum of her hand.

The anaesthetist, wearing a mask and hat, scrubs before donning a sterile gown and gloves. With the patient sitting up and positioned for a spinal, her back is cleaned with 0.5% chlorhexidine. The anaesthetist would then perform a spinal with 2.6ml 0.5% hyperbaric bupivacaine and 300µg of diamorphine. The patient is positioned with a left tilt of 30° and an infusion of phenylephrine is commenced at 50µg/min and titrated to maintain the patient's blood pressure. The block is checked, and once it has reached T5, the surgeons are allowed to start preparing the abdomen.

Prophylactic antibiotics are given prior to the skin incision. Continuous monitoring of the patient is the key to anticipate and prevent adverse events. Following delivery, a slow bolus of 5 international units of oxytocin is administered. The patient and the baby are then moved into recovery after the operative procedure from where they will be sent to the post-natal ward.

Case scenario 2

A 36-year-old woman presents at 37 weeks' gestation in her third pregnancy in labour. Her past medical and obstetric history are unremarkable. She has had no problems during the pregnancy, but reports headaches over the past 2 days. Her blood pressure is 192/124mmHg and urinalysis demonstrates 3+ of protein. A diagnosis of pre-eclampsia is made.

What would you do next?

The patient needs to be moved to the labour ward HDU and bloods sent to the laboratory for a full blood count, urea and electrolytes, coagulation screen and group and antibody screen. A large-bore venous cannula and an arterial cannula should be placed and the patient commenced on magnesium and labetalol infusions.

Her blood pressure remains elevated, and she is in pain. What would be your analgesic option?

After confirmation that her platelet count and coagulation are normal, an epidural for labour analgesia would be a good choice. It is loaded with 15ml 0.1% bupivacaine with 2µg/ml fentanyl and a patient-controlled epidural is started. The aim is to provide good pain control and stabilise her blood pressure.

Unfortunately, despite an oxytocin infusion, she fails to progress and her cardiotocograph trace is non-reassuring, so a decision is

made to take her for a Caesarean section. What would be your anaesthetic plan for this patient?

On assessment, her epidural block should be extending bilaterally and if it has helped in easing off the labour pain, a decision to proceed with an epidural top-up is reasonable. Following transfer to theatre and the application of full monitoring, the epidural should be topped up using a mixture of 19ml 2% lidocaine, 1:200,000 adrenaline and 1ml 8.4% sodium bicarbonate given as a 3ml test dose and then in aliquots over 5 minutes. The block should extend from S5-T5 bilaterally and the obstetricians can then proceed with a Caesarean section. Fluid administration is limited to avoid overload.

Following delivery, 5 international units of oxytocin is given intravenously followed by a 10 international unit/hr infusion. The uterine tone remains low, and blood loss continues. What other drugs can you use?

The surgeons should continue to manually stimulate the uterus. The intravenous fluid infusion is increased to keep up with losses. Since the patient is pre-eclamptic there should be concerns about drug-induced hypertension. Ergometrine should be avoided; instead carboprost 250µg intramuscularly can be used.

After three doses the uterine tone improves. The procedure is complete and estimated blood loss is around 1000ml. The patient is haemodynamically stable. What would you do next?

At the end of the procedure 3mg diamorphine is administered through the epidural catheter prior to its removal. The patient should return to the labour ward HDU for ongoing monitoring of her blood pressure and blood loss.

Further reading

1. The Eighth Report of the Confidential Enquiries into Maternal Deaths in the United Kingdom. *Br J Obstet Gynaecol* 2011; 118s1: 1-203.

2. Rucklidge M, Hinton C. Difficult and failed intubation in obstetrics. *Contin Educ Anaes Crit Care Pain* 2012; 12: 86-91.

3. National Institute for Health and Care Excellence. NICE guideline CG 132. Caesarean section. London, UK: NICE, 2011.

4. Russell IF. A comparison of cold, pinprick and touch for assessing the level of spinal block at Caesarean section. *Int J Obstet Anesth* 2004; 13: 146-52.

5. Nejdlova M, Johnson T. Anaesthesia for non-obstetric procedures during pregnancy. *Contin Educ Anaes Crit Care Pain* 2012; 12: 203-6.

6. The Royal College of Obstetricians and Gynaecologists. Green-top Guideline No. 52. Postpartum haemorrhage, prevention and management. The Royal College of Obstetricians and Gynaecologists, 2011.

7. The Royal College of Obstetricians and Gynaecologists. Good Practice No.11. Classification of urgency of Caesarean section - a continuum of risk. The Royal College of Obstetricians and Gynaecologists, 2010.

8. The Magpie Trial Collaborative Group. Do women with pre-eclampsia, and their babies, benefit from magnesium sulphate? The Magpie Trial: a randomised placebo-controlled trial. *Lancet* 2002; 359: 1877-90.

9. Allam J, Malhotra S, Hemingway C, Yentis SM. Epidural lidocaine-bicarbonate-adrenaline versus levobupivacaine for emergency Caesarean section: a randomised controlled trial. *Anaesthesia* 2008; 63: 243-9.

29 Paediatric anaesthesia

Charles Pairaudeau and Antonia Mayell

Introduction

While serious comorbidity is rare in children presenting for the most commonly performed surgical procedures, an understanding of the anatomical and physiological differences between adults and children is crucial for the safe conduct of paediatric anaesthesia. These differences are most marked in neonates (less than 28 days old), infants (under 1 year) and preschool children, hence these are the groups focused on below. By the age of approximately 6 years, normal physiological values are similar to those of adults and anatomical differences, besides those of scale, are minimal.

Airway

Anatomy and physiology

The larynx sits more anteriorly and one to two vertebral levels higher compared with adults and older children. The tongue and epiglottis are also both proportionally larger. The former has a tendency to fall posteriorly in the supine position during anaesthesia causing airway obstruction, while the latter can obstruct the view at laryngoscopy. The head and occiput are also larger in proportion to the rest of the body, resulting in a tendency for the head and neck to flex when the child is supine. The narrowest portion of the airway is at the level of the cricoid cartilage, as opposed to the distal trachea in adults. The trachea is short, approximately 5cm in a 6-month-old.

Changes in the diameter of the large airways due to oedema or secretions, even by as little as 1-2mm, can represent a significant percentage reduction in airway patency in small children. This will result in a disproportionate decrease in airflow for a given inspiratory effort, as the relationship between airway diameter and flow is non-linear.

Implications for anaesthesia

Optimal positioning for bag mask ventilation and intubation in the very young child requires a neutral position of the head and neck, as opposed to the 'sniffing' position, which may result in complete or partial airway obstruction. Even without a pillow, the head and neck may be excessively flexed in the supine position. A folded towel placed under the shoulders and/or body of the child, lifting the torso relative to the head and neck, may be the best way to achieve this correct neutral alignment. Mask ventilation requires careful positioning of the operator's fingers, taking care not to compress the soft tissues under the chin which may impede ventilation. The jaw thrust manoeuvre is useful to bring the tongue forward and off the posterior oropharynx. Round as opposed to anatomical masks often give a better seal in neonates and infants.

The use of straight instead of curved laryngoscope blades is popular with those who intubate neonates and small children. A right paraglossal approach is used with this blade, placing the tip under the epiglottis (as opposed to in the vallecular) lifting it out of the way.

Concerns about the pressure effects of endotracheal tube cuffs on the tracheal wall have meant that traditionally, uncuffed tubes have been used in paediatric anaesthesia. A correctly sized uncuffed tube will give only a small leak while exerting minimal pressure on the tracheal mucosa. They also have the advantage of having a greater internal diameter for a given external diameter, thereby decreasing the work of breathing during spontaneous ventilation. Cuffed tubes, however, are increasingly used in modern practice due to improved low-pressure/high-volume cuff designs.

Careful positioning and fixation of endotracheal tubes is needed to prevent inadvertent endobronchial intubation. Formulae are available to calculate the expected tube size and length at the lips. Tracheal tubes are sized according to the internal diameter of the tube; a size 3 tube means the internal diameter is 3mm. In a newborn, a size 3 or smaller tube may be needed. The tube is usually inserted to a depth of 7-9cm at the lips. For a 1-year-old child, usually a size 4 tube is used and inserted to a depth of about 12cm at the lips. Above 1 year, the approximate size of the tube required can be calculated using the following formula:

Size of the tube = (Age/4) + 4

And the length at the lips is calculated using the following formula:

Length = (Age/2) + 12

A range of supraglottic airway devices are now available in paediatric sizes. They are often used for preschool and older children, but less frequently for infants and neonates due to their higher rate of failure in these populations and the increased need for controlled ventilation in the very young.

The use of the lateral position during the recovery phase can aid in maintaining a clear airway after removal of an endotracheal tube or a supraglottic airway device without the need for a shoulder roll, and has the added benefit that secretions or blood will tend to drain away from the glottis due to gravity.

Respiratory system

Anatomy and physiology

The ribs are arranged more flatly relative to the transverse plane, so the 'bucket handle' mechanism which allows adults to increase their tidal volumes is largely absent. Babies and infants therefore increase minute ventilation (tidal volume x respiratory rate) mainly by increasing their respiratory rate. Most of the work of breathing is carried out by the diaphragm which has a different muscle fibre composition to adults and is therefore more susceptible to fatigue.

The normal respiratory rate in an infant is up to 60 breaths per minute, with similar tidal volumes to adults of around 7ml/kg. Minute ventilation is thus higher on a per kilo basis and lung compliance is also higher. Functional residual capacity (FRC) is low and is similar to closing capacity even when awake. Desaturation can therefore occur rapidly when FRC is reduced, as happens under anaesthesia. This is compounded by the effect of a higher resting oxygen consumption which can be over twice that of adults.

Neonates and infants, particularly those who were born prematurely, are prone to postoperative apnoea. The rate of laryngospasm in small children is also higher than it is in adults.

Implications for anaesthesia

Pre-oxygenation may not be tolerated by small children, so rapid control of the airway after induction is essential. The high minute ventilation speeds the process of gas induction.

The period between starting a gas induction and obtaining IV access carries an increased risk, as the options for managing laryngospasm, should it occur, are more limited. Insertion of a supraglottic airway device or endotracheal tube is therefore deferred until after IV access has been obtained, in case airway manipulation induces laryngospasm.

Without the use of positive pressure ventilation and positive end-expiratory pressure (PEEP), the reduction in FRC under anaesthesia means that neonates and infants are prone to desaturate, as their closing capacity becomes higher than the FRC and significant atelectasis ensues. When intermittent positive pressure ventilation (IPPV) is employed, pressure-controlled modes have the advantage of compensating for a tube leak and minimising the risk of barotrauma or volutrauma. Acceptable intubating conditions can often be achieved under deep inhalational anaesthesia alone, avoiding the need for neuromuscular blockade.

Older children will often breathe quite adequately with a supraglottic airway device or endotracheal tube. Anaesthetic circuits need to have sufficiently low resistance and dead space if a spontaneously breathing technique is used. The Jackson Rees modification of Ayre's T-Piece (the Mapleson F circuit) is frequently used for this purpose in those under 20kg, but paediatric circle systems are available and provide an acceptable alternative.

Infants having procedures requiring long-acting opiates, or those with other risk factors such as prematurity, need to be looked after postoperatively in an area where they can be monitored for apnoeas.

Cardiovascular system

Healthy children have robust circulatory systems which allow them to compensate well for the vasodilatory effects of general anaesthesia. In situations where there are large stresses on the cardiovascular system, such as meningococcal sepsis or acute severe blood loss, a consequence of this resilience is that hypotension occurs very late, often as a preterminal sign. The absence of a low blood pressure is therefore a very poor predictor of impending critical illness in children. Other symptoms and signs should therefore be sought in the assessment of the sick child, such as an abnormal cry, poor urine output, sunken eyes or fontanel, tachycardia and prolonged capillary refill time.

Circulating volume and cardiac output are higher on a ml/kg basis in infants compared with adults. The stroke volume is fixed, so maintenance of cardiac output is dependent on heart rate; hence, bradycardia is tolerated poorly. Children are more prone to becoming bradycardic in response to vagal stimuli.

Intravenous access can be difficult to obtain in children, particularly toddlers.

Implications for anaesthesia

It is useful to have two anaesthetists present during a gas induction, one to maintain face mask anaesthesia and one to secure IV access. The space between the fourth and fifth metacarpals often yields venous access, even if no vein is visible externally. Intraosseous access may be the quickest route by which access to the circulation can be obtained in an emergency situation.

Fast circulation times mean that the peak effect of IV induction agents will be obtained rapidly. A smooth induction can therefore be easily achieved with IV induction, with the avoidance of airway difficulties due to 'light' anaesthesia. The high cardiac output ensures that redistribution to the tissues will occur equally quickly however; therefore, the offset of action is fast as well.

Some practitioners use antimuscarinics, such as atropine or glycopyrrolate, as prophylaxis against bradycardia before vagally-stimulating procedures such as intubation or ocular surgery. Whether this is done or not, it is prudent to always have the correct dose of such an agent drawn up in the event that a vagal bradycardia arises. It is important to remember, however, that small children will become bradycardic in response to hypoxia, and that the remedy in these instances is urgent restoration of oxygenation, rather than pharmacological treatment of the bradycardia.

Doses of fluids and drugs should be calculated based on an up-to-date body weight. It is easy to give an excessive amount of fluid to young children if a bag and giving set is attached directly to a cannula. If fluid is to be given during surgery, consider using a volumetric pump, burette or manual boluses via a syringe.

Other considerations

A high surface area to volume ratio means that there is a greater propensity for hypothermia than in adults. Many of the same methods of minimising heat loss can be used, but an increased ambient temperature in the operating theatre is frequently needed in the very young.

Prolonged or inefficient bag mask ventilation can cause gastric distention which may impede respiratory mechanics by diaphragmatic splinting. It may also increase the risk of aspiration and postoperative nausea or vomiting. In cases where this is suspected, the stomach may be deflated with an orogastric tube.

Infants and neonates are prone to hypoglycaemia due to their limited glycogen stores, so frequent monitoring and the use of peri-operative glucose infusions may be needed.

A detailed discussion of pharmacology in children is beyond the scope of this book. Points of note, however, include that the minimum alveolar concentration (MAC) peaks at the age of about 12 months, and then falls with increasing age. The induction dose of propofol is also proportionately higher than in adults, due to a larger central volume of distribution. Neonates and infants are relatively sensitive to non-depolarising neuromuscular blocking drugs, but require larger doses of suxamethonium due to greater extracellular fluid volumes.

Common cases in neonates

Necrotising enterocolitis (NEC) is a condition of the bowels which mostly occurs in premature babies in the first few weeks of life. It may present with intolerance to feeds, abdominal distention and features of sepsis. The condition can be managed conservatively with antibiotics, but a proportion of patients will require surgical intervention. The majority will have, or be recovering from, respiratory distress syndrome.

A congenital diaphragmatic hernia (CDH) is a condition where abdominal viscera are present in the chest cavity due to a defect in the diaphragm. Most cases are now identified from routine antenatal ultrasound scans. The underlying lung is abnormal with a high pulmonary vascular resistance and hence there is a tendency for reversion back to a foetal circulation. Surgery is usually delayed until around the second post-natal day to provide time to optimise ventilation. This is likely to deteriorate in the period immediately after the repair, as while the mechanical problem will have been solved, the abnormal pathology in the lung will persist. The repair is usually carried out through an upper abdominal incision.

Anaesthetic considerations

The majority of babies with these conditions will already be intubated and ventilated on the neonatal intensive care unit (NICU) and have lines *in situ*. In cases of NEC, the patient may be unstable and require ongoing fluid resuscitation and inotropes. Those with congenital diaphragmatic hernias have a high incidence of other congenital abnormalities, the presence or absence of which should be noted in the pre-op visit.

High-dose opiate techniques (e.g. fentanyl 10-25µg/kg) are useful for these cases, as this minimises cardiovascular instability and obtunds the stress response to surgery. Modulation of the stress response may help to reduce post-op catabolism in those with NEC and help prevent pulmonary vasoconstriction in those with CDH. As the patients will remain intubated, concerns regarding apnoeas and delayed recovery are not relevant.

'Lung-protective' ventilation is continued from the NICU; this involves limiting tidal volumes and peak pressures, if necessary, tolerating a degree of hypercarbia. Hyperoxia should be avoided because of the association with retinopathy and bronchopulmonary dysplasia.

Common surgical procedures in infants

Pyloric stenosis is a condition of unknown aetiology where the pylorus of the stomach becomes thickened. It usually presents between 3-12 weeks of age and has a male predominance of 4:1. The resulting gastric outflow obstruction causes non-bilious projectile vomiting after feeds. Consequently, dehydration, with a hypochloraemic metabolic alkalosis, ensues. Surgical correction is by a pyloromyotomy, a procedure which involves division of the muscle of the pylorus down to the submucosa.

During the pre-operative phase, the main concerns are volume depletion, acid base disturbance and electrolyte derangements. If there is a severe volume deficit, 0.9% saline boluses are used to restore the circulating volume. An infusion of a dextrose-saline solution is then started to replace the intracellular deficits. A nasogastric (NG) tube is passed pre-operatively in all cases; losses from this are replaced like-for-like with 0.9% saline.

Pyloromyotomy should take place only once fluid resuscitation is complete, as evidenced by normalised biochemical measurements; in particular, chloride, bicarbonate and sodium.

The main concern on induction, because of the inability of the stomach to empty properly, is aspiration. The NG tube should be carefully suctioned before inducing anaesthesia. A rapid sequence induction is advocated by many anaesthetists, but inhalational induction is also felt to be safe if the NG tube is aspirated effectively.

A combination of paracetamol and local anaesthetic infiltration provides effective analgesia. Postoperatively, these children need to be monitored for apnoeas because of their age and the fact that they may have a residual cerebrospinal fluid alkalosis which can further increase the risk of apnoea.

Common procedures in older Infants and children

The most commonly performed cases in district general hospitals are ENT procedures, such as adenotonsillectomy and grommets, which are covered in Chapter 22. Other common procedures include dental extractions, urological operations, ophthalmic surgery such as correction of strabismus, and orthopaedic procedures which typically include closed reduction of fractures or their fixation with K-wires. A common elective orthopaedic procedure is the correction of talipes equinovarus or 'club foot' which is usually performed at the age of around 6 months.

Dental procedures

Dental anaesthesia is commonly provided for two main groups of children. Community dental surgeons perform extractions on over 30,000 children per year in the United Kingdom for dental caries. Older children present for dental extractions and exposure and bonding of adult teeth, as part of their orthodontic treatment.

Urological procedures

Urological procedures such as circumcision and orchidopexy are often performed as day cases. A typical technique would be IV or inhalational induction of general anaesthesia, with placement of a laryngeal mask airway (LMA) followed by a caudal block. A caudal block involves injection of local anaesthetic solution into the sacral canal which is the distal continuation of the epidural space. The injection is performed through the gap between the non-fused laminae of the 5th sacral vertebra, which is called the sacral hiatus. This block is straightforward to perform in children, and has a high rate of success and a low incidence of complications. A volume of 0.5ml/kg of 0.25% bupivacaine will produce a block of the lumbosacral nerve roots and is therefore ideal for procedures such as these. Alternatively, for circumcision, a penile nerve block can be used. Without the continued use of regular doses of medications such as paracetamol and ibuprofen after discharge, there is likely to be a period of suboptimal analgesia at home when the block wears off. Parents should therefore be given clear advice about the need for continuing analgesia and its timing. This is particularly important now that codeine phosphate can no longer be given in children under 12 years in the UK. This is due to concerns about variation in its metabolism in children causing respiratory depression in some cases.

Ophthalmic procedures

Surgery for strabismus presents two main challenges. The first is the oculocardiac reflex which has the potential to cause severe bradycardia.

The second is a high incidence of postoperative nausea and vomiting which may delay discharge. The oculocardiac reflex can be managed expectantly with an antimuscarinic agent or alternatively these can be given in response to any episode of low heart rate, after asking the surgeon to release traction on the extraocular muscles. Hypercapnia is associated with an increased incidence of the oculocardiac reflex, so controlled ventilation is recommended with either a reinforced endotracheal tube or an LMA. Maintaining a deeper plane of anaesthesia also seems to have a protective effect, but this may come at the expense of delayed recovery.

Multi-agent antiemetic prophylaxis will reduce the level of nausea and vomiting, but a significant proportion of children are still likely to experience this to some extent after this procedure.

Orthopaedic procedures

Simple reduction of fractures and uncomplicated K-wire fixation can be performed using an LMA and a spontaneous breathing technique. Paracetamol and ibuprofen postoperatively usually provide good analgesia.

Talipes equinovarus is a more involved procedure which usually requires the infant to be positioned prone and has more postoperative pain. A tourniquet is used, but there is the potential for blood loss after its release; hence, suitable IV access should be in place and a pre-op group and screen performed. A suitable technique may therefore be controlled ventilation via a reinforced endotracheal tube and a catheter placed in the caudal space for a postoperative local anaesthetic infusion.

Case scenario 1

A 3-year-old boy weighing 15kg presents for a right inguinal hernia repair. He has no past history of note. On the ward he is playing normally, but has a constantly runny nose and mild cough.

How would you manage this child?

Pre-operative management

- His symptoms raise the concern that he could be developing an upper respiratory tract infection, with the potential for complications such as laryngospasm during induction and the recovery phase due to increased airway reactivity.
- In the absence of adverse features such as systemic upset, purulent secretions or pyrexia, it may be acceptable to proceed with surgery.
- The pre-operative visit should be used as an opportunity to build rapport with the child and parents.
- Routine pre-operative investigations are not needed in this case, other than baseline ward observations and body weight.
- Sedative premedication is given relatively infrequently, due to difficulties in timing the peak effect of the drug with the anaesthetic room visit and possible delayed discharge. Oral midazolam 0.5mg/kg disguised in Calpol® can be used if necessary.
- Ensure that topical local anaesthetic cream such as Ametop® or EMLA® is applied over potential IV access sites.

Intra-operative management

- In UK practice, it is common to have a parent or guardian present at induction, but they should not feel obliged to be present if they are particularly anxious themselves.
- IV cannulation should be attempted in an area where local anaesthetic cream has been applied while the child is distracted by a parent or staff member.

- If successful, IV induction with propofol 3-4mg/kg and fentanyl 0.5-1µg/kg can be used. Lidocaine 10mg per 100mg of propofol can be added to reduce the pain on injection.
- If unable to obtain IV access, a gas induction with sevoflurane can be performed (warn parents about involuntary movements during the excitatory phase).
- Once adequately anaesthetised, insert a laryngeal mask airway and use a spontaneous breathing technique via a Mapleson F circuit.
- Perform a caudal block for analgesia with 0.25% levobupivacaine before the surgery starts.
- Give ondansetron 0.1mg/kg and dexamethasone 0.1mg/kg as prophylaxis for postoperative nausea and vomiting.
- Ensure the cannula is flushed with saline at the end of the case to ensure there is no residual drug left in the dead space.

Postoperative management

- Disconnect any giving sets and bandage the cannula before the child emerges to minimise the chance of it becoming displaced.
- Prescribe multimodal analgesia with paracetamol and ibuprofen.
- Advise parents to give these regularly for the first few days postoperatively.
- Patients for this surgery would normally go home as a day case.

Further reading

1. Wilkinson K, Gibson J. Anaesthesia for common conditions in infancy. *BJA CEACCP* 2003; 3: 79-82.
2. Adewale L. Anatomy and assessment of the pediatric airway. *Pediatr Anesth* 2009; 19: 1-8.
3. Webber S, Barker I. Paediatric anaesthetic pharmacology. *BJA CEACCP* 2003; 3: 50-3.
4. Adewale L. Anaesthesia for paediatric dentistry. *BJA CEACCP* 2012; 12: 288-94.

30 Airway and respiratory problems

Christina Tourville

Introduction

This chapter looks at the most common airway and respiratory-related problems and ways to manage them. The National Audit Project of major airway incidents in the United Kingdom estimated the incidence of peri-operative major airway incidents as 1 in 22,000 general anaesthetics. Airway and respiratory problems are also the second most common complication in the postoperative period. It is therefore very important to plan, and be vigilant, for these complications throughout the intra-operative period and into the postoperative period.

Hypoxia

This occurs when a patient's oxygen levels are lower than would be expected for them; for example, a patient with COPD may have saturations normally of 88-92%.

Causes

- Airway obstruction.
- Respiratory depression.
- Laryngospasm.
- Endobronchial intubation.
- Bronchospasm.
- Inadequate ventilation, e.g. reduced lung volumes due to pneumoperitoneum.
- Anaphylaxis.

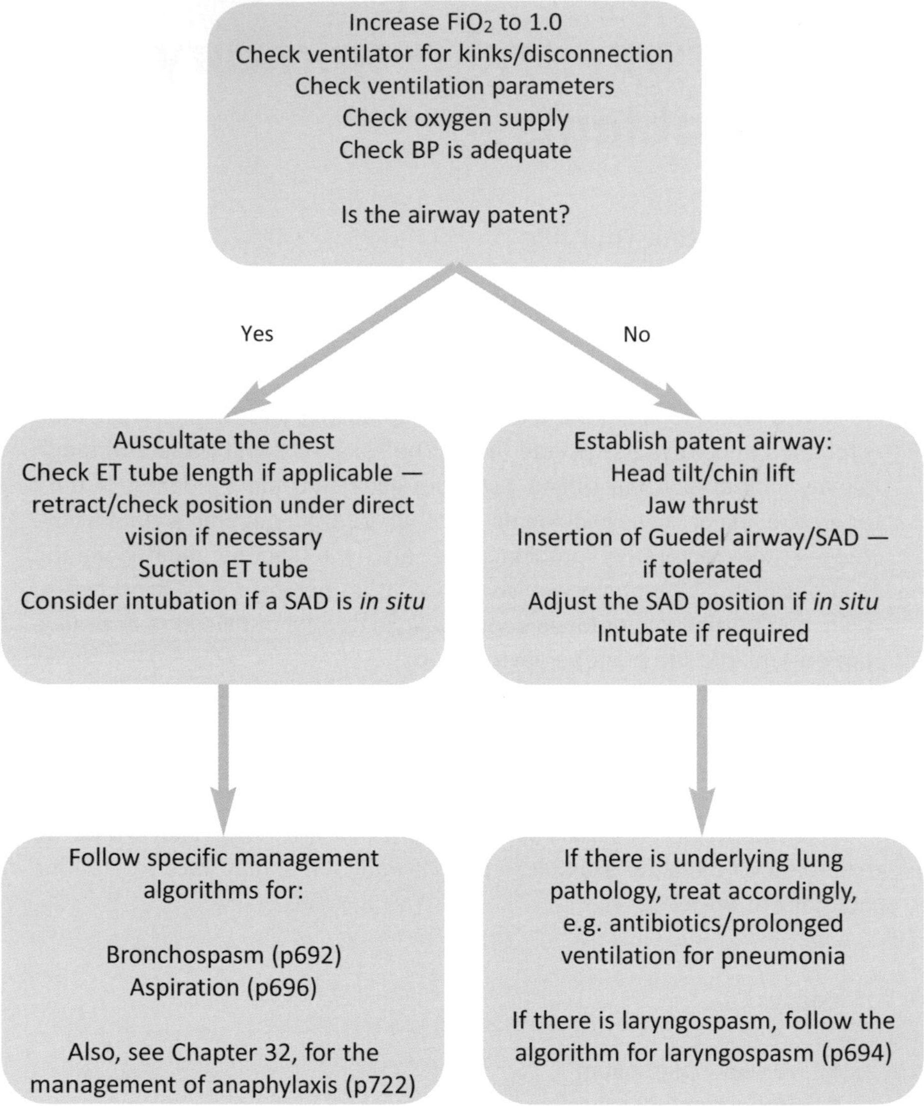

Figure 30.1. An algorithm for the management of hypoxia.

- Aspiration.
- Pneumothorax.
- Underlying lung pathology, e.g. pneumonia, COPD.
- Reduced peripheral perfusion due to hypotension.
- Equipment problems, e.g. oxygen failure, kinked ventilator tubing.

Management

The initial management remains the same, no matter the cause. This should include: an increase in FiO_2 to 1.0, a quick visual check of machine tubing to look for kinks/disconnection and checking the ventilator parameters if the patient is ventilated. The key to further management is differentiating whether or not there is a patent airway. If the problem occurs due to an obstructed larynx or upper airway, the key management is to open the airway by whatever means. Once the airway patency is confirmed then the source of the problem should be identified, e.g. the lungs themselves, the endotracheal tube or the supraglottic airway device (SAD).

An algorithm for the management of hypoxia is outlined in Figure 30.1.

Prevention

Hypoxia can potentially be prevented. The important measures include maintenance of a clear and appropriate airway (e.g. endotracheal [ET] tube if there is a high risk of laryngospasm), provision of adequate depth of anaesthesia and FiO_2, secure fixation of your chosen airway device and regular auscultation of the chest once intubated to prevent ET tube migration.

Hypercapnia

This occurs when levels of CO_2 in arterial blood or in expired gases are higher than expected (usually $PaCO_2$ >6.0kPa or 45mmHg or end-tidal concentration of CO_2 [$EtCO_2$] >6.0kPa).

Causes

Inadequate removal of CO_2 due to:

- Respiratory depression (N.B. could be due to CNS pathology or medication).
- Hypoventilation.
- Severe bronchospasm (N.B. raised CO_2 in asthma indicates a life-threatening exacerbation).
- V/Q mismatch within the lung, e.g. PE, pneumonia.
- Chronic hypercarbia, e.g. COPD, fibrosis, obesity hypoventilation, obstructive sleep apnoea (OSA), neuromuscular disorders, severe kyphoscoliosis.
- Rebreathing expired CO_2, e.g. due to exhausted sodalime.

OR

Increased production of CO_2 due to:

- Hypermetabolic states, e.g. sepsis, hyperthyroidism.
- Malignant hyperthermia.
- Deflation of arterial tourniquet causes a transient rise in $EtCO_2$.

Management

The key to managing such patients is to differentiate between those patients that are anaesthetised and those that are not. This allows appropriate management to be instituted. If the patient is not anaesthetised, the causes include respiratory depression due to drugs (some of which can be reversed) and due to CNS pathology (for which further imaging is required). If the patient is anaesthetised, management is centred on improving ventilation and looking for other causes of increased CO_2 production, e.g. malignant hyperthermia.

An algorithm for the management of hypercapnia is outlined in Figure 30.2.

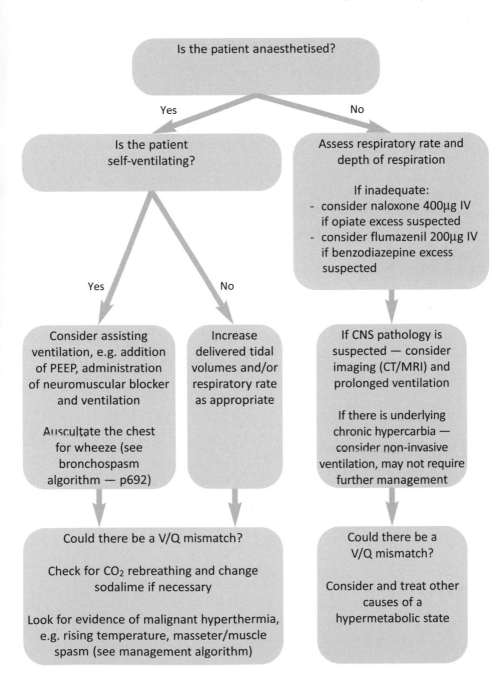

Figure 30.2. An algorithm for the management of hypercapnia.

Prevention

The mainstay of prevention of hypercarbia is to ensure adequate ventilation, be it spontaneous or invasive. This includes appropriate ventilator settings and regular maintenance of sodalime levels. It also includes the usage of appropriate dosages of sedative drugs, as well as anticipating those patients that are at higher risk of hypoventilation peri-operatively, e.g. those with OSA, COPD, neuromuscular disorders. The latter patients can then be considered for peri-operative non-invasive ventilation.

Hypocapnia

This occurs when there are low levels of CO_2 in arterial blood ($PaCO_2$ <4.5kPa) or there is a low concentration of end-tidal CO_2 ($EtCO_2$ <4.0kPa).

Causes

Increased removal of CO_2:

- Excessive invasive ventilation (i.e. large tidal volumes, high respiratory rate).
- Hyperventilation due to anaesthetic factors, e.g. light anaesthesia or pain.
- Hyperventilation due to patient factors, e.g. anxiety, asthma, underlying metabolic acidosis.

Decreased production/delivery of CO_2 and likely to cause hypocapnia:

- Partial airway obstruction/oesophageal intubation.
- Hypoperfusion and hypotension.

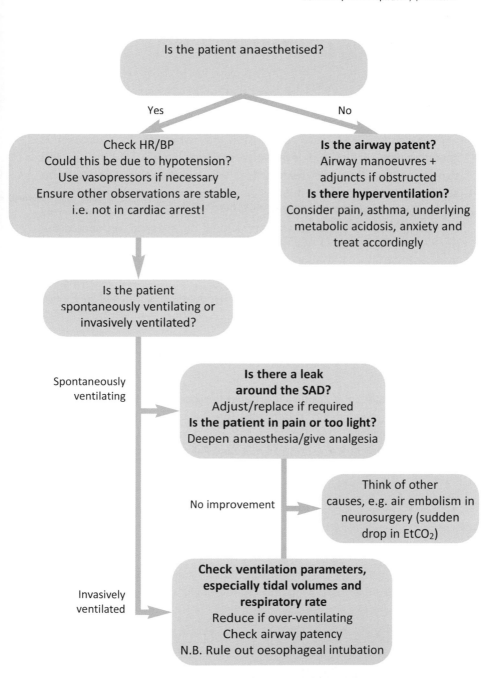

Figure 30.3. An algorithm for the management of hypocapnia.

- Air embolism.
- Cardiac arrest.

Management

Management will vary according to whether the patient is spontaneously ventilating or invasively ventilated. If the patient is breathing spontaneously, then the reason for the hyperventilation should be addressed, for example, if there is an inadequate depth of anaesthesia, pain or an underlying metabolic acidosis. If the patient is invasively ventilated, then ventilator parameters should be checked, as should the position of the endotracheal tube. More infrequent causes should be excluded, such as air embolism or cardiac arrest.

An algorithm for the management of hypocapnia is outlined in Figure 30.3.

Prevention

In the spontaneously ventilating patient, hypocarbia can be prevented by adequate anaesthetic depth and analgesia. In patients who are invasively ventilated, care should be taken with appropriate tidal volumes and respiratory rates. Ensuring cardiovascular stability can also address one potential cause for the development of hypocarbia.

Bronchospasm

Bronchospasm occurs when bronchial smooth muscle contracts, causing bronchiolar narrowing and characteristic expiratory wheeze.

Causes

- Underlying lung pathology, e.g. asthma, COPD.

- Anaphylaxis.
- Aspiration.

Management

The first step in management is identification that bronchospasm is occurring. Characteristic symptoms and signs include: shortness of breath, tachypnoea, audible expiratory wheeze, desaturation, increased airway pressures and difficulty in providing manual ventilation. Once this has been established, management will include applying 100% oxygen and nebulised bronchodilators (salbutamol +/- ipratropium). Further management will then be determined by the suspected underlying cause, e.g. adrenaline in anaphylaxis.

An algorithm for the management of bronchospasm is outlined in Figure 30.4.

Prevention

In patients with underlying lung disease, e.g. asthma or COPD, there are a number of preventative measures that can be taken. It is very important that such patients continue their usual medications peri-operatively and that they are optimised prior to surgery where possible. If there is evidence of an active exacerbation in such patients, then elective surgery should be postponed until this has improved. It may also be appropriate to consider a pre-operative nebuliser to try to prevent bronchospasm from occurring intra-operatively. The technique of anaesthesia can also be adapted, for example, providing regional anaesthesia where possible or through the use of ketamine (which has bronchodilator properties) or avoidance of histamine-releasing medications such as atracurium, morphine and fentanyl.

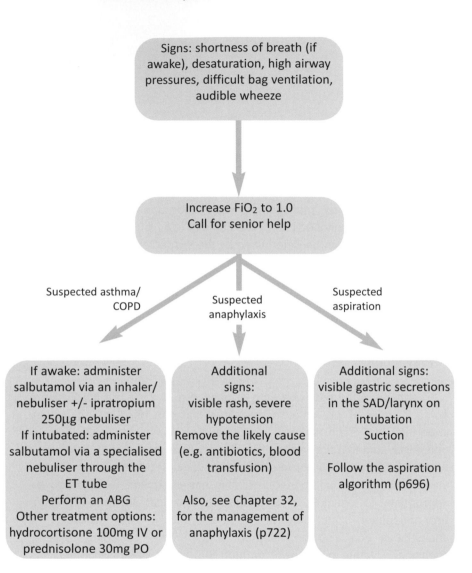

Figure 30.4. An algorithm for the management of bronchospasm.

Laryngospasm

This occurs when contraction of laryngeal muscles causes complete/partial airway obstruction.

Causes

- Inadequate anaesthesia.
- Painful stimulus under anaesthesia.
- Secretions touching the vocal cords.
- Removal/insertion of the SAD prematurely, i.e. without adequate anaesthesia.

Management

There are two main aspects to managing laryngospasm. The first aspect is to try to remove the stimulus for laryngospasm, e.g. removing the airway device, suctioning secretions or temporarily stopping surgery. The second aspect is then to deepen anaesthesia and attempt to break the spasm. This can be achieved through airway manoeuvres, such as a jaw thrust, or through the use of propofol and a neuromuscular blocker.

An algorithm for the managemont of laryngospasm is outlined in Figure 30.5.

Prevention

The main methods of prevention include ensuring adequate depth of anaesthesia and through the anticipation of particular procedures that will be very stimulating, such as the first incision of an abscess. You can then pre-empt this point by giving a bolus of propofol, fentanyl or alfentanil prior to the stimulus. A target-controlled infusion (TCI) of remifentanil during the stage of extubation may also help to prevent laryngospasm during extubation.

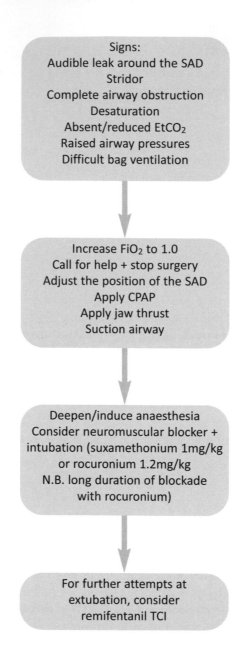

Figure 30.5. An algorithm for the management of laryngospasm.

Aspiration

This occurs when gastric fluid/contents or oral secretions pass below the level of the vocal cords.

Causes

- Patient factors: insufficient fasting, known reflux/hiatus hernia, achalasia, abdominal pathology, e.g. bowel obstruction, pre-operative vomiting, obesity, gastric irritation with blood, pregnancy, pain especially if opiates are required.
- Anaesthetic factors: the use of opiates at induction can precipitate vomiting in susceptible patients, use of a supraglottic airway device, light anaesthesia and patient coughing, inflation of the stomach during mask ventilation, inadequate tracheal cuff position/pressure.
- Surgical factors: procedures that increase the risk of regurgitation and aspiration include laparoscopic procedures, laparotomy, procedures that require a steep Trendelenburg position, e.g. certain gynaecological/urological procedures.

Management

The initial management when aspiration is suspected is to tip the patient head-down as soon as possible to attempt to suction the aspirate. If a supraglottic airway device is *in situ*, then this should be removed. It will then be necessary to perform a rapid sequence induction (RSI) with cricoid pressure and intubation. If it is possible, the endotracheal tube should be suctioned prior to intermittent positive-pressure ventilation (IPPV). Subsequent management will then be determined by the severity of the aspiration and may include admission to the HDU/ITU for prolonged ventilation and antibiotics.

An algorithm for the management of aspiration is outlined in Figure 30.6.

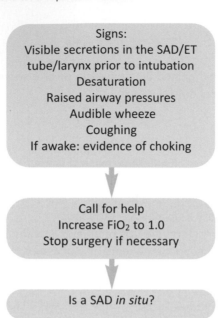

Signs:
Visible secretions in the SAD/ET tube/larynx prior to intubation
Desaturation
Raised airway pressures
Audible wheeze
Coughing
If awake: evidence of choking

Call for help
Increase FiO₂ to 1.0
Stop surgery if necessary

Is a SAD *in situ*?

Yes · No

Yes:
Deepen anaesthesia
Suction oropharynx/larynx
Tip trolley head down

Bag valve ventilation via a mask
Rapid sequence induction with cricoid pressure
ET tube suctioning
(ideally prior to IPPV)

No:
Tip trolley head down + attempt suction
Rapid sequence induction with cricoid pressure
ET tube suctioning
(ideally prior to IPPV)

Monitor sats closely
Auscultate chest
Once surgery complete:
Consider chest X-ray +/- antibiotics
Depending on severity:
- either extubate and monitor closely — if adverse signs are present, manage the patient in the HDU/ITU
  OR
- continue IPPV in the ITU

Figure 30.6. An algorithm for the management of aspiration.

Prevention

In order to prevent aspiration, it is very important to identify those patients that are at higher risk of aspiration. In such patients, you can premedicate with agents such as prokinetics (e.g. metoclopramide), proton-pump inhibitors (e.g. omeprazole), H_2 receptor antagonists (e.g. ranitidine) or sodium citrate (immediately prior to induction of anaesthesia). In such patients, intubation +/- RSI should be performed. If an NG tube is *in situ*, this should be suctioned prior to induction to further reduce this risk. Care should also be taken at extubation as high-risk patients are still at increased risk at extubation; for example, some would advocate extubation in the left lateral position.

Case scenario 1

A 65-year-old man is undergoing a laparoscopic hernia repair under general anaesthesia. During the intra-operative period, soon after inflating the peritoneal cavity with carbon dioxide in the head-down position, his peripheral oxygen saturation decreases to 90%.

How would you manage hypoxia in this patient?

Immediate action is to increase the inspired oxygen concentration to 100% and call for help if appropriate. The inspired/expired oxygen concentration, $EtCO_2$ and other vital parameters such as heart rate and blood pressure should be checked. One should quickly rule out any problems at the anaesthetic machine end and in the breathing system, and then check the patient's airway and breathing. The chest should be auscultated for bilateral air entry.

The most likely cause could be endobrochial intubation due to pneumoperitoneum, displacing the mediastinum upwards leading to the movement of the tracheal tube towards the right main bronchus. The diagnosis is confirmed by unilateral air entry. A pneumothorax is one of the differential diagnoses.

Management involves deflating the cuff, withdrawing the endotracheal tube under vision to ensure that the cuff of the tube is just beyond the cords. Then the cuff is reinflated and ventilation commenced and confirmed with a normal $EtCO_2$ trace.

Further reading

1. 4th National Audit Project of The Royal College of Anaesthetists and The Difficult Airway Society. Major complications of airway management in the United Kingdom, Report and Findings, March 2011.

2. Hines R, Barash PG, Waltrous G, O'Connor T. Complications occurring in the postanesthesia care unit: a survey. *Anesth Analg* 1992; 74: 503.

3. Popat M, Mitchell V, Dravid R, *et al*. Difficult Airway Society guidelines for the management of tracheal extubation. *Anaesthesia* 2012; 67: 318-40.

31 Cardiovascular problems

Christina Tourville

Introduction

The common cardiovascular problems in the peri-operative period are associated with changes in the cardiac rhythm and blood pressure.

Hypotension

Hypotension is defined as a drop in systolic blood pressure (BP) of more than 20% from the patient's baseline/previous value. Many sources define this as a systolic BP of less than 90mmHg.

Causes

BP is determined by cardiac output and systemic vascular resistance: $BP = CO \times SVR$. Therefore, any factor that affects these components has the potential to cause hypotension:

- Patient factors: the use of ACE inhibitors/alpha receptor blockers, e.g. losartan; pathophysiological processes, e.g. sepsis; inadequate steroid replacement if the patient is on significant doses of steroids pre-operatively, e.g. prednisolone 10mg; acute cardiac event, e.g. MI; hypovolaemia.
- Anaesthetic factors: high doses of volatiles/IV induction agents/ opiates, spinal/epidural anaesthesia, development of anaphylaxis/ arrhythmias.

Check HR and oxygen saturations
(if either abnormal, treat as per algorithms)
Could the BP cuff be misreading, e.g. incorrect sizing?
Check radial pulse — if present, systolic BP is usually >80mmHg

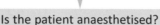

Is the patient anaesthetised?

Yes   No

- Give a vasopressor, e.g. metaraminol 0.5mg
- Check end-tidal volatile concentration — reduce if necessary (caution if levels at approx. 1 MAC)
- Has a spinal just been given? May require vasopressor boluses to stabilise BP
- Has an epidural just been given?
- Could the catheter be intrathecal or intravenous?

- Full history and examination
- Check operative site if applicable for evidence of haemorrhage
- If concerns re: acute cardiac event, perform a 12-lead ECG
- Give fluids if there is evidence of dehydration, e.g. prolonged capillary refill time, poor urine output
- Give vasopressors
- Perform an arterial blood gas, especially looking at Hb, oxygenation, lactate, base excess

No improvement

No improvement

- Call for help, alert surgeons
- Increase fluids
- Give vasopressors
- Could this be due to the patient's pre-operative medications? (N.B. could include pre-operative steroids)
- May require vasopressor infusion + invasive monitoring
- Differential diagnoses to consider:
  - underlying sepsis in emergency surgery
  - anaphylaxis
  - haemorrhage
  - arrhythmias
  - underlying cardiac disease, e.g. ACS (check ECG)
  - bone cement implantation syndrome if applicable

Figure 31.1. An algorithm for the management of hypotension.

- Surgical factors: patient positioning, e.g. deckchair positioning, uncontrolled bleeding, bone cement implantation syndrome in orthopaedic procedures.

Management

It is very important to determine whether the cause of the hypotension is likely to be related to the anaesthetic (e.g. following a spinal anaesthetic), the patient (e.g. existing comorbidities or potential cardiac event) or as a complication of the surgery (e.g. haemorrhage). Treatment can then be targeted appropriately. If this is difficult to determine, then further investigations may be required while management is ongoing.

An algorithm for the management of hypotension is outlined in Figure 31.1.

Prevention

Pre-operative measures include the avoidance of certain medications known to potentiate hypotension under anaesthesia, e.g. ACE inhibitors. It is also very important to initiate adequate pre-operative resuscitation, e.g. IV fluids in septic patients. In unstable patients or those in whom non-invasive BP may be unreliable, arterial line insertion and invasive BP measurement should be considered. In such patients, it is also important to be careful with dosages of IV induction agents and volatile concentrations. It is possible to predict certain points at which hypotension may occur, e.g. at induction or after spinal insertion. Hypotension can therefore be pre-empted with a bolus/infusion of a vasopressor such as metaraminol.

Hypertension

This occurs with an increase in a patient's BP by >20% from a baseline/previous reading. Hypertension is commonly defined as a BP of greater than 140/90mmHg.

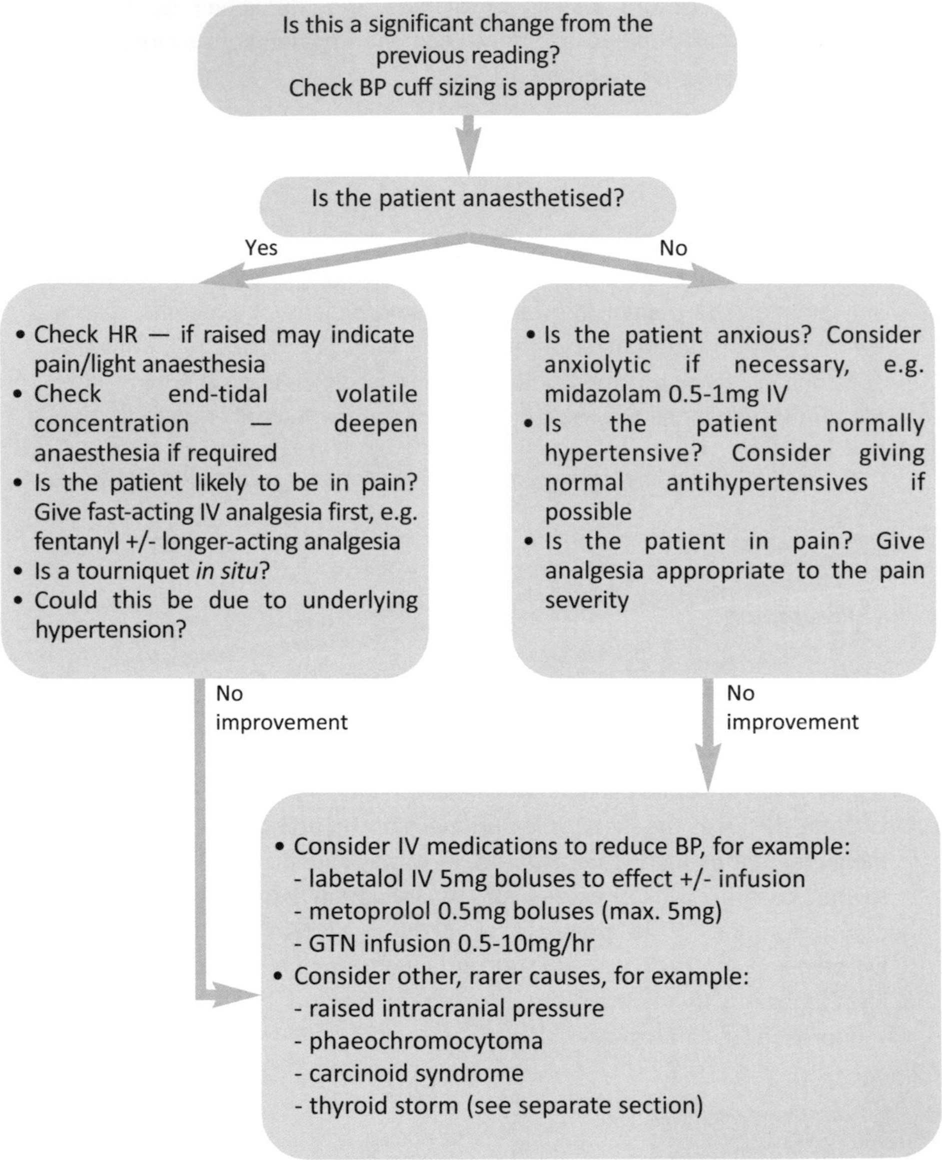

Is this a significant change from the previous reading?
Check BP cuff sizing is appropriate

Is the patient anaesthetised?

Yes   No

- Check HR — if raised may indicate pain/light anaesthesia
- Check end-tidal volatile concentration — deepen anaesthesia if required
- Is the patient likely to be in pain? Give fast-acting IV analgesia first, e.g. fentanyl +/- longer-acting analgesia
- Is a tourniquet *in situ*?
- Could this be due to underlying hypertension?

- Is the patient anxious? Consider anxiolytic if necessary, e.g. midazolam 0.5-1mg IV
- Is the patient normally hypertensive? Consider giving normal antihypertensives if possible
- Is the patient in pain? Give analgesia appropriate to the pain severity

No improvement

No improvement

- Consider IV medications to reduce BP, for example:
  - labetalol IV 5mg boluses to effect +/- infusion
  - metoprolol 0.5mg boluses (max. 5mg)
  - GTN infusion 0.5-10mg/hr
- Consider other, rarer causes, for example:
  - raised intracranial pressure
  - phaeochromocytoma
  - carcinoid syndrome
  - thyroid storm (see separate section)

Figure 31.2. An algorithm for the management of hypertension.

Causes

- Patient factors: underlying hypertension (may have omitted antihypertensives pre-operatively), anxiety, underlying endocrine disturbance, e.g. phaeochromocytoma/thyroid storm, raised intracranial pressure (mechanism to increase brain perfusion).
- Anaesthetic factors: light anaesthesia, pain, excess dose of vasopressors, response to intubation.
- Surgical factors: tourniquet pain (develops 30-60 minutes after inflation and is resistant to IV analgesia), manipulation of specific structures, e.g. the adrenal glands.

Management

It is very useful to divide management according to whether the patient is anaesthetised or not. If they are anaesthetised, initial steps will include deepening of the anaesthetic and the administration of analgesics with a rapid onset of action. If the patient is not anaesthetised, options will include analgesia and anxiolysis. If these measures do not work, then antihypertensives should be given according to the needs of the patient. This may involve short-acting IV agents, e.g. labetalol or the patient's own antihypertensive medication.

An algorithm for the management of hypertension is outlined in Figure 31.2.

Prevention

If the patient is already hypertensive pre-operatively, then this ideally should be optimised pre-operatively. This can be achieved by continuing the patient's normal medications or referral to primary care to start antihypertensives in patients with a BP of >180/110mmHg or if there is evidence of end-organ damage. For urgent/emergency surgery, you may need to commence antihypertensives, e.g. amlodipine 5mg orally. It is also worth considering a pre-operative anxiolytic in anxious/hypertensive patients if this is appropriate. Particular aspects of a procedure may be particularly painful or stimulating, e.g. first incision of an abscess. This can therefore be pre-empted with a bolus of propofol or a fast-acting opiate, e.g. alfentanil.

Tachycardia

This occurs when the heart rate is greater than 90 bpm.

Causes

- Patient factors: anxiety, hypoxia, hypercarbia, pyrexia, sepsis, compensatory tachycardia due to hypotension (e.g. due to haemorrhage), endocrine abnormalities including hypoglycaemia/thyrotoxicosis/thyroid storm/phaeochromocytoma, electrolyte abnormalities (e.g. hyperkalaemia/hypomagnesaemia), pulmonary embolus, and the omission of the patient's normal anti-arrhythmics.
- Anaesthetic factors: light anaesthesia, pain, metabolic disturbance, e.g. malignant hyperthermia, anaphylaxis.
- Surgical factors: uncontrolled haemorrhage, surgical stimulation and pain, hypovolaemia.

Management

It is important to look at the patient's heart rate in conjunction with their BP. If the BP is high, then this may suggest light anaesthesia or pain that can be quickly addressed. If the BP is low, this may indicate hypovolaemia or shock that can be addressed initially with IV fluids +/- vasopressors. If there is a corresponding drop in oxygen saturation, then 100% O_2 should be administered. If the tachycardia continues or recurs, then it is vital to differentiate between a narrow and a broad complex tachycardia as the management of each will be very different (as detailed in the appropriate sections).

An algorithm for the management of tachycardia is outlined in Figure 31.3.

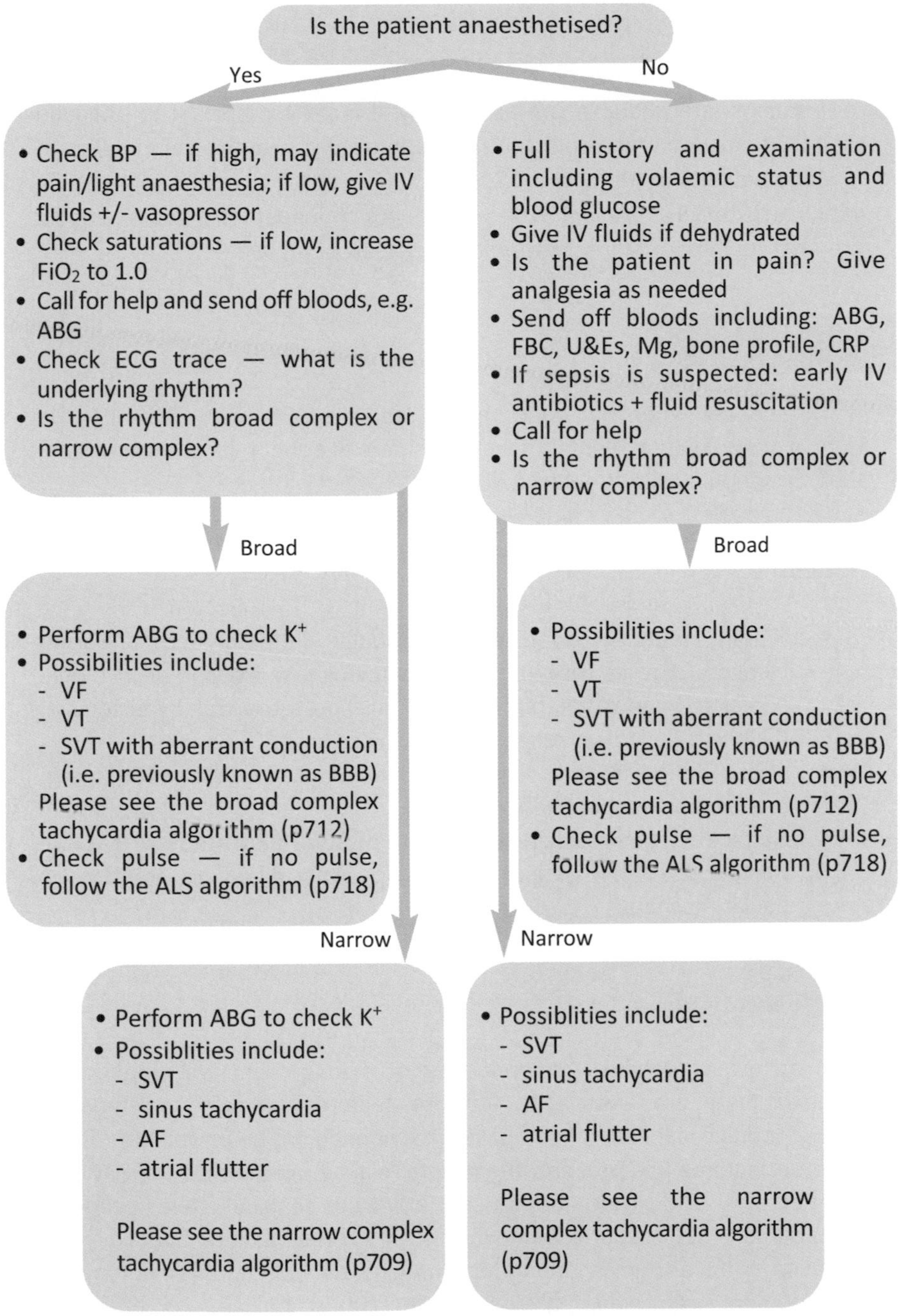

Is the patient anaesthetised?

Yes   No

Yes branch:

- Check BP — if high, may indicate pain/light anaesthesia; if low, give IV fluids +/- vasopressor
- Check saturations — if low, increase FiO_2 to 1.0
- Call for help and send off bloods, e.g. ABG
- Check ECG trace — what is the underlying rhythm?
- Is the rhythm broad complex or narrow complex?

No branch:

- Full history and examination including volaemic status and blood glucose
- Give IV fluids if dehydrated
- Is the patient in pain? Give analgesia as needed
- Send off bloods including: ABG, FBC, U&Es, Mg, bone profile, CRP
- If sepsis is suspected: early IV antibiotics + fluid resuscitation
- Call for help
- Is the rhythm broad complex or narrow complex?

Broad (Yes):

- Perform ABG to check K^+
- Possibilities include:
  - VF
  - VT
  - SVT with aberrant conduction (i.e. previously known as BBB)
  Please see the broad complex tachycardia algorithm (p712)
- Check pulse — if no pulse, follow the ALS algorithm (p718)

Broad (No):

- Possibilities include:
  - VF
  - VT
  - SVT with aberrant conduction (i.e. previously known as BBB)
  Please see the broad complex tachycardia algorithm (p712)
- Check pulse — if no pulse, follow the ALS algorithm (p718)

Narrow (Yes):

- Perform ABG to check K^+
- Possiblities include:
  - SVT
  - sinus tachycardia
  - AF
  - atrial flutter

  Please see the narrow complex tachycardia algorithm (p709)

Narrow (No):

- Possiblities include:
  - SVT
  - sinus tachycardia
  - AF
  - atrial flutter

  Please see the narrow complex tachycardia algorithm (p709)

Figure 31.3. An algorithm for the management of tachycardia.

Prevention

If patients are unstable pre-operatively, it is very important to optimise their fluid balance and electrolytes pre-operatively. It is also very important in these patients to perform a 12-lead ECG in order to accurately identify which arrhythmia is present. Adequate depth of anaesthesia and analgesia are also very important in preventing tachycardia.

Bradycardia

This occurs when the heart rate is less than 60 bpm. This may be normal in particular patients; however, if there is concomitant hypotension, then this should be corrected quickly.

Causes

- Patient factors: good cardiovascular fitness, use of beta-blockers/digoxin, hypothermia, hypothyroidism, existing heart block, complete heart block, raised intracranial pressure with hypertension (Cushing's triad), electrolyte abnormalities.
- Anaesthetic factors: deep anaesthesia, medications, e.g. remifentanil, metaraminol.
- Surgical factors: certain procedures trigger reflex bradycardia, e.g. peritoneal stretch during laparoscopy, anal dilatation, traction on ocular muscles.

Management

In an awake patient, the principles of management will depend on whether there are associated adverse features (namely hypotension, altered consciousness, chest pain or evidence of heart failure). If no adverse features are present, then there is time available to identify and correct the underlying cause. If adverse features are present, management will include removal of any precipitating causes, e.g. deflation of the abdomen during laparoscopy, as well as pharmacological management with either glycopyrrolate 100µg boluses to effect or atropine 500-600µg IV.

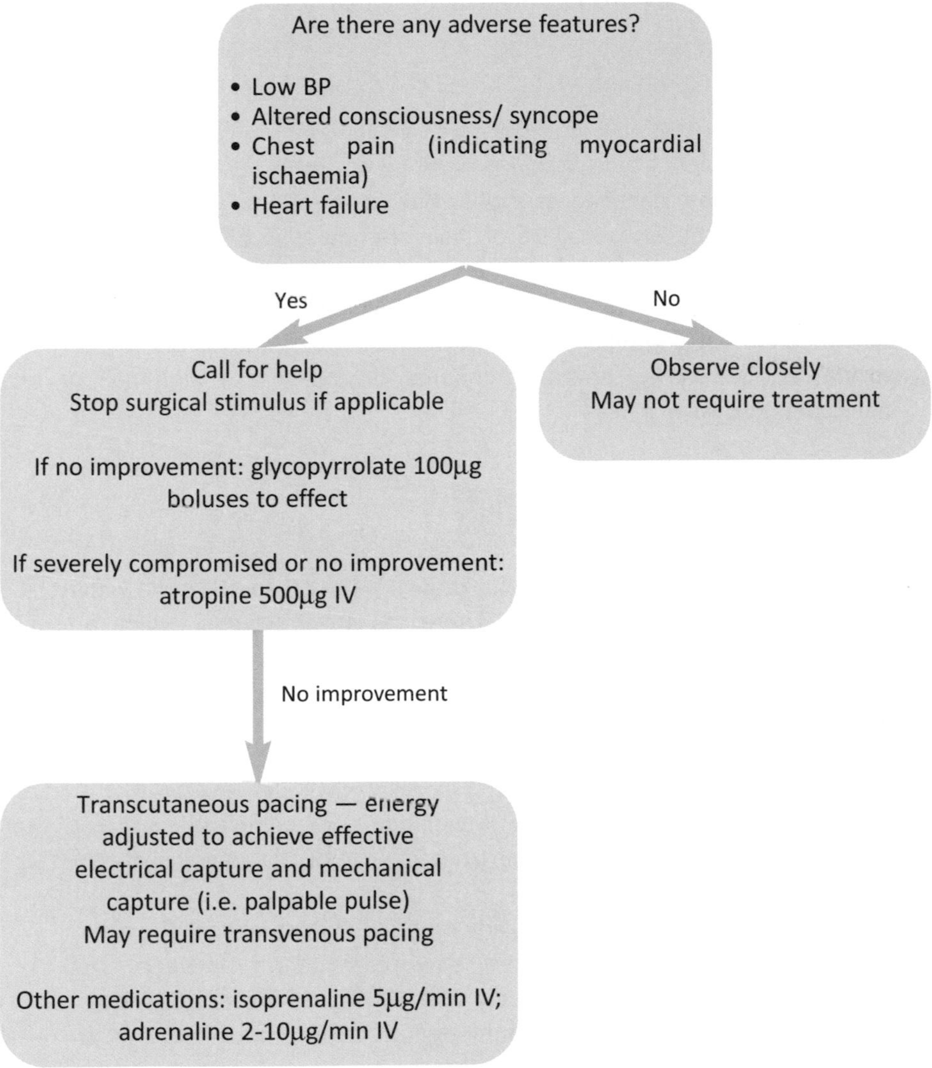

Are there any adverse features?

- Low BP
- Altered consciousness/ syncope
- Chest pain (indicating myocardial ischaemia)
- Heart failure

Yes

No

Call for help
Stop surgical stimulus if applicable

If no improvement: glycopyrrolate 100µg boluses to effect

If severely compromised or no improvement: atropine 500µg IV

Observe closely
May not require treatment

No improvement

Transcutaneous pacing — energy adjusted to achieve effective electrical capture and mechanical capture (i.e. palpable pulse)
May require transvenous pacing

Other medications: isoprenaline 5µg/min IV; adrenaline 2-10µg/min IV

Figure 31.4. An algorithm for the management of bradycardia.

An algorithm for the management of bradycardia is outlined in Figure 31.4.

Prevention

Patients can be identified as higher risk for developing bradycardias and heart block through analysis of their pre-operative ECG. If there is bifascicular or trifascicular block, a cardiology opinion should be sought pre-operatively for elective surgery. There are also certain procedures that carry a risk of causing reflex bradycardia. It is therefore advisable to have pacing facilities in the operating theatre for patients at high risk of significant bradyarrhythmias.

Narrow complex tachycardia

This occurs when a patient's heart rate is greater than 100 bpm with a QRS width of less than 0.12ms. There are several types, which are detailed below.

Causes

- Sinus tachycardia: regular P waves and QRS complexes.
- Supraventricular tachycardia (AVNRT or AVRT): regular rhythm, P waves not easily visible.
- Atrial fibrillation (AF): irregularly irregular rhythm, absent P waves.
- Atrial flutter: regular rhythm, saw-tooth pattern between QRS complexes, atrial rate typically 200-400 bpm (typically 300 bpm), may be regular/irregular numbers of QRS complexes that are conducted, e.g. 3:1 block, 2:1 block.

Management

Management should initially follow the previous "Tachycardia" section, which includes assessment of the patient's volaemic status and treatment with IV fluids +/- vasopressors.

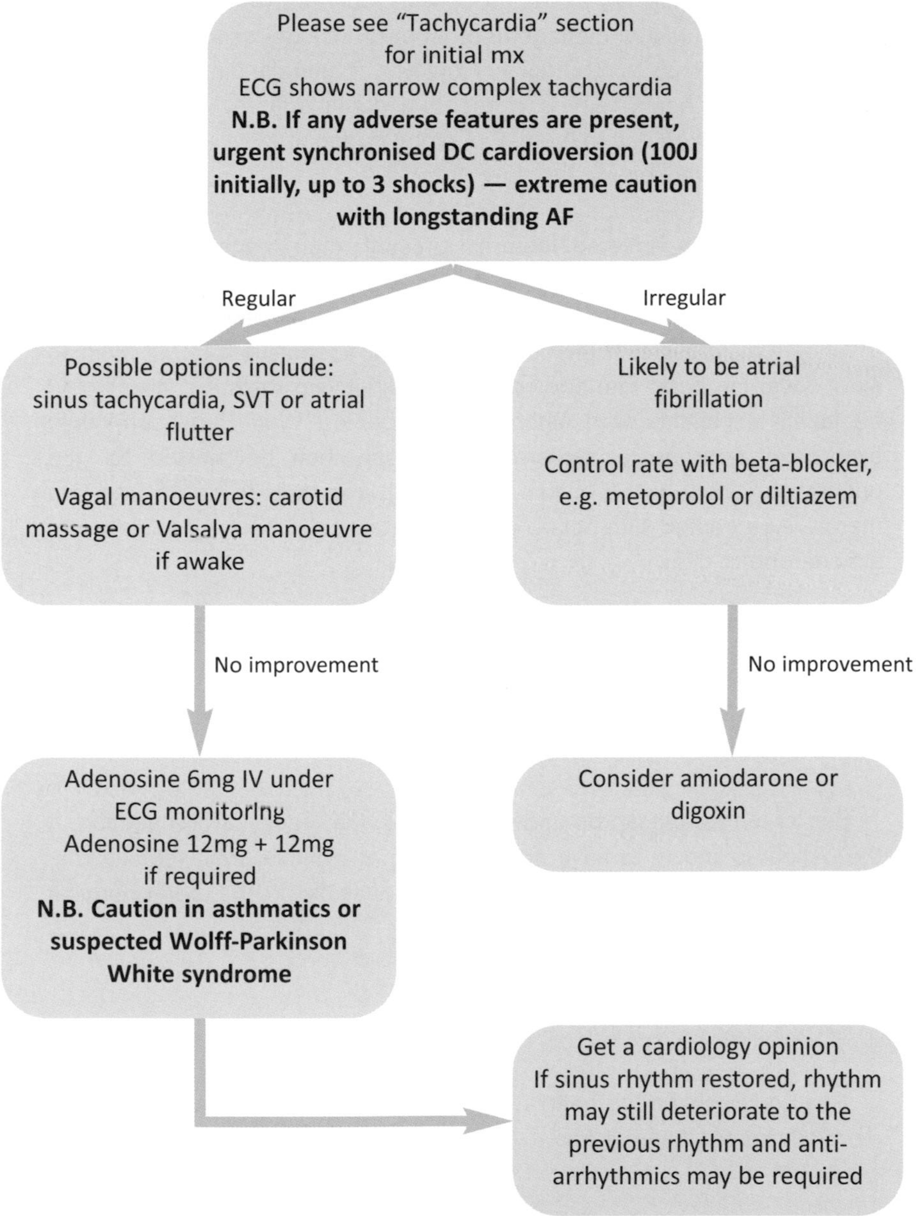

Figure 31.5. An algorithm for the management of narrow complex tachycardia.

If the arrhythmia is associated with adverse features (detailed previously), immediate management should include synchronised DC cardioversion for up to 3 shocks. However, if longstanding (present for longer than 48 hours) AF is present, a cardiology review should be speedily undertaken due to the risk of embolisation of clots within the heart following cardioversion.

If there are no adverse features present, then management differs according to whether the rhythm is regular or irregular. If the rhythm is regular, vagal manoeuvres can be attempted, such as carotid massage or a Valsalva manoeuvre. If this is not effective, adenosine can be given to slow down the heart rate and reveal the underlying rhythm. Care should be taken in patients with asthma or suspected Wolff-Parkinson-White syndrome. Appropriate anti-arrhythmics can then be started for the underlying rhythm. If the rhythm is irregular, it is likely to be AF and can therefore be treated with beta-blockers, certain calcium channel blockers, amiodarone or digoxin.

An algorithm for the management of narrow complex tachycardia is outlined in Figure 31.5.

Prevention

Similar measures can be undertaken as in the "Tachycardia" section. If the patient is known to have an underlying arrhythmia, their regular anti-arrhythmics should be continued where possible in the peri-operative period.

Broad complex tachycardia

This occurs when the heart rate is greater than 100 bpm with a QRS duration greater than 0.12ms.

Causes

- Ventricular tachycardia (VT) or polymorphic VT.
- Ventricular fibrillation (VF).
- Supraventricular tachycardia (SVT) with aberrant conduction, i.e. SVT with bundle branch block (BBB).

Management

As broad complex tachycardias can be seen during cardiac arrest, it is very important to assess for the presence of a pulse and manage accordingly. The management of cardiac arrest will be covered in a later section.

If a pulse is present, irregular or regular tachycardias should be differentiated. If a regular arrhythmia is present, then this is likely to represent VT or SVT with aberrant conduction. Advanced Life Support (ALS) guidelines state that if VT is suspected, it should be treated as such with amiodarone unless there is evidence of previous aberrant conduction, e.g. LBBB. In this situation, SVT with aberrant conduction is treated as per SVT.

If an irregular arrhythmia is present, this could be polymorphic VT, AF with aberrant BBB or pre-excited AF. As it can be extremely difficult to differentiate between these rhythms, a cardiology opinion should be sought in the first instance.

An algorithm for the management of broad complex tachycardia is outlined in Figure 31.6.

Prevention

Similar measures can be used as outlined in the "Tachycardia" section. It is also very important to check the patient's electrolytes pre-operatively.

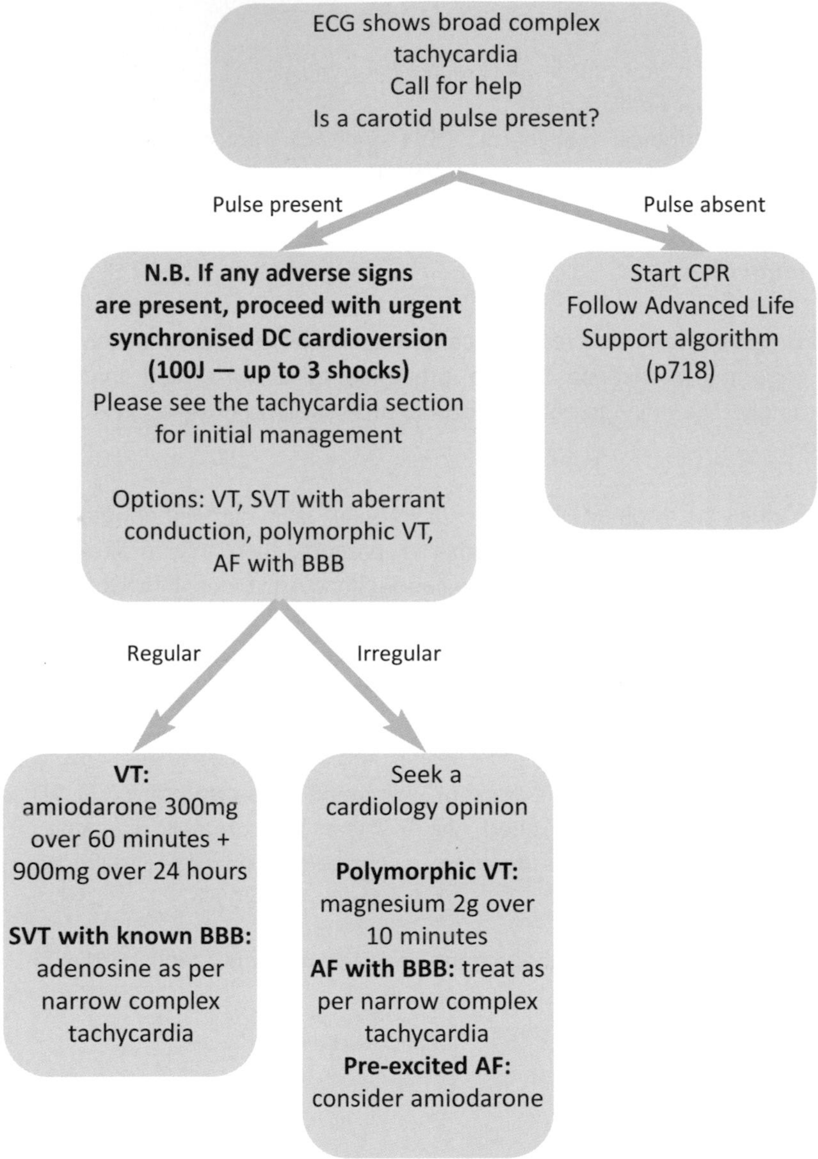

Figure 31.6. An algorithm for the management of broad complex tachycardia.

Pulmonary embolus (PE)

This occurs with the presence of a clinically significant blood clot present within the pulmonary arterial circulation that has embolised from elsewhere in the body, most commonly associated with a deep vein thrombosis (DVT) of the leg. This can be further subdivided into three classes:

- Massive PE — causes cardiovascular instability.
- Submassive PE — no cardiovascular instability but evidence of right heart dysfunction, e.g. RV dilatation on echo, R heart strain on ECG.
- PE — no cardiovascular instability.

Causes

- Patient causes: prolonged immobility, long-haul flights, inherited thrombophilia disorders, e.g. Factor V Leiden, use of oral contraceptive pill, pregnancy, obesity.
- Surgical causes: pelvic surgery, lower limb fractures, long procedures, head-up positioning during surgical procedures due to increased venous stasis.
- Medical causes: dehydration, sepsis, ITU admission, presence of DVT.

Symptoms and signs

- Symptoms: central chest pain, shortness of breath, haemoptysis, collapse.
- Signs: tachypnoea, respiratory distress, reduced peripheral oxygen saturations, tachycardia, hypotension (if large, proximal clot), cardiac arrest.

Management

- Give O$_2$ as required.
- If there is evidence of cardiovascular instability, i.e. hypotensive or during cardiac arrest, consider thrombolysis (tenecteplase 500-600μg/kg IV bolus or alteplase 50mg IV bolus) — bear in mind the contraindications to thrombolysis (Table 31.1). If thrombolysis is contraindicated, a pulmonary embolectomy can be performed but

Table 31.1. Relative and absolute contraindications to thrombolysis.

Relative contraindications	Absolute contraindications
Uncontrolled hypertension	Known intracranial neoplasm or vascular malformation
Major surgery within 3 weeks	Recent surgery to spinal cord or brain
Concurrent use of anticoagulants, e.g. warfarin	Evidence of active bleeding
Pregnancy	Allergy to thrombolytic agents or previous administration of alteplase
Age >75 years	Evidence of abnormal coagulation, e.g. liver disease
Traumatic or prolonged CPR (>10 minutes)	Recent closed head or facial injury with evidence of fractures or brain injury
Recent internal bleeding (within 3 weeks)	Ischaemic stroke <3 months ago
	Suspected aortic dissection

this is only performed at cardiothoracic centres and still carries significant risk.
- If the patient is cardiovascularly stable, give a treatment dose of low-molecular-weight heparin (e.g. enoxaparin 1.5mg/kg OD), unfractionated heparin or fondaparinux initially, and commence warfarin.

Prevention

- Recognition of high-risk patients peri-operatively and appropriate measures taken, e.g. TEDs, intermittent pneumatic calf compression devices, e.g. Flowtron® boots, prophylactic low-molecular-weight heparin.
- Risk of venous thromboembolism (VTE) scoring systems used at regular intervals throughout the inpatient stay.
- Early recognition and treatment of DVT.

Acute coronary syndrome

This occurs when blood flow to the coronary arteries is reduced which causes cardiac ischaemia. This can then cause unstable angina, non-ST elevation MI (NSTEMI) or ST elevation MI (STEMI).

ST elevation MI occurs when there is ST elevation >0.2mV in two or more contiguous chest leads or >0.1mV in two or more contiguous limb leads or new-onset LBBB.

Non-ST elevation MI is indicated by ischaemic chest pain with none of the above ECG changes (may have other ECG changes, e.g. T wave inversion) but with a raised troponin result.

Unstable angina has a similar clinical picture to NSTEMI, but troponin levels are normal.

Causes

- Reduced oxygen delivery to the myocardium, e.g. due to atherosclerosis of coronary arteries, vasoconstriction of the coronary arteries, anaemia.
- Increased oxygen demand of the myocardium that cannot be met, e.g. exercise, intercurrent illness, arrhythmias.

Symptoms and signs

- Symptoms: crushing central chest pain classically with radiation into the left arm or neck, shortness of breath, palpitations, sweating, anxiety, collapse.
- Signs: tachycardia, tachypnoea, sweating, abnormal ECG trace, hypotension.

Management

If the patient is awake, give O_2 if needed to maintain oxygen saturations above 95%, morphine/diamorphine if chest pain is present, GTN, aspirin 300mg and clopidogrel 300mg (discuss with the surgical team if a large operation is planned or has been carried out), perform bloods including troponin, and arrange a cardiology review.

If the patient is anaesthetised and shows ECG changes:

- Increase FiO_2 to 1.0.
- If hypotensive give a vasopressor.
- Inform the surgeon.
- If a NG tube is present, give aspirin 300mg and clopidogrel 300mg.
- Arrange a cardiology review post-op.

It is very important to discuss other management options with the cardiologists. Procedural options include percutaneous coronary intervention (PCI) or a coronary artery bypass graft (CABG).

Pharmacological options include thrombolysis (if STEMI and no nearby facilities for PCI); glycoprotein IIb/IIIa inhibitors, e.g. tirofiban or eptifibatide; fondaparinux or unfractionated heparin.

Prevention

If a patient has known ischaemic heart disease, continue their normal cardiac medications where possible peri-operatively. In patients with known or suspected ischaemic heart disease, maintain BP within 20% of their baseline and avoid additional stresses to the heart, such as tachycardia or arrhythmias.

Cardiac arrest

This is indicated by cardiovascular collapse and the absence of a central pulse.

Reversible causes

- 4 Hs — Hypovolaemia, Hypothermia, Hypoxia, Hypo/hyperkalaemia.
- 4 Ts — Thrombus, Tamponade, Tension pneumothorax, Toxins.

Prevention

Cardiac arrest may be prevented through early identification and treatment of deteriorating patients. Once cardiac arrest is confirmed, a successful outcome is more likely when chest compressions and appropriate defibrillation are given early (Figure 31.7).

Adult Advanced Life Support

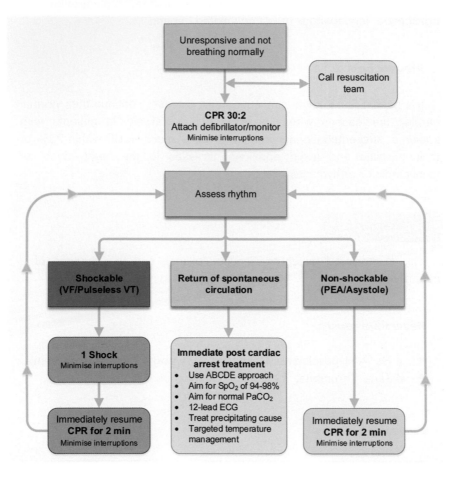

Figure 31.7. Advanced Life Support management algorithm. *Reproduced with permission from the Resuscitation Council (UK).*

Case scenario 1

A 28-year-old pregnant patient with a diagnosis of a ruptured ectopic pregnancy is anaesthetised for a laparotomy. Her pre-operative blood pressure was 110/84mmHg and heart rate was 98 per minute. Soon after induction of general anaesthesia her blood pressure reading is 74/34mmHg and heart rate is 110 per minute.

How would you manage this situation?

In this case, immediate action would be to confirm the hypotension and take measures to increase the blood pressure using vasoconstrictors and intravenous fluids. The team should be informed and appropriate help requested. The inspired oxygen concentration should be increased and the patient should be checked that she is ventilated, and this should be confirmed by capnography. Due to a low cardiac output, $EtCO_2$ decreases proportionately. Metaraminol is administered in boluses of 0.5mg or as an intravenous infusion to maintain blood pressure. Elevating the lower limb increases venous return and helps to improve cardiac output. Venous access should be secured with a wide-bore (16-14G) intravenous cannula. A litre of warm lactated Ringer's solution should be infused rapidly. To control haemorrhage this patient needs immediate surgical intervention; therefore, in this situation it is advisable to proceed with the surgery.

This patient was hypovolaemic prior to induction. On induction, vasodilatory and myocardial depressant effects of the induction agents led to severe hypotension. There is a possibility of ongoing blood loss as well.

In a similar situation where the patient is hypovolaemic due to bleeding, the surgeon should be scrubbed, gowned and ready prior to induction of general anaesthesia. The only way to control haemorrhage is clamping the bleeding vessel.

Further reading

1. Hartle A, McCormack T, Carlisle J, *et al.* The measurement of adult blood pressure and management of hypertension before elective surgery: Joint Guidelines from the Association of Anaesthetists of Great Britain and Ireland and the British Hypertension Society. *Anaesthesia* 2016; 71(3): 326-37.

2. Management of massive and submassive pulmonary embolism, iliofemoral deep vein thrombosis, and chronic thromboembolic pulmonary hypertension - AHA scientific statement. *Circulation* 2011; 123: 1788-830.

3. Hardmann JG. Complications during anaesthesia. In: Aitkenhead AR, Rowbothom DJ, Smith G, Eds. *Textbook of Anaesthesia*, 5th ed. Churchill Livingstone, 2006: 367-99.

4. https://www.resus.org.uk/resuscitation-guidelines/.

32 Metabolic problems

Christina Tourville

Introduction

This chapter looks at a range of metabolic problems that can arise perioperatively. These include anaesthetic emergencies such as anaphylaxis and malignant hyperthermia, while also covering commoner problems such as hypoglycaemia and hyperglycaemia.

Anaphylaxis

This is classified as a generalised, severe Type I hypersensitivity reaction resulting in immunoglobulin E (IgE) antibody production and cardiovascular collapse. The incidence in the UK is estimated at between 1:10,000-1:20,000.

Anaphylactoid reactions are clinically indistinguishable from anaphylactic reactions but do not result from sensitising IgE antibodies.

Causes

The commonest causes for anaphylaxis in anaesthesia are as follows:

- Neuromuscular blocking agents (cause 60% of cases related to anaesthesia): suxamethonium > rocuronium > atracurium.
- Latex (20% of cases).
- Antibiotics (15%): penicillins are most likely (N.B. 8% cross-reactivity with cephalosporins).
- Colloids (4%): the risk is greatest with gelatins; hyperosmolar solutions can cause histamine release directly.

- Induction agents: thiopental > propofol > etomidate.
- Benzodiazepines.
- Opioids: morphine is implicated most commonly.
- Antiseptics/disinfectants: increasing in incidence, with reactions ranging from contact dermatitis to life-threatening anaphylaxis.
- Other agents: radiocontrast agents, protamine, bone cement.

Signs and symptoms

Symptoms include rash, shortness of breath, palpitations, dizziness, abdominal pain or urticaria. Signs include urticarial rash, hypotension, tachycardia, airway oedema, stridor, desaturation or raised airway pressures (if intubated).

Management

The key to management of suspected anaphylaxis is rapid recognition and treatment with adrenaline. Good team working is essential with the use of a structured approach. Help should be summoned.

Immediate management involves the following approaches:

- Stop administration of all agents likely to have caused the anaphylaxis.
- Airway, breathing and circulation approach.
- Administer 100% oxygen and secure the airway with a tracheal tube if not already secured.
- Elevate the patient's legs to improve the venous return to the heart.
- Give epinephrine (adrenaline). The adult dose is 50µg intravenously (0.5ml of 1:10,000). The intramuscular dose is 0.5-1mg (0.5-1ml of 1:1000).
- Start a rapid intravenous infusion; in adults, 500-100ml of lactated Ringer's solution.
- Secondary management includes antihistamines (chlorpheniramine 10-20mg by slow intravenous infusion), hydrocortisone 100-500mg by slow IV. Bronchodilators such as salbutamol may be required for persistent bronchospasm.

- Paediatric doses for chlorpheniramine are: 6-12 years = 5mg, 6 months to 6 years = 2.5mg, <6 months = 0.25mg/kg.
- Paediatric doses for hydrocortisone are: 6-12 years = 100mg, 6 months to 6 years = 50mg, <6 months = 25mg.
- Measure serum tryptase levels at 3 times: shortly after the onset of the reaction, 1-2 hours post-reaction and 24 hours post-reaction (serum or clotted blood required — usually the same tube as a liver function text sample).

Following successful management, the decision should be made whether to proceed with the surgery or to abandon the surgery. In most cases, the patient may need a transfer to intensive care for further management.

Prevention

Identifying patients who are at high risk for allergies, such as those with atopy, and avoidance of particular medications is one way to prevent anaphylaxis. The other method is to pay close attention to a patient's allergy status, hence the reason for why this is confirmed during the WHO Surgical Safety checklist. If the patient is awake, consider early intubation and ventilation to avoid significant airway compromise.

Hypoglycaemia

This is defined as a blood glucose level less than 4mmol/L.

Causes

- In diabetic patients (more common): diabetic medications, critical illness, excess insulin dose.
- In non-diabetic patients: starvation, exercise, pregnancy, hypoadrenalism, hypopituitarism, insulin-producing tumours of the pancreas, e.g. islet cell adenoma (insulinoma), non-beta cell tumours, e.g. malignant mediastinal or retroperitoneal tumours, autoimmune hypoglycaemia.

Symptoms and signs

Symptoms include shaking, anxiety, drowsiness, lethargy or weakness. Some diabetic patients have awareness of hypoglycaemia and know the signs of it developing. Signs include tremor, tachycardia, reduced GCS or confusion, coma, delayed recovery from anaesthesia or seizures in extreme hypoglycaemia.

Management

- Assess the patient in the ABCDE manner and treat accordingly.
- Stop any IV medications that may be causing hypoglycaemia, e.g. insulin infusion.
- Give oral glucose, e.g. Glucogel®, sugary food or drink, if the patient is awake.
- Give IV 10% dextrose 100ml over 10-15 minutes if the patient is unable to take orally.
- If there is no improvement, repeat the above twice.
- Consider glucagon 1mg IM if the blood glucose remains low.
- Once the blood glucose is within the normal range, consider administering long-acting carbohydrates, e.g. two biscuits, a slice of toast/bread.
- Review the patient's diabetic medications and adjust the dosages as necessary.

Prevention

The main method of prevention is to take extra care to monitor blood glucose levels regularly in diabetic patients, especially those who are nil by mouth, critically ill or are on a variable rate intravenous insulin infusion (VRIII). Blood glucose levels should also be checked routinely in any patients who are newly confused/unconscious.

Hyperglycaemia

This is defined as a blood glucose level of greater than 11.1mmol/L.

Causes

- The commonest cause is diabetes and its associated complications (diabetic ketoacidosis [DKA] and hyperosmolar non-ketotic coma [HONKC]).
- Drugs such as corticosteroids and antipsychotics (olanzapine/duloxetine) and thiazide diuretics.
- Pancreatic disorders, e.g. pancreatitis, pancreatic carcinoma.
- Other endocrine disorders, e.g. hyperthyroidism, Cushing's syndrome.
- Central nervous system disorders, e.g. intracranial bleeds, encephalitis, meningitis.

Signs and symptoms

Symptoms include polyuria, polydipsia, blurred vision or it can be asymptomatic. Signs include evidence of dehydration or a reduced GCS if severe.

Management

- Assess the patient in the ABCDE manner and treat accordingly.
- Perform an arterial blood gas (ABG) if there is evidence of critical illness and escalate care as necessary.
- If the capillary blood glucose (CBG) is >12mmol/L or the patient is likely to be fasted for long periods and is unable to take normal oral hypoglycaemics, consider commencing a VRIII with hourly checks of CBG and concomitant administration of IV fluids in line with CBG as per local hospital guidelines (e.g. 5% dextrose if CBG <17mmol/L, 0.9% saline if CBG >17.1mmol/L).

- If there is evidence of DKA, commence aggressive IV fluid resuscitation and an insulin infusion of 0.1units/kg/hr (convert to VRIII once the acidosis and ketosis have resolved). The patient may require care in a high dependency unit if the DKA is severe.
- If there is evidence of hyperosmolar non-ketotic coma (usually in Type 2 diabetics), commence IV fluid resuscitation (less aggressive than with DKA) and a VRIII.
- Stop or reduce the dose of medications that may cause hyperglycaemia.
- If the patient is a known diabetic, their medication should be reviewed and discussed with the diabetes team as it may require adjustment.
- Monitor potassium if IV insulin is used.

Prevention

It is important to try to minimise pre-operative fasting times in diabetics to reduce the number of missed doses of their oral hypoglycaemics. Once hyperglycaemia has developed, it should be managed promptly as it can have a number of negative effects, such as increasing wound infection rates.

Electrolyte imbalance — hyponatraemia

This occurs with a serum sodium (Na^+) level of less than 135mmol/L. The causes are best classified according to the patient's volaemic status.

Causes

- Hypovolaemia: GI losses, e.g. due to diarrhoea/vomiting, renal losses, e.g. thiazide diuretics, cerebral salt wasting.
- Normovolaemia: syndrome of inappropriate antidiuretic hormone secretion (SIADH), hypothyroidism, Addison's disease, primary polydipsia, pseudohyponatraemia (e.g. due to hyperlipidaemia, hyperproteinaemia).
- Hypervolaemia: heart failure, cirrhosis, advanced renal failure.

Symptoms and signs

Symptoms can include nausea, lethargy, headache or confusion. Signs can include a reduced GCS, coma or seizures. The development of serious complications is largely determined by the speed of onset of the hyponatraemia.

Management

- Assess the patient in the ABCDE manner.
- Note the chronicity of hyponatraemia, i.e. if it is chronically low and the patient is asymptomatic, Na^+ levels may not need to be corrected acutely.
- Stop any causative medications.
- Further investigations include urine and plasma osmolality, and urinary Na^+ levels.
- If the patient is hypovolaemic, give IV fluid resuscitation, aim to correct Na^+ by 4-8mmol/L per day.
- If the patient is hypervolaemic, treat the underlying cause.
- If the patient is normovolaemic:
  - send bloods for thyroid function tests and a short synacthen test;
  - SIADH is suggested by a raised urinary Na^+, low plasma osmolality and raised urine osmolality;
  - cerebral salt wasting is suggested by hypovolaemia and raised urine osmolality.

Electrolyte imbalance — hypernatraemia

This is defined as a serum Na^+ level of greater than 145mmol/L.

Causes

- Due to a loss of water: GI losses, insensible/sweat losses, central or nephrogenic diabetes insipidus, osmotic diuresis, e.g. due to mannitol, uncontrolled diabetes, dehydration.
- Due to excess Na^+: hypertonic saline administration.

Signs and symptoms

These can include thirst, irritability, restlessness, lethargy, spasticity or hyperreflexia.

Management

- Assess the patient in the ABCDE manner.
- For chronic hypernatraemia, give 5% dextrose IV at 1.35ml/kg/hr (aim to lower by 10mmol/L per 24 hours).
- For acute hypernatraemia, give 5% dextrose IV at 3-6ml/kg/hour (aim to lower by 1-2mmol/L per hour).
- If diabetes insipidus is suspected, administer desmopressin intranasally or intravenously.

Electrolyte imbalance — hypokalaemia

This is defined as a serum potassium (K^+) of less than 3.5mmol/L (severe if <2.5mmol/L).

Causes

- Inadequate K^+ ingestion: alcoholism, eating disorders, refeeding syndrome.
- Excess K^+ excretion: GI losses, e.g. diarrhoea; drugs, e.g. diuretics, theophylline, steroids; osmotic diuresis, e.g. mannitol, hyperglycaemia; Cushing's syndrome; genetic disorders, e.g. Bartter's syndrome, congenital adrenal hyperplasia.

Signs and symptoms

Symptoms include lethargy, muscle weakness or muscle cramps in severe hypokalaemia. Signs can include arrhythmias, cardiovascular instability or respiratory muscle weakness. It may also be completely asymptomatic. ECG changes include reduced T-wave amplitude, ST depression, prominent U waves and a prolonged QT interval.

Management

- Perform a full examination including a 12-lead ECG.
- Identify and treat the cause.
- If asymptomatic with a normal ECG and K^+ is >3.0mmol/L, give oral K^+ replacement, e.g. Sando-K®. If there is no improvement or the patient is nil by mouth (NBM), consider IV replacement, e.g. 0.9% saline with 40mmol KCl.
- If severe or there are ECG changes, commence IV replacement, e.g. 0.9% saline with 40mmol potassium chloride (aiming to replace 10-20mmol per hour); this can also be given via a central vein (40mmol potassium chloride over 1 hour).
- Long-term management with a potassium-sparing diuretic may be necessary, e.g. spironolactone, amiloride.

Electrolyte imbalance — hyperkalaemia

This occurs with a serum K^+ of greater than 5.0mmol/L (severe if >6.5mmol/L).

Causes

- Increased K^+ release from cells:
  - metabolic acidosis;
  - hyperglycaemia or insulin deficiency;
  - increased tissue breakdown, e.g. crush injury, rhabdomyolysis, tumour lysis syndrome following cytotoxic or radiation treatment, extensive burns;
  - drugs, e.g. beta-blockers, suxamethonium;
  - red cell transfusion;
  - pseudohyperkalaemia, e.g. due to haemolysis on venepuncture;
  - rare causes, e.g. hyperkalaemic periodic paralysis.

729

- Reduced urinary K$^+$ secretion:
  - renal hypoperfusion due to hypovolaemia;
  - drugs, e.g. NSAIDs, ACEIs, K$^+$-sparing diuretics;
  - acute or chronic renal failure.

Signs and symptoms

Symptoms can include severe muscle weakness or palpitations. Signs can include arrhythmias or conduction abnormalities. ECG signs include peaked T waves, a shortened QT interval, progressive lengthening of the PR interval and QRS complexes, and this eventually progresses to ventricular tachycardia/ventricular fibrillation/asystole.

Management

- Assess the patient in the ABCDE manner and establish the cause.
- If ECG changes are present or K$^+$ is >6.5mmol/L:
  - IV calcium chloride 10ml 10% solution or calcium gluconate 10ml 10% solution;
  - IV infusion of insulin 10 IU and 50ml 50% dextrose;
  - salbutamol 250µg nebuliser repeated as necessary;
  - sodium bicarbonate or loop diuretics may be considered;
  - haemodialysis if required.
- Longer-acting treatment is calcium resonium PO 15g QDS.

Thyroid storm

This is a rare, life-threatening syndrome that involves severe clinical manifestations of thyrotoxicosis, accompanied by a high mortality (10-30%).

Causes

- Usually precipitated by thyroid or non-thyroid surgery, infection, trauma, acute iodine load or parturition.

- It can develop in any patient with longstanding untreated hyperthyroidism.

Signs and symptoms

Symptoms can include anxiety, agitation, palpitations and abdominal pain. Signs include tachycardia, arrhythmias, heart failure, hyperpyrexia (>39.4°C), confusion, psychosis or coma.

Diagnosis

- Signs and symptoms suggestive of thyroid storm.
- Low thyroid-stimulating hormone (TSH), raised free T4 and/or T3.
- May have hyperglycaemia.

Management

- Assess the patient in the ABCDE manner and treat the underlying trigger.
- Propranolol (usually 60-80mg PO QDS or 0.5-1mg IV) at a dose to control the heart rate. Other bota-blockers can also be used, e.g. esmolol, metoprolol, or calcium channel blockers, e.g. diltiazem.
- Either propylthiouracil (200mg 4-hourly) or methimazole (20mg PO 4-6-hourly) or carbimazole to block hormone synthesis.
- 1 hour after propylthiouracil/methimazole, give iodine as a saturated solution of potassium iodide (SSKI) 5 drops PO, QDS or Lugol's iodine 10 drops TDS.
- Hydrocortisone 100mg TDS to reduce T4-T3 conversion.
- Bile acid sequestrants, e.g. cholestyramine 4g PO QDS to reduce enterohepatic cycling.

Malignant hyperthermia

This is a genetic disorder which affects the ryanodine receptor in skeletal muscle and causes excessive calcium release. It is precipitated by volatile anaesthetic agents and suxamethonium. The incidence is 1:100,000 general anaesthetics.

Signs

- Hyperthermia with rapidly rising temperature, tachycardia, arrhythmias, muscle rigidity (masseter or generalised), rising expired CO_2 levels and myoglobinuria.

Management

Immediate management:

- Stop all trigger agents.
- Call for help. Allocate specific tasks to team members.
- Install a clean, vapour-free breathing system and hyperventilate with 100% oxygen.
- Maintain anaesthesia with intravenous agents.
- Abandon/finish the surgery as soon as possible.
- Muscle relaxation with a non-depolarising neuromuscular blocking drug.

Monitoring and treatment:

- Give dantrolene as a 2.5mg/kg immediate IV bolus. Repeat 1mg/kg boluses as required to a maximum 10mg/kg, e.g. for a 70kg adult, the initial bolus is 9 vials dantrolene 20mg (each vial mixed with 60ml sterile water); and then further boluses of 4 vials dantrolene 20mg, repeated up to 7 times.
- Initiate active cooling, avoiding vasoconstriction.

Further management depends on the associated biochemical abnormalities:

- Treatment of hyperkalaemia with calcium chloride, glucose/insulin and sodium bicarbonate.
- Arrhythmias should be treated with magnesium sulphate/ amiodarone/metoprolol. Calcium channel blockers should be avoided as they can interact with dantrolene.

- Metabolic acidosis should be managed with hyperventilation and administration of sodium bicarbonate.
- Myoglobinaemia can be managed with forced alkaline diuresis (mannitol/furosemide and $NaHCO_3^-$). The patient may require renal replacement therapy later.
- Disseminated intravascular coagulation should be treated with fresh frozen plasma (FFP), cryoprecipitiate and platelets.

Monitoring and investigations:

- Check plasma creatine kinase (CK) as soon as possible.
- Core and peripheral temperature, $EtCO_2$, SpO_2, ECG, invasive blood pressure, central venous pressure (CVP), ABG, urea & electrolytes (U&Es) (potassium), full blood count (FBC) (haematocrit/platelets), and coagulation should be monitored continuously.

The differential diagnosis includes sepsis, phaeochromocytoma and thyroid storm.

Subsequently, the patient should be referred to the malignant hyperthermia unit for further follow-up and investigations.

Case scenario 1

A 38-year-old female patient underwent an elective subtotal thyroidectomy. Her current medication included carbimazole 20mg OD and methylcellulose eye drops. Ten hours postoperatively she becomes agitated and complains of nausea. She is febrile (temperature 39.5°C) and tachycardic.

How would you manage this patient?

As this patient had a subtotal thyroidectomy 10 hours ago and she has been on carbimazole, this suggests that she had a toxic goitre. Therefore, she is at risk of developing a thyroid storm postoperatively. Management involves supportive measures and specific drug therapy outlined below.

Supportive measures

An airway, breathing and circulation approach should be used and 100% oxygen administered. Venous access should be secured and cold intravenous fluids administered (a litre of crystalloid infused rapidly and further IV fluids should be given as required). Paracetamol 1g IV should be given 6-hourly to control the temperature. This patient should be managed in an intensive care unit or in the post-anaesthesia care unit.

Specific drug therapy

- Propylthiouracil 200mg, 4-hourly, given orally or via a nasogastric tube.
- Lugol's iodine (potassium iodide) 10 drops TDS, given orally, or sodium iodide 0.25g IV. It should not be given until an hour after the administration of antithyroid drugs. It acts immediately and prevents a further release of thyroid hormones.
- Esmolol 0.5mg/kg as a bolus dose over 1 minute, followed by 50-200µg/kg/minute as an infusion, or propranolol 1-5mg IV up to 10mg should be used to control the sympathetic effects.
- Hydrocortisone 100mg IV should be administered every 6-hourly.
- Plasma exchange may be needed.
- Ionotropes and vasopressors may rarely be required.

Further reading

1. The Association of Anaesthetists of Great Britain and Ireland (AAGBI) safety guideline 4. Suspected anaphylactic reactions associated with anaesthesia. *Anaesthesia* 2009; 64: 199-211.
2. The Association of Anaesthetists of Great Britain and Ireland (AAGBI). Malignant hyperthermia crisis. http://www.aagbi.org/sites/default/files/MH%20guideline%20for%20web%20v2.pdf.
3. Anaphylactic and analphylactoid reactions. In: Gaba DM, Fish KJ, Howard SK, Burden A, Eds. *Crisis Management in Anesthesiology*, 2nd ed. Elsevier Saunders, 2015.

33 Neurological problems

Christina Tourville

Introduction

Common neurological problems during the peri-operative period include seizures and postoperative confusion. Seizures can be presenting features of local anaesthetic toxicity.

Seizures

These are abnormal synchronous discharges from cortical neurons manifested clinically by changes in motor control, sensory perception, behaviour, and/or autonomic function. Physical manifestations vary according to the area of the brain involved. Status epilepticus is continuous seizure activity for greater than 5 minutes or failure to regain consciousness between two or more seizures.

Types of seizure

- Focal: neuronal firing within a specific area of the cortex which causes specific manifestations, for example, temporal lobe epilepsy, can cause secondary generalised seizures if discharges then spread across the brain.
- Generalised: abnormal neuronal discharge in both hemispheres simultaneously, for example, absence seizures or generalised tonic-clonic seizures.

Causes

- Neurological: epilepsy, head injury, transient ischaemic attack (TIA), stroke, cerebral vascular disease, hydrocephalus, space-occupying lesions, meningitis, encephalitis, cerebral anoxia, e.g. following cardiac arrest.
- Non-neurological: hyponatraemia, hypoglycaemia, hypocalcaemia, hypomagnesaemia, chronic renal failure, hyperthyroidism, alcohol withdrawal, drug toxicity, eclampsia.

Management

- Ensure the airway is clear and that breathing is adequate. Continue to assess in the ABCDE manner.
- Give O_2 and establish full monitoring (ECG/NIBP/SpO$_2$), and check the capillary glucose level.
- Place the patient in the recovery position and call for help.
- Obtain IV access if not already present.
- If the seizure continues for longer than 5 minutes, administer IV lorazepam 0.1mg/kg (usual dose 4mg in adults) or IV diazepam 0.2mg/kg (usual dose 10mg in adults), which can be repeated once more if required.
- If there is no IV access, administer IM or buccal midazolam 10mg or rectal diazepam 10mg.
- If there is no improvement, administer IV phenytoin 20mg/kg as a 25-50mg/min infusion (ensuring full ECG monitoring). Other options include fosphenytoin, valproate or levetiracetam infusions.
- If there is no improvement, intubate and ventilate, and administer a propofol or thiopentone infusion.
- Aim to identify and treat the cause where possible, e.g. performing a CT of the head to rule out cerebral pathology.

N.B. In suspected eclampsia, the first-line treatment is 4g magnesium sulphate ($MgSO_4$) over 10 minutes followed by a maintenance infusion of 1g/hr for 24 hours. Further boluses of 2g $MgSO_4$ can be given if necessary but serum Mg levels should be monitored.

Prevention

In epileptic patients, it is very important to minimise starvation time and also ensure that antiepileptic medications are taken pre-operatively. This may require parenteral administration if the patient is unable to take it orally or if the patient is likely to miss multiple doses. In such patients, it is also important to use with caution any medications that are known to interact with antiepileptics, or those that are pro-convulsant, e.g. opioids (meperidine, pethidine, fentanyl, alfentanil, morphine).

Postoperative confusion

This occurs when there is a reduction in cognitive function when compared to the pre-operative state.

This can be further subdivided into:

- Postoperative delirium: a reduction and fluctuation in mental status with reduced attention and disordered awareness of their environment, but this is not temporally related to emergence from anaesthesia.
- Postoperative cognitive dysfunction: a reduction in cognitive function temporally associated with surgery.

Postoperative confusion is associated with increased morbidity and mortality in patients who have sustained a hip fracture.

Causes

- Neurological: underlying cognitive dysfunction, e.g. dementia; cerebrovascular disease, e.g. peri-operative stroke; raised intracranial pressure; pain.
- Cardiovascular: arrhythmias, hypotension and reduced cerebral perfusion.
- Respiratory: hypoxia, hypercarbia.
- Metabolic: hypoglycaemia, hyponatraemia, anaemia, alcohol withdrawal.

- Pharmacological: residual effects of general anaesthetic agents, e.g. ketamine; side effects, e.g. opiates, newly-added medications.
- Other: urinary retention, use of urinary catheter, malnutrition.

Management

- Assess the patient in the ABCDE manner and check observations (including ECG).
- Attempt to establish the underlying cause if possible.
- Optimise the environment and provide adequate analgesia.
- If the patient is agitated or aggressive, i.e. posing a danger to themselves or staff, consider sedation, e.g. haloperidol 0.5-1mg IV every 10-15 minutes until their behaviour is controlled.
- Perform an arterial blood gas (ABG) if possible to check PaO_2, $PaCO_2$, Na^+ levels and blood glucose.
- May require non-invasive or invasive ventilation if there is evidence of respiratory failure.
- Consider a CT of the head if there is a suspicion of stroke/raised ICP.

Prevention

Elderly patients can be particularly prone to confusion and delirium if their normal medications are disrupted peri-operatively. Therefore, ensuring ongoing administration of medications and minimising starvation time is very important. If there is a history of alcohol abuse, medications should be prescribed to help prevent withdrawal. Peri-operative review by a geriatrician may also help to reduce the incidence of postoperative delirium. Intra-operatively, the avoidance of significant hypotension in patients at risk of cerebrovascular disease is also important.

Local anaesthetic toxicity

This occurs with systemic absorption of toxic doses of local anaesthetic agents. There are multiple factors involved in the likelihood of developing toxicity. A key factor is the site of injection, with high-risk sites listed below.

The sites of injection according to the degree of absorption/risk of toxicity are as follows:

- Intercostal and paracervical block (highest risk).
- Caudal.
- Epidural.
- Brachial plexus block.
- Sciatic and femoral nerve blocks.
- Subcutaneous infiltration (lowest risk).

Symptoms and signs

Symptoms can include peri-oral tingling/paraesthesia, tinnitus, a metallic taste or dizziness.

Signs can be divided into two groups:

- Neurological: confusion, twitching, tremors progressing to grand mal seizures.
- Cardiovascular: arrhythmias, hypotension, cardiac arrest.

Management

A crucial step in management is the recognition of this emergency and stopping the injection of local anaesthetic. The aims of management thereafter are to control the signs and symptoms through supportive management (e.g. intubation and ventilation if there is a reduced GCS) and advanced life support management if cardiac arrest ensues. Definitive management is IV 20% lipid emulsion 1.5ml/kg followed by an infusion at 15ml/kg/hr.

After 5 minutes, if cardiovascular stability has not been restored, a further two bolus doses can be repeated at 5-minute intervals and the infusion rate can be doubled. The maximum cumulative dose is 12ml/kg.

Prevention

Care should be taken at all times when using large amounts of local anaesthetic and the calculation of the maximum dosing should be performed. It is also very important to always aspirate for blood before injection and to inject in 5ml aliquots. There should be extra vigilance during higher-risk blocks.

Case scenario 1

A 35-year-old female, with a past history of intravenous drug abuse is on the emergency list for incision and drainage of an abscess on the left forearm. Following discussion with the patient and surgeon, a decision has been taken to perform the surgery under an axillary nerve block. Using a nerve stimulator, after eliciting the twitches at 0.5mA of current, you have started injecting 0.5% levobupivacaine. Soon after injecting 4ml of local anaesthetic, the patient says that she feels light-headed and has tingling around her lips and tongue, and becomes semi-conscious.

How would you manage this patient?

These symptoms are most likely due to accidental intravascular injection of local anaesthetic.

Management should be as follows:

- Stop injecting the LA.
- Call for help.
- Maintain the airway, administer 100% oxygen and assess breathing; if necessary, secure the airway with a tracheal tube and establish intravenous access with a wide-bore cannula.
- Control seizures with a benzodiazepine, thiopental or small incremental doses of propofol.

- Monitor the heart rate, rhythm, blood pressure and $EtCO_2$ if ventilated.
- Administer an intravenous bolus injection of Intralipid® 20%, 1.5ml/kg over 1 minute (~100ml for an average adult) and start an IV infusion of Intralipid® 20% at 15ml/kg/hour.
- Further boluses can be administered if cardiovascular instability persists.

Further reading

1. Perks A, Cheema S, Mohanraj R. Anaesthesia and epilepsy. *Br J Anaesth* 2012; 108: 562-71.
2. The Association of Anaesthetists of Great Britain and Ireland (AAGBI) safety guideline. Management of severe local anaesthetic toxicity. https://www.aagbi.org/sites/default/files/la_toxicity_2010_0.pdf.
3. Orena EF, King AB, Hughes CG. The role of anesthesia in the prevention of postoperative delirium: a systematic review. *Minerva Anesthesiol* 2016; 82(6): 669-83.

34 General critical care management

Alistair Burns and Nick Talbot

Introduction

Patients within the critical care environment receive extensive input from a multidisciplinary team. Much of this essential care is delivered with little or no input from the intensive care physician. To adequately encompass all of the multifaceted duties fulfilled by the various team members would require a dedicated text and as such will not be covered here. This chapter aims to review the role of the physician in ensuring that essential aspects of care are fulfilled for all critical care patients.

When considering the methods employed by physicians to achieve this goal it is important to appreciate the relative excess of clinical information commonly generated for any one critical care patient. Interventions, investigations and monitoring modalities all yield clinical data. Presented on mass this information may overwhelm the clinician resulting in omissions of care. To minimise this effect, checklists and care bundles may be employed to aid the clinician in ensuring that all essential aspects of care are delivered to all patients.

Care bundles

Care bundles consist of a number of elements which when instituted in unison have a demonstrable improvement on patient outcomes. Higher levels of evidence may not necessarily support all individual elements of a care bundle. As such, bundles often incorporate implementations supported by lower levels of evidence or expert opinion. Regardless of the weight of evidence behind any individual component, the effectiveness of a bundle relies upon adherence to all aspects at all times, unless a clear overriding reason exists. At this time, non-compliance is an active decision rather than an act of omission.

Two bundles widely utilised within critical care will be discussed in greater depth. These are the ventilator care bundle and the central line bundle.

The ventilator care bundle

Ventilator-acquired pneumonia (VAP) is a significant cause of morbidity and mortality within the critical care patient population. As well as having significant implications for the patient, VAP is responsible for prolonging ventilator requirements and delaying discharge from the ICU with associated resource and cost implications.

The ventilator care bundle was widely implemented with the aim of reducing VAP. The bundle drew five simple and cost-effective actions from a broad basis of research (Table 34.1). These interventions were felt to represent those interventions with the strongest evidence base.

The central line bundle

Central venous catheters (CVCs) are commonly utilised within the critical care setting as a method of vascular access, drug delivery, monitoring and organ support. CVCs disrupt skin integrity and are responsible for precipitating localised infection, bacteraemia and sepsis. As with VAP, the associated morbidity and mortality are detrimental to the patient and have cost and resource implications for the ICU.

Table 34.1. Actions of a ventilator care bundle.

Action	Rationale
30-45° head elevation	The use of a semi-recumbent nursing position may reduce silent oesophageal reflux and subsequent micro-aspirations. The passage of gastric contents into the respiratory tract induces chemical irritation and provides a mechanism for bacterial translocation. The semi-recumbent position has the secondary benefit of aiding respiratory mechanics.
Daily sedation breaks	Daily sedation breaks aid with respiratory weaning. The resulting reduction in ventilator requirements reduces the overall patient exposure to the risks of VAP.
Oral hygiene	The use of oropharyngeal decontamination with 2% chlorhexidine mouth wash or an equivalent agent minimises colonisation of the oropharynx and subsequent transmission of organisms to the lower respiratory tract.
Tracheal tube cuff pressure monitoring	Inadequate cuff pressures <20cmH$_2$O may permit leakage of secretions into the respiratory tract. Conversely, excessive pressures >30cmH$_2$O may result in necrosis and long-term complications. Regular monitoring of cuff pressures should be employed to guard against both possibilities. The design of the cuff is also a point of contention, with some suggestion that cuffs requiring only partial inflation may result in a greater occurrence of micro-aspirations.
Subglottic aspiration	Suggested for patients requiring periods of ventilation in excess of 72 hours. Subglottic drainage may help minimise the passage of contaminated secretions from above the cuff into the lower respiratory tract.
Stress ulcer prophylaxis	Often included within the ventilator care bundle, the utilisation of pharmacological stress ulcer prophylaxis may in fact increase the risk of VAP. It is discussed in greater detail within the checklists subsection.

Significant emphasis has been placed upon reducing line-related infections and in using the central line care bundle (Table 34.2).

The care bundle covers five main domains.

Table 34.2. Five main domains of a central line care bundle.

Action	Rationale
Catheter selection	Single-lumen catheters reduce infective complications versus multi-lumen catheters. Where multiple lines are required, however, a multiple lumen device is still advocated.
Site selection	Catheters are typically placed in the subclavian, internal jugular and femoral veins. The subclavian approach demonstrates the lowest rates of catheter-related line infection (<1%) with femoral lines resulting in the highest rate (>6%). The risks of infection should, however, be balanced against the procedural risks of utilising each site.
Asepsis	Appropriate skin decontamination with a 2% chlorhexidine solution minimises the possibility of seeding micro-organisms from the patient's skin at the time of insertion. The use of full aseptic precautions including mask, gown, gloves and a large drape minimise the risks of contamination during the procedure.
Dressing	Subsequent application of a sterile transparent dressing minimises the potential for micro-organism contamination during catheter manipulations whilst permitting observation of the insertion site for evidence of localised infection.
Note keeping	Completion of a standardised CVC insertion record serves as a suitable means of documentation whilst prompting compliance with the other components of the care bundle.

Checklists

Checklists may also be employed within the intensive care setting. These may contain components of one or more care bundles as well as other aspects of patient care. Unlike care bundles, checklists do not necessarily carry a proven benefit to outcome, nor do they require the same all or nothing compliance. The role of the checklist within critical care is akin to that of the pilot's pre-flight check. It provides a framework for the clinician to ensure that all key aspects of patient care are considered.

FASTHUG

The most widely utilised critical care checklist is that of FASTHUG. The mnemonic, which stands for Feeding, Analgesia, Sedation, Thromboprophylaxis, Head-up, Ulcer Prophylaxis and Glucose control was developed as a tool for clinicians to employ during routine review of any critical care patient. An adapted mnemonic of FLATHUG adds the component of lines whilst combining analgesia and sedation.

FLATHUG components

Each component of the FLATHUG (Table 34.3) reflects an area of ICU management where careful monitoring and intervention yields proven benefits.

Table 34.3. Components of the FLATHUG checklist for general supportive therapy.

Component	Rationale
Feeding	Nutritional requirements and available routes of delivery may vary greatly during the course of admission. Over- and under-feeding are associated with poor outcomes as is prolonged parenteral delivery. Regular re-evaluation by the multidisciplinary team is necessary to ensure adequate delivery by the most appropriate available route.

Continued overleaf

Table 34.3 *continued*. Components of the FLATHUG checklist for general supportive therapy.

Component	Rationale
Lines	Line sepsis is a significant cause of morbidity and mortality. Regular evaluation of all access points permits timely removal of unnecessary lines and a reduction in line-related sepsis.
Analgesia/ sedation	As discussed above, sedation breaks aid in ventilation weaning and a reduction in the duration of ventilator requirement. Consideration should be given to the provision of appropriate analgesia in all patients but particularly where opioid-based sedation is to be discontinued as part of a sedation break.
Thromboprophylaxis	Critical illness and prolonged immobility are major risk factors for the development of thromboembolic events. Appropriate utilisation of mechanical deep vein thrombosis prevention devices and pharmacological prevention should be employed where appropriate.
Head-up position	A component of the ventilation care bundle with the rationale as discussed above.
Ulcer prophylaxis	The stress response associated with critical illness induces hypoperfusion of the gastric mucosa and failure of protective gastrointestinal mechanisms. Subsequent development of gastric stress ulceration may lead to significant bleeding with associated mortality, morbidity and prolonged critical care admission. The use of pharmacological agents such as proton pump inhibitors or H_2 receptor antagonists minimise such complications.

Conversely, the increased gastric pH removes a barrier to microbial growth and may contribute to the development of VAP. Regular review should ensure timely cessation of treatment where full enteral nutrition is instituted or prophylaxis is no longer deemed necessary. |

Continued overleaf

Table 34.3 *continued*. Components of the FLATHUG checklist for general supportive therapy.	
Component	Rationale
Glucose control	Critical illness is associated with deranged metabolism and poor glucose control. Hyperglycaemia may affect all patients, not only those with diabetes. Hyperglycaemia predicts poor outcome within these patients and evidence exists to suggest that appropriate control improves outcome. Although some studies advocated tight control of blood glucose below 6mmol/L, concern exists regarding the potential for severe hypoglycaemia. As such, insulin infusions are commonly utilised to ensure that target ranges of 6-11mmol/L are maintained.

Nutrition

Malnutrition in critical care patients is associated with an increased rate of complications, increased length of stay, dependency on mechanical ventilation and increased mortality. Nutritional support aims to alter the clinical course and improve the outcome of critical illness through the provision of calories, protein, electrolytes, vitamins, minerals, trace elements, and fluids, whilst avoiding associated complications (Table 34.4).

Carbohydrates are metabolised to simple sugars, in particular, glucose. Some tissues including red blood cells are obligate utilisers of glycolysis for energy production. Without exogenous glucose, hepatic glycogen stores are depleted and gluconeogenesis generates glucose from lipids, proteins and lactate. The early stages of acute illness are predominantly a catabolic state and during this time relative insulin resistance may develop. This may precipitate hyperglycaemia, which is pro-inflammatory and worsens outcomes. The optimal blood glucose range is between 6-10mmol/L.

Proteins are needed to provide a substrate for amino acid gluconeogenesis and spare muscle breakdown, promoting a positive nitrogen balance. During the recovery phase, the provision of nutritional substrates supports anabolic reconstitution.

Lipids are a concentrated energy source and provide free fatty acids, the preferred substrate of the myocardium under aerobic conditions. Free fatty acids also modulate inflammatory responses and are important in cellular membrane function. In addition, the fatty acids, linoleic acid and α-linoleic acid are essential and cannot be synthesised.

Nutritional support may be delivered enterally (via the intestine) or parenterally (intravenously). If the gut can be used, enteral feeding is preferred, as early enteral nutrition may reduce infectious complications, reduce the risk of gut failure and is cheaper than parenteral nutrition.

The guidance in this chapter is derived from the European Society of Parenteral and Enteral Nutrition/Canadian guidelines. These were developed by an interdisciplinary expert group, discussed and accepted at a consensus conference. The recommendations are focused on patients with at least one organ failure, acute illness and an inflammatory response. There is a relative paucity of evidence over nutrition in intensive care, owing to the heterogenous nature of this group of patients and consequent difficulties in comparing outcomes across a wide range of illness severities. Therefore, the majority of the recommendations are level C, or expert opinion.

Table 34.4. Nutritional requirements in a healthy 70kg adult.

Calories	25-35kcal/kg per day total energy
Protein	0.8-1.5g/kg per day (0.13-0.24g/kg/day nitrogen)
Fluid	30-35ml/kg
Electrolytes, vitamins and trace elements	Sodium, potassium, chloride, magnesium, phosphate, selenium, copper, zinc, manganese, vitamin A, vitamin C, vitamin E, vitamin K, amongst others

Whilst underfeeding or starvation is associated with increased morbidity and mortality, the provision of excessive calories should be avoided in critical illness, particularly in the early stages. Prospective observational studies have shown that survival odds are greater in those patients receiving 33-66% of their target energy intake compared to those receiving 66-100%. The National Institute for Health and Care Excellence (NICE) recommends that in critical illness, feeding should be started at no more than 50% of the daily energy and protein needs, and increased as tolerated over the next 24-48 hours. During this period of time the full requirements for fluid, electrolytes and trace elements should be met.

It is also important to ensure that the patient is haemodynamically stable before commencing feeding as there are case reports of gut ischaemia that may have been precipitated by making demands on the gut that the cardiovascular system is unable to meet.

There is also a difficulty in determining the pre-existing nutritional status of the patient and therefore the target energy intake. Bedside anthropometric measures such as the triceps skin-fold thickness may be obscured by oedema; laboratory tests such as albumin and transferrin are deranged in acute illness and the basal metabolic rate increases in critical illness. The gold standard test is indirect calorimetry but this requires specialist equipment.

One practical method of determining a target energy intake in critical care patients is the Ireton-Jones formula. This takes age, gender and weight and then makes adjustments for the presence of trauma, burns and ventilation status to produce an estimated basal metabolic rate. This will only provide an estimate and there are no data that the use of such formulas improves outcomes.

Enteral feeding

All patients not expected to be on a full oral diet within 3 days should receive enteral nutrition. Enteral feeding within 48 hours of admission is associated with a reduction in infective complications and a reduced length of critical care admission.

Enteral feeding is most commonly delivered to the stomach. Access to the stomach may be via a nasogastric tube or percutaneous endoscopic gastrotomy (PEG). Nasogastric tube placement should be confirmed radiologically before starting feeding as it can be misplaced into the chest. Incorrect placement can have catastrophic consequences and deaths from enteral feed being delivered into the chest have occurred.

Nasogastric tube placement may be confirmed by a nasogastric aspirate with a pH measuring less than 5.5. This method is not commonly used in the critical care setting as many patients are on gastric stress ulcer prophylaxis with consequently a high gastric juice pH. The gold standard therefore is a chest X-ray (Figure 34.1).

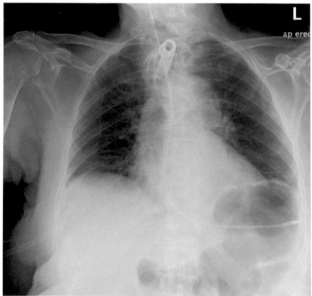

Figure 34.1. Chest X-ray demonstrating the correct position of nasogastric tube placement. The radio-opaque NG tube can be seen to bisect the carina and the tip is seen below the level of the diaphragm.

Jejunal feeding tubes can be placed endoscopically or surgically. There is no significant difference in the efficacy of jejunal feeding versus gastric feeding, so jejunal feeding tubes are best reserved for patients unable to tolerate gastric feeding.

At present, enteral feeding is usually commenced at a low rate, approximately 25ml/hour and increased as tolerated over subsequent days. Successful enteral feeding is commonly defined as feeding at >40ml/hour with gastric aspirates <400ml every 4 hours, although recently the value of routinely measuring gastric aspirate volumes has been called into question. Motility or prokinetic agents may improve tolerance to enteral feeding, but their routine use is not recommended and motility agents have not been shown to reduce the risk of ventilator-associated pneumonia.

The composition of enteral feeding is outlined in Table 34.5.

Table 34.5. Composition of enteral feeding.

Isotonic to plasma
Calorie density 1000kcal/L (4200kJ/L)
Protein 40g/L
Carbohydrate 123g/L
Fat 39g/L
Water 850ml/L
Electrolytes and trace elements:
       Na^+ 44mmol/L
       Ca^{++} 20mmol/L
       Fe^{++} 0.3mmol/L
       K^+ 39mmol/L
       Phosphate 23mmol/L
       Zn 0.18mmol/L
       Cl^- 35mmol/L
       Mg^{++} 9mmol/L
       Cu 0.03mmol/L
Vitamins A, D, E, K, thiamine, riboflavin, niacin, B6, folic acid, B12, biotin, C

Immune modulators

Immune modulators are 'functional' substrates added to enteral nutrition; these include arginine nucleotides, omega-3 fatty acids and glutamine. No benefit and indeed harm may arise from using immune modulators in patients with severe sepsis. Glutamine reduces mortality, hospital length of stay and improves wound healing in burns patients and reduces infection rates in trauma patients.

Complications associated with enteral feeding

The complications associated with enteral feeding are outlined in Table 34.6.

Table 34.6. Complications associated with enteral feeding.

Complication	Prevention strategy
Aspiration	Head of bed elevated to 30°, confirm correct feeding tube placement radiographically
Diarrhoea	Remove precipitating drugs (e.g. antibiotics, PPI), exclude *Clostridium difficile*, fibre added to feed
Refeeding syndrome	Monitor for electrolyte abnormalities, replace phosphate, potassium, magnesium
Dehydration	Enteral feed alone will not necessarily meet daily water requirements Supplemental enteral water or intravenous fluids

Parenteral nutrition

Parenteral nutrition can provide a means to supply nutrients when enteral feeding is contraindicated or has proven unsuccessful. All patients not expected to be on normal nutrition within 3 days should receive parenteral nutrition within 24-48 hours if enteral nutrition is contraindicated or not tolerated. Parenteral nutrition may also supplement enteral nutrition if patients are not reaching target feeding after 2 days.

Parenteral nutrition is usually supplied as a single bag administered continuously to meet the daily nutritional requirements of the individual patient. It is normally delivered into a large central vein, subclavian or internal jugular, such that vessel tolerance to the hyperosmolar solution is not a limiting step. Dedicated lumens are preferred to minimise the risk of infection and strict asepsis must be observed. Tunnelled lines are recommended for those needing parenteral nutrition for more than 30 days.

The composition of total parenteral nutrition is outlined in Table 34.7.

Table 34.7. Composition of total parenteral nutrition.

Volume 2000ml
Nitrogen 8g
Total calories 1400kcal
Glucose 600kcal
Lipid 600kcal
Electrolytes:

Na^+ 42mmol/L

Ca^{++} 4mmol/L

Acetate 55mmol/L

K^+ 32mmol/L

Phosphate 14mmol/L

Cl^- 49mmol/L

Mg^{++} 4.4mmol/L

The complications associated with parenteral feeding are outlined in Table 34.8.

Table 34.8. Complications associated with parenteral feeding.	
Complication	**Prevention strategy**
Related to line insertion	Ultrasound guidance
Catheter-related bloodstream infection	Strict asepsis, dedicated lumen for parenteral nutrition
Electrolyte abnormalities	Daily monitoring of electrolytes
Liver dysfunction	Cyclical feeding, reduce lipid content
Rebound hypoglycaemia	Avoid abrupt withdrawal of parenteral nutrition

Refeeding syndrome

Patients who resume nutritional intake after a period of starvation are at risk of refeeding syndrome. Intracellular and therefore total body stores of phosphate, magnesium and potassium are depleted in starvation despite serum levels remaining normal. When nutrition is reinstated, glucose availability causes insulin levels to rise and this causes cellular uptake of these ions, resulting in hypophosphataemia, hypomagnesaemia and hypokalaemia. Abnormal sodium, fluid balance and thiamine deficiency may also occur. Depletion of adenosine triphosphate (ATP) and 2,3-DPG causes failure of cellular energy metabolism. This can precipitate cardiac arrhythmias, respiratory failure, paraesthesia and coma.

Refeeding syndrome can be fatal if not recognised and treated promptly. The risk factors for refeeding syndrome are outlined in Table 34.9.

Table 34.9. Risk factors for refeeding syndrome.

Any one of the following	Any two of the following
Body mass index (kg/m^2) <16	Body mass index <18.5
Unintentional weight loss >15% in the past 3-6 months	Unintentional weight loss >10% in the past 3-6 months
Little or no nutritional intake for >10 days	Little or no nutritional intake for >5 days
Low levels of potassium, phosphate, or magnesium before feeding	History of alcohol misuse or drugs, including insulin, chemotherapy, antacids, or diuretics

If refeeding syndrome is suspected or detected, then the rate of feeding should be slowed and electrolytes measured and replaced. Consultation with the dietician is recommended.

Case scenario 1

A 67-year-old female is admitted to the intensive care unit with severe upper abdominal pain, nausea and vomiting. She requires multi-organ support and is intubated and ventilated, and a central venous line is placed for vasopressor therapy. A raised amylase is indicative of pancreatitis and this is subsequently confirmed on CT imaging of the abdomen with a small area of pancreatic necrosis and pseudocyst formation.

What are the key issues regarding her general supportive care?

She should be managed using a ventilation care bundle, central line care bundle and sepsis care bundle. At the daily review, the FLATHUG checklist should be employed. Nutritional support should be initiated within 24-48 hours as this patient is unlikely to resume normal feeding within 3 days. Nasogastric enteral feeding would be the first-line route of feeding. Historically, pancreatitis had delayed initiation of enteral nutrition, but this is not currently recommended practice. If the pseudocyst enlarges and results in gastric outlet obstruction, she may require nasojejunal feeding.

Further reading

1.   Horner D, Bellamy M. Care bundles in intensive care. *BJA CEACCP* 2012; 12: 199-202.

2.   Vincent JL. Give your patient a fast hug (at least) once a day. *Crit Care Med* 2005; 33: 1225-9.

3.   Kreymann K, Berger MM, Deutz NEP, *et al.* ESPEN guidelines on enteral nutrition: intensive care. *Clin Nutr* 2006; 25: 210-23.

4.   Marik PE, Zaloga GP. Early enteral nutrition in acutely ill patients: a systematic review. *Crit Care Med* 2001; 29: 2264-70.

5.   Rice TW, Wheeler AP, Thompson BT, *et al.* Initial trophic vs full enteral feeding in patients with acute lung injury: the EDEN randomized trial. *JAMA* 2012; 307: 795-803.

6.   Seres D. Nutrition support in critically ill patients: an overview, 2014. http://www.uptodate.com/contents/nutrition-support-in-critically-ill-patients-an-overview.

7.   The NICE-SUGAR Study investigators. Intensive versus conventional glucose control in critically ill patients. *N Engl J Med* 2009; 360: 1283-97.

35 Sepsis

Tom Billyard

Introduction

Sepsis is a syndrome brought about by an exaggerated immune response to infection. It leads to 100,000 hospital admissions per year in the United Kingdom, can affect multiple body systems and is fatal in 35% of cases. The body's immune system goes into overdrive as it tries to fight the infection. As a result, the blood supply to vital organs such as the brain, heart and kidneys may get compromised and without treatment, it can lead to multiple organ failure and death.

What is sepsis?

Sepsis is a syndrome caused by an exaggerated response to infection, usually bacterial, fungal or occasionally viral. The presence of an infective microorganism leads to activation of the immune system in several stages. This then results in an inflammatory response, which causes the sepsis syndrome.

The first stage of the inflammatory response is vasodilatation. This is intended to increase blood flow to the infected area to aid delivery of immune cells to the infection. Vasodilatation is directly caused by the action of various inflammatory compounds including tumour necrosis factor, prostaglandins and the inflammatory interleukins. In sepsis, the vasodilatory response is excessive, leading to blood pooling in dilated vascular beds and reduced venous return to the heart. This is the main cause of hypotension and shock in sepsis.

Following vasodilatation, the second inflammatory stage is an increase in vascular permeability, which has the effect of allowing large molecules to leave the circulation into the interstitium. This means that antibodies and leucocytes are able to gain access to the infective microorganisms. However, the increased capillary permeability means that other plasma proteins, particularly albumin and fluid, also leak from the circulation. This causes tissue oedema and further worsens the reduced venous return, exacerbating the hypotension and shock. While the tissue oedema is not generally harmful, one area where it can cause problems is in the lung. Fluid leaks into the alveolar spaces, which impedes gas diffusion. This can lead to hypoxaemia.

The final stage is the infiltration of leucocytes into the infected tissue. This proliferation of cells, along with other effects of sepsis, leads to a significant increase in tissue oxygen demand. In severe sepsis, the total body oxygen demand can increase up to twelve times the baseline value. This means that a large increase in cardiac output and, hence, oxygen delivery, is required to meet this demand. This is often not possible, particularly in view of reduced venous return and its consequent effect on stroke volume, meaning that anaerobic respiration will start to occur.

Other inflammatory effects

Fever is a common indicator of infection. It is generated by the hypothalamus raising the body's thermoregulatory set point in response to inflammatory markers, particularly prostaglandin E_2. Prostaglandin E_2 release is triggered by the presence of bacterial endotoxins and other inflammatory mediators.

The coagulation system is activated by capillary endothelial damage, and also by the action of the inflammatory interleukins, IL1 and IL6, as well as tissue necrosis factor, inducing tissue factor in the endothelium. Tissue factor activates the coagulation cascade leading to microthrombus formation in the capillaries. This can eventually block capillaries leading to compromise of the blood supply and potentially tissue necrosis.

This activation of the clotting cascade and widespread microthrombosis will consume clotting factors, platelets and fibrinogen, leading to impaired coagulation. This gives the clinical picture of disseminated intravascular coagulation (DIC) where, despite this activation of the clotting cascade, uncontrolled bleeding can occur because clotting factors are not available where they are needed.

Diagnosis of sepsis

There is no simple test for the identification of sepsis; it is a clinical diagnosis. A good level of knowledge of sepsis and a high index of suspicion are the most important tools.

A number of screening tools have been developed, all based on the international Surviving Sepsis Campaign guidelines. These use a staged decision-making tool to decide on the likelihood of sepsis and its severity.

Stage one

Does the patient have at least two signs or symptoms of the systemic inflammatory response syndrome (SIRS)?

- Temperature <36°C or >38.3°C.
- Respiratory rate >20 per minute.
- Heart rate >90 per minute.
- Acute confusion or reduced conscious level.
- Glucose >7.7mmol/L.

Stage two

Could the patient have an infection?

Consider:

- Pneumonia.
- Urinary tract infection.

- Abdominal pain or distension.
- Meningitis.
- Cellulitis/wound infection.

If the answer to stage one and stage two is yes, the patient has sepsis.

Stage three

Is this severe sepsis? Are any of the following present?

- Systolic blood pressure <90mmHg or MAP <65mmHg.
- Lactate >2mmol/L.
- Heart rate >130 per minute.
- Respiratory rate >25 per minute.
- Oxygen saturation <91%, or requiring oxygen to maintain >91%.
- Drowsy or unresponsive.
- Purpuric rash.
- If the blood test results are available:
  - bilirubin >34µmol/L;
  - INR >1.5;
  - platelets <100 x 10^9/L;
  - creatinine >177µmol/L.

If the answer to stage three is yes to any point, the patient has severe sepsis.

Septic shock

Septic shock is defined by the presence of:

- Lactate >4mmol/L at any time.
- Hypotension persisting after 30ml/kg IV fluids.

Management of sepsis

Severe sepsis is a medical emergency; the overall mortality of severe sepsis is approximately 35% and the mortality risk is strongly associated with the time between onset and commencing treatment. Observational studies have shown each hour of delay in the administration of appropriate antibiotics is associated with an 8% increase in the risk of mortality.

Immediate treatment

On recognising severe sepsis, the immediate management is aimed at addressing organ dysfunction, as well as definitive treatment of the infection.

In the United Kingdom, the Sepsis Six has been widely adopted for the early treatment of severe sepsis. This has been endorsed in guidelines from both the Royal College of Physicians and the Royal College of Emergency Medicine.

The Sepsis Six:

- Administer high-concentration oxygen via a face mask.
- Take blood cultures, and consider other cultures depending on the likely source.
- Administer intravenous antibiotics appropriate to the likely infective source.
- Intravenous fluid resuscitation — up to 30ml/kg crystalloid solution in divided boluses.
- Measure haemoglobin and lactate.
- Measure urine output hourly.

The standard of care is that the Sepsis Six should be completed within 1 hour of the recognition of severe sepsis. Retrospective observational studies of the six aspects have shown that where they are completed within 1 hour, there is a significant reduction in mortality with a number needed to treat to prevent one death of 4.6.

Each item in the sepsis six is important; the rationale behind each is oulined below.

Administer high-concentration oxygen

Oxygen delivery is often impaired in sepsis. Administration of oxygen will address the effects of pulmonary alveolar fluid by increasing the concentration gradient and thereby reversing the impaired diffusion. By doing this the blood oxygen content is increased and this in turn will increase oxygen delivery.

Blood cultures and other cultures depending on the likely source

Cultures to identify the causative organism are a central part of treating infection. They allow the de-escalation of antibiotics to narrow-spectrum agents and they also allow for the identification of organisms that may not be treated by the initial choice of antibiotics. Blood cultures are mandatory in sepsis and other cultures should be performed depending on the likely source of the infection; sputum, urine and cerebrospinal fluid are common examples. Ideally, cultures should be taken before the administration of antibiotics to maximise the chance of a positive result. It is important, however, that the administration of antibiotics is not delayed, so that if taking cultures is likely to take a long time, antibiotics can be given first.

Administer intravenous antibiotics

Antibiotics are the only definitive treatment for infection. A delay in administration is associated with increased mortality in severe sepsis. Broad-spectrum antibiotics that will cover the likely organisms involved in the infection should be given; this will be dictated by the local infection and resistance patterns and each hospital will have an antibiotic policy that reflects this. Once the culture results are available, the spectrum of the antibiotics used can be narrowed — this is known as de-escalation. In severe sepsis, antibiotics must be given intravenously to ensure effective tissue levels are achieved quickly.

Intravenous fluid resuscitation

The vascular system becomes dilated and leaks fluid. Both of these will reduce the effective circulating volume and hence the cardiac output, reducing oxygen delivery. Intravenous fluids will act to refill the vascular system and restore cardiac output. Large volumes are sometimes required but the aim in the first hour should be to give up to 30ml/kg of fluid. This should be given as divided doses to avoid worsening pulmonary oedema; the patient's existing state of health will guide how large and how quickly each bolus should be given. Changes in heart rate, lactate, urine output and blood pressure will guide the effectiveness of fluid resuscitation.

There has been some controversy over the best fluid to use in resuscitation in severe sepsis. Despite their theoretical advantage, no trial has ever proven the superiority of colloid over crystalloid solutions. For this reason it is generally recommended to use crystalloid solutions initially.

Measure haemoglobin and lactate

Haemoglobin concentration is one of the major determinants of blood oxygen content and hence oxygen delivery. It is important, therefore, to optimise the blood haemoglobin level. This does not mean that every patient needs a transfusion; the adverse effects of blood transfusion will outweigh the benefits above a certain level. Lactate is a byproduct of anaerobic respiration, so a rise in lactate indicates failure of oxygen delivery. Lactate should be measured regularly in the resuscitation of sepsis and a lactate persistently above 2mmol/L or a rising lactate is a cause for concern.

Measure the urine output hourly

The kidneys are sensitive to reduced cardiac output as glomerular filtration rate and, hence, urine output, is proportional to renal blood flow. At normal blood pressures the kidneys can autoregulate to maintain renal blood flow but they cannot do this once the blood pressure drops too low. Because of this, urine output is a sensitive marker of reduced cardiac output and is detectable before other markers, such as lactate, change. A urine output of <0.5ml/kg body weight is a cause for concern and may indicate the need for further resuscitation.

Further treatment

In a substantial number of cases of severe sepsis, carrying out the Sepsis Six will be enough; the blood pressure will improve and the organ dysfunction will start to resolve. These patients can be managed on a standard hospital ward with continuation of their antibiotics, de-escalating when appropriate.

However, there will be a subgroup of severe sepsis patients who develop septic shock and do not respond to the initial resuscitation measures. These patients can be spotted by noting persistent hypotension, poor urine output, ongoing raised lactate or other manifestations or organ dysfunction that does not improve. Patients with septic shock will need more advanced forms of organ support and should be admitted to a critical care unit as soon as possible.

Cardiovascular support

Invasive monitoring is useful in septic shock. An arterial line will allow accurate monitoring of blood pressure and provides an easy route for regular blood sampling to monitor lactate, oxygenation and other markers of organ dysfunction. A central venous line will allow monitoring of central venous pressure and the administration of vasoactive infusions.

Some patients with septic shock will benefit from the administration of further intravenous fluids beyond the initial 30ml/kg. This should be guided by some kind of haemodynamic monitoring. The international Surviving Sepsis Campaign recommends the use of central venous pressure (CVP) monitoring with fluids administered to achieve a CVP of 8-12mmHg. The use of CVP monitoring is controversial with an increasing body of evidence showing that the CVP is a poor reflection of the circulating volume status. Increasingly, many experts are recommending the use of non-invasive cardiac output monitoring, such as the oesophageal Doppler or pulse contour analysis devices, to assess the response to fluid challenges and therefore optimise the patient's filling status.

If the patient remains hypotensive once they have been optimally filled, vasopressors should be added to increase the blood pressure. These act by constricting the arterial system, increasing afterload and by constricting the venous system, which will increase venous return to the heart. Currently, the first-line vasopressor of choice is noradrenaline (norepinephrine), which must be administered via a central venous line. Noradrenaline is run as an infusion to raise the blood pressure to a mean arterial pressure (MAP) target of 65mmHg. Some patients with longstanding hypertension may require a higher MAP target, as their organs, particularly the kidneys, will have adapted to a higher blood pressure. A vasopressin infusion may be used alongside noradrenaline, especially if noradrenaline alone does not achieve the target MAP.

If, once optimum filling and the target MAP have been achieved and there are still signs of insufficient cardiac output (these could include raised lactate, organ dysfunction or a low mixed venous oxygen saturation), an inotrope can be used to increase cardiac output. Dobutamine is the drug of choice currently; it is generally effective but can be arrhythmogenic at higher doses. There is no proven benefit to increasing cardiac output to supranormal levels.

Respiratory support

Respiratory failure is common in sepsis and can be caused by many factors. This can simply be a pneumonia that causes severe sepsis, and the pneumonia itself interferes with oxygenation and leads to respiratory failure. However, respiratory failure is common in sepsis of other causes; it is generally due in these cases to an increase in pulmonary capillary endothelial permeability. This leads to fluid accumulation in the alveolar air spaces, which impairs gas diffusion, causing hypoxic and hypercapnic respiratory failure. Ultimately, this manifests as the acute respiratory distress syndrome (ARDS).

Once severe respiratory failure occurs, it is likely that respiratory support will be required. Initially, supplemental oxygen may be adequate, but eventually the impaired gas exchange and increased work of breathing will mean that mechanical support is needed. Non-invasive ventilation can be used but is rarely successful in ARDS, meaning that intubation and invasive ventilation will be required. This should be performed with low tidal volumes (6ml/kg); plateau pressures of less than 30cm of water and an adequate amount of positive end-expiratory pressure. Ventilation in ARDS is complex and a detailed description is beyond the scope of this chapter.

Renal support

Renal failure is common in sepsis, usually from hypoperfusion leading to acute tubular necrosis. It may be short-lived and improve once the blood pressure is raised. However, in a proportion of cases, renal failure will be severe enough to be life-threatening. The prime indications for renal replacement therapy in sepsis are hyperkalaemia, metabolic acidosis and severe fluid overload. In the United Kingdom, renal replacement therapy is usually provided as continuous veno-venous haemofiltration (CVVH) with or without haemodialysis. Continuous therapies provide efficient solute clearance with the added advantage of precise hour-to-hour control of fluid removal. CVVH is usually provided using a large-bore dual-lumen catheter situated in a central vein. It is associated with a low complication rate and does not require high levels of anticoagulation.

Some experts have advocated the use of high-volume CVVH in sepsis to remove bacterial endotoxins to reduce the immune response to sepsis. This has been investigated in several trials but high-volume CVVH has not been shown to improve mortality compared to standard therapy.

Other therapies

Nutrition
Enteral feeding should be started as soon as possible unless contraindicated. Trials have shown that it is not necessary, and may be harmful, to achieve full calorie targets within the first few days of feeding. Gut failure in sepsis is common and generally manifests as failure to absorb feed, resulting in high-volume aspirates from the nasogastric tube. The use of prokinetic agents (e.g. metoclopramide or domperidone),

avoidance of constipation and post-pyloric feeding can all help to raise the success rate of enteral feeding.

In the event of complete failure of enteral feeding, parenteral nutrition can be used. However, it is associated with significant risks and should not be started in the first week of illness, provided that the patient was not previously malnourished.

Numerous substances, especially glutamine and selenium, have been suggested as immunomodulatory and can be added to feeds in sepsis. The clinical trials conducted so far have not shown a mortality benefit and therefore the Surviving Sepsis Campaign does not currently recommend immunonutrition.

Corticosteroids

The role of corticosteroids remains uncertain. Despite early trials showing promise, later studies have shown little difference in outcome using steroids. Current guidelines suggest using corticosteroids only in shocked patients where the administration of fluids and vasopressors has failed to correct the shock. The dose of vasopressor at which steroids are indicated is unclear and varies between clinicians. There is no role for using the adrenocorticotropic hormone (ACTH) stimulation test to determine a need for steroid supplementation.

Glucose control

Tight control of glucose levels has been shown to improve mortality in ICU patients. However, pragmatic studies have shown that attempting to control blood glucose in the optimum range, 4-8mmol/L, leads to an unacceptably high number of hypoglycaemic episodes with consequent harm. Because of this, it is now recommended to start an insulin infusion when the blood glucose exceeds 10mmol/L on two consecutive readings, then aim for a blood glucose level between 6 and 10mmol/L. This carries the benefits of glucose control while minimising the risk of hypoglycaemia.

Thromboprophylaxis

Because of the way in which sepsis activates the clotting system, as well as the potential for prolonged immobility, patients with severe sepsis are at high risk of deep vein thrombosis and consequent pulmonary embolism. Prophylaxis with low-molecular-weight heparin (LMWH) should be started early in the hospital admission; the use of once-daily LMWH has been shown to be superior to twice-daily unfractionated heparin. In patients admitted to critical care, this should be supplemented with mechanical prophylaxis; sequential pneumatic compression devices have been shown to be superior to compression stockings.

Stress ulcer prophylaxis

Gastrointestinal stress ulcers occur commonly in severe illness and, if a coagulopathy develops, it can be a source of significant bleeding. For this reason ulcer prophylaxis should be commenced on admission using agents, which reduce gastric acid secretion, i.e. H_2 receptor antagonists or proton pump inhibitors. The current Surviving Sepsis guidelines recommend proton pump inhibitors for first-line use. It is important to be aware that raising the gastric pH can increase bacterial colonisation of the gastrointestinal tract by reducing its effectiveness as a barrier. This can increase the risk of ventilator-associated pneumonia.

Case scenario 1

A 61-year-old man presents to hospital with a 3-day history of a productive cough and difficulty in breathing. On examination, he is drowsy and finds it difficult to cooperate. His respiratory rate is 32 breaths/minute, oxygen saturation is 86% on air and there are coarse inspiratory crackles heard over most of the left side of the chest. His hands and feet are warm to the touch, his radial pulse is palpable and the heart rate is 125. His blood pressure is 86/47mmHg. His tympanic temperature is 38.9°C.

How would you manage this patient?

This patient most likely has pneumonia. However, this is complicated by the development of the systemic syndrome of sepsis. Based on the stage-wise approach, the presence of cardiovascular compromise means that this is severe sepsis. We need to treat this patient based on the Sepsis Six principles. These include:

- Administer high-concentration oxygen via a face mask.
- Take blood cultures, and consider other cultures depending on the likely source.
- Administer intravenous antibiotics appropriate to the likely infective source.
- Intravenous fluid resuscitation — up to 30ml/kg crystalloid solution in divided boluses.
- Measure haemoglobin and lactate.
- Measure urine output hourly.

The patient should be moved into a critical care environment (HDU/ ITU) for further care and evaluation.

Further reading

1. Surviving Sepsis Campaign: International Guidelines for Management of Severe Sepsis and Septic Shock: 2012, 3rd ed (published in Critical Care Medicine and Intensive Care Medicine, February 2013). http://www.survivingsepsis.org/Guidelines/Pages/default. aspx.

2. Yende S, Austin S, Rhodes A, *et al*. Long-term quality of life among survivors of severe sepsis: analyses of two international trials. *Crit Care Med* 2016; 44: 1461-7.

3. Montull B, Torres A, Reyes S, *et al*. Community-acquired pneumonia with severe sepsis: etiology and prognosis. *Eur Resp J* 2013; 42(Suppl 57): 293.

4. Angus DC, Van der Poll T. Severe sepsis and septic shock. *N Engl J Med* 2013; 369(9): 840-51.

5. Sarmah P, Green N, Youssef H. Sepsis in emergency surgical patients: is management optimal? *Int J Surg* 2015; 23: S73.

36 Ventilatory support

Nick Talbot and Alistair Burns

Introduction

The main function of the lung is to transfer oxygen to the bloodstream, to fuel aerobic respiration and to remove the waste product, carbon dioxide.

In a normal spontaneous breath, during inspiration the diaphragm contracts and flattens and the external intercostal muscles move the ribs upwards and outwards. These actions together increase the intrathoracic volume and as a consequence the pressure within the thorax becomes less than that of the atmosphere at the mouth. This causes air to be drawn down a pressure gradient from the mouth, via the trachea and major conducting bronchi, eventually reaching the alveoli where it can participate in gas exchange. Whilst energy must be expended for inspiration, expiration is typically a passive process. The lung tissue has intrinsic elastic properties and it wishes to collapse back to what is termed the functional residual capacity (FRC). Functional residual capacity is the position the chest wall will adopt at the end of a tidal volume breath. In this position the elastic forces causing the lung to be pulled inward are in equilibrium with the elastic forces trying to make the chest wall spring outward. As the volume in the thorax decreases, so the pressure increases and gas is expelled from the alveoli towards the upper airway.

Transfer of gas from the alveoli to the blood and vice versa occurs by passive diffusion down a partial pressure gradient. The partial pressure of oxygen in the alveoli is higher than that of the venous blood entering the pulmonary capillary. Consequently, oxygen then moves from the alveolar space into the pulmonary capillary and from here it diffuses into red blood cells and is bound to haemoglobin.

Oxygen is a poorly soluble gas and only a small amount can be dissolved in the blood. Therefore, haemoglobin is necessary to vastly increase the oxygen-carrying capacity of the blood. Carbon dioxide is present in the pulmonary capillary at a higher partial pressure than that found in the alveoli so it diffuses from the blood into the alveoli.

Lung compliance

Compliance describes how easily lung can be distended and is measured in ml/cmH$_2$O. This relationship is non-linear as the lungs exhibit a phenomenon termed hysteresis; greater pressure changes are required to yield a given volume change during inspiration than in expiration. Work must be done to overcome the elastic lung tissue. The wall tension in the airways is highest at small volumes and more work must be done to inflate collapsed alveoli than would be needed to further expand a patent one.

The lungs are suspended in the pleural cavity and this produces a negative intrapleural pressure. Due to the weight of lung tissue, this intrapleural pressure is not uniform throughout. It is lower (more negative) in non-dependent areas (the apices when standing) and higher (less negative) in dependent areas (basally when standing). The intrapleural pressure is transmitted to alveoli such that at FRC those alveoli at the apex are relatively more inflated than those at the base of the lung. This produces regional differences in ventilation. The apices are held open throughout the respiratory cycle to a greater degree than the bases and therefore have less capacity to expand and participate in ventilation. This can be seen more clearly when we examine the position of the apices and the base on the compliance curve (Figure 36.1).

The higher intrapleural pressure causes apical lung units to be held open throughout respiration and the change in volume in these units are less compared to the basal lung units. Basal lung units operate on a steeper part of the compliance curves and therefore exhibit a greater change in volume for a given change in pressure. The compliance curve

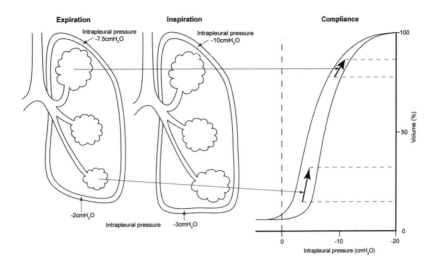

Figure 36.1. Regional differences in lung ventilation and compliance curve.

also demonstrates that basal lung units are more vulnerable to collapse should they be exposed to more positive intrapleural pressure. At positive intrapleural pressures the gradient of the curve becomes flat meaning very little change in volume will take place.

As the bases operate on a steeper part of the compliance curve, they expand more readily and are responsible for a greater proportion of alveolar ventilation. This is appropriate, as owing to gravity and hydrostatic pressure these regions of the lung are better perfused. Starting from a lower alveolar volume and being acted upon by a less negative intrapleural pressure also makes the alveoli vulnerable. They have the least pressure gradient from alveoli to mouth and subsequently are the most likely to be compressed during active expiration. The volume of lung at which dependent airways begin to close is termed the closing volume. In young healthy subjects, the closing volume is 10% of vital capacity. As we age, the closing volume can approach the functional residual capacity. At 40 years of age, dependent airways will close when supine at the end of a tidal volume breath. At age 65, they will close even when erect.

Air spaces must be patent to contribute to ventilation. If they are not, the capillaries serving these lung units will not participate in gas exchange. This venous blood then returns to the left heart and causes venous admixture to the systemic circulation; this phenomenon is known as shunt. Many of the strategies used in ventilatory support aim to recruit collapsed alveoli and prevent the collapse of threatened alveoli, thus increasing the available surface area for gas exchange (Table 36.1).

Table 36.1. Aims of ventilatory support in critical care patients.

- Improve oxygenation.
- Aid carbon dioxide clearance.
- Reduce work of breathing.
- Protect the airway if an endotracheal tube or a tracheostomy is present.
- Minimise the risk of complications.

Respiratory failure

Respiratory failure represents impaired gas exchange and may be classified as Type 1 or Type 2.

Type 1 respiratory failure is a low arterial oxygen tension (paO_2 <8kPa, hypoxaemia) with a normal or low arterial carbon dioxide tension. This failure of adequate oxygenation is caused by a mismatch between the ventilation (V) and perfusion (Q) of lung units. Owing to the underlying pathology, certain lung units are unable to participate in gas exchange. This mismatch may represent lung units that are ventilated but are not perfused as in pulmonary embolism (alveolar dead space) or at the other end of the spectrum, lung units that are perfused but are not ventilated (shunt). Shunting of blood may occur when alveoli are flooded with fluid as in pneumonia or pulmonary oedema. Deoxygenated blood perfusing these lung units is unable to participate in gas exchange and subsequently mixes with blood that has been successfully oxygenated. This lowers the final arterial oxygen tension of blood entering the left atrium. Type 1 respiratory failure may also occur if there is a diffusion defect caused by parenchymal lung disease, such as lung consolidation or acute respiratory distress syndrome (ARDS). Carbon dioxide is 20 times more soluble than oxygen and therefore diffuses through tissues far more quickly, making it less susceptible to diffusion defects.

Type 2 respiratory failure is a low arterial oxygen tension (paO_2 <8kPa, hypoxaemia) with a concomitant elevation in arterial carbon dioxide tension (paO_2 >6kPa, hypercapnia). Type 2 respiratory failure represents a failure of alveolar ventilation across all lung units. As a consequence, both oxygen and carbon dioxide are affected. Type 2 respiratory failure can be thought of as failure of the respiratory pump and may be caused by a lesion at any level in the normal maintenance of respiration. It may be owing to a central cause (i.e. sedative drug overdose, stroke), neuromuscular disease (i.e. Guillain-Barré syndrome), airway obstruction (i.e. COPD, asthma, obstructive sleep apnoea) or a mechanical chest wall deformity (i.e. kyphoscoliosis, flail chest).

Oxygen

Oxygen is present in room air at 21%. This can also be denoted as a fraction of inspired oxygen or FiO_2 0.21. Depending on the method of delivery it is possible to administer oxygen at anywhere between 21% and 100%.

It is important to know the concentration of oxygen that a patient is breathing when assessing the need for ventilatory support. Due to the shape of the oxygen-haemoglobin dissociation curve (Figure 36.2), there is little benefit in providing supplemental oxygen to a patient with saturations of 94-100% on room air. These saturations lie on the upper flat part of the curve and in most clinical situations the oxygen content of the blood will not be improved by increasing the FiO_2. Conversely, a patient with saturations of 98% breathing 100% oxygen may have markedly abnormal respiratory physiology.

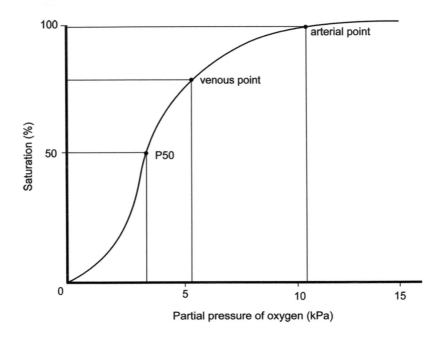

Figure 36.2. Oxygen-haemoglobin dissociation curve.

The upper flat part of the oxygen-haemoglobin dissociation curve means that a fall in PaO_2 of 15 to 10 will not significantly reduce the oxygen content of the blood. Conversely, there is little benefit to increasing the PaO_2 above 11kPa, as at this level nearly all of the haemoglobin molecules are saturated. It can be seen on the oxygen-haemoglobin dissociation curve that in a healthy person breathing room air with an oxygen concentration of 21%, they will achieve oxygen saturation close to 100%

and a PaO_2 around 11kPa. Atmospheric pressure at sea level means that 21% oxygen equates to a partial pressure of 21kPa oxygen in air. This difference between atmospheric (21kPa) and arterial partial pressures of oxygen (11kPa) is due to humidification of the air, mixing with carbon dioxide and true shunt. This creates a 'rule of thumb' that the PaO_2 should be approximately 10kPa less than the FiO_2. Hence, if a patient is breathing 40% oxygen, it is expected that their PaO_2 should be around 30kPa. If they have saturations of 98% and a PaO_2 of 10kPa, then their blood oxygen content is abnormally low.

Oxygen is a drug and complications can arise from its use and misuse. In the emergency setting, high-flow oxygen should be given initially. Later it can be titrated to achieve a given saturation. Administration of high concentrations of oxygen for prolonged periods of time can cause lung injury.

Oxygen delivery devices can be broadly classified into variable performance and fixed performance devices. Variable performance devices will deliver a concentration of oxygen that is dependent on the patient's respiratory effort. Examples include nasal cannulae and simple face masks. Such devices are comfortable to wear and do not greatly impede the ability to communicate, but they can only deliver low concentrations of oxygen and the FiO_2 is unpredictable. The presence of a reservoir bag can increase the FiO_2 to around 0.85 (85%) provided the bag does not empty on maximum inspiration. If a specific concentration of oxygen is required, then a Venturi device can be incorporated into a face mask. The Venturi device features vents, which entrain air when an oxygen supply is passed through the device. This produces a fixed ratio of oxygen to air, which will generate a given FiO_2. This is useful in patients with a chronically raised carbon dioxide who are at risk of CO_2 narcosis if exposed to high concentrations of oxygen.

Ventilatory support

Ventilatory support can be provided either using a non-invasive technique or an invasive technique. Non-invasive techniques include continuous positive airway pressure and bi-level non-invasive ventilation. Tracheal intubation and invasive ventilation may be required to treat hypercapnia-associated ventilatory failure. The indications for ventilatory support are shown in Table 36.2.

Table 36.2. Indications for ventilatory support.

- Respiratory rate >30/min.
- Vital capacity <10-15ml/min.
- Hypoxaemia, PaO_2<8kPa.
- Hypercapnia with respiratory acidosis pH <7.2.
- Shunt fraction 15-20%.
- Exhaustion.

Continuous positive airway pressure (CPAP)

CPAP is a form of ventilatory support where the airway pressure is maintained at a level higher than atmospheric pressure. It is achieved by applying positive pressure to the expiratory limb of a breathing system. CPAP is used in a patient taking spontaneous breaths and may be delivered by a tightly fitting facial mask, hood and nasal mask or delivered via an endotracheal tube or tracheostomy. The indications for CPAP are shown in Table 36.3.

Table 36.3. Indications for CPAP.

- Type 1 respiratory failure.
- Cardiogenic pulmonary oedema.
- Obstructive sleep apnoea.
- Diaphragmatic splinting.
- Weaning from mechanical ventilation.

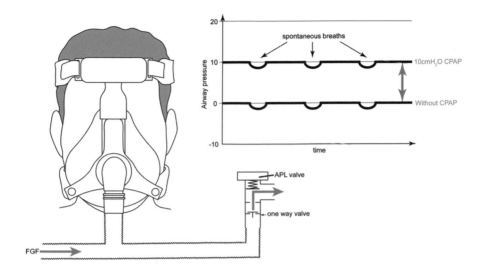

Figure 36.3. Continuous positive airway pressure (CPAP) mask.

In the CPAP circuit shown (Figure 36.3), a fresh gas flow (FGF) higher than the patient's peak inspiratory flow is delivered into a tightly fitting mask with an attached adjustable pressure limiting (APL) valve set to 10cmH$_2$O. The airway and patent alveoli are thus held 10cmH$_2$O above atmospheric pressure. By holding the airway at a higher mean pressure, CPAP increases the functional residual capacity, reduces alveolar collapse and recruits collapsed lung units, producing a reduction in shunt and increasing compliance. These measures increase the available surface area for diffusion. In patients with a high intrinsic positive end-expiratory pressure (PEEP), CPAP reduces the pressure gradient from the alveoli to the mouth, requiring a less negative intrapleural pressure and reducing the work of breathing.

Bi-level non-invasive ventilation

Bi-level non-invasive ventilation (NIV) is the delivery of inspiratory and expiratory pressure to support spontaneous respiration. NIV is commonly delivered via a tightly fitting face mask or nasal mask, with an engineered fixed leak, in addition to the leak that exists between the mask and facial tissues. Expiratory positive airway pressure (EPAP) is applied during expiration and while the nomenclature is different this fulfils the same role as CPAP in maintaining the airway pressure above atmospheric pressure. Inspiratory positive airway pressure (IPAP) is delivered above the EPAP baseline and can improve tidal volumes and consequently alveolar ventilation. During expiration the pressure in the system returns to EPAP and expiratory gases are vented from the leak.

Inspiration may be triggered, detected by a drop in circuit pressure as the patient draws breath, or mandatory, where the breath is delivered dependent on the respiratory rate programmed into the ventilator. There is good evidence to support the use of NIV in patients with Type 2 respiratory failure secondary to exacerbation of COPD. NIV has been shown to decrease mortality, intubation rate, in-hospital length of stay and treatment failure in this specific group of patients. NIV may also be considered in patients deemed unsuitable for intubation and invasive ventilation. The contraindications for CPAP/bi-level NIV are outlined in Table 36.4.

Table 36.4. Contraindications for CPAP/bi-level NIV.

- Cardiac or respiratory arrest.
- Severely impaired consciousness.
- Facial surgery, trauma or deformity.
- High aspiration risk.
- Prolonged duration of mechanical ventilation anticipated.
- Recent oesophageal anastomosis.

Invasive mechanical ventilation

In addition to the respiratory reasons for ventilatory support outlined above, there are non-respiratory indications for invasive ventilation (Table 36.5).

Table 36.5. Non-respiratory indications for invasive mechanical ventilation.

- Airway protection.
- Avoidance of movement, i.e. unstable C-spine fracture, for diagnostic imaging.
- Control of intracranial pressure.
- Major circulatory instability, hypothermia, acidosis.
- Need for repeat surgery in a short time frame.

Mechanical ventilation depends upon inspiratory motive force to generate a tidal volume and a means of determining when inspiration and expiration should occur. Negative pressure ventilators generate a negative pressure around the outside of the chest causing the pressure in the alveoli to fall. These ventilators are rarely used in general intensive care. Intermittent positive pressure ventilation (IPPV) creates a positive pressure at the airway and this is the driving force for inspiration.

The ventilator or the patient may determine the onset of inspiration. In a paralysed patient unable to make any respiratory effort, inspiration will depend upon the time since the last breath. The desired respiratory rate or frequency can be dialled into the ventilator and additional control may be taken over the proportion of the time spent in inspiration and expiration. This may be set as the Inspiratory: Expiratory (I:E) ratio or inspiratory time (Ti) versus expiratory time (Te). This describes continuous mandatory ventilation as the ventilator controls both the onset of inspiration and expiration.

If the patient is able to make respiratory efforts, then this can be detected and used to determine the onset of inspiration. If the ventilator does no work to assist inspiration, the breath is referred to as spontaneous. The breath may still be accommodated if sufficient gas flow is present in the breathing system. If the ventilator is set up to detect and contribute to the work of inspiration, then the resulting breath can be referred to as a triggered supported breath.

The means by which the positive pressure breath is delivered can be controlled through either setting a desired tidal volume (volume control) or a desired inspiratory pressure (pressure control). In volume control mode, the tidal volume is the independent variable and the resultant measured pressure is dependent on the compliance within the breathing system and the patient's lungs. Volume control ventilation utilises a constant gas flow, which together with the inspiratory time will produce a given tidal volume. In pressure control ventilation, the pressure delivered is the independent variable and the tidal volume achieved becomes the dependent variable. The decelerating flow pattern seen in pressure control ventilation produces a non-linear increase in tidal volume, which is more comfortable for sedated patients and may reduce ventilator asynchrony.

Expiration can be initiated by either a predetermined period of time passing, by reaching a flow threshold (in pressure control mode) or by reaching a pressure limit whereby the ventilator will alarm and cycle to expiration to prevent barotrauma in a patient making asynchronous efforts or coughing.

The complications of invasive ventilation are outlined in Table 36.6.

Table 36.6. Complications of invasive ventilation.

- Barotrauma.
- Volutrauma causing pneumothorax.
- Ventilator-associated pneumonia.
- Reduction in cardiac output.
- Complications associated with endotracheal intubation: need for sedation, dental/palate injury, tracheal stenosis.

Acute respiratory distress syndrome

Acute respiratory distress syndrome (ARDS) is a disease of the lung parenchyma. It is characterised by inflammation, cytokine release, loss of surfactant, oedema and fibrotic changes resulting in impaired gas exchange.

ARDS may be caused by pulmonary or extrapulmonary insults. Diagnosing it requires an arterial blood gas, chest X-ray/CT (Figure 36.4) and fulfilling the four criteria described below (Table 36.7).

Table 36.7. Criteria for diagnosing ARDS.

Berlin criteria for ARDS — expert consensus opinion from the ESICM

1. Acute onset (within 1 week).
2. Bilateral opacities consistent with pulmonary oedema on thoracic imaging.
3. Presentation not fully explained by cardiac failure or fluid overload.
4. P/F ratio as below with a minimum of 5cmH$_2$O PEEP.

Severity	PaO$_2$/FiO$_2$ (mmHg)	PaO$_2$/FiO$_2$ (kPa)	Mortality (%)
Mild	200 - 300	26.6 - 40	27
Moderate	100 - 200	13.3 - 26.6	32
Severe	<100	<13.3	45

ESICM = European Society of Intensive Care Medicine; P/F = PaO$_2$/FiO$_2$.

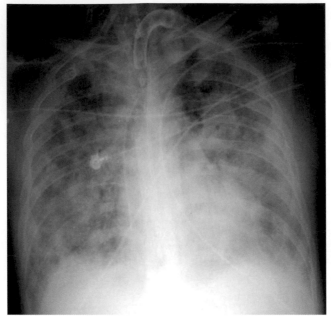

Figure 36.4. Chest X-ray demonstrates patchy bilateral lung infiltrates throughout both lung fields and the presence of a tracheostomy tube.

Lung protective ventilation

Whilst mechanical ventilation is the treatment for life-threatening respiratory failure, it can itself be harmful. The ARDSnet trial showed a better mortality outcome when using a lung protective ventilation strategy.

The volumes of patient's lungs are related to their height and therefore their predicted body weight (PBW). Being overweight or underweight may change actual body weight but has no impact on lung volume. The ARDSnet ventilation strategy (Table 36.8) therefore advocated the use of smaller tidal volumes (6ml/kg PBW), versus the 10ml/kg that had been the mainstay of treatment previously.

Table 36.8. ARDSnet ventilation strategy.

- Set tidal volume 6ml/kg predicted body weight (not actual weight).
- Set frequency to achieve similar minute ventilation to conventional ventilation.
- Aim for a SpO_2 of 88-95%.
- Minimum PEEP 5cmH$_2$O and increase PEEP with increases in FiO_2.
- Achieve plateau pressures <30cmH$_2$O.
- pH target 7.30-7.45.
- Inspiratory time < expiratory time.

Extracorporeal membrane oxygenation (ECMO)

In refractory respiratory failure it is possible to use an extracorporeal circuit for gas exchange, resting the lungs in the hope that the underlying insult can be given time to recover. A peripheral extracorporeal veno-arterial circuit incorporating a gas permeable membrane of sufficient surface area can be used to both oxygenate blood and remove CO_2. Very large blood flows are required through such devices and consequently large cannulae must be placed both intravenously and intra-arterially. As with all extracorporeal circuits anticoagulation is necessary. The CESAR study conducted at a single centre in the UK demonstrated ECMO to be a safe technique in the treatment of severe respiratory failure, but did not demonstrate a survival benefit compared to ARDSnet lung protective ventilation.

Case scenario 1

A 72-year-old man with known congestive cardiac failure presents with signs and symptoms of acute pulmonary oedema. His arterial blood gas (ABG) analysis demonstrates a PaO_2 of 6.7kPa on room air and $paCO_2$ of 5.4kPa.

How would you proceed?

His arterial blood gas analysis reveals a Type 1 respiratory failure. Supplementary oxygen delivered via a face mask may adequately correct this. If he remains hypoxaemic on oxygen he would be a suitable candidate for continuous positive airway pressure (CPAP).

Case scenario 2

A 66-year-old lady with an extensive smoking history presents with increasing dyspnoea and productive cough with yellow sputum. The chest X-ray is consistent with an infective exacerbation of COPD. She is receiving 85% oxygen via a non-rebreathing mask in the emergency department. Her ABG shows Type 2 respiratory failure with a PaO_2 of 22kPa and $paCO_2$ of 8.3kPa.

How would you proceed?

This lady may be retaining CO_2 due to a loss of hypoxic drive. Titration of her inspired oxygen concentration to achieve saturations of 88-92% would be an appropriate first step. If the CO_2 remains elevated despite this she should be considered for non-invasive ventilation.

Case scenario 3

A 28-year-old male presents with a suspected overdose. He is unresponsive to painful stimuli.

What would you do next?

This gentleman is unresponsive to painful stimuli and is unresponsive (U) on the AVPU scale. This equates to a GCS of 3. As a result his airway is threatened and it would be appropriate to intubate and ventilate him to protect his airway and then manage him in an intensive care setting.

Further reading

1. Bersten A, Soni N, Eds. *Oh's Intensive Care Manual*, 6th ed. Butterworth Heinemann Elsevier, 2009.
2. Mackenzie I, Ed. *Core Topics in Mechanical Ventilation*. Cambridge University Press, 2008.
3. West J. *Respiratory Physiology: the Essentials*, 8th ed. Lippincott Williams and Wilkins, 2008.
4. The ARDSnet Investigators. Ventilation with lower tidal volumes as compared with traditional tidal volumes for acute lung injury and the acute respiratory distress syndrome. *N Engl J Med* 2000; 342: 1301-8.

37 Management of chronic pain

Akilan Velayudhan and Alireza Feizerfan

Introduction

Pain is one of the most important warning signs of human experience during a threat to the normal physiologic homeostasis in the body. Pain is described by the International Association for the Study of Pain (IASP) as an "unpleasant sensory and emotional experience associated with actual or potential tissue damage, or described in terms of such damage". The experience of pain is very complex and it is initiated by a noxious (unpleasant) stimulus, which consequently results in perception of pain in the brain. The perception of the pain not only depends on the degree of tissue insult but also depends on the emotional state, cognitive perception, memory and cultural influences related to the patient. That is why the experience of the pain is unique for each individual.

Anatomy and physiology of pain

To understand the physiology of pain better, we can simplify it as below (Figure 37.1):

- Nociceptors in the periphery detect the noxious stimulus.
- Primary afferent neurons transfer the generated pain signals from the periphery to the spinal cord.
- Secondary afferent neurons transfer the pain signals from the spinal cord to the thalamus.
- Tertiary afferent neurons interconnect the thalamus to the midbrain and cortical centres in the brain.

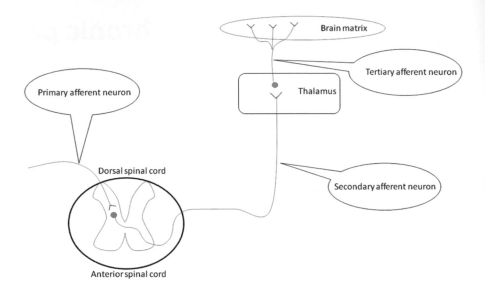

Figure 37.1. Pain pathways.

Nociceptors

Nociception is the neural process of encoding noxious stimuli. The neural process starts from the site of tissue injury where a noxious stimulus is detected, transduced and encoded by peripheral pain receptors called "nociceptors". Nociceptors are high-threshold sensory receptors of the pain system and are the free nerve endings of C and Aδ fibres.

C fibres are unmyelinated with a slow conduction velocity (<3m/sec). C fibres are responsible for detecting a thermal, chemical and mechanical stimulus and they are associated with prolonged burning and a dull pain sensation. On the other hand, Aδ fibres are myelinated and they transfer the stimulus faster than C fibres (5-30m/sec). Aδ fibres have a role in withdrawal reflexes and they respond to mechanical and thermal stimuli.

Another group of peripheral nerve fibre is the Aβ fibre. These fibres are thickly myelinated, hence they transmit sensation very fast. Aβ fibres carry light touch with an important role in the pain mechanism, which will be discussed later. Table 37.1 gives an overview of different nerve fibres.

Table 37.1. Peripheral nerve fibres with a role in nociception.		
Fibre type	**Aδ**	**C**	**Aβ**
Diameter	2-5μm	0.4-1.2μm	5-12μ
Conduction velocity	12-30m/sec	0.5-2m/sec	30-70m/sec
Type of sensation	Sharp pain, temperature, pinprick, well localised	Dull pain, temperature, mechanoreceptor, diffuse sensation	Light touch, pressure

Acute tissue insult such as heat, cold, chemical or mechanical injury causes a release of a wide range of inflammatory mediators from the damaged tissue or by activated mast cells and neutrophils. Some of these mediators are adenosine triphosphate (ATP), bradykinin, prostanoids, hydrogen (H^+), potassium (K^+), histamine and serotonin. The released substances interact with their corresponding receptors on the Aδ and C fibre nerve endings, leading to a change in the membrane potential. Once the membrane potential reaches the pain threshold, depolarisation and an action potential develop within the Aδ and C fibres. A generated action potential (which now is the pain signal) rapidly travels up within the primary afferent neurons up into the spinal cord.

Other features that are observed following tissue damage are:

- Activation of the cyclo-oxygenase (COX) enzyme leading to peripheral inflammation.
- Release of pro-inflammatory substances (interleukin-1B, interleukin-6, nerve growth factor, tumour necrosis factor-alpha) via macrophages causing systemic inflammation.
- Activation of the sympathetic nervous system and release of noradrenaline.

All these changes further activate the silent C fibres, reduce the pain threshold, increase the pain fibres and receptor excitability, leading to a state called "peripheral sensitisation" and hyperalgesia. Sensitisation is a generic term which describes hyperexcitability and increased responsiveness of the nociceptors to a noxious stimuli. Hyperalgesia is a clinical term and is "increased pain" from a stimulus that normally provokes pain.

Primary afferent neurons and the spinal cord

Peripheral pain fibres join and ascend as a primary afferent neuron (PAN). A PAN's cell body is located in the dorsal root ganglion just before they enter into the spinal cord. Once the PAN enters into the dorsal horn of the spinal cord, it synapses ipsilaterally with the secondary afferent neuron (SAN).

A developed action potential travels into the spinal cord via PANs. This action potential should be transferred from PANs to the SANs. Transfer of the action potential occurs via a release of excitatory substances such as substance P and glutamate. Secreted excitatory substances attach to their relevant receptors at the post-synaptic membrane, generating an action potential within the SANs, ready for transfer to the brain.

The dorsal horn of the spinal cord is divided into various layers named the Rexed laminae. There are multiple and complex synapses between PANs, SANs, interneurons and descending inhibitory pathways in different parts of the Rexed laminae; hence, the spinal cord can be termed a "switch board" where pain transmission is processed. While excitatory mechanisms facilitate the transmission of nociception to the brain, inhibitory mechanisms within the spinal cord dampen and impede the transmission. These inhibitory mechanisms consist of:

- Inhibitory GABAergic and glycinergic interneurons.
- Descending inhibitory pathways from the brain, via serotonin and noradrenaline release.
- Production of endogenous opioids.
- Gate control theory.
- Higher order brain functions responsible for distraction and cognitive function.

The balance between excitatory and inhibitory functions determines the overall transmission of noxious stimuli to the brain.

Secondary afferent neurons

After synapse with the PANs, most of the SANs cross over to the contralateral part of the spinal cord and ascend to the brain via various tracts. These tracts are:

- Lateral spinothalamic tract. This tract terminates at the thalamus and is responsible for carrying sensory and discriminative components of the pain by which a person can identify and sense the type and location of the pain.
- Medial spinothalamic tract. This terminates at the medulla and midbrain (reticular formation, periaqueductal grey matter, hypothalamus) and is responsible for carrying the affective (emotional) and aversive (unpleasantness) component of the pain.
- Spinoreticular, spinomesencephalic and parabrachial tracts. These tracts are particularly important in arousal, mood and modulation of the pain signal.

Tertiary afferent neurons and the pain matrix

Tertiary afferent neurons are the fibres which connect the thalamus to various parts of the brain such as the midbrain, limbic system and the somatosensory cortex. These pain centres collectively are called the "pain matrix".

Physiology of pain within the brain is a complex topic and is beyond the scope of this book.

The pain matrix is the brain network responding to nociception. It incorporates multiple areas in the brain, which collaboratively are activated by nociception. With advances in imaging technology such as functional MRI scanning and positron emission tomography, it has been possible to identify important regions in the brain (thalamus, mid/anterior insula, anterior cingulated cortex and prefrontal cortex, periaqueductal gray matter, rostroventromedial medulla, reticular formation, hypothalamus and amygdala) responsible for pain physiology. These areas have a different role in pain perception such as somatosensory discrimination, mood, the motivational component of pain, coping mechanisms, fight or flight and autonomic responses such as sweating/nausea/vomiting/palpitations.

Inhibitory pain mechanisms

We mentioned earlier that the overall balance between the excitatory and inhibitory mechanisms in the spinal cord determine the degree of pain transmission to the brain (Figure 37.2). These mechanisms are:

- Inhibitory GABAergic and glycinergic interneurons. Release of these substances would reduce the excitability in the SANs. Overall, the pain signals may be reduced or even be stopped from propagation to the brain.
- Descending inhibitory pathways from the brain. Higher brain centres project neural pathways descending to the spinal cord. Activation of the pain matrix releases serotonin and noradrenaline via these descending pathways which overall reduce the transmission of the pain signals from PANs to the SANs. That is why some

antidepressants such as amitriptyline and selective serotonin reuptake inhibitors (SSRIs) are effective in controlling some painful conditions.

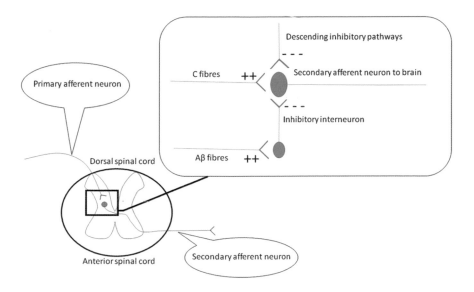

Figure 37.2. Effect of excitatory and inhibitory pain fibres on secondary afferent neurons.

- Endogenous opioids. Endogenous opioids are produced by neurons within the central nervous system. Endogenous opioids act on opioid receptors, which are abundant in the central nervous system. Secretion of endogenous opioids produce analgesia similar to the way a patient receives morphine.
- Gate control theory. Imagine you accidentally hit your hand on the door frame. You would most likely first look at your hand making sure the injury is not serious and then start rubbing it. The rubbing part or 'light touch' reduces the intensity of the pain. This process has been explained by Melzack and Wall, proposing an inhibitory function at the level of the spinal cord. Light touch sensation, which is a non-noxious stimulus, is carried by Aβ fibres to the spinal cord.

The non-noxious stimuli, such as rubbing your hand, would stimulate the inhibitory interneurons in the dorsal horn of the spinal cord and would reduce the severity of noxious signal transmission from PANs to the SANs. This phenomenon is called the gate control theory.

- Higher order brain functions responsible for distraction and cognitive function. This is a very powerful non-pharmacological mechanism that can control the pain, yet its effectiveness varies between individuals.

A mother's approach to her toddler who sustains a simple injury is a perfect example of remembering the inhibitory pathways. Once a child hurts himself and starts crying, his mother assesses her child to make sure that there is no major injury. With reassurance she starts rubbing or kissing the sore part of the toddler, utilising the gate control theory. A mother starts drawing the child's attention to something interesting utilising a distraction technique and she may give a little treat (chocolate, crisps) which releases endorphins, activating the descending inhibitory pathways.

Visceral pain

Visceral pain by definition is a pain which is sensed as arising from internal organs of the body such as the heart, great vessels, lung, gastrointestinal organs, peritoneum, reproductive organs and urological structures. Key features with the visceral pain include:

- Diffuse localisation.
- Described as a deep or dull sensation.
- Unreliable association with pathology.
- Referred sensation.
- Autonomic changes (changes in heart rate, blood pressure, nausea, vomiting, syncope).

These features are due to the unique pain pathways originating from viscera comparing to the ones from the periphery. The viscera are largely innervated by C fibres which project to the spinal cord as PANs via the autonomic nervous system. Once the PANs enter the spinal cord, they arborise extensively and enter multiple spinal segments above and below the segment of entry with a diffuse synaptic contact with various other somatic nerves. That is why the visceral pain is sensed as diffuse and extensive with referred pain. An example of this pain is secondary to myocardial infarction, which is felt as dull and crushing across the chest with referred pain in the limbs or even the face.

Neuropathic pain

Neuropathic pain is a type of pain caused by a lesion or disease of the nerves in the peripheral or central nervous system. Examples are diabetic neuropathic pain due to chronic dysfunction of the peripheral nervous system, post-stroke pain due to lesions in the central nervous system or neuropathic pain due to nerve damage secondary to a bony fracture or an injury. Neuropathic pain has different clinical features to nociceptive pain. Typically, the patient describes the pain as shooting, burning, tingling, electrical or lancinating in nature. Pain may be constant or paroxysmal and there may be sensory changes such as hyperalgesia and/or allodynia (painful response to a normally innocuous stimulus). Neuropathic pain usually is not responsive to conventional analgesics such as NSAIDs and opioids, and they require antineuropathic medications.

Assessment of patients with chronic pain

A clinical history and examination will form an important aspect in the diagnosis and management of patients with chronic pain. Patients with chronic pain most often present with multiple-site pain, hence, it is helpful to address the most distressing problem or chief complaint that has brought them to the clinic. Following that, it is valuable to explore the necessary components of the history of presenting complaints in the mnemonic, OPQRST: the O represents the Onset of pain, P stands for Provocation (aggravates the pain) or Palliative factors (relieves the pain), Q for the quality of the pain, in other words describing the nature of the pain such as aching, burning, throbbing, etc., R for region (anatomical location, any radiation, etc.), S for the severity of the pain which can be assessed by using numerous pain scores (e.g. a numerical pain score of 0-10), and T for temporal factors such as the time of day and duration, etc.

The medication history will provide important information about the patient's general ill health, including anxiety, depression and analgesics that have been tried before. In addition, it will inform us if there are any specific considerations to be taken into account when performing interventions, for example, if they are on anticoagulants, etc.

Social history will focus more on the patient's occupation and how the pain interferes with their profession and level of job satisfaction. This information may provide some prognostic clue about their return to work. Also, enquiring about their hobbies and daily activities will provide some information about their functionality and their support system. The social history should also encompass any history of substance abuse, as this will have a significant impact on the outcome of any intervention.

Clinical examination should be tailored to their chief complaint. Table 37.2 describes a template for a pain-directed physical examination.

Table 37.2. Template for a pain-directed clinical examination.

- General appearance.
- Gait.
- Range of motion.
- Tenderness (e.g. muscle, bone, tendon, scar).
- Provocative test (e.g. Tinel's test, straight leg raise [SLR], Spurling's test).
- Sensory exam (i.e. anaesthesia or hypoaesthesia, allodynia, hyperalgesia).
- Motor exam (e.g. muscle bulk, symmetry, strength, spasm, abnormal movement, reflexes).
- Vascular exam (e.g. skin temperature, colour, sweating, oedema, pulses, venodilation, ulcers, stasis).
- Other relevant examinations: head and neck, chest, abdomen, back, peripheries, etc.

The laboratory evaluations include relevant blood tests pertinent to painful conditions such as rheumatoid arthritis, lupus, diabetes and HIV. Neurodiagnostic studies such as electromyograms, nerve conduction studies and radiological investigations such as an X-ray, CT scan and MRI will provide valuable information guiding the appropriate management of patients with chronic pain.

In summary, clinical encounters with patients who have chronic pain will pose many challenges. A methodological approach in their evaluation will aid the overall management and improve patient satisfaction.

Management of chronic pain (Figure 37.3)

Pharmacological management of pain

The most commonly used pharmacological agents are: paracetamol alone or in combination with codeine or tramadol, NSAIDs, antidepressants, anticonvulsants, opioids, local anaesthetics, steroids as an injection therapy and other rarely used drugs such as ketamine, clonidine and capsaicin.

Nociceptive pain is treated with either paracetamol alone or as a combination therapy with codeine or tramadol, NSAIDs and if pain is persistent, opioids can be considered.

Neuropathic pain is treated with first-line antineuropathic medications such as antidepressants or anticonvulsants and for persistent pain, opioids, local anaesthetic and other rarely used drugs mentioned above can be considered.

NSAIDs such as ibuprofen, naproxen, diclofenac, ketorolac and piroxicam are used because of their anti-inflammatory and analgesic action. They act via inhibition of the cyclo-oxygenase enzyme reducing prostaglandin, prostacyclin and thromboxane production. Inhibitors of the cyclo-oxygenase-2 (COX-2) enzyme, such as parecoxib and celecoxib, can be used for their potential relative lack of gastrointestinal side effects.

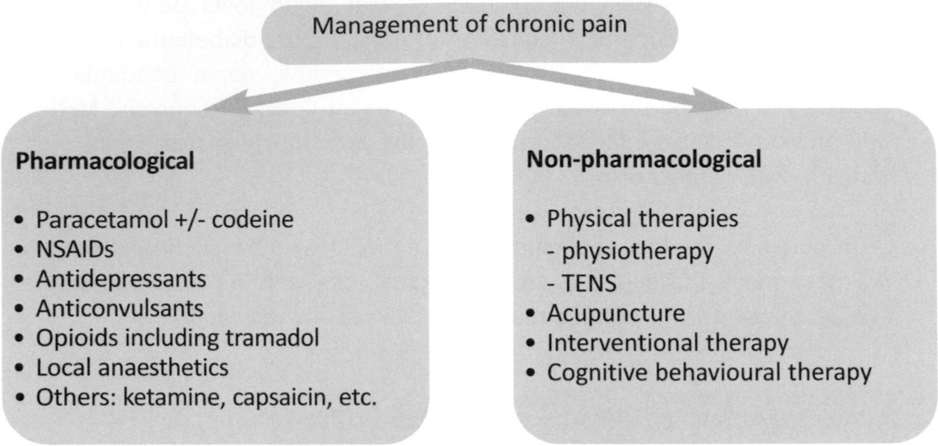

Figure 37.3. Summary of chronic pain management.

Antidepressants such as tricyclic (e.g. amitriptyline) and selective serotonin reuptake inhibitors (e.g. fluoxetine) are usually used for their analgesic effects but at a lower dosage compared to the mood-altering doses. The proposed analgesic effect is due to blockade of the reuptake of noradrenaline and serotonin in the central nervous system; thereby, they enhance the descending inhibitory action in the spinal cord in addition to monoaminergic effects elsewhere in the CNS.

Anticonvulsant drugs such as gabapentin and pregabalin are commonly used in clinical practice. They exert their analgesic effect via functional blockade of voltage-gated calcium channels, which results in reduced neuronal hyperexcitability seen in neuropathic pain.

Opioid use, in particular strong opioids, for the management of chronic non-malignant pain is surrounded with controversy in relation to their short- and long-term side effects. The British Pain Society recommends the use of strong opioids only after the consideration of adjuvant analgesics and other available treatment options. Opioid receptors are coupled with inhibitory G-proteins and their activation closes the voltage-sensitive calcium channels and stimulation of potassium efflux. These changes lead to hyperpolarisation and a reduction of neuronal excitability and nociceptive afferent transmission.

Other agents

Tramadol is a centrally-acting, synthetic, non-narcotic analgesic, which has two mechanisms of action: a low-affinity binding to μ-opioid receptors and weak inhibition of norepinephrine and serotonin reuptake.

Topical agents such as lidocaine 5% is used for localised neuropathic pain. They exert their analgesic effect transdermally delivering small amounts of lidocaine sufficient to block sodium channels on the small pain fibres locally. Another topical agent is capsaicin, a vanilloid compound isolated from chili peppers believed to elevate the pain threshold through the depletion of substance P from the membranes.

Non-pharmacological pain management

Transcutaneous electrical nerve stimulation (TENS) is one of the simplest non-invasive treatments available widely. TENS functions via stimulating the peripheral nerve fibres at different amplitudes and frequencies utilising the gate control theory. This technique provides a short-term improvement in pain and is often used as an adjunct to help patients undergo rehabilitation exercises.

Acupuncture is a complementary therapy and is used as a modality for the treatment of both acute and chronic pain. It involves placement of fine needles into body locations known as acupoints. There are several postulated mechanisms of actions. One of these actions is the endogenous release of naturally occurring opiates: dynorphin, endorphin and encephalin which modulate the pain transmission.

Interventional pain management involves performing invasive procedures using local anaesthetics and steroids. Invasive procedures can be either used as a diagnostic modality helping to identify the origin of the pain, or as a therapeutic modality, such as radiofrequency denervation to reduce the pain level. Patients with complex refractory pain conditions may benefit from advanced interventional techniques such as intrathecal pumps and spinal cord stimulators.

Psychological and behavioural modalities play an important role in the multidisciplinary management of chronic pain. Psychological factors such as mood, beliefs about pain and coping style all play a significant role in an individual's adjustment to chronic pain. Cognitive behavioural therapy (CBT) involves modifying negative thoughts related to pain and a focus on increasing a person's activity level and productive functioning.

Case scenario 1

A 25-year-old male patient presents to the pain clinic with a 3-month history of worsening low back pain and radiation of pain to the right leg. He describes the pain as a constant ache in the lower back associated with an intermittent burning and shooting pain along the leg. He gives a history of spinal claudication pain. He has been commenced on regular paracetamol with codeine and NSAIDs by his primary care doctor, with no pain relief. On examination, he has a positive right-sided straight leg raise test and a reduced ankle reflex with no sensory changes.

What would be the next appropriate management strategy to help him with his pain?

Patients presenting with back pain should have a focused history and physical examination to place them into one of three broad categories:

- Non-specific low back pain.
- Back pain potentially associated with radiculopathy or spinal stenosis.
- Back pain potentially associated with another specific spinal cause.

The history should also include assessment of red flag signs and psychosocial risk factors which predict risk for chronic disabling back pain.

In this clinical example, the patient has back pain potentially associated with radiculopathy and requires further investigation with MRI. Depending on the MRI findings (evidence of any spinal canal stenosis and nerve root impingement), the treatment options would be either pharmacological or non-pharmacological.

The pharmacological options can be considered if there is no significant nerve root impingement, which would then include either antidepressants or anticonvulsants, as a first-line treatment option for neuropathic pain.

On the other hand, if there is moderate to severe nerve root impingement, either an epidural steroid or surgical exploration can be considered. The patient should be encouraged to remain active with intensive physiotherapy and also be provided with information about effective self-care options.

Case scenario 2

A 65-year-old male patient had an elective right total knee replacement secondary to osteoarthritis under spinal anesthesia 24 hours ago. He is reporting severe uncontrolled knee pain preventing him from participating in physiotherapy. He is a retired gardener without any comorbidity. He gives a history of gastritis and intolerance to NSAIDs. The nurse looking after the patient states that the patient's original drug chart is missing and the locum night doctor rewrote a new drug chart and prescribed regular paracetamol for analgesia.

The patient describes his pain as the worst ever pain in his life with a pain score of 10 out of 10 on a numeric rating scale, even without movement. Clinical assessment does not find any surgical complications and the diagnosis is an inadequate analgesic regime.

What would be the next appropriate analgesic management?

Large joint arthroplasties, particularly total knee replacement, can be very painful during the first few post-procedure days. At the same time it is crucial for the patient to be mobile and active, and participate in daily physiotherapy for rehabilitation and avoid complications; hence, beside ethical reasons, it is very important to provide adequate analgesia for this group of patients. Paracetamol and NSAIDs should be the first-line treatment managing most of the somatic pain. However, this combination is usually insufficient and opioids should be prescribed and titrated according to the response for total knee replacement surgery.

The patient in this scenario is unable to tolerate NSAIDs; hence, regular paracetamol and regular long-acting opioids should be the combination used according to the local hospital policy. This combination aims to control the background pain secondary to the surgery. However, this combination may be insufficient for dynamic pain, which is generated during activities such as physiotherapy, so it is beneficial to prescribe an immediate-release opioid formulation for breakthrough pain.

After prescription of the new analgesic regime, the patient should be reviewed regularly to assess the pain and response to the medications. If it is required, the opioid dose should be readjusted according to the response.

Following an effective pain regime, the patient was discharged home on the third postoperative day. The patient was referred to the pain clinic 3 months later due to severe knee pain unresponsive to opioids. Now the patient is reporting that the post-surgical pain gradually got better and it was under control with regular paracetamol 2 weeks after the surgery. However, he gradually developed a burning sensation and sharp pain anterior to the surgical scar and he has found it difficult to kneel. Even simple touch to the knee or rubbing trousers to the affected area elucidates a disturbing annoying pain.

On clinical examination there is a healed surgical scar with normal skin colour and temperature, and a full range of movement with no joint effusion. Normal motor power and cutaneous sensation in the lower limb are noted. There is hypersensitivity and allodynia around the medial border of the knee joint. The blood test and X-ray investigation are normal.

What is the diagnosis and what would be the next step in management?

The clinical finding suggests post-surgical neuropathic pain, which is possibly due to damage to the cutaneous sensory fibres or saphenous nerve. Neuropathic pain is unresponsive to paracetamol, NSAIDs and opioids and hence antineuropathic agents are indicated. Some of these agents are tricyclic antidepressants, gabapentin, pregabalin or duloxetine. Starting off with antineuropathic agents and referral to the chronic pain clinic is an ideal initial management.

Further reading

1. Basic principles of chronic pain. In: Brook P, Connell J, Pickering T, Eds. *Oxford Handbook of Pain Management.* Oxford University Press, 2011: 143-57.

2. Pharmacological therapies. In: Brook P, Connell J, Pickering T, Eds. *Oxford Handbook of Pain Management.* Oxford University Press, 2011: 159-77.

3. Ringkamp M, Raja SN, Campbell JN, Meyer RA. Peripheral mechanisms of cutaneous nociception. In: McMahon S, Koltzenburg M, Tracey I, Turk DC. *Wall and Melzeck's Textbook of Pain*, 6th ed. Elsevier Saunders, 2013: 1-30.

4. Ng KFJ. Neuropathic pain. In: Tsui S, Chen PP, Ng KFJ. *Pain Medicine - A Multidisciplinary Approach.* Hong Kong University Press, 2010: 235-51.

5. Feizerfan A, Sheh G. Transition from acute to chronic pain. *Br J Anaesth CEACCP* 2015; 15: 98-102.

Index

A

B

C

D

E

F

goal-directed therapy (GDT) 244-7
goitres 285-6, 452-6
Guedel airway 392-3
gynaecological surgery 639

H

haem biosynthesis disorder 296-9
haematology, in pregnancy 648-9
haemoglobin 258, 765, 777-8
haemophilia 263
haemorrhage 256-7
    emergency surgery 632-4, 642-3
    massive 258-60
    peri-operative 269-70, 719
    post-partum 661-3
halothane 20-1, 24-7, 32-5, 344
halothane hepatitis 33
Hartmann's procedure 618-19
Hartmann's solution 242-3
head and neck procedures 435-60
    dental procedures 436-41
    maxillofacial trauma 444-8
    radical neck dissection 448-52
    thyroidectomy 452-6
head tilt, airway opening 391-2
head-up position 149-50
heparin 226-7, 335, 380
hernia, diaphragmatic 675-6
hip replacement 382-5
history taking 197-200
hormone replacement therapy (HRT) 216
hydrocephalus 511
hyperaldosteronism 290-1
hypercapnia 685-8

I

J

K

L

M

N

O

P

R

S

T

U

V

W

X

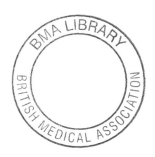

Other books in the series

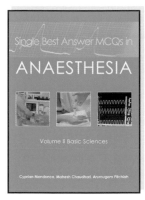

Single Best Answer MCQs in Anaesthesia
Volume II — Basic Sciences

Cyprian Mendonca MD FRCA *Consultant Anaesthetist, University Hospitals Coventry and Warwickshire, Coventry, UK,* **Mahesh Chaudhari MD FRCA FFPMRCA** *Consultant Anaesthetist, Worcestershire Royal Hospital, Worcester, UK,* **Arumugam Pitchiah MD FRCA** *Specialty Registrar, Welsh School of Anaesthesia, Wales, UK*

Paperback
ISBN: 978-1-903378-83-0
210pp; 149mm x 210mm

e-formats
epub:
ISBN: 978-1-908986-84-9
mobi:
ISBN: 978-1-908986-85-6
web pdf:
ISBN: 978-1-908986-86-3
Retail price:
GBP £30
USD $59.95
EUR €45

This book comprises six sets of single best answer practice papers. Each set contains 30 single best answer questions on physiology, pharmacology, clinical measurement and physics. The scenarios are based on the application of a wide knowledge of basic sciences relevant to the clinical practice of anaesthesia. The best possible answer to a given question is substantiated by detailed explanation drawn from recent journal articles and textbooks of anaesthesia and basic sciences. These questions enable the candidates to assess their knowledge in basic sciences and their ability to apply it to clinical practice. Alongside the previously published book Single Best Answer MCQs in Anaesthesia (Volume I — Clinical Anaesthesia, ISBN 978-1-903378-75-5), this book is an ideal companion for candidates sitting postgraduate examinations in anaesthesia, intensive care medicine, and pain management. It is also a valuable educational resource for all trainees and practising anaesthetists.

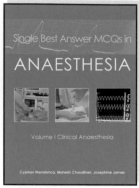

Single Best Answer MCQs in Anaesthesia Volume I — Clinical Anaesthesia

Cyprian Mendonca MD FRCA *Consultant Anaesthetist, University Hospitals Coventry and Warwickshire, Coventry, UK,* **Mahesh Chaudhari MD FRCA FFPMRCA** *Consultant Anaesthetist, Worcestershire Royal Hospital, Worcester, UK,* **Josephine James FRCA** *Consultant Anaesthetist, Heart of England Foundation Trust and Programme Director, Warwickshire School of Anaesthesia, Regional Advisor, West Midlands south region, Birmingham, UK*

Paperback
ISBN: 978-1-903378-75-5
210pp; 149mm x 210mm

e-formats
epub:
ISBN: 978-1-908986-63-4
mobi:
ISBN: 978-1-908986-64-1
web pdf:
ISBN: 978-1-908986-65-8
Retail price:
GBP £30
USD $59.95
EUR €45

The single best answer format of questions is invaluable in assessing a trainee's clinical skills and problem-solving abilities. It allows the trainee to demonstrate application of their knowledge to clinical practice.

This book comprises six sets of practice papers. Each set contains 30 single best answer questions which cover topics including clinical anaesthesia, pain and intensive care. The questions are based on the recent changes introduced to the written part of the final FRCA examination. The best possible answer to a given clinical scenario is substantiated by a detailed explanation drawn from recent review articles and textbooks in clinical anaesthesia.

These questions will enable candidates to assess their clinical knowledge and skills in problem-solving, data interpretation and decision making. This book is essential study material for candidates sitting postgraduate examinations in anaesthesia and intensive care medicine. It is not only an essential guide for trainees but also an invaluable educational resource for all anaesthetists.

The Structured Oral Examination in Clinical Anaesthesia

Practice examination papers

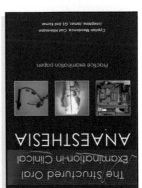

Cyprian Mendonca MD, **FRCA** *Consultant Anaesthetist, University Hospitals Coventry and Warwickshire, Coventry, UK*
Carl Hillemann **FRCA** *Consultant Anaesthetist, University Hospitals Coventry and Warwickshire, Coventry, UK*
Josephine James **FRCA** *Consultant Anaesthetist, Heart of England Foundation Trust and Programme Director, Warwickshire School of Anaesthesia, Regional Advisor, West Midlands south region, Birmingham, UK,* **Anil Kumar FRCARCSI** *Specialist Registrar, Warwickshire School of Anaesthesia, UK*

Paperback
ISBN: 978-1-903378-68-7
576pp; 149mm x 210mm

e-formats
epub:
ISBN: 978-1-908986-45-0
mobi:
ISBN: 978-1-908986-46-7
web pdf:
ISBN: 978-1-908986-47-4

Retail price:
GBP £35
USD $70
EUR €55

This book comprises structured questions and answers that closely simulate the structured oral examination (SOE) format of The Royal College of Anaesthetists' final FRCA examination. The style of exam questions has changed over the years and this book matches the most recent changes in this updated exam. It consists of ten sets (chapters) of complete SOE papers. Each SOE set (chapter) includes one long case, three short cases and four different applied basic science topics (anatomy, physiology, pharmacology and clinical measurement). As this book is presented in the format of complete examination papers, it will enable candidates to assess their knowledge and skills. It will also assist trainers in setting up mock exams. With thorough revision of this book, trainees can confidently sit their exams. The authors have been organising final FRCA viva courses for the past five years, running four exam preparation courses a year, attended by about 200 trainees each year. This book includes updated knowledge based on the syllabus and more recent questions asked in the FRCA examination. It is, therefore, essential study material for trainees and a great educational tool for trainers. This book will also help candidates all over the world to pass highly competitive postgraduate examinations in anaesthesia. It is an invaluable educational resource for all anaesthetists.

Winner of a HIGHLY COMMENDED AWARD in the Anaesthesia category of the 2010 BMA Medical Book Competition

The Objective Structured Clinical Examination in Anaesthesia

Practice papers for Teachers and Trainees

Cyprian Mendonca MD FRCA *Consultant Anaesthetist, University Hospitals Coventry and Warwickshire, Coventry, UK*, **Shyam Balasubramanian MD FRCA** *Consultant Anaesthetist, University Hospitals Coventry and Warwickshire, Coventry, UK*

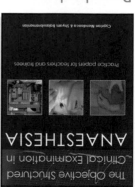

Paperback
ISBN: 978-1-903378-56-4
398pp; 149mm x 210mm

e-formats

epub:
ISBN: 978-1-908986-18-4

mobi:
ISBN: 978-1-908986-19-1

web pdf:
ISBN: 978-1-908986-20-7

Retail price:
GBP £35
USD $70
EUR €55

The Objective Structured Clinical Examination (OSCE) is a highly reliable and valid tool for the evaluation of trainees in anaesthesia. It enables examiners and trainees to assess a number of competencies in an organised way. Performance in the OSCE is considered to be a fair reflection of the level of knowledge and skill attained during anaesthesia training. Apart from having a wide and deep knowledge on the subject, trainees are expected to have the capacity to demonstrate their competency in a short period of time allotted for each station.

The authors of this book have a rich experience in successfully conducting OSCE courses in the United Kingdom. The sample OSCE sets in the book closely simulate the style and content of the Royal College of Anaesthetists' examination format. The book contains 100 OSCE stations with answers based on key practical procedures, clinical skills, communication skills, data interpretation, anaesthetic equipment and the management of critical incidents on a simulator. This book will also help candidates all over the world to pass highly competitive postgraduate examinations in anaesthesia. It is an invaluable educational resource for all anaesthetists.